Essentials of
Life Cycle
Nutrition

Edited by:

Judith Sharlin, PhD, RD
Senior Lecturer
Department of Nutrition and Dietetics
Simmons College

Sari Edelstein, PhD, RD
Associate Professor
Department of Nutrition and Dietetics
Simmons College

JONES AND BARTLETT PUBLISHERS

Sudbury, Massachusetts

BOSTON   TORONTO   LONDON   SINGAPORE

World Headquarters

Jones and Bartlett Publishers
40 Tall Pine Drive
Sudbury, MA 01776
978-443-5000
info@jbpub.com
www.jbpub.com

Jones and Bartlett Publishers
Canada
6339 Ormindale Way
Mississauga, Ontario L5V 1J2
Canada

Jones and Bartlett Publishers
International
Barb House, Barb Mews
London W6 7PA
United Kingdom

Jones and Bartlett's books and products are available through most bookstores and online booksellers. To contact Jones and Bartlett Publishers directly, call 800-832-0034, fax 978-443-8000, or visit our website, www.jbpub.com.

Substantial discounts on bulk quantities of Jones and Bartlett's publications are available to corporations, professional associations, and other qualified organizations. For details and specific discount information, contact the special sales department at Jones and Bartlett via the above contact information or send an email to specialsales@jbpub.com.

The authors, editor, and publisher have made every effort to provide accurate information. However, they are not responsible for errors, omissions, or for any outcomes related to the use of the contents of this book and take no responsibility for the use of the products and procedures described. Treatments and side effects described in this book may not be applicable to all people; likewise, some people may require a dose or experience a side effect that is not described herein. Drugs and medical devices are discussed that may have limited availability controlled by the Food and Drug Administration (FDA) for use only in a research study or clinical trial. Research, clinical practice, and government regulations often change the accepted standard in this field. When consideration is being given to use of any drug in the clinical setting, the health care provider or reader is responsible for determining FDA status of the drug, reading the package insert, and reviewing prescribing information for the most up-to-date recommendations on dose, precautions, and contraindications, and determining the appropriate usage for the product. This is especially important in the case of drugs that are new or seldom used.

Production Credits
Publisher: David Cella
Acquisitions Editor: Katey Birtcher
Associate Editor: Maro Gartside
Editorial Assistant: Teresa Reilly
Senior Production Editor: Renée Sekerak
Marketing Manager: Grace Richards
Manufacturing and Inventory Control Supervisor: Amy Bacus
Composition: Auburn Associates, Inc.
Cover and Title Page Design: Kristin E. Parker
Assistant Photo Researcher: Emily Howard
Cover Image: © Monkey Business Images/ShutterStock, Inc.
Printing and Binding: Malloy, Inc.
Cover Printing: Malloy, Inc.

Library of Congress Cataloging-in-Publication Data
Essentials of life cycle nutrition / edited by Judith Sharlin, Sari Edelstein.
    p. ; cm.
  Includes bibliographical references and index.
  ISBN 978-0-7637-7792-0
  1. Nutrition—Textbooks. 2. Life cycle, Human—Textbooks. I. Sharlin, Judith. II. Edelstein, Sari.
  [DNLM: 1. Nutritional Physiological Phenomena. 2. Dietary Therapy. 3. Food. 4. Human Development–physiology.
  QU 145 E785 2010]
  QP141.E87 2010
  612.3—dc22
                                                                                    2009050589

6048
Printed in the United States of America
14 13 12 11 10   10 9 8 7 6 5 4 3 2 1

DEDICATION

The editors would like to dedicate this edition of *Essentials of Life Cycle Nutrition* to I. David Todres, MD, who died on September 26, 2008, after fighting a courageous battle with lymphoma. David was the beloved husband of Judith Sharlin, friend and colleague of Sari Edelstein, and co-author of one of the chapters in this book. Born in South Africa, David was one of the founders of the neonatal and pediatric intensive care units in Massachusetts General Hospital (MGH), where he worked for 37 years. Until the time of his death, he served as chief of the pediatric ethics unit at MGH and was a professor at Harvard Medical School. A loving and devoted husband and father, David expressed his gentle patience, humility, and kindness every day. He combined humor, wisdom, care, and concern in both his professional and personal lives. David was one of those few special people who inspired others, by example, to be the most ethical, humane, and compassionate people they could be. A deeply spiritual and optimistic person, David also loved travel, literature, art, politics, and religion. David's legacy will be remembered in the thousands of children's lives he saved and in the scores of students and residents he mentored. With his wild curls, charming South African accent, wisdom, and gentle kindness, David made an indelible impression on anyone he touched . . . he is deeply missed.

CONTENTS

CHAPTER **5**   **Special Topics in Prenatal and Infant Nutrition: Failure to Thrive**. **83**
Claire Blais, RD, LDN, CNSD

Special Section: Genetics and Inborn Errors of Metabolism
Laura Harkness, PhD, RD; Sara Snow, MS, RD

CHAPTER **6**   **Special Topics in Toddler and Preschool Nutrition:**
Vitamins and Minerals in Childhood **98**
Aaron Owens, MS, RD

CHAPTER **9** **Special Topics in Adult Nutrition: Chronic Disease Nutritional Assessment** 197

Jennifer L. Bueche, PhD, RD, CDN

CHAPTER **10** **Special Topics in Adults and Chronic Diseases: Nutrition and Public Health** 218

Judith Sharlin, PhD, RD

PREFACE

Essentials of Life Cycle Nutrition provides a unique learning experience, a unique reference, and a unique start for students learning about nutrition throughout the life cycle. It also provides a comprehensive reference for those of us already in practice. The book stands alone in its interwoven coverage of public health nutrition, with subjects as diverse as media influences on eating, skipping breakfast, sociodemographic moderators of dietary intake, tobacco use and nutritional status, and clinical nutrition; it includes a wide array of diverse topics, including inborn errors of metabolism, and cancer. Contemporary issues such as fruit juice consumption, nutritional needs of athletes, and dietary supplements as ergogenic aids are addressed across the life cycle as well as by using a multidisciplinary approach. This book gives students current knowledge, helps them evaluate emerging knowledge, and prepares them to uncover new knowledge for the public, their clients, and themselves as they journey together throughout the life cycle.

The book is divided into two sections. The first section brings us from the prenatal period to adolescence and covers virtually every topic imaginable. The first chapter covers nutrition during pregnancy, the essential nutrients and potential complications. Chapter 2 gives students insight into the growth, and development of normal infants, along with some of their nutrition "issues," such as food safety and the effect of early diet on health outcomes. As outlined in Chapter 3, toddlers have different issues as they begin to explore their world and express food preferences; food habits begin to be formed and are influenced by caregiver behaviors. Chapter 4 emphasizes that school-aged children have different needs and are influenced by a wide variety of outside forces, including role models and television and other media. Although caregivers have a large influence, these children begin to make their own food choices and may be grazers or picky eaters. Adolescents, discussed in Chapter 4, are an understudied group with many nutrition issues; they, too, are influenced by media but also by their peers. Adolescents also make many of their own food choices and may skip breakfast or consume fast food and added sugars, often in the form of sweetened beverages. Poor food choices contribute to rising obesity and the appearance of nutrition-related chronic diseases formerly seen only in adults, such as metabolic syndrome and type 2 diabetes. As students learn about nutritional needs of infants, children, and adolescents, they also learn how to help these groups improve their nutritional status.

Chapters 5 through 8 discuss special nutrition considerations for infants, children, and adolescents. Eating disorders, failure to thrive, food allergies, and the nutrition needs of children with disabilities are all covered in these chapters. Highlighted are pediatric vegetarianism, childhood obesity, and dietary needs of athletes. Very specialized topics, such as inborn errors of metabolism, are also included.

Section 2 covers adults. Chapters 9 to 11 include information on chronic nutrition-related diseases, such as coronary heart disease, hypertension, diabetes, kidney disease, cancer, osteoporosis, HIV/AIDS, and obesity. Evidence analysis for evidence-based practice in these diseases is included, as are prevention strategies. Chapter 11 is devoted to physical activity and weight management issues. Chapters 12 and 13 are dedicated to nutritional issues of the elderly; all topics ranging from special nutritional needs to nutritional problems, from activities of daily living to polypharmacy, and from risks of malnutrition to nutrition intervention are included in these chapters. Chapters 14 and 15 discuss professionalism and ethical issues, the final preparation for students to join us as colleagues.

This book has many exciting features that not only enhance its usefulness as a teaching tool but also pave the way in developing future clinicians and scientists at the cutting edge of nutritional sciences:

Evidence-Based Practice: This section contains articles where readers can transform the written word into a peer-reviewed study or clinical trial. I tell my students that we don't want to know their opinion, we want to know their informed opinion. But how do they shape these opinions? Only by reading about evidence-based studies and medicine and by conducting studies themselves can students learn the importance of evidence-based practice. The American Dietetic Association, with its Evidence Analysis Library, is a leader in presenting practitioners with the concept of evidence-based practice. This text complements this effort and enhances our students' familiarity with this important subject.

Cultural Diversity Sidebar: Cultural differences that involve the nutrition and health differences and similarities among ethnic groups are highlighted. This is a wonderful opportunity for students to learn more about what I call "diseases that discriminate": Obesity, cardiovascular disease, and diabetes are all most common in minority populations. Why? Are differences genetic or are they related to lifestyle or to health care? What are the gaps in nutrition research in different groups? How do you work with people from cultures or ethnicities that are different from your own to improve their health or nutritional status? This feature will help students answer these questions, develop their professionalism, and improve their practice.

Critical Thinking Sidebar: Found throughout the chapters, the points considered assist the reader in critical thinking concepts of different sections of the text. Perhaps the most important thing a student can learn is to analyze and evaluate, examine and reason, reflect and decide. Why? In order to solve complex real-world problems, weigh evidence and make conclusions, learn to ask the right questions, and develop informed opinions to share with others.

Case Studies and Nutritional Management: These sections are provided to demonstrate chapter concepts. Case studies actively involve students in learning and simulate or represent actual problems they will face as professionals. Students can work alone or in groups to develop solutions, as they would in the workplace. Thus, case studies help develop knowledge and skills of students in a wide variety of subjects and improve critical thinking skills, public speaking, and group interactions.

Issues to Debate: These issues include withholding and withdrawing nutrition, the ethical implications of nutritional care, and right-to-die case law. It is critical that students learn the physiologic, moral, ethical, and legal issues surrounding these emotionally charged issues. Debate and discussion with others help students understand these issues as they apply across the life span; it also helps nutrition students learn how they will interact with other health professionals.

Website Resources: Websites are provided not only for present use as students work through the material presented, but also for use by the students when they become the teachers. The Internet has opened virtually all information to all people at all times. No health professional can work without it. However, there are no filters on or standard for materials posted on the Web. It is important to help students understand this and to help them use appropriate materials. The websites provided in this book provide reliable and accurate information.

For students, *Reader Objectives* guide them stepwise through the chapter, and *Key Terms* sidebars throughout the chapters assist with new terminology and concepts. Also included are *Special Sections,* which are designed to heighten curiosity and give insight to a particular issue. *Chapter Summaries* crystallize the most important elements of the chapters and help bring the chapter contents into perspective.

For instructors, there is a separate *Instructor's Manual* with multiple-choice questions and answers to case studies, as well as PowerPoints available electronically for all chapters.

Carol E. O'Neil, PhD, MPH, LDN, RD
Theresa A. Nicklas, DrPH

ABOUT THE EDITORS

Judith Sharlin, PhD, RD

BA University of California, Berkeley
BS University of California, Berkeley
MS Boston University
PhD Tufts University

Dr. Judith Sharlin is a senior lecturer in the Department of Nutrition and Dietetics at Simmons College. Before coming to Simmons College, Dr. Sharlin co-directed the Graduate Nutrition Communications Program at Boston University and owned and operated a catering and baking business. She is the author or editor of multiple books, including a national award-winning cookbook and nutrition guide, *The Romantic Vegetarian* (1984) as well as *Life Cycle Nutrition: An Evidenced-Based Approach* (2009). She is also the author of many research articles and chapters including topics on food consumption behavior and cardiovascular risk, weight management, diet and chronic disease risk, and end-of-life nutrition. She has lectured nationally on these topics. Dr. Sharlin competes as a U.S. Masters swimmer and ranks as a "Top Ten" record holder in New England.

Sari Edelstein, PhD, RD

BS Florida State University
MS Florida International University
PhD University of Florida

Dr. Sari Edelstein is Associate Professor in the Department of Nutrition and Dietetics at Simmons College. She teaches both Food Science and Food Service classes. Before coming to Simmons College, Dr. Edelstein was previously in private practice and served as a hospital Food Service Director and Chief Dietitian. She is the author of many research articles on such topics as ethics, yoga, the glycemic index, and athletic performance, as well as the author or editor of multiple books, including *Nutrition in Public Health*, 2nd and 3rd ed. (2005, 2010); *Life Cycle Nutrition: An Evidence-Based Approach* (2009); *Nutrition: Rapid References for Nurses* (2007); *Managing Food and Nutrition Services* (2008); N*utrition Guide for Dietitians* (2009); and *Food, Cuisine and Cultural Competency* (2010).

CONTRIBUTORS

Claire Blais, RD, LDN, CNSD
Massachusetts General Hospital

Lisa S. Brown, PhD, RD
Simmons College

Jennifer L. Bueche, PhD, RD, CDN
State University of New York

Victoria Hammer Castellanos, PhD, RD
Florida International University

Karen Chapman-Novakofski, RD, LDN, PhD
University of Illinois at Urbana-Champaign

Sari Edelstein, PhD, RD
Simmons College

Karen M. Funderburg, MS, RD, LD
University of Oklahoma Health Sciences Center

Laura Harkness, PhD, RD
Nestle

Edna Harris-Davis, MS, MPH, RD, LD
Georgia East Central Health District

Roschelle Heuberger, PhD, RD
Central Michigan University

Pamela S. Hinton, PhD
University of Missouri

Rachelle Lessen, MS, RD, IBCLC
The Children's Hospital of Philadelphia

Reed Mangels, PhD, RD
University of Massachusetts

Migy K. Mathews, MD
The Donald W. Reynold Department of
   Geriatric Medicine
University of Oklahoma Health Sciences Center

Theresa A. Nicklas, DrPH
Baylor College of Medicine

Liesje Nieman, RD, CNSD, LDN
The Children's Hospital of Philadelphia

Carol O'Neil, PhD, MPH, LDN, RD
Louisiana State University

Aaron Owens, MS, RD
ECI Infant Development Program

Barbara Robinson, MPH, RD, CNSD
Hasbro Children's Hospital
Brown Medical School

Jennifer Sabo, RD, LDN, CNSD
The Children's Hospital of Philadelphia

Angela Sader, RD, LD, MBA
Beverly Enterprises, Inc.

Judith Sharlin, PhD, RD
Simmons College

Sara Snow, MS, RD
Nestle

Inger Stallmann-Jorgensen, MS, RD, LD
Medical College of Georgia

I. David Todres, MD
Massachusetts General Hospital
Harvard Medical School

Stella Lucia Volpe, PhD, RD, LDN, FACSM
University of Pennsylvania

Nutrition Requirements During Pregnancy

Lisa S. Brown, PhD, RD

With a Special Section: Unusual Complications of Pregnancy

CHAPTER OUTLINE

Reader Objectives

After studying this chapter and reflecting on the contents, you should be able to

1. Discuss the rationale for healthy nutrition during pregnancy.
2. Summarize the growth changes that occur during fetal development.
3. Discuss the common nutrition-related problems that can occur during pregnancy.
4. Explain the complications of pregnancy.
5. Summarize how life-style choices can affect fetal development.

What a woman eats when she is pregnant can have profound and lasting effects on her child's health. The expression "you are what you eat" applies, but in this case, it is this: "You are what your mother eats." During the prenatal period, the fetus has the enormous task of evolving in only 9 short months from a single-celled, fertilized egg to a human infant. In order to accomplish this, the fetus must have all of the necessary resources available in the proper quantities and at the exact times they are needed. Despite the daunting nature of the task, mothers have been producing healthy infants for thousands of years, demonstrating the amazing adaptability of both the mother and her child. The capacity of the mother's body to create the necessary conditions for fetal growth is one of the great miracles of life. There are limits, however, and the health of the child may suffer in obvious and not-so-obvious ways if certain thresholds for nutrients are not met.

Although a pregnant body has an amazing ability to compensate for nutrient deficiencies and excesses, a woman cannot provide essential nutrients for her child if she herself is deficient in them. Many factors influence a mother's nutritional status during her pregnancy. The mother's own health before conception, her health during pregnancy, her life-style choices, and environmental exposures can all change what and how much she eats and limit precious nutrients available for the growing fetus.

It is important that knowledgeable health care providers are available to support the mother-to-be with strategies to help her achieve the most balanced diet possible, thus ensuring the health of both mother and child. This chapter examines normal prenatal nutritional requirements and common factors that may compromise the mother's ability to provide ideal nutrition for her growing fetus.

Nutritional Status Prior to Pregnancy

The period when a woman is pregnant is often looked at in isolation and is not put in a larger context of the mother's overall health. Although this has been the traditional approach to pregnancy, there is a growing movement to look at human nutrition using the life-course approach, which is promoted by the World Health Organization (WHO). Using the life-course approach, a woman is followed from her own conception through death, and factors that have influenced her health since she herself was in utero are considered when assessing risk of developing chronic diseases for both the mother and her offspring (Darnton-Hill et al., 2004).

The Fetal Origins Hypothesis

The mother's health before and during pregnancy may be affected by genetics, as well as malnutrition, acute and chronic disease, exposure to environmental toxins, and a number of other factors. The fetal origins hypothesis proposes that certain genes in the fetus may or may not be "turned on" depending on the environment that the mother is exposed to while pregnant (Hampton, 2004). For example, if a mother is exposed to severe food restriction during pregnancy, as was the case in the Dutch famine during World War II, her developing fetus will adapt genetically to thrive in an environment of severe energy restriction. The child's genetic programming will be sensitized to store fat more efficiently compared with that of people not exposed to famine in utero. If the environmental conditions the child is born into do not match the famine conditions, the child will accumulate fat more quickly than desired and be at higher risk for obesity, diabetes, and cardiovascular disease. Findings from the Dutch famine and other cohorts support the fetal origins hypothesis, and research is ongoing to confirm the process by which this may have occurred (Roseboom et al., 2006; Thompson, 2007).

In the World Health Organization's life-course approach to disease prevention, the passing on of excess risk for chronic disease from mother to child based on prenatal environmental exposures is known as the intergenerational effect. The intergenerational effect is thought to be one reason behind the clustering of chronic disease risk factors in families of lower socioeconomic status. Women in lower socioeconomic classes are more likely to be exposed to extreme environmental conditions and have substandard health care that exacerbates problems. Interventions should seek to maximize the mother's health before and during pregnancy to improve the short- and long-term health of her children.

Maternal Preconception Weight Status

Many aspects of the mother's health and life-style before pregnancy have been shown to affect her subsequent pregnancies with potential to impact the health of her children, but one area of particular concern is the mother's weight before pregnancy. The dramatic increase of overweight and obesity in women in the United States has forced many health care providers to focus their counseling on weight management before and during pregnancy. Preconception obesity has been associated with a substantial increase in risk for pregnancy complications, such as gestational diabetes and preeclampsia, as well as a significant increase in birth defects (Chu et al., 2007; Hauger et al., 2008; Stothard et al., 2009).

Both maternal obesity (body mass index [BMI] > 30) and maternal overweight status (BMI = 25 to 29.9) have been shown to increase the risk of birth defects. One study from the Centers for Disease Control and Prevention (CDC) found that babies born to mothers who were overweight at the time of conception had a higher risk of birth defects than those born to normal-weight women, and twice the risk of heart abnormalities. Mothers who were obese prior to conception were more than 3 times as likely to have babies with spina bifida or the abdominal malformation omphalocele (Watkins et al., 2003).

A mother who is underweight prior to becoming pregnant also puts her baby at higher risk for complications, mainly because of the association between underweight status and malnutrition (Ehrenberg et al., 2003). As discussed earlier, maternal malnutrition during pregnancy may influence fetal programming, priming the child to be more susceptible to heart disease, diabetes, and high blood pressure later in life. Malnutrition may be due to illness, food insecurity, or other factors, and both the malnutrition and the underlying cause need to be addressed to maximize positive outcomes for both mother and baby.

Regardless of nutritional status, a BMI of less than 18.5 has been associated with a higher risk of preterm delivery (Hauger et al., 2008). Underweight women should be carefully monitored to ensure that they are meeting their nutritional needs during pregnancy, and weight-gain goals should be emphasized. Supplements may need to be customized to ensure that the mother-to-be meets her nutritional requirements. Referrals to social service programs to help the mother obtain food, health insurance, and housing assistance may be necessary if malnutrition is caused by food insecurity.

In some cases, underweight status before pregnancy and/or failure to gain appropriate weight during pregnancy may be a sign of either a preexisting eating disorder or one that has developed during pregnancy. "Pregorexia" is a recently coined term used to describe the practice of overly restricting energy intake and/or overexercising during pregnancy to minimize weight gain. The pregorexic mother disregards prenatal health guidelines in an effort to control her weight, with potentially dangerous short- and long-term effects for her baby, placing her baby at risk for poor growth and vitamin deficiencies. One study found that women with eating disorders were significantly more likely than those without to be at risk for fetal growth restriction, preterm labor, anemia, genitourinary tract infections, and labor induction (Bansil et al., 2008).

● **Learning Point** In 2009 the Institute of Medicine changed the guidelines for weight gain during pregnancy. See these guidelines in Table 1.1.

Preexisting Conditions

In some cases, the mother may have a preexisting medical condition that may jeopardize the fetus's health long before the child is born. Mothers with multiple sclerosis, type 1 diabetes, and other serious health conditions can have healthy, successful pregnancies, but they need to be carefully monitored by specialists as well as by a health care team that is typically led by the obstetrician/gynecologist.

Public Health Campaigns to Improve Preconception Nutritional Status

Ideally, most women will plan ahead and begin to adopt healthful behaviors compatible with a healthy pregnancy long before they are necessary. In reality, the majority of pregnancies are not planned, and thus health care providers need to take every opportunity to encourage women to adopt healthful practices that will support a healthy pregnancy.

A few social marketing campaigns have been mounted over the years, designed to educate women of childbearing age about behaviors related to positive pregnancy outcomes, thus maximizing the health of their children if pregnancy occurs. One example is the March of Dimes campaign to encourage supplementation with folic acid for all women of childbearing age. The campaign had limited success, and many experts concluded that these public health messages were ultimately far less effective than fortification of the food supply with folic acid (Bower et al., 2005). The March of Dimes discontinued this campaign and is currently focusing its education and prevention efforts more broadly on reducing behaviors in women associated with premature birth.

General Preconception Health and Nutrition Recommendations for Women

Preconception planning for all women should include advice to begin prenatal multivitamin/mineral supplements even before conception to build stores and ensure adequate intake of valuable nutrients. In addition to a standard prenatal supplement, most women could likely benefit from taking fish oil to build stores of essential fatty acids before becoming pregnant.

Life-style interventions should include advising women to stop smoking before they become pregnant. Alcohol and caffeine consumption should be moderated prior to conception, and drinking of alcohol should be discontinued altogether if a women suspects that she is pregnant.

Other good practices to prepare for a healthy pregnancy include evaluating the safety of all medications the mother takes, whether prescription or over the counter, to determine whether they are safe to take during pregnancy. Alternate medications that are determined to be safe during pregnancy should be identified, and women should work with their doctors to switch to these alternates if necessary in the case of prescription medications.

A woman who needs to lose weight prior to conception should be very careful not to over-restrict micronutrients to a point that she becomes deficient. She should be careful not to compromise the health of the fetus by following a strict diet plan before becoming pregnant. The focus of preconception weight loss should be on cutting empty-calorie foods and increasing low-calorie, nutrient-dense foods such as fruits and vegetables, whole grains, and low-fat meats and dairy. Increasing exercise may also help the woman lose weight prior to becoming pregnant and have benefits after she becomes pregnant in helping her cope with some of the unpleasant side effects associated with pregnancy.

Nutrient Needs During Pregnancy

The needs for most nutrients are increased during pregnancy to meet the high demands of both the growing fetus and the mother, who herself goes through a period of growth to carry the child and prepare for lactation. In this section, we discuss the general need for increased macronutrients and micronutrients **(Figure 1.1)**.

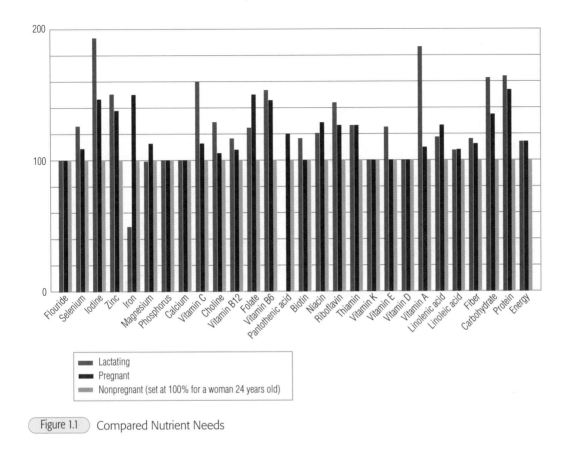

Figure 1.1   Compared Nutrient Needs

Total Energy

It is often said that a pregnant woman is "eating for two." Although this is technically correct, mothers-to-be often overestimate their need for additional calories, especially early in the pregnancy. For most women, the extra energy needs are easily met by adding a small snack or two during the day. Eating smaller amounts of food more frequently also has the benefit of helping with some of the uncomfortable side effects of pregnancy, including nausea and heartburn. The focus should be on increasing the consumption of nutrient-dense foods and minimizing empty-calorie foods that may provide the extra energy needed but do not provide micronutrients that are needed in much higher amounts compared with increased caloric needs.

Before 2002, the advice for pregnant women was to increase their energy intake by approximately 300 kcal/day in the second and third trimesters (Institute of Medicine, 1990). In 2002 the Institute of Medicine (IOM) revised the Dietary Reference Intake (DRI) recommendations for energy intake during pregnancy. The new recommendations are higher in total calories and more specific in how increased calorie needs should be distributed over the trimesters of pregnancy. The new recommendations advise no additional calories for the first trimester, add 340 kilocalories for the second trimester, and add 452 kilocalories for the third trimester (Panel on Macronutrients, Institute of Medicine, 2002).

In a comprehensive study released in 2004, Butte et al. reported that additional energy needs not only should differ by trimester but also should be tailored based on the mother's preconception BMI. Butte et al. (1994) outlined the additional energy needs during pregnancy by trimester: In the first trimester, the underweight woman should increase her usual energy intake by an additional 150 kcal/day. In the second trimester, the underweight woman should add 200 kcal/day to her usual intake, whereas the normal-weight woman should add 350 kcal/day extra, and the overweight/obese woman should add 450 kcal/day of extra energy. In the third trimester, the underweight woman should add 300 kcal/day to

TABLE 1.1	2009 Institute of Medicine Guidelines for Prenatal Weight Gain	
Weight Category	**Total Weight Gain (lbs)**	
Underweight: BMI under 18.5	28–40 lb	
Normal weight: BMI 18.5–24.9	25–35 lb	
Overweight: BMI 25–29.9	15–25 lb	
Obese: BMI greater or equal to 30.0	11–20 lb	
Source: Adapted from Institute of Medicine		

TABLE 1.2	Average Weight Distribution of Weight Gained During Pregnancy
Weight	**Distribution**
7.5 pounds	Average baby's weight
7 pounds	Extra stored protein, fat, and other nutients
4 pounds	Extra blood
4 pounds	Other additional body fluids
2 pounds	Breast enlargement
2 pounds	Uterine enlargement
2 pounds	Amniotic fluid
1.5 pounds	The placenta
Source: Adapted from Institute of Medicine	

her usual energy intake, the normal-weight woman should add 500 kcal/day, and the overweight/obese woman should add 350 kcal/day.

Although the Butte et al. study and the DRI recommendations provide general guidelines for caloric intake during pregnancy, the most accurate way to monitor whether the mother is getting the appropriate energy intake is to monitor her weight gain. A variety of factors may alter the woman's need for additional calories, with level of physical activity being the most influential, just as it is for nonpregnant women. Physical activity during pregnancy is discussed later in this chapter (see Tables 1.1 and 1.2).

Protein

Healthy fetal development is dependent on the availability of adequate protein, which provides the basic building blocks necessary for formation of enzymes, antibodies, muscle, and collagen. Collagen is used as the framework for skin, bones, blood vessels, and other body tissue. During pregnancy, the mother must consume adequate protein to meet the needs of her growing fetus in addition to meeting her own increased needs as she physically grows in size to carry her baby. To accommodate the high demand, the mother's body adapts during pregnancy to conserve protein. Hormones signal the body that she is in a state of anabolism, which causes her body to retain nitrogen for protein synthesis.

The DRI for protein for a nonpregnant woman is 0.8 g/kg/day, which comes to approximately 54 g/day for a 150-pound woman. The 2002 DRI for pregnant women recommends 1.1 g/kg/day of body weight or an additional 25 g/day to meet the needs of pregnancy. According to the National Health and Nutrition Examination Survey (NHANES), the average daily protein intake for a women aged 20 to 39 in the United States is 74 grams, and thus protein needs should easily be met by most American women, even during times of elevated need such as pregnancy (Centers for Disease Control and Prevention, 2004).

Despite the generally high level of protein intake within the United States, several special populations should be carefully monitored for adequate protein intake and quality during pregnancy: vegetarians, vegans, low-income women experiencing food insecurity, and women experiencing severe nausea and vomiting.

When evaluating the mother's protein status, several factors should be taken into account. The mother may be consuming an adequate number of calories but taking in insufficient protein, leading to a protein deficiency. Conversely, the mother may consume adequate protein but may still have a protein deficiency if her calorie intake is too low. To meet the increased energy needs of pregnancy, some amino acids may be used for energy, thus leading to a protein deficiency. Finally, the quality of the mother's protein intake should be accounted for. If the mother does not consume high-quality sources of protein, meaning sources that include all essential amino acids, such as meat, eggs, poultry, fish, and dairy, she should be encouraged to consume a variety of plant-based foods to ensure that all essential amino acids are available to the fetus.

A woman who chooses a vegan diet eats no dairy products, meat, fish, or poultry, placing her at high risk for protein deficiency both before and during pregnancy. She must consume all essential amino acids from plant sources to create the protein necessary for her fetus's growth. Although it is possible for a vegan mother to have a healthy pregnancy, careful planning and monitoring to ensure that she is meeting her increased protein needs is essential. Lacto-ovo vegetarians who do not eat red meat, poultry, or fish should also be screened for protein deficiency, although they are at a much lower level of risk because of consumption of high-quality protein in the form of milk, cheese, yogurt, and eggs.

Low-income women are also at high risk for protein deficiency during pregnancy because of potential issues with food insecurity. A woman who is food insecure may lack adequate resources to obtain protein-rich, nutrient-dense foods, which often cost more compared with less nutritious foods. It is important to help food-insecure women identify low-cost protein sources, such as canned tuna, beans, eggs, and limited amounts of meat. Woman experiencing food insecurity should also be referred to nutrition assistance programs such as the Supplemental Nutrition Assistance Program (SNAP) for Women, Infants, and Children (WIC), formerly known as the Food Stamps program, and local food pantries.

Lipids and Fats

The mother-to-be must include enough fat in her diet to meet the needs of her growing baby. Lipids, including sterols, phospholipids, and triglycerides, which are primarily made up of fatty acids, are another basic building material of body tissue and integral to body functioning. Lipids are essential for the formation of cell membranes and hormones and are necessary for proper eye and brain development, especially during the prenatal period and into the first few years of the child's life (Innis & Friesen, 2008).

Fat is also a source of concentrated calories and may be beneficial to women at risk of energy malnutrition while pregnant. Women who are not at risk should avoid excess fat because it can easily lead to undesired weight gain; moderation is essential. There is no separate RDA/DRI for fat intake during pregnancy, and the recommendation remains 20% to 35% of total calories, the same as for the general population. Fat intake during pregnancy should emphasize sources that provide the essential fatty acids and choline, a component of phospholipids necessary for healthy brain function.

Essential Fatty Acids

The essential fatty acids linoleic acid (omega-6) and linolenic acid (omega-3) are necessary for optimal formation of the brain and eyes and also play a key role in the body as precursors of hormone-like substances called eicosanoids. Eicosanoids are used to signal a number of local reactions within the human body necessary for basic functioning. Reactions such as muscle relaxation and blood vessel constriction are signaled by eicosanoids. Immune functions such as the inflammatory response to injury and infection that signals initiation of fever, aggregation of antibodies, and pain are also controlled by eicosanoids (Connor, 2000).

Although omega-6 fatty acids are used to create proinflammatory eicosanoids, omega-3 fatty acids are used to create anti-inflammatory versions. When the body has sufficient access to both essential fatty acids, it is able to create balanced amounts of each type, allowing for optimal immune function. This balance is possible only when the two essential fatty acids are consumed through diet or supplements in adequate amounts. Although omega-6 fatty acids are plentiful in the American diet through meat and vegetable oils, omega-3 fatty acids are relatively insufficient. This imbalance would theoretically lead to the ability to mount a pro-inflammatory response without an equal ability to slow and stop it. Omega-3 fatty acid deficiency has also been linked with lower intelligence quotient (IQ) scores in infants and with lower scores of visual acuity, as well as an increased risk of depression in adults; it is suspected to be one potential reason for an increased risk of chronic diseases with an inflammatory component such as cardiovascular disease (Horrocks and Yeo, 1999; Bourre, 2007; Connor, 2000).

The amount of these essential fatty acids available to the fetus is based on how much of each the mother eats. If a mother-to-be consumes a typical American diet, the fetal tissue will have a high concentration of omega-6. Omega-3 fatty acids are generally deficient in the standard American diet and consumed in a 1:10 ratio with omega-6 fatty acids (Briefel & Johnson, 2004). This deficiency may be even more pronounced in pregnant women, who may avoid seafood, one of the richest sources of omega-3, because of fears of mercury contamination.

Supplementation with omega-3 fatty acids increases the availability to the fetus and should be recommended to every woman who is currently pregnant or is planning to become pregnant. The mother should be advised to continue to supplement with omega-3 fatty acids during lactation.

The revised 2002 RDA/DRI recommendation for essential fatty acids is an adequate intake (AI) of 13 g/day of omega-6 and 1.4 g/day of omega-3. It further states that the ratio of the two fatty acids should be no more than 5:1. Because of a lack of data, the AI for essential fatty acids likely does not represent ideal levels for each nutrient and will almost certainly change as more information becomes available.

Choline

When selecting appropriate dietary fat sources, mothers-to-be should be advised to include good sources of choline. Choline is a component of phospholipids and is needed for synthesis of lecithin, a structural component of cell membranes and an essential constituent of the human brain and nervous system. Choline is also necessary to make the neurotransmitter acetylcholine. During fetal development, choline supports the structure and function of the brain and spinal cord. In animal models, choline deficiency during pregnancy in the mother has been associated with impaired memory in her children (Zeisel, 2006).

The AI for pregnant and lactating women is 450 mg/day, increased from 425 mg/day in nonpregnant women of childbearing age. Good sources of choline are whole, reduced-fat, and low-fat milk; liver; eggs; and peanuts. Choline intake in the United States has declined over the past few decades because Americans avoid eating egg yolk and reduce the amount of milk and dairy products they consume to lower cholesterol intake.

Fiber

Fiber is a very important component of the prenatal diet. The development of the fetus is not dependent on an adequate supply of fiber, but a high-fiber diet significantly increases the comfort of the pregnant mother by helping to reduce constipation, a common side effect of pregnancy. Although the AI for pregnant women is 28 g/day, according to NHANES 1988–91, the average intake for a nonpregnant American woman of childbearing age is only approximately 13 g/day (Alaimo et al., 1994).

Although the American diet is generally low in fiber, leading to adverse effects on health, including constipation, hemorrhoids, and diverticulitis, it is even more important that pregnant women get enough fiber because they are at higher risk for these problems. Higher fluid needs, reduced exercise, and hormonal changes within the woman's body designed to allow the baby more room for growth may all contribute to problems with constipation and hemorrhoids during pregnancy. Pregnant women should be given the standard advice to reduce these problems, including increasing noncaffeinated fluids, moderate exercise, and high fiber intake. Fruits, vegetables, beans, whole grains, seeds, and nuts are all good dietary sources of fiber.

● **Learning Point** See what MyPyramid recommends for pregnant and breast-feeding women at: http://www.mypyramid.gov/mypyramidmoms/

Carbohydrate

Dietary carbohydrate is broken down to form glucose, also known as blood sugar. The rapid growth of the fetus requires that ample amounts of energy in the form of glucose be available to the fetus at all times. The recommended daily allowance (RDA) for carbohydrate during pregnancy is 175 g/day, increased from 130 g/day for nonpregnant women. Most Americans eat enough carbohydrate to meet normal and pregnancy requirements with a mean intake of approximately 260 g/day for women of childbearing age (Centers for Disease Control and Prevention, 2004).

Pregnant women should be advised that a low-carbohydrate diet is dangerous during pregnancy and could place the baby at risk for poor growth. A mild restriction of dietary carbohydrate may be recommended if the mother is diabetic. If a mother enters pregnancy with preexisting diabetes or develops it while she is pregnant, she will need to work closely with her health care team to make sure that she provides enough, but not too much, glucose to ensure optimal growth of her baby. Gestational diabetes is discussed in more detail later in this chapter.

Vitamin A

Vitamin A, a fat-soluble vitamin, and beta carotene, which can be used in the body as either an antioxidant or a precursor to vitamin A, are critical during fetal development because of their involvement in growth, vision, protein synthesis, and cell differentiation. Beta carotene is found in fruits and vegetables, and preformed vitamin A can be found in animal products, including fish, meat, and milk. Despite the important role vitamin A plays in the body, the RDA for pregnant women of 770 μg/day is only slightly higher than the RDA for nonpregnant women. This is due to the high risk of birth defects associated with excessive doses of preformed vitamin A early in pregnancy (Miller et al., 1998).

Although it is unlikely that the mother-to-be will overconsume vitamin A from food sources alone, close attention should be paid to choosing a prenatal vitamin supplement that contains no more than the usual RDA for vitamin A. To minimize risks associated with excess intake, a significant percentage of the vitamin A content in the supplement should come from beta carotene instead of providing it all as preformed vitamin A (Strobel et al., 2007). Beta carotene is not converted to vitamin A unless the body determines the need, and thus it is a safer form to consume.

Vitamin D

Vitamin D may be obtained through diet and supplements or can also be made by the body when skin is exposed to ultraviolet rays. Vitamin D is necessary to help build and maintain strong bones and teeth and is very important during fetal development for this reason. Recent research shows that babies born during the late summer and early fall are taller and have wider bones (Sayers & Tobias, 2008). There is also mounting evidence that vitamin D plays a key role in preventing common cancers, autoimmune diseases, type 1 diabetes, heart disease, and osteoporosis. Furthermore, studies have shown that vitamin D deficiency is common in the United States, suggesting that most Americans would benefit from supplements (Holick, 2008).

Fatty fish (mackerel, sardines, salmon), liver, egg yolks, and fortified milk are all good dietary sources of vitamin D. Vegans, women with lactose intolerance or milk allergies, women who dislike dairy products, and women who avoid the sun may be at particular risk for vitamin D deficiency. The RDA for vitamin D in pregnant and nursing women is currently 200 IU (5 μg/day), although this is considered much too low by experts in the field. Michael Holick, MD, PhD, one of the leading researchers on vitamin D, recommends 1,000 IU daily for everyone over the age of 1 year. Alternatively, if the latitude provides adequate year-round ultraviolet light, vitamin D needs can be met by exposure of the arms and legs to sunlight for 5 to 10 minutes three times a week. Women in the United States living north of Atlanta, Georgia; women with darker skin tones; and women who use a lot of sunblock or who limit their sun exposure should be strongly advised to supplement with additional vitamin D beyond that provided by the prenatal supplement.

Calcium

Although calcium is also necessary for proper bone formation in conjunction with vitamin D, the RDA/DRI for pregnant women is the same as it is for nonpregnant women: 1,000 mg/day for women over 18 years old. Dietary sources include milk, yogurt, and cheese, as well as sardines with bones and some leafy green vegetables. Vegan women and women who consume fewer than 3 servings of dairy per day should be advised to take a separate calcium supplement during pregnancy to make sure they are getting enough. Alternatives to cow's milk such as soy, rice, and almond milk should be checked to make sure that they are fortified with calcium. These products must be shaken well because the calcium has a tendency to settle on the bottom on the containers. Consuming adequate calcium while pregnant and breast-feeding may not affect the baby's bone density, but it will protect the mother's bones from losing too much of the calcium that she will give to her baby if dietary calcium is not enough.

B Vitamins

The RDA/DRI for most B vitamins is higher during pregnancy compared with that of nonpregnant women in the same age category. B vitamins are primarily used as cofactors in energy metabolism, and the need for these vitamins is increased proportional to the increase in energy needs during pregnancy. Deficiency of most B vitamins is rare because of their availability in a wide variety of food sources and their presence in prenatal supplements. Two B vitamins, folate and B12, should be given special attention, however, because of their unique roles during fetal development and potential for deficiency in a pregnant woman.

Vitamin B12

Vitamin B12 is essential for the production of red blood cells, the manufacturing of genetic material, and healthy functioning of the nervous system. The RDA is 2.4 μg/day in nonpregnant women, compared with 2.6 μg/day in pregnant women. Deficiencies in pregnant and breast-feeding women may cause neurologic damage in their children. Deficiency of B12 at the start of pregnancy may increase risk of birth defects such as neural tube defects and may contribute to preterm delivery (Molloy et al., 2008). The only natural dietary sources are animal products, including meats, dairy products, eggs, and fish (clams and oily fish are very high in B12), but like other B vitamins, B12 is added to commercial dried cereals and included in adequate amounts in prenatal supplements.

Folate

Folate, available also in its synthetic form folic acid, is a B vitamin that is used in the manufacturing of neurotransmitters and is particularly important during early pregnancy because of its essential role in synthesizing DNA in the cells. The RDA for folic acid in nonpregnant women of childbearing age is 400 μg/day and increases to 600 μg/day during pregnancy. Good food sources include avocado, bananas, orange juice, dry cereal, asparagus, fruits, green leafy vegetables, and dried beans and peas.

In preconception and early pregnancy, 400 μg of folic acid in supplement form appears to be adequate for the prevention of neural tube defects, the most common of which are spina bifida and anencephaly. Spina bifida occurs when there is an incomplete closure of the spinal cord and spinal column, and anencephaly is severe underdevelopment of the brain. Neural tube defects occur during the first 28 days of pregnancy, usually before a woman even knows that she is pregnant, making the timing of folate supplementation of particular importance. Additional folate introduced after this critical period will not reverse prior damage done by a lack of the nutrient (Molloy et al., 2008).

As with other nutrients, the fetus has priority for folate over the mother's needs, potentially leaving the mother deficient after delivery unless her intake is sufficient to meet both of their needs. The extra folate in most prenatal vitamins is to prevent the mother from becoming deficient as the pregnancy progresses, both for her own health and to prevent birth defects if a pregnancy occurs within a few months of delivery.

The U.S. Public Health Service recommended in 1992 that all women of childbearing age consume 400 μg of folic acid daily (Centers for Disease Control and Prevention, 1992); however, surveys suggested that the overwhelming majority of U.S. women were not doing so. To deal with the public health crisis of neural tube defects, the Food and Drug Administration mandated folic acid supplementation in enriched grain products. Supplementation, which began in 1998, was estimated to increase the daily folate intake of the average American by approximately 100 μg (Honein et al., 2001).

Monitoring has shown that fortification has been effective in reducing the incidence of neural tube defects; they have decreased by 70% in the United States since the program began. Although prevention of neural tube defects was the primary justification, folic acid fortification has been effective in reducing cardiovascular events as well. During the same period, stroke and stroke deaths declined by 15% (Yang et al., 2002). Despite concern about potential adverse effects, such as a masking of B12 deficiency, no problems have been identified as a result of the fortification, and controversy remains over whether the level should be increased in the United States to match the model used in Canada and Europe.

Iron

Iron is a trace mineral that is vital for fetal growth and development because it plays a key role as a cofactor for enzymes involved in oxidation-reduction reactions, which occur in all cells during metabolism. Iron is also necessary as the component of hemoglobin that allows red blood cells to carry oxygen needed throughout the body. Perhaps most important, iron is essential for normal neurodevelopment during fetal and early childhood development. Iron deficiency in infancy and early childhood is associated with impaired memory function and changes in temperament that may mimic attention deficient disorder. Memory deficits persist even after normal iron levels are achieved (Georgieff, 2008). Worldwide, inadequate dietary iron intake is the most common nutrient deficiency, and women are at particularly high risk because of a regular loss of iron during monthly menses.

Pregnancy places an even higher demand for iron on the woman's body, both as her own blood volume expands to carry the pregnancy and as her child demands iron for normal development. The DRI for iron during pregnancy is 27 mg/day, and is particularly vital to meet this recommendation during the second and third trimesters. During the last 3 months, the baby is accumulating iron for use during early life. Studies show that if adequate iron is not available during the prenatal period and first 6 months of life, there can be lifelong neurologic effects that cannot be reversed even if iron is supplemented at adequate levels in early childhood (Beard, 2008).

Fetal iron stores are meant to last the child until approximately 6 months of life. After the age of 6 months, the American Academy of Pediatrics recommends a good dietary source of iron be introduced into the infant's diet to help support the accelerated growth of the child during the first year of life. The best method for combating iron deficiency in pregnancy is to promote high intakes before pregnancy so that there will be at least 300 mg of iron stored as a woman enters pregnancy.

Mothers should be encouraged to take a prenatal vitamin with adequate iron to meet their needs, although high amounts of supplemented iron are associated with constipation and upset stomach for many pregnant women. If a woman enters pregnancy iron replete, prenatal supplements do not have to contain as high a level of iron as for a woman who enters pregnancy iron deficient. Lower levels of iron in the multivitamin/mineral will minimize unpleasant side effects.

For women who require high amounts of iron during pregnancy, several measures can be suggested to decrease associated discomfort. It is important to give these women strategies to improve their tolerance of the high iron levels in prenatal supplements, as iron intolerance is a primary reason that mothers stop taking their vitamins. Many women find taking their prenatal vitamin just before bed and/or with food helps them tolerate the high level of iron better. Taking the iron with a source of vitamin C will improve absorption and may help the mother to reduce the amount of extra iron she needs to take. Finally, eating sources of iron that are highly bioavailable, such as red meat, or snacking on iron-fortified cereal will also help to increase iron intake. Women who snack on dry cereal should be advised to have with it juice or another vitamin C source, instead of dairy products, which inhibit the absorption of iron.

Magnesium

Magnesium is a cofactor in over 300 enzymes in the body. Dietary magnesium inadequacy has been demonstrated to be common among American women and is associated with an increased risk of miscarriage, fetal growth retardation, maternal hospitalizations, and preterm delivery (Durlach, 2004). Inadequacy of magnesium has also been identified as a risk factor for the development of both gestational diabetes and type 2 diabetes (Barbagallo et al., 2007). After birth, it has been associated with an increased risk of Sudden Infant Death Syndrome (SIDS) and increased referrals to the neonatal intensive care unit (NICU). Most prenatal vitamins contain only 10% to 25% of the RDA for magnesium, and thus emphasis should be put on consuming good dietary sources. The best dietary sources include peanuts, bran, wheat germ, nuts, and legumes. Acute therapeutic intravenous magnesium is sometimes used to treat preeclampsia and premature labor (Thapa & Jha, 2008). Other studies have shown a potential benefit of supplementing magnesium at the RDA level in the reduction of leg cramps in pregnancy, although the association is not conclusive (Young & Jewell, 2002).

Zinc

The RDA for zinc during pregnancy is 11 mg/day, increased from 8 for nonpregnant women. Adequate zinc is extremely important during the first trimester, when organs are formed and may play a role in assisting in immune system development (Shah & Sachdev, 2006). Zinc deficiency is common worldwide, and supplementation within the RDA is advised during pregnancy. Because red meat is the best source of zinc, it may be more difficult for vegans and vegetarians to get enough. Furthermore, phytates found in a plant-based diet can interfere with zinc absorption. For vegetarian and vegan women, a supplement that includes 15 mg of zinc is advised throughout the pregnancy.

Iodine

Although overt deficiency of iodine is uncommon in the United States because of fortification of table salt, iodine deficiency affects more than 2 billion people worldwide and is the leading cause of mental retardation. Women in the United States are at risk, however, of consuming inadequate amounts of iodine caused by variable levels in commonly eaten foods. Given the nutrient's important role in fetal development, supplementation is recommended for pregnant and lactating women (Pearce, 2007).

The RDA for pregnant women is 220 µg of iodine per day. Mothers who do not get enough can put their baby at greater risk for mental retardation, as well as growth, hearing, and speech problems. Women consuming a low-salt diet during pregnancy, especially those trying to manage edema and/or pregnancy-induced hypertension, are at particular risk for iodine insufficiency.

In a recent study done by scientists at the Boston University Iodine Research Laboratory, researchers determined that a large percentage of prenatal vitamins do not include any iodine (Leung et al., 2009). They found that of 223 prenatal multivitamins in the United States, both prescription and over the counter, only half of them contained iodine. Of the vitamins that listed iodine, many fell short of the amount stated on the label. Prenatal multivitamins that contain potassium iodide instead of kelp were more likely to contain adequate amounts. Pregnant women are advised to take a prenatal supplement containing iodine, preferably one that uses potassium iodide as the source.

Fetal Development

A healthy pregnancy lasts an average of 40 weeks, with a normal range of 38 to 42 weeks. There are 3 distinct stages of fetal development during which the baby must complete specific developmental tasks. The zygote period is the first stage, beginning at conception and lasting approximately 2 weeks. The embryonic period goes from 2 to 8 weeks, and the fetal period lasts from 8 weeks until birth.

Weeks of pregnancy are counted from the first day of the woman's last period, and thus a woman is considered pregnant approximately 2 weeks before she actually conceives the baby. After conception, the fertilized egg, also known as the zygote, makes its way to the uterus, where it implants and begins its rapid growth.

The Embryonic Phase

The embryonic stage begins shortly after implantation of the zygote in the wall of the uterus and lasts until the 8th week. This period often begins before a woman even knows she is pregnant, but it is a critical stage of fetal development. During this time, the embryo's cells are dividing rapidly to form the basic body systems. By 8 weeks after conception, the embryo is only approximately 1.25 inches long, but it already has a complete central nervous system, a beating heart, a digestive system, fingers, toes, and the beginning of facial features.

The Fetal Phase

Fetal development begins after the 8th week. Early in this period the fetus continues to develop all of the necessary body systems and begins to take on a more human appearance. Distinguishable genitals, hair, nails, and vocal cords form. The kidneys begin to process bodily fluids, and the liver begins to function. Bones also begin to harden early in the fetal period.

Although far from ready for birth, by the 28th week of gestation, most babies born can survive outside the womb with intervention to aid breathing until the lungs are more mature.

During the final 12 weeks of gestation, brain and eye development proceed at a fast rate. The fetus also builds bone mass and gains fat stores to help him or her survive outside of the protective environment of the womb. The immune system begins to mature during this time, and lungs develop to a point where the baby can breathe without external intervention after approximately 37 weeks' gestation. Finally, the fetus spends the last several weeks of gestation laying stores of nutrients to help support functioning during early life until he or she is able to transition to a more varied diet at 6 months of age.

Critical Periods of Nutrient Intake During Embryonic and Fetal Development

Given the fast rate of growth and the enormous complexity of the task, it is easy to see how deficiency of any nutrient needed during a specific phase of development could impact this delicate process. Although deficiency of almost any micronutrient or macronutrient will certainly impact the course of development, several in particular have been identified with specific birth defects if the nutrient is not present during a very narrow window of time. Several others are suspected to cause less-overt problems if the nutrient is deficient during a critical period.

Folic acid deficiency during the first 4 weeks of development, when the central nervous system is forming, is perhaps the most devastating nutrient deficiency because it may result in neural tube defects. Deficiency of iodine during brain development can also have dramatic and obvious permanent effects, such as mental retardation. The effects of other nutrient deficiencies may be less dramatic but may nonetheless have a significant impact in the child's health over the course of the lifetime. For example, a deficiency of vitamin D during the fetal period can result in undermineralized bones, and a deficiency of iron during brain development may lead to permanent alteration of memory function (see the sections on each specific nutrient for more information).

Even when adequate nutrients are available for the child's physical development, during the last several weeks in the womb, the fetus builds stores of nutrients, including fat, vitamin D, vitamin B12, and iron to help the baby through its early development outside of its mother. If nutrient supplies are not adequate in the mother during pregnancy, the infant will need to consume these nutrients in ample amounts after birth, which may tax the immature digestive system.

Common Problems Associated with Pregnancy

How a woman experiences pregnancy is very different from woman to woman. Even for the same woman, the experience may be very different from pregnancy to pregnancy. A number of factors contribute to the mother's experience with pregnancy, including how the mother feels about being pregnant; her physical reaction to pregnancy; any health conditions that she has or develops; her physical environment, including availability of food, housing, and health care; and finally, other demands that cause stress for the mother (e.g., her job or other kids). This section discusses some of the common physical side effects of pregnancy, as well as some of the more serious health problems that may develop as a result of the pregnancy.

Nausea and Vomiting of Pregnancy and Food Aversions and Cravings

During pregnancy, the mother's body goes through many changes to accommodate the new life growing inside her. Many women experience side effects of these changes that influence her ability to eat as healthfully as she might like. Hormonal shifts caused by the pregnancy are thought to be responsible for the majority of these side effects, but controversy remains regarding whether some common conditions related to pregnancy are physiologic or psychological phenomena (Markl et al., 2008). Regardless of their origin, it is important to help pregnant women struggling with problems like nausea, vomiting, food aversions, and cravings to minimize the impact of these factors and maximize nutrition for the health of both mother and baby (Keller et al., 2008).

Nausea and Vomiting of Pregnancy

One of the most common side effects of pregnancy is known as "nausea and vomiting of pregnancy" (NVP), more commonly known as "morning sickness." Ironically, morning sickness is usually not limited to the morning, although that may be when a woman experiences it most acutely. Up to 80% of pregnant women experience NVP at some point, usually beginning between the 4th and 7th weeks after their last period and ending for most women by the 20th week. For 10% of those that have it, however, it remains an ongoing battle throughout the pregnancy (Quinla & Hill, 2003).

Nutrition Requirements During Pregnancy

The underlying causes of nausea and vomiting of pregnancy remain unclear, but hormonal shifts are hypothesized to be one potential cause. Estrogen, progesterone, and human chorionic gonadotropin (hCG) have all been investigated for possible mechanisms of action (Davis, 2004). Progesterone, for example, which is released during pregnancy, has been suggested to cause delayed gastric motility, which can cause nausea. One study found that when progesterone was given to nonpregnant women they developed nausea and vomiting similar to the symptoms of NVP (Walsh et al., 1996).

The most severe version of NVP is known as hyperemesis gravidarum, which is estimated to affect approximately 1 in every 200 pregnant women. Although there is no standard definition, the condition is characterized by persistent vomiting, dehydration, ketosis, electrolyte disturbances, and weight loss of more than 5% of body weight (Ismail & Kenny, 2007).

Although normal NVP is actually associated with positive outcomes for the baby, hyperemesis can be dangerous to both the mother and the child. NVP has been associated in several studies with improved pregnancy outcomes, including fewer miscarriages, preterm deliveries, and stillbirths, as well as fewer instances of fetal low birth weight, growth retardation, and mortality. One potential explanation for this is that NVP is a mechanism designed to increase the mother's intake of simple carbohydrates, which alleviates her symptoms and supplies increased amounts of glucose to the growing fetus (Furneaux et al., 2001). In contrast, hyperemesis gravidarum has been associated with increased adverse effects for both the mother and fetus. The mother is more likely to experience splenic avulsion, esophageal rupture, Mallory-Weiss tears, pneumothorax, peripheral neuropathy, and preeclampsia. The fetus is at increased risk for fetal growth restriction and mortality (Ismail & Kenny, 2007).

Dietary modifications are the first line of treatment for women with mild nausea and vomiting. Several measures are often used in combination to help manage symptoms until they pass on their own. Most women find that it helps to eat small, frequent meals. Avoidance of smells and food textures that cause nausea also helps, keeping in mind that what triggers the nausea may be different for each woman. Usually, bland-tasting, cold foods that are high in carbohydrates and low in fat are best tolerated. Eating high-carbohydrate foods first thing in the morning often helps and may be most useful even before the woman gets out of bed. Sour and tart liquids such as lemonade often are tolerated better than water. It may also help if the woman avoids the smell of food until mealtime, as smells often trigger nausea.

Other treatments include acupressure bands, ginger, and special supplements made specifically for NVP, such as "Pregipops" and "Pregidrops." Supplementation with vitamin B6 has also been associated with relief of symptoms, and several trials have tested both the effectiveness and safety of this treatment (Sahakian et al., 1991; Tiran, 2002).

Cravings and Aversions

Although food cravings and their flip-side food aversions are thought of as a common condition of pregnancy, not all women experience these sensations. One study found that food cravings occurred in only 61% of pregnant women, whereas aversions occurred even less frequently, appearing in 54% of pregnant women (Bayley et al., 2002). There is little understanding of what causes craving and aversions, and not all experts agree that they are a real phenomenon and not simply a psychological manifestation.

One plausible explanation for cravings and aversions during pregnancy is changes in smell and taste. One study found that abnormal smell and/or taste perception was reported by 76% of pregnant women surveyed. Increased smell sensitivity was found to be very common in early pregnancy, occurring in 67% of respondents. Abnormal taste sensitivity was reported by 26% of women in the study, who often described increased bitter sensitivity and decreased salt sensitivity. The results of this study suggest that abnormal smell and/or taste perception is experienced by a large majority of pregnant women and may underlie food aversions and cravings during pregnancy (Nordin et al., 2004).

Another theory behind the development of craving is that some women who deprive themselves when they are not pregnant think of pregnancy as a time to treat themselves to foods they typically avoid and indulge themselves—because, after all, they are "eating for two."

There are also several less plausible theories behind the prevalence of food cravings and aversions during pregnancy. One states that food cravings are nature's way of helping the mother meet her nutritional needs. For example, the woman may need sodium to help manage her increased fluid volume during pregnancy, and thus she may crave salty foods. Although this is an interesting idea, there is no evidence that potential nutrient shortfalls are translated into food cravings in the body.

Common Problems Associated with Pregnancy

A similar theory regarding food aversions is that they are a protective mechanism during pregnancy designed to steer the mother away from dangerous foods. For example, a woman may have an aversion to drinking coffee when pregnant, which is beneficial because limiting caffeine intake during pregnancy may aid in fetal mental and physical development and decreases risk of infant death. Many women also develop aversions to the taste and smell of cigarettes while pregnant, which increases compliance with smoking cessation during the prenatal period (Pletsch & Kratz, 2004). Although there is no evidence that aversions are developed as a protective mechanism, this remains a persistent myth.

Pregnant women can indulge their cravings so long as they are meeting their needs nutritionally. The craved-for food also should be screened to ensure that it is not contraindicated by special dietary restrictions, such as a high-carbohydrate food for a woman with gestational diabetes. Finally, the concept of moderation must be emphasized to keep the mother's weight gain within the IOM guidelines based on her pre-pregnancy BMI. Mothers-to-be should be advised to keep portions small and to try to eat only healthier versions. For example, a woman who craves ice cream may want to indulge in a reasonable half cup of low-calorie ice cream or frozen yogurt instead of a pint of premium high-calorie ice cream.

Reflux

Reflux, also known as heartburn, occurs when acid from the stomach makes its way through the lower esophageal sphincter, causing a burning sensation in the lower esophagus. It is a very common problem during pregnancy and is often one of the first symptoms of pregnancy, appearing within the first month after conception for many women. Occurring early in pregnancy, reflux is likely caused by hormonal changes, perhaps even before most women have gained any pregnancy weight. Later in pregnancy, the pressure of the baby pushing upward against the mother's stomach may exacerbate the problem (Ali & Egan, 2007).

Most health authorities agree that calcium carbonate supplements like Tums are safe to use during pregnancy and helpful for alleviating symptoms (Richter, 2005). Other measures encompass standard advice for anyone with reflux, including keeping upright for 1 to 2 hours after eating, eating smaller meals, drinking between meals instead of with the meal to avoid overfilling the stomach, elevating the head of the bed a few inches, and avoiding trigger foods. Although trigger foods differ from person to person, the most common are coffee, acidic foods such as tomato sauce, minty foods, and chocolate. Other novel approaches to managing reflux include drinking water to wash down the acid and chewing sugarless (non-mint-flavored) gum to generate saliva to help wash down the acid.

Reflux is not serious for most women and will go away within a few months post pregnancy. In very rare cases, the mother may need to be prescribed a stronger medication to manage her reflux. This decision should be made based on the mother's level of discomfort.

The Interaction of Life-style and Pregnancy

Life-style behaviors such as physical activity, smoking, and alcohol consumption have a strong impact on pregnancy. When a pregnancy is planned, it is easier to modify harmful behaviors ahead of time, but women are often unexpectedly pregnant. Furthermore, many life-style choices are coping mechanisms used to handle stress. Pregnancy may place extra stress on the mother, making it even more difficult to give up harmful practices. It is important to help the mother develop a strong support system to help her cope with the stress of pregnancy as well as stress she may face after delivery to help her give up harmful behaviors and adopt positive ones that will benefit both her child's health and her own. This section discusses some of the common life-style choices that may impact pregnancy.

Physical Activity, Safety, and Energy Needs

There are many good reasons for women to exercise during pregnancy. Exercise during pregnancy helps to reduce some of the common complaints of pregnancy, including backaches, constipation, and bloating and swelling. It improves mood and may help mothers sleep better. It also promotes the strength, muscle tone, and endurance that may be helpful during labor and recovery. The American College of Obstetricians and Gynecologists (ACOG) recommends that pregnant women without medical or obstetric complications engage in 30 minutes or more of moderate exercise a day on most, if not all, days of the week (ACOG Committee on Obstetric Practice, 2002).

Expert organizations, including the ACOG and the National Academy of Sports Medicine, have agreed that most women can safely engage in a level of physical activity similar to their activity level prior to pregnancy, as long as weight gain and infant development are not compromised (ACOG, 1994). Women who maintain a moderate to high level of physical activity during pregnancy will have relative caloric needs higher than less-active women who are in the same stage of pregnancy. Moderate to high levels of physical activity have been associated with lower infant birth weights compared with infants of more sedentary women, but this is likely because the higher caloric needs of the active women were not met during pregnancy (Penney, 2008). If the mother is gaining appropriate weight, indicating that she is meeting her caloric needs, the birth weight of the baby should not be affected, regardless of the amount of physical activity.

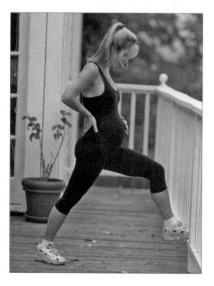

Some caution should be observed when helping mothers decide on an exercise program during pregnancy. Women with medical or obstetric complications should be encouraged to avoid vigorous physical activity. Contraindications to exercise during pregnancy put forth by ACOG include pregnancy-induced hypertension, preterm rupture of membranes, preterm labor during the prior or current pregnancy, incompetent cervix or cerclage placement, persistent second- or third-trimester bleeding, placenta previa, and intrauterine growth retardation. Relative contraindications include chronic hypertension, thyroid function abnormality, cardiac disease, vascular disease, and pulmonary disease.

Pregnant women should be advised to avoid contact sports such as soccer and high-impact sports and those that require advanced balance, which may be affected later in pregnancy. Examples include horseback riding, skiing, and gymnastics.

Pregnant women should also be warned to be careful when engaging in flexibility exercises. During pregnancy, a hormone called relaxin is produced that is designed to help loosen joints so that the baby has room to grow and to make labor easier. The relaxing of ligaments caused by the release of relaxin increases risk of injury, especially during flexibility exercises, and thus women should be advised not to overdo stretching.

Food Safety

Food safety should be a concern for every American at all times, but pregnant women, young children, individuals with compromised immune systems, and older individuals need to take extra precautions to avoid exposure to food-borne pathogens.

Infection from a food-borne illness may cause harm to both the mother and her fetus and should be avoided if possible. Women become more susceptible to infection with the hepatitis E virus, *Coxiella burnetii*, *Listeria monocytogenes,* and *Toxoplasma gondii,* which are intracellular pathogens that take advantage of hormonal shifts during pregnancy that down-regulate cell-mediated immune functions (Smith, 1999).

All pregnant women in the United States are currently advised to avoid foods that are considered health risks for pregnant women and developing babies. These include any meat, seafood, or egg item that is raw or undercooked and any unpasteurized food, including milk, cheeses made from unpasteurized milk like brie and feta, and unpasteurized juice. Women are advised to wash all fruits and vegetables thoroughly before eating them and to avoid any that cannot be properly washed or are known to carry food-borne illness, such as alfalfa sprouts.

Special precautions have been set forth by the American Food and Drug Administration Center for Food Safety and Applied Nutrition to reduce risk of contamination with *Listeria monocytogenes (http://www.fda.gov/Food/ResourcesForYou/HealthEducators/ucm083320.htm). L. monocytogenes* is of particular concern because it can grow at refrigerator temperatures, whereas most other food-borne bacteria do not. Measures to reduce exposure include avoiding unpasteurized foods and heating ready-to-eat foods until they are steaming to kill the bacteria. For example, it is recommended that hot dogs and luncheon meats should be eaten only if they are reheated until steaming hot.

The Center for Food Safety and Applied Nutrition (CFSAN) recommends that pregnant women avoid the following foods:

Sushi or sashimi. Raw fish (including oysters, clams, mussels, and scallops) or foods made with raw fish are more likely to contain parasites or bacteria than foods made from cooked fish.

Swordfish, tilefish, king mackerel, and shark. These fish can contain high levels of methylmercury, a metal that can be harmful to the unborn baby. Other cooked fish/seafood is considered safe, but women should try to vary their seafood. Up to 12 ounces (2 average meals) a week of a variety of fish and shellfish that are lower in mercury appear to be safe during pregnancy. Five of the most commonly eaten fish that are low in mercury are shrimp, canned light tuna, salmon, pollock, and catfish. Albacore ("white") tuna has more mercury than canned light tuna.

Raw sprouts (including alfalfa, clover, radish, and mung bean). Bacteria can get into sprout seeds through cracks in the shell before the sprouts are grown. After this occurs, these bacteria are nearly impossible to wash out. Sprouts grown in the home are also risky if eaten raw. Many outbreaks have been linked to contaminated seed. If pathogenic bacteria are present in or on the seed, they can grow to high levels during sprouting—even under clean conditions.

Unpasteurized or untreated juice. These juices are normally in the refrigerated sections of grocery stores, health food stores, cider mills, or farm markets.

Mothers should also be advised to wash their hands regularly.

Alcohol

No level of alcohol consumption is considered safe during pregnancy. Alcohol can pass freely through the placenta, and thus if the mother drinks, so does her unborn child. Consumption of alcohol during pregnancy is associated with higher risk of birth defects and miscarriage. At high levels, alcohol may cause fetal alcohol syndrome (FAS), which is the leading cause of preventable mental retardation (Chiriboga, 2003).

FAS is characterized by mental retardation, malformations of the skeletal system, malformation of the heart and brain, growth problems, central nervous system problems, poor motor skills, increased mortality, and problems with learning, memory, social interaction, attention span, problem solving, speech, and/or hearing. Children with FAS can often be identified by characteristic facial features, including small eyes, a short or upturned nose, flat cheeks, and thin lips. These features fade as the child gets older, but other effects do not (National Organization on Fetal Alcohol Syndrome, n.d.).

It is important for mothers to understand that although FAS is usually caused by binge drinking or regular alcohol consumption during pregnancy, any alcohol intake during pregnancy may contribute to fetal damage and place the child at risk of fetal alcohol spectrum disorder (FASD). The term "FASD" is used to encompass the full spectrum of birth defects that are caused by prenatal alcohol exposure. FASD is usually split into two levels of damage: fetal alcohol syndrome, which represents the most severe damage, and fetal alcohol effects, used to describe lesser damage caused by more moderate drinking.

According to the Fetal Alcohol Spectrum Disorders Center for Excellence, fetal alcohol effects are manifestations of moderate drinking during pregnancy. Physical and neurological deficiencies may be a result of fetal alcohol effects. The effect that fetal alcohol exposure has on the developing brain explains common mental and behavioral impairments characteristic of fetal alcohol exposure, such as learning disabilities, poor school performance, poor impulse control, and problems with memory, attention, and judgment.

Illegal Drug Use

Just as with alcohol, there is no safe level of illegal drug consumption during pregnancy. Illegal drug use during pregnancy may result in miscarriage, low birth weight, premature labor, placental abruption, and fetal death. Mothers suspected of using illegal drugs during pregnancy should be referred to their doctor, who should prescribe appropriate treatment (Floyd et al., 2008).

> ● **Learning Point** More research is needed on the life-style of the father and fetal health, especially in the areas of paternal alcohol and drug use.

Cigarette Smoking

According to the American Lung Association, smoking during pregnancy is estimated to account for 20% to 30% of low-birth-weight babies, up to 14% of preterm deliveries, and about 10% of all infant deaths. Furthermore, even exposure to secondhand smoke can increase risk. Smoking during pregnancy has also been associated with an increased risk for colds, lung problems, learning disabilities, and physical growth problems for exposed children after birth.

It is strongly advised that pregnant women quit smoking for the duration of the pregnancy. Studies show that approximately half of all women who smoke are able to do this, but half are not. One study looked at the profile of women who did not quit smoking and found that they were more likely to have been heavy smokers prior to pregnancy and had more psychosocial problems compared with women who quit (Pickett et al., 2009). If a woman is not able to quit smoking, she should be encouraged to cut her usual amount to the lowest possible level.

Helping the mother-to-be deal with the stressors in her life may help her quit smoking. In addition to putting her in contact with food, housing, and counseling resources, there are public health resources available to help women stop smoking in addition to help she may get from her doctor. The American Lung Association has the following suggestions for pregnant women who wish to quit smoking: Ask for help from health care providers, family, and friends. Make a list of reasons for wanting to quit, for yourself as well as for the baby. Set a quit date—the sooner the better. If you are not ready to set a date, you can begin to cut down on smoking, and then you can make a plan to stop all smoking in the near future. Try the four Ds: delay, deep breathe, drink water, and do something else. If you slip and go back to smoking, you should first find out what caused the slip, and then you can keep trying to quit again until you succeed. The only failure is if you stop trying.

Caffeine

Caffeine is one of the most widely consumed pharmacologically active substances in the world. It is found in various drinks, chocolate, and some medications. Caffeine is an important concern during pregnancy because it crosses the placenta to the baby, whose metabolism is still maturing and cannot fully process it. Some studies have shown that there may be an increased risk of miscarriage among women who consume more than 300 mg/day, the equivalent of a medium cup of coffee at most fast-food restaurants. Other potential adverse outcomes include preterm labor and low-birth-weight babies (Kuczkowski, 2009).

Although most doctors advise women that they can drink caffeine in moderation while pregnant, keeping under 300 mg/day, it is safer to avoid caffeine altogether if possible. If a woman must have caffeine, she should be advised to limit herself to 1 cup per day of coffee, tea, or soda. To reduce the common side effects of headache, ideally women would gradually reduce their intake prior to pregnancy. A stepwise reduction during pregnancy will also help to manage headaches that will likely result from sudden stoppage of caffeine consumption.

SPECIAL SECTION: UNUSUAL COMPLICATIONS OF PREGNANCY

Pica

A pregnant woman may occasionally crave nonfood items such as ice, dirt, clay, paper, and even paint chips, a condition known as pica. It has been theorized, although never proved, that pica may signal iron deficiency (Mills, 2007). Expectant mothers may also get the urge to eat flour or cornstarch, which despite being food items are a problem in large amounts. Too much can lead to blocked bowels and crowd out the nutrients the baby needs by causing the mother to feel full. A woman with pica or an unhealthy craving such as cornstarch should resist eating these items and should speak to her doctor right away.

Preeclampsia

Preeclampsia is a syndrome that is characterized by dangerously high blood pressure and protein in the urine. It is often accompanied by edema, sudden weight gain, headaches, and changes in vision. It occurs only during pregnancy and up to 6 weeks postpartum, usually appearing in the late second or the third trimester. According to the National Heart, Lung, and Blood Institute (NHLBI), the condition appears in 5% to 8% of pregnancies in the United States.

Preeclampsia, pregnancy-induced hypertension, and eclampsia (formerly known as toxemia) are closely related conditions. Pregnancy-induced hypertension is generally considered the mildest manifestation, whereas eclampsia is one of the most serious complications of severe preeclampsia. Left untreated, eclamptic seizures can result in coma, brain damage, or maternal or infant death. HELLP syndrome, which stands for hemolysis, elevated liver enzymes, and lowered platelets, is another of the most severe forms of preeclampsia, usually affecting the liver and causing stomach and right shoulder pain.

HELLP syndrome occurs in 4% to 12% of the women who have preeclampsia. It is particularly dangerous because it may occur even before the mother develops the classic symptoms of preeclampsia. It is often mistaken for the flu or gallbladder problems (Haram et al., 2009).

Complications of preeclampsia in the fetus include prematurity, growth restriction, and death. Fetal growth restriction results from reduced blood flow to the placenta, which compromises the supply of nutrients to the baby and can result in a shortage of food and subsequent starvation. As a result, the baby may be small for its gestational age. This shortage of nutrients available through the placenta places the baby at serious risk, and premature birth may result naturally or be induced for the protection of both mother and child (Sibai et al., 2005). According to the March of Dimes, preeclampsia is a leading cause of premature birth in the United States. Worldwide, preeclampsia and other hypertensive disorders of pregnancy are leading causes of maternal and infant death.

There are several known risk factors for preeclampsia, two of which should be of particular concern given changing trends in the profile of pregnant women in the United States over the past few decades: a BMI of 30 or higher and a maternal age of over 40 or under 18 years. Other risk factors include a previous history of preeclampsia, a history of chronic high blood pressure, diabetes or kidney disorder, a family history of the disorder, carrying multiple fetuses, polycystic ovarian syndrome, and lupus or other autoimmune disorders, such as rheumatoid arthritis, sarcoidosis, or multiple sclerosis.

Several nutritional interventions have been associated with reduced risk of developing preeclampsia. Increased intake of fiber and calcium has been positively associated with reduced risk in several studies (Hofmeyr et al., 2007; Wallis and Saftlas, 2008). Women who are at risk should be encouraged to consume adequate dairy products and fruits and vegetables before and during pregnancy.

The role of nutrient deficiencies has also been examined. One study showed that women with low levels of the mineral selenium were 4 times more likely to have preeclampsia than women with higher levels (Rayman et al., 2003). The researchers also found that low selenium was associated with an increased risk of premature delivery. Selenium is found in whole grains, fortified cereal, and Brazil nuts.

Gestational Diabetes

"Gestational diabetes" is the term used for diabetes diagnosed during pregnancy whether or not it is thought to be directly caused by the pregnancy. It is present in about 5% of all pregnancies and is usually detected between 24 and 28 weeks by an oral glucose tolerance test (Lucas, 2001). In some cases, type 2 diabetes is originally diagnosed during pregnancy. In this case, the diabetes is referred to as gestational diabetes until the mother is no longer pregnant. If the blood sugar fails to return to normal levels after the baby is delivered, the mother will then be diagnosed with type 2 diabetes.

Women of certain ethnic backgrounds appear to have a higher genetic predisposition, increasing rates to as high as 7% to 9% within certain populations. Women who identify themselves as Hispanic, African-American, Native American, Asian, Pacific Islander, or Indigenous Australian are at an elevated risk. Women who were obese prior to pregnancy, who have been diagnosed with polycystic ovarian syndrome, and who have thyroid disorders are also at higher risk (Cheng and Caughey, 2008).

Under normal conditions, the mother's body adapts during pregnancy to ensure that a constant supply of glucose is available to her baby by becoming slightly insulin resistant. If the mother's body is not able to control this natural phenomenon adequately, she may develop gestational diabetes, creating an overabundance of glucose in her bloodstream. To compensate for the extra supply of glucose, the fetus begins to overproduce insulin in order to manage its own blood sugar level. Insulin is a growth hormone, and a high level of fetal production leads to excessive infant growth and high birth weight.

Untreated gestational diabetes is associated with a higher risk of stillbirth and macrosomia, usually defined as a birth weight of over 10 pounds. When the infant is abnormally large, the mother is at a high risk for a caesarian section, which carries with it all of the complications of any major surgery (Schmidt et al., 2001). In addition, children born via caesarean section are more likely to develop asthma and allergies, potentially because of a lack of exposure to the normal vaginal flora that helps immunize them (Bager et al., 2008).

A macrosomic (large) baby is also at high risk for birth complications such as shoulder dystocia, which occurs when the baby's shoulders are too large to move through the birth canal. Shoulder dystocia can lead to permanent nerve damage for the infant and may be a potentially life-threatening situation. In addition to the physiological complications associated with delivery of a large infant, there are other potential adverse outcomes. If the baby is overproducing insulin at the time of delivery, there is a serious risk of subsequent low blood sugar for the infant after the umbilical cord is cut and the constant supply of glucose is no longer present. There is a significantly higher rate of neonatal intensive care unit admissions for infants of diabetic mothers who have poor blood sugar control. Prevention is very effective in reducing most risks associated with gestational diabetes.

Women who are diagnosed with gestational diabetes can usually keep their blood sugar within a reasonable range with a mild restriction of carbohydrate in their diet. If the mother has tried dietary modifications but blood sugars remain above optimal levels, medication may be indicated. Insulin therapy is the accepted treatment for gestational diabetes if a mother fails diet and life-style therapy.

Even if the mother's blood sugar returns to normal after the birth, it is important to continue to follow up. Women with gestational diabetes are at high risk for developing the disease during subsequent pregnancies. Furthermore, studies show that as many as 70% of all women with gestational diabetes will eventually be diagnosed with type 2 diabetes (Kim et al., 2002). Prevention efforts after the birth include stressing the importance of maintaining or achieving a healthy weight, regular exercise, and a diet that emphasizes complex carbohydrates.

Summary

Pregnancy is a critical time of human development, and anything that compromises the fetal environment may have important and lasting effects on the child's future health. It is important as a society to prioritize helping women understand the impact that their life-style choices have on their children. Maximizing the health of the pregnant mother will ensure her child the best start at life possible.

Nutrition is a vital component of fetal development, as the baby cannot build with materials he or she does not have. Limiting exposure to damaging substances such as nicotine, caffeine, food-borne bacteria, and alcohol will also aid in the child's development. Helping women deal with unpleasant side effects of pregnancy as well as more serious ones should be a focus of prenatal support. Finally, encouraging healthful life-style practices during pregnancy such as moderate exercise and healthy eating will impact not only the child's long-term health, but potentially the mother's as well.

Issues to Debate

1. Does the public have a responsibility to assist pregnant women in receiving good nutrition?
2. What are the long-term consequences of a lack of assistance programs for pregnant women?
3. Most of the discussion in this chapter has revolved around the nutritional health of the fetus, but what is the effect of poor nutrition during pregnancy on the mother?

Case Studies

(Answers to all case studies are in the Instructor's Manual available at jbpub.com.)

Case Study 1

Nadine is a 37-year-old African-American woman. She is at 28 weeks' gestation and has 3 children already. Her routine glucose screen at 24 weeks was high; she has not yet had a follow-up glucose tolerance test to determine if she has gestational diabetes.

Her weight is 244 lb; height is 5'6". Her mother has type 2 diabetes. Her first baby weighed 9 lb, her second baby weighed 9 lb, 4 oz. She has a hectic job as a day-care provider. She often skips meals.

1. How likely is it that Nadine will be diagnosed with gestational diabetes? What are her risk factors?
2. Assuming Nadine is diagnosed with gestational diabetes, what recommendations would you make in terms of her nutrition management?
3. Below is a 24-hour recall for Nadine. Help Nadine modify her diet to better control her blood sugar.

Continues

Sample 24-hour recall:

8:30 am	1.5 cups orange juice, 2 slices toast (white bread)
11:00 am	candy bar
12:30 pm	2 slices pepperoni pizza (14")
5:30 pm	20 banana chips
8:45 pm	2 cups red beans and rice

Case Study 2

Maria is a 27-year-old woman with a 2-year-old child who is now 14 weeks pregnant with her second child. She weighs 160 lb and her height is 4'11".

Maria gained 80 pounds with her first pregnancy and has never lost most of the weight. She is at home all day with her child, while her husband works 2 jobs. Maria drinks 4 cups of coffee and 3 cans of diet cola a day because she is so tired all the time. She also drinks fruit punch with her son when they have meals. She has not been taking her prenatal vitamin because she feels that it upsets her stomach and constipates her. She and her son often eat at fast-food restaurants or have packaged food like boxed macaroni and cheese or frozen chicken nuggets because those are foods her son likes to eat. She eats very few fruits and vegetables, and she drinks no milk, although she eats some American cheese.

Maria would like to eat better, but doesn't know what she should do. She has also heard that exercise during pregnancy is a good idea because it will help keep her back and legs from aching, and she would like to try it.

1. What recommendations would you make in terms of life-style management for Maria?
2. How would you modify her diet? Based on the Institute of Medicine guidelines, how much weight should Maria gain during this pregnancy?
3. How should the weight gain break down by trimester? What recommendations can we give her to slow her weight gain?
4. Assuming that Maria and her family are at the federal poverty line, what nutrition programs are they eligible for?

Case Study 3

Arunima is a 25-year-old woman born in India. She is 8 weeks pregnant with her first child. For the past month she has been very nauseous, though not vomiting, and has not been eating much. She weighs 110 lb and her height is 5'4"; she has lost 2 lb since she became pregnant. She does not work outside the home, and her husband works as a store manager. She is a strict vegetarian (vegan).

1. Discuss interventions that may help manage Arunima's nausea.
2. At 12 weeks the nausea passes and Arunima is hungry! What recommendations would you make in terms of nutrition management for Arunima? As a vegan, what elements of her diet do we need to be concerned about? How can you modify her diet to make sure she gets the nutrients she needs?

Websites

American Lung Association http://www.lungusa.org/
Exercise During Pregnancy http://www.acog.org/publications/patient_education/bp119.cfm
Fetal Alcohol Spectrum Disorders Center for Excellence www.fascenter.samhsa.gov/
National WIC Association www.nwica.org/
Supplemental Nutrition Assistance Program www.fns.usda.gov/fsp/
World Health Organization http://www.who.int/nutrition/publications/fetomaternal/en/
March of Dimes http://www.marchofdimes.com/21209_11560.asp
The National Partnership for Smoke-Free Families http://www.smokefreefamilies.tobacco-cessation.org/

References

Nutrition Requirements During Pregnancy

ACOG Committee on Obstetric Practice. (2002). ACOG committee opinion. Exercise during pregnancy and the postpartum period. No. 267, January. *Obstetrics and Gynecology, 99*(1), 171–173.

Alaimo, K., McDowell, M. A., Briefel, R. R., Bischof A. M., Caughman, C. R., Loria, C. M., et al. (1994). Dietary intake of vitamins, minerals, and fiber of persons ages 2 months and over in the United States: Third National Health and Nutrition Examination Survey, Phase 1, 1988–91. *Advance Data, 14*(258), 1–28.

Ali, R. A., & Egan, L. J. (2007). Gastroesophageal reflux disease in pregnancy. *Best Practice and Research. Clinical Gastroenterology, 21*(5), 793–806.

American College of Obstetricians and Gynecologists. (1994). *Exercise During Pregnancy and the Postpartum Period.* ACOG Technical Bulletin 189. Washington, DC: American College of Obstetricians and Gynecologists.

Bager, P., Wohlfahrt, J., & Westergaard, T. (2008). Caesarean delivery and risk of atopy and allergic disease: Meta-analyses. *Clinical and Experimental Allergy, 38*(4), 634–642.

Bansil, P., Kuklina, E. V., Whiteman, M. K., Kourtis, A. P., Posner, S. F., Johnson, C. H., et al. (2008). Eating disorders among delivery hospitalizations: Prevalence and outcomes. *Journal of Women's Health, 17*(9), 1523–1528.

Barbagallo, M., Dominguez, L. J., & Resnick, L. M. (2007). Magnesium metabolism in hypertension and type 2 diabetes mellitus. *American Journal of Therapeutics, 14*(4), 375–385.

Bayley, T. M., Dye, L., Jones, S., DeBono, M., & Hill, A. J. (2002). Food cravings and aversions during pregnancy: Relationships with nausea and vomiting. *Appetite, 38*(1), 45–51.

Beard, J. L. (2008). Why iron deficiency is important in infant development. *Journal of Nutrition, 138*(12), 2534–2536.

Bourre, J. M. (2007). Dietary omega-3 fatty acids for women. *Biomedicine and Pharmacotherapy, 61*(2–3), 105–112.

Bower, C., Miller, M., Payne, J., & Serna, P. (2005). Promotion of folate for the prevention of neural tube defects: Who benefits? *Paediatric and Perinatal Epidemiology, 19*(6), 435–444.

Briefel, R. R., & Johnson, C. L. (2004). Secular trends in dietary intake in the United States. *Annual Review of Nutrition, 24*, 401–431.

Butte, N. F., Wong, W. W., Treuth, M. S., Ellis, K. J., & Smith, E. (2004). Energy requirements during pregnancy based on total energy expenditure and energy deposition. *American Journal of Clinical Nutrition, 79*(6), 1078–1087.

Centers for Disease Control and Prevention. (1992). Recommendations for the use of folic acid to reduce the number of cases of spina bifida and other neural tube defects. *Morbidity and Mortality Weekly Review, 41*, 1–8.

Centers for Disease Control and Prevention. (2004). Trends in intake of energy and macronutrients—United States, 1971–2000. *Morbidity and Mortality Weekly Review, 53*(4), 80–82. Retrieved from http://www.cdc.gov/mmwr/preview/mmwrhtml/mm5304a3.htm

Cheng, Y. W., & Caughey, A. B. (2008). Gestational diabetes: Diagnosis and management. *Journal of Perinatology, 28*(10), 657–664. Epub 2008, July 17.

Chiriboga, C. A. (2003). Fetal alcohol and drug effects. *Neurologist, 9*(6), 267–279.

Chu, S. Y., Callaghan, W. M., Kim, S. Y., Schmid, C. H., Lau, J., England, L. J., et al. (2007). Maternal obesity and risk of gestational diabetes mellitus. *Diabetes Care, 30*(8), 2070–2076.

Connor, W. E. Importance of n-3 fatty acids in health and disease. (2007). *American Journal of Clinical Nutrition, 71* (1 Suppl), 171S–175S.

Darnton-Hill, I., Nishida, C., & James, W. P. (2004). A life course approach to diet, nutrition and the prevention of chronic diseases. *Public Health Nutrition, 7*(1A), 101–121.

Davis, M. (2004). Nausea and vomiting of pregnancy: An evidence-based review. *Journal of Perinatal and Neonatal Nursing, 18*(4), 312–328.

Durlach, J. (2004). New data on the importance of gestational Mg deficiency. *Journal of the American College of Nutrition, 23*(6), 694S–700S.

Ehrenberg, H. M., Dierker, L., Milluzzi, C., & Mercer, B. M. (2003). Low maternal weight, failure to thrive in pregnancy, and adverse pregnancy outcomes. *American Journal of Obstetrics and Gynecology, 189*(6), 1726–1730.

Floyd, R. L., Jack, B. W., Cefalo, R., Atrash, H., Mahoney, J., Herron, A., et al. (2008). The clinical content of preconception care: Alcohol, tobacco, and illicit drug exposures. *American Journal of Obstetrics and Gynecology, 199*(6 Suppl 2), S333–S339.

Furneaux, E. C., Langley-Evans, A. J., & Langley-Evans, S. C. (2001). Nausea and vomiting of pregnancy: Endocrine basis and contribution to pregnancy outcome. *Obstetrical and Gynecological Survey, 56*(12), 775–782.

Georgieff, M. K. (2008). The role of iron in neurodevelopment: Fetal iron deficiency and the developing hippocampus. *Biochemical Society Transactions, 36*(Pt 6), 1267–1271.

Hampton, T. (2004). Fetal environment may have profound long-term consequences for health. *JAMA: Journal of the American Medical Association, 292*, 1285–1286.

Haram, K., Svendsen, E., & Abildgaard, U. (2009). The HELLP syndrome: Clinical issues and management. A review. *BMC Pregnancy and Childbirth, 9*(1), 8.

Hauger, M. S., Gibbons, L., Vik, T., & Belizán, J. M. (2008). Prepregnancy weight status and the risk of adverse pregnancy outcome. *Acta Obstetricia et Gynecologica Scandinavica, 87*(9), 953–959.

Hofmeyr, G. J., Duley, L., & Atallah, A. (2007). Dietary calcium supplementation for prevention of pre-eclampsia and related problems: A systematic review and commentary. *BJOG 114*(8), 933–943. Epub 2007, June 12.

Holick, M. F. (2008). The vitamin D deficiency pandemic and consequences for nonskeletal health: Mechanisms of action. *Molecular Aspects of Medicine, 29*(6), 361–368.

Honein, M. A., Paulozzi, L. J., Mathews, T. J., Erickson, J. D., & Wong, L. C. (2001). Impact of folic acid fortification of the U.S. food supply on the occurrence of neural tube defects. *JAMA: Journal of the American Medical Association, 285*(23), 2981–2986.

Horrocks, L. A., & Yeo, Y. K. (1999). Health benefits of docosahexaenoic acid (DHA). *Pharmacological Research, 40*(3), 211–225.

Innis, S. M., & Friesen, R. W. (2008). Essential n-3 fatty acids in pregnant women and early visual acuity maturation in term infants. *American Journal of Clinical Nutrition, 87*(3), 548–557.

Institute of Medicine. (2009). *Nutrition During Pregnancy.* Washington, DC: National Academy of Sciences Press.

Ismail, S. K., & Kenny, L. (2007). Review on hyperemesis gravidarum. *Best Practice and Research Clinical Gastroenterology, 21*(5), 755–769.

Keller, J., Frederking, D., & Layer, P. (2008). The spectrum and treatment of gastrointestinal disorders during pregnancy. *Nature Clinical Practice Gastroenterology and Hepatology, 5*(8), 430–443.

Kim, C., Newton, K. M., & Knopp, R. H. (2002). Gestational diabetes and the incidence of type 2 diabetes: A systematic review. *Diabetes Care, 25*(10), 1862–1868.

Kuczkowski, K. M. (2009). Caffeine in pregnancy. *Archives of Gynecology and Obstetrics.* February 24. Epub ahead of print.

Leung, A. M., Pearce, E. N., & Braverman, L. E. (2009). Iodine content of prenatal multivitamins in the United States. *New England Journal of Medicine, 360*(9), 939–940.

Lucas, M. J. (2001). Diabetes complicating pregnancy. *Obstetrics and Gynecology Clinics of North America, 28*(3), 513–536.

Markl, G. E., Strunz-Lehner, C., Egen-Lappe, V., Lack, N., & Hasford, J. (2008). The association of psychosocial factors with nausea and vomiting during pregnancy. *Journal of Psychosomatic Obstetrics and Gynaecology, 29*(1), 17–22.

Miller, R. K., Hendrickx, A. G., Mills, J. L., Hummler, H., & Wiegand, U. W. (1998). Periconceptional vitamin A use: How much is teratogenic? *Reproductive Toxicology, 12*(1), 75–88.

Mills, M. E. (2007). Craving more than food: The implications of pica in pregnancy. *Nursing for Women's Health, 11*(3), 266–273.

Molloy, A. M., Kirke, P. N., Brody, L. C., Scott, J. M., & Mills, J. L. (2008). Effects of folate and vitamin B12 deficiencies during pregnancy on fetal, infant, and child development. *Food and Nutrition Bulletin, 29*(2 Suppl), S101–S111; discussion S112–S115.

Nordin, S., Broman, D. A., Olofsson, J. K., & Wulff, M. (2004). A longitudinal descriptive study of self-reported abnormal smell and taste perception in pregnant women. *Chemical Senses, 29*(5), 391–402.

Panel on Macronutrients, Institute of Medicine. (2002). *Report on Dietary Reference Intakes for Energy, Carbohydrate, Fiber, Fat, Fatty Acids, Cholesterol, Protein, and Amino Acids.* Washington, DC: Institute of Medicine.

Pearce, E. N. (2007). National trends in iodine nutrition: Is everyone getting enough? *Thyroid, 17*(9), 823–827.

Penney, D. S. (2008). The effect of vigorous exercise during pregnancy. *Journal of Midwifery and Women's Health, 53*(2), 155–159.

Pickett, K. E., Wilkinson, R. G., & Wakschlag, L. S. (2009). The psychosocial context of pregnancy smoking and quitting in the Millennium Cohort Study. *Journal of Epidemiology and Community Health, 63*(6), 474–480.

Pletsch, P. K., & Kratz, A. T. (2004). Why do women stop smoking during pregnancy? Cigarettes taste and smell bad. *Health Care for Women International, 25*(7), 671–679.

Quinla, J. D., & Hill, D. A. (2003). Nausea and vomiting of pregnancy. *American Family Physician, 68*(1), 121–128.

Rayman, M. P., Bode, P., & Redman, C. W. (2003). Low selenium status is associated with the occurrence of the pregnancy disease preeclampsia in women from the United Kingdom. *American Journal of Obstetrics and Gynecology, 189*(5), 1343–1349.

Richter, J. E. (2005). Review article: The management of heartburn in pregnancy. *Alimentary Pharmacology and Therapeutics, 22*(9), 749–757.

Roseboom, T., de Rooij, S., & Painter, R. (2006). The Dutch famine and its long-term consequences for adult health. *Early Human Development, 82*(8), 485–491.

Sahakian, V., Rouse, D., Sipes, S., Rose, N., & Niebyl, J. (1991). Vitamin B6 is effective therapy for nausea and vomiting of pregnancy: A randomized, double-blind placebo-controlled study. *Obstetrics and Gynecology, 78*(1), 33–36.

Sayers, A., & Tobias, J. H. (2008). Estimated maternal ultraviolet B exposure levels in pregnancy influence skeletal development of the child. *Journal of Clinical Endocrinology and Metabolism, 94*(3), 765–771.

Schmidt, M. I., Duncan, B. B., Reichelt, A. J., Brachtein, L., Matos, M. C., Costa e Forti, A., et al. (2001). Gestational diabetes mellitus diagnosed with a 2-h 75-g oral glucose tolerance test and adverse pregnancy outcomes. *Diabetes Care 24*(7), 1151–1155.

Shah, D., & Sachdev, H. P. (2006). Zinc deficiency in pregnancy and fetal outcome. *Nutrition Reviews, 64*(1), 15–30.

Sibai, B., Dekker, G., & Kupferminc, M. (2005). Pre-eclampsia. *Lancet, 365*(9461), 785–799.

Smith, J. L. (1999). Foodborne infections during pregnancy. *Journal of Food Protection, 62*(7), 818–829.

Stothard, K. J., Tennant, P. W., Bell, R., & Rankin, J. (2009). Maternal overweight and obesity and the risk of congenital anomalies: A systematic review and meta-analysis. *JAMA, 301*(6), 636–650.

Strobel, M., Tinz, J., & Biesalski, H. K. (2007). The importance of beta-carotene as a source of vitamin A with special regard to pregnant and breastfeeding women. *European Journal of Nutrition, 46*(Suppl 1), I1–I20.

Thapa, K., & Jha, R. (2008). Magnesium sulphate: A life saving drug. *JNMA: Journal of Nepal Medical Association, 47* (171), 104–108.

Thompson, J. N. (2007). Fetal nutrition and adult hypertension, diabetes, obesity, and coronary artery disease. *Neonatal Network, 26*(4), 235–240.

Tiran, D. (2002). Nausea and vomiting in pregnancy: Safety and efficacy of self-administered complementary therapies. *Complementary Therapies in Nursing and Midwifery, 8*(4), 191–196.

Wallis, A. B., & Saftlas, A. F. (2008). A gram of prevention: A modest increase in fiber consumption may reduce risk of preeclampsia. *American Journal of Hypertension, 21*(8), 849–850.

Walsh, J. W., Hasler, W. L., Nugent, C. E., & Owyang, C. (1996). Progesterone and estrogen are potential mediators of gastric slow-wave dysrhythmias in nausea of pregnancy. *American Journal of Physiology, 270*(3 pt 1), G506–G514.

Watkins, M. L., Rasmussen, S. A., Honein, M. A., Botto, L. D., & Moore, C. A. (2003). Maternal obesity and risk for birth defects. *Pediatrics, 111*(5 Part 2), 1152–1158.

Yang, Q., Botto, L. D., Erickson, J. D., Berry, R. J., Sambell, C., Johansen, H., et al. (2006). Improvement in stroke mortality in Canada and the United States, 1990 to 2002. *Circulation, 113*(10), 1335–1343.

Young, G. L., & Jewell, D. (2002). Interventions for leg cramps in pregnancy. *Cochrane Database of Systematic Reviews,* (1), CD000121.

Zeisel, S. H. (2006). The fetal origins of memory: The role of dietary choline in optimal brain development. *Journal of Pediatrics, 149*(5 Suppl), S131–S136.

Normal Infant Nutrition

Rachelle Lessen, MS, RD, IBCLC

Sari Edelstein, PhD, RD

CHAPTER OUTLINE

Growth

Adequate Growth in Infancy • Development of Growth Charts

Early Feeding

Colic

Food Safety

Safe Handling of Infant Formula • Safe Handling of Complementary Foods

Nutrient Requirements

Energy • Protein • Fatty Acids • Iron • Zinc • Vitamin D • Supplemental Nutrients • Vegetarianism

Complementary Feeding

Transitioning from All Milk to Family Foods • Feeding Guidelines • Complementary Foods and Growth • Meal Patterns and Nutrient Intakes

Feeding Skills and Neuromuscular Development

Reflexes • Advanced Motor Skills • Chewing Ability • Determinants of Food Acceptance • Caregiver Behaviors • Effect of Feeding Mode in Infancy • Feeding Relationship • Portion Size

After studying this chapter and reflecting on the contents, you should be able to

1. Compare growth differences between breast-fed and formula-fed infants.
2. Describe the impact of early diet on later development of obesity, diabetes, and food allergies.
3. Discuss adequate intake of key nutrients in the first year of life, including energy, protein, fatty acids, iron, zinc, and vitamin D.
4. Describe caregiver behaviors that can impact normal transitioning from an all-milk infant diet to a diet of family foods.
5. Compare and contrast actual complementary feeding patterns with recommended guidelines.

Early childhood is an important time for the development of food preferences and eating patterns. Establishment of lifelong eating habits begins in infancy and is based on a complex integration of physiologic and psychological events, including food preferences, food availability, parental modeling, praise or reward for food consumption, and peer behaviors (Stang, 2006).

Growth

Adequate Growth in Infancy

In general, if a mother is well nourished and is exclusively breast-feeding, her milk will provide adequate nutrition for her infant to grow at an appropriate rate. The American Academy of Pediatrics (AAP) Committee on Nutrition and the American Dietetic Association, authorities on breast-feeding for nutrition professionals, have strongly recommended the breast-feeding of infants (American Dietetic Association, 2003; AAP, 2005). According to these sources, breast-feeding offers both the mother and the infant several advantages, which may include:

- a sense of bonding between mother and infant.
- a convenient and economical choice of feeding.
- an aid in maternal weight loss from accumulated pounds as a result of pregnancy due to the caloric burden of the production of human milk.
- a mechanism by which the maternal uterus contracts during feeding and returns to normal size.
- availability of colostrum to the newborn. Colostrum, or "first" milk, is clear to yellowish in color. Colostrum contains antibodies transmitted from the mother and has a higher concentration of protein, vitamin A, and vitamin E and less fat and carbohydrate than later mature human milk. Colostrum is replaced with mature human milk at approximately 2 to 10 days after the birth of the infant.
- availability of additional immunologic properties for the newborn, such as protection from bacterial infection and allergy.
- newborn milk digestibility, as human milk is low in electrolyte composition and higher in fat and protein in the latter portion of the feeding, which aids in feeding satiety. Also, breast milk is higher in whey than in casein and thus has been associated with easier digestibility.
- iron availability; although maternal breast milk has a lower total amount of iron, the bioavailability of the iron is greater for the infant.

In addition to these potential benefits, human milk has unique nutritional characteristics, such as the high ratio of whey to casein, a high proportion of nonprotein nitrogen, and fatty acids essential for brain and retinal development. It is not known at what point human milk is no longer sufficient for sustained growth, but it is unlikely that complementary foods are required before 6 months of age. Although it is commonly believed that insufficient calories and protein in human milk limit growth, it is probably more likely that other factors, such as iron and zinc, affect growth. This applies to infants in both disadvantaged and affluent populations (Dewey, 2001).

Feeding mode has been found to impact weight gain and body composition during the period of exclusive or predominant milk feeding in early infancy. In a prospective cohort study of 40 exclusively breast-fed infants and 36 exclusively formula-fed infants, weight gain was greater in the formula-fed group (Butte, Wong, Hopkinson, Smith, & Ellis, 2000). Changes in body composition and weight were both age dependent and gender dependent. Daily intakes of energy, protein, fat, and carbohydrates were positively associated with weight gain and fat-free mass from birth through 12 months, but not after that. Formula-fed infants took in greater volumes and consumed significantly more energy, protein, fat, and carbohydrates.

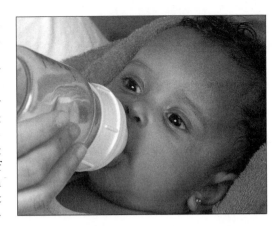

Development of Growth Charts

The nutritional status of children is assessed by plotting height and weight on **growth charts** to determine adequacy of nutrient intake, particularly calories and protein. The growth charts currently in use by the Centers for Disease Control and Prevention (CDC) have been available since 2000 and are an improvement over the previous charts from 1977 (see Appendix 1). The growth charts for children from birth through 3 years are based on data from the National Health and Nutrition Examination Survey (NHANES III) with supplemental birth data from Wisconsin and Missouri. These national survey data represent the combined size and growth patterns of breast-fed and formula-fed infants in the U.S. general population from 1971 to 1994. They replace data based on primarily formula-fed infants from 1929 to 1975 from the Fels Longitudinal Study, which contained few breast-fed infants (National Center for Health Statistics, 2000). These data do not reflect differences in racial or ethnic groups that could affect growth and include all infants and children in the United States regardless of race or ethnicity. The most important influences on growth potential appear to be economic, nutritional, and environmental (National Center for Health Statistics, 2000).

Growth charts: Used to assess nutritional status of children by plotting height and weight and comparing with reference data.

Current growth charts do not accurately reflect the growth patterns of breast-fed infants (Dewey, 2001). From 1988 to 1994, when NHANES III data were collected, less than 50% of all infants born in the United States were exclusively breast-fed at birth, and only about 10% were exclusively breast-feeding at 6 months (Ryan, Wenjun, & Acosta, 2002). There is considerable evidence to show that growth rates differ for breast-fed and formula-fed infants. Formula-fed infants typically weigh 600 to 650 g more at 12 months than breast-fed infants. Average weight of breast-fed infants is noticeably lower than formula-fed infants from 9 to 12 months, whereas length is not significantly different. Thus, breast-fed infants appear leaner and may even be diagnosed with failure to thrive because of a downward trend in percentiles on the growth chart (Dewey, 2001). However, one study found no decrease in weight gain observed in exclusively breast-fed children in the first year of life (Kramer et al., 2002).

The World Health Organization (WHO) conducted a 6-year multicenter international study to develop new growth charts derived from the growth of exclusively or predominantly breast-fed infants based on the assumption that optimal infant growth occurs in infants from healthy populations who are exclusively breast-fed for the first 6 months of life with continued breast-feeding until 2 years of age. The WHO Child Growth Standards (de Onis, Garza, Onyango, & Borghi, 2007) show how every child in the world should grow when free of disease and when their mothers follow healthy practices such as breast-feeding and not smoking. The standards depict normal human growth under optimal environmental conditions and can be used to assess children everywhere, regardless of ethnicity, socioeconomic status, and type of feeding (de Onis et al., 2007). Compared with the CDC growth charts, the WHO growth standards have been found to be a better tool for monitoring growth and identifying early overweight and excess weight gain in infants and young children (Ponce-Rivera et al., 2008; vanDijk & Innis, 2009).

Early Feeding

Colic

Infantile colic is characterized by paroxysms of uncontrolled crying or fussing in an otherwise healthy and well-nourished infant. The crying and fussing behavior can be described by the rule of threes: It starts at 3 weeks of age, crying lasts more than 3 hours a day for at least 3 days a week, and it lasts for more than 3 weeks. Colic resolves spontaneously without any further sequelae. Some attribute this behavior to psychogenic causes like tension in the maternal-infant bond or to maternal smoking or alcohol consumption, whereas other models focus on possible allergens in breast milk or infant formula as a causative agent (Schach & Haight, 2002).

Colic can be particularly distressing not only for the infant but for the parents as well. Colic occurs in both breast-fed and formula-fed infants. Breast-feeding is not protective against colic, and it is estimated that at 6 weeks the overall prevalence of colic in all infants is 24% (Clifford, Campbell, Speechley, & Gorodzinsky, 2002). Colic appears earlier and resolves earlier in formula-fed infants. Lucas and St. James-Robert (1998) conducted a study comparing colic behavior of formula-fed and breast-fed infants. They found that at 2 weeks 43% of the formula-fed infants showed signs of intense crying and colic behavior, but only 16% of the breast-fed infants demonstrated these symptoms. By 6 weeks distressed behavior was seen in 31% of the breast-fed infants but in only 12% of the formula-fed infants.

In searching for a remedy for this stressful condition, attempts to modify the infant's diet may be implemented. Cow's-milk protein may contribute to the etiology of colic, and removal of the protein may alleviate the symptoms. Use of a hypoallergenic formula for non–breast-fed infants may be recommended (Canadian Paediatric Society, 2003). Switching to a low-lactose formula or a formula with fiber was not found to be helpful in reducing colic symptoms.

A hypoallergenic maternal diet for breast-feeding mothers may reduce colicky symptoms in some infants. For some, removal of all cow's milk from the mother's diet can provide relief for the colicky breast-fed infant. Other common allergens that may produce colic symptoms in an infant include proteins from peanuts, eggs, soy, wheat, tree nuts, and strawberries. Hill et al. (2005) conducted a randomized, controlled trial of breast-feeding infants younger than 6 weeks with colic. Mothers in the experimental group excluded dairy, soy, wheat, eggs, peanuts, tree nuts, and fish from their diets. After 1 week 74% of mothers in the experimental group reported a 25% reduction in crying or fussy behavior versus 37% of the mothers in the control group.

Lust and colleagues (1996) hypothesized that maternal intake of cruciferous vegetables would cause colic symptoms in the breast-fed infant. A mailed questionnaire was used to collect information on maternal diet and colic in infants under 4 months of age. A positive relationship was seen between colic and consumption of cabbage, cauliflower, broccoli, cow's milk, onion, and chocolate. Symptoms were self-reported, and analysis failed to show a dose-response relationship between colic symptoms and frequency of the foods consumed by the mother. Mothers reported that they avoided cruciferous vegetables, milk, dried beans, spicy foods, chocolate, and caffeine either on the advice of a friend or because of a past experience related to the mother's perception of the infant's reaction to the food. Clifford et al. (2002) found that maternal intake of caffeinated beverages was not associated with colic symptoms.

As an alternative to transitioning an infant from breast milk to a hypoallergenic formula when symptoms persist, a unique protocol treatment at the Davis Medical Center at the University of California called for a maternal elimination diet followed by the use of Pancrease MT 4 enzymes with all meals and snacks (Schach & Haight, 2002). Pancrease is a digestive enzyme that further breaks down protein in the digestive track before it enters the bloodstream, thereby minimizing the potential for allergens to appear in human milk and elicit an allergic reaction in the infant. Symptoms of colic, as well as blood in the stool, were reduced after the mothers began the treatment.

Research on Colic

Studies have failed to show a clear link between dietary factors in either breast milk or formula as the cause of infant colic. Evidence suggests that dietary interventions may be helpful for some infants, especially those with a family history of atopic disease and severe colic. Most studies on the impact of dietary changes on colic have had a small sample size and were not blinded or controlled. Colic always improves over time, and any intervention is susceptible to a placebo effect affecting the outcome. Speculations as to the origins of colic abound, and treatment options are limited.

Food Safety

Safe Handling of Infant Formula

Infant formula should be prepared with careful attention to manufacturers' instructions for use and storage. Bottle-fed infants are at an increased risk for exposure to food-borne pathogens, particularly if the bottles are left at room temperature for several hours. Freshly expressed, but not previously frozen, breast milk contains live white cells that destroy pathogens and can remain at room temperature for up to 8 hours before feeding. All bottles, nipples, and other feeding equipment should be properly cleaned and disinfected between uses.

Powdered infant formula products are not sterile and can be a source of potentially devastating illness and infection in infants. At greatest risk are neonates in the first 28 days of life, premature infants, low-birth-weight infants, and immunocompromised infants. Intrinsic contamination of powdered infant formula products with *Enterobacter sakazakii* and *Salmonella* has been a cause of significant disease, causing severe developmental sequelae and death (Centers for Disease Control, 2002). The Infant Formula Act of 1980 (revised 1986) requires formula makers to use "good manufacturing practice" but does not guarantee or require sterility (Baker, 2002). Formula manufacturers are urged to develop a sterile powdered product for high-risk infants. Even low concentrations of *E. sakazakii* in powdered infant formula can cause serious harm due to the potential for exponential multiplication during preparation and holding at ambient temperatures. Good hygienic practices, such as hand washing, using sanitized containers, and preparing only the amount needed for one feeding and using it immediately, have been recommended to minimize risk (European Food Safety Authority, 2004). The U.S. Food and Drug Administration (FDA) issued warnings regarding the use of powdered infant formula in neonatal intensive care units. No events have been reported for healthy full-term infants in home settings or involving the use of sterile liquid infant formula products (FDA Talk Paper, 2002).

Nitrates

Infant methemoglobinemia leads to cyanosis in infants with few other clinical symptoms and is caused by nitrates in food or water that are converted to methemoglobin-producing nitrites before or after ingestion. The resulting compound, methemoglobin, cannot bind oxygen and results in hypoxemia. Absorbed nitrate that has not been converted to nitrite can be readily excreted in the urine without adverse effects. The greatest risk to infants comes from well water contaminated with nitrates (Greer, Shannon, the Committee of Nutrition, & the Committee on Environmental Health, 2005). It is estimated that 2 million families drink water from private wells that fail to meet federal drinking water standards for nitrate, and 40,000 infants younger than 6 months live in homes that have nitrate-contaminated water supplies. Breast-fed infants whose mothers consume water with high nitrate nitrogen concentrations are not at increased risk, because nitrate concentration does not increase in human milk.

Nitrates also occur naturally in plants and may be concentrated in foods such as green beans, carrots, squash, spinach, and beets. Some commercially prepared infant foods are voluntarily monitored for nitrate content, and because of exceedingly high levels in spinach, this product is often labeled as not to be given to infants younger than 3 months. Concerns for home-prepared foods are unfounded because there is no nutritional indication for introduction of complementary foods before 6 months. The risk of methemoglobinemia decreases with age as the infant's gastric pH level approaches lower levels typical of later childhood, and fetal hemoglobin, which more readily oxidizes to methemoglobin, is replaced by adult hemoglobin after 3 months.

Safe Handling of Complementary Foods

Infants are at risk of exposure to food-borne pathogens when complementary foods are not prepared using safe food-handling techniques. Contamination of food with microbes is recognized as the leading cause of diarrheal disease and ill health in infants. A wide range of symptoms, including diarrhea, vomiting, abdominal pain, fever, and jaundice, occurs with potentially severe and life-threatening consequences. Two particular areas of food preparation are of concern because they allow the survival and growth of pathogens to disease-causing levels. The first is preparation of food several hours before consumption along with storage at ambient temperatures favoring the growth of pathogens and/or toxins. The second concern is insufficient cooling of foods or inadequate reheating to reduce or eliminate pathogens (Motarjemi, 2000). General food safety guidelines for both commercially prepared and homemade infant food should be followed.

Nutrient Requirements

Energy

It is difficult to estimate energy requirements for infants and young children. The 1985 Food and Agriculture Organization/WHO/United Nations Organization (FAO/WHO/UNO) recommendations for energy intake were derived from the observed intakes of healthy, thriving children. This assumes that the natural ad libitum feeding of infants and toddlers reflects desirable intake. However, the observed energy intake of infants and toddlers may not be optimal and may reflect outside influences such as type of feedings and caregiver behaviors. The FAO/WHO/UNO recommendations for energy were based on data compiled from the literature predating 1940 and up to 1980 and included an extra 5% allowance for presumed underestimation of energy intake (Institute of Medicine [IOM], 2002).

Experts questioned the validity of the 1985 FAO/WHO/UNO recommendations for energy intake, and in 1996 experts concluded that the guidelines were too high. Energy requirements for infants and toddlers based on actual energy expenditure and energy deposition, rather than observed intake, would more accurately reflect true energy needs. Energy requirements of infants and young children need to support a rate of growth and body composition consistent with good health. Satisfactory growth is an indicator that energy needs are being met.

The WHO/United Nations Children's Fund (UNICEF) compiled data from 21 studies of children in developing countries to estimate the amount of energy received from breast milk and to determine how much energy would be required from complementary foods to meet children's needs for growth. To ensure that children receive sufficient calories, foods must be prepared with an adequate energy density and served an appropriate number of times per day. Both energy density and meal frequency independently affect the child's total energy consumption.

Dewey (2000a) expressed concern that the improper introduction of complementary foods has the potential to adversely affect breast milk intake and breast-feeding duration. Providing excess energy in the form of complementary foods can reduce the intake of breast milk. Breast-fed infants reduce their intake of human milk when non–breast milk foods and fluids are introduced. Although it appears that the timing of breast-feeding in relation to complementary foods (e.g., offering complementary foods before or after breast-feeding) does not seem to affect overall breast milk intake, there is a paucity of information on the effect of the introduction of complementary foods on breast-feeding.

Protein

It is not difficult to meet the protein needs of infants. Exclusively breast-fed infants receive adequate protein for at least the first 6 months of life. The most recent recommended adequate intake (AI) of protein for infants from birth to 6 months is 1.5 g/kg/day and reflects the observed mean intake of infants who are fed mostly human milk (IOM, 2002). This value is derived from various studies in which the volume of human milk consumed is measured by test weighing, and the average protein content of human milk was determined using values from several studies.

DuPont (2003) reported that total protein in breast milk varies greatly during the course of lactation, providing from less than 2.0 g/kg/day in the first weeks of life to approximately 1.15 g/kg/day at 4 months, less than the AI recommendations of the IOM. Dewey, Cohen, Rivera, Canahuati, and Brown (1996) reported that protein intake of breast-fed infants decreases from 2.0 g/kg/day at 1 month to 1.0 g/kg/day at 6 months as protein concentration in milk decreases and average breast milk intake increases slightly. According to Dewey et al., estimated daily protein intake of a 6-month-old breast-fed infant is 8.0 to 8.4 g/day, lower than the calculated AI of 9.1 g/day.

Protein content of infant formula is greater than that of human milk, but no study has shown that the amount of protein in human milk has deleterious effects. Multiple studies have shown that infants fed human milk have improved immune function and fewer illnesses than formula-fed infants. The casein and whey in infant formula are different from those present in human milk; therefore, the digestibility, absorption, and functionality of these proteins differ. The IOM (2001) states that digestibility and comparative protein quality need to be considered when determining the amount of protein to be included in infant formula based on various protein sources. Protein requirements for formula-fed infants may be greater due to their less-efficient utilization and retention of protein than breast-fed infants. Dewey, Cohen, et al. (1996) found that giving and additional 20% protein to 4- to 6-month-old exclusively breast-fed infants did not improve weight or length gain, and no differences were found in growth rate based on protein intake.

The amount of protein required for growth is highest in early infancy and decreases over time. At 1 month of age 64% of protein intake is used for growth, decreasing to 24% at 6 to 12 months. Daily increments in body protein gains in male breast-fed infants decreased from 1.0 g/kg/day at 1 month to 0.2 g/kg/day at 6 months. Protein needs for growth in early infancy are influenced by birth weight as well. Infants with higher birth weights generally grow at a slower rate and would require less protein than infants born at a lower birth weight, who experience faster rates of weight gain (Dewey, Beaton, Fjeld, Lonnerdal, & Reeds, 1996). Protein requirements (both total protein and protein per kilogram of body weight) for infants older than 6 months are lower than the requirements for younger infants. High-protein follow-up formulas are not indicated or necessary for infants consuming a variety of foods (Dewey, 2000b).

Calculations for protein requirements for infants aged 7 through 12 months are based on the relationship between protein intake and nitrogen balance. Studies examining protein losses, requirements for maintenance, and protein deposition were used to derive the Dietary Reference Intake (DRI)/Recommended Daily Allowance (RDA) values for older infants of 1.5 g/kg/day, which do not differ greatly from the AI for younger infants. Higher protein intake would be indicated for a child requiring catch-up growth or recovering from an infection. Infants older than 6 months may receive a significant portion of their protein needs from complementary foods.

An adequate growth rate has traditionally been used as the determinant for sufficient protein intake. Dewey, Beaton, et al. (1996) reported that other measures of protein intake, such as immune function and behavioral development, may become compromised long before growth falters. Observed differences in growth rates between infants who are breast-fed and infants who are formula-fed raise the question of whether maximal growth rate is synonymous with optimal growth rate. Higher intakes of protein in formula-fed infants have been a cause for concern because the liver and kidney need to metabolize and excrete the increased levels of plasma amino acids and urea nitrogen, which could have long-term consequences for immature organs.

Fatty Acids

Both human milk and currently available infant formula contain generous amounts of the essential fatty acids, linoleic and alpha-linolenic acid. Cow's milk contains very little, and infants and toddlers who drink cow's milk often have low levels of these fatty acids. Corn, soybean, or safflower oil can be added to the diet of a child who has been weaned from breast milk or formula to provide these nutrients (Butte, Cobb, Dwyer, et al., 2004).

> **LCPUFA (long-chain polyunsaturated fatty acids):** A category of dietary fats important in brain and retinal growth; normally present in human milk, they are now added to infant formula.

In addition to the essential fatty acids linoleic and alpha-linolenic acid, there is growing concern that infants also need long-chain polyunsaturated fatty acids (**LCPUFAs**) in their diets. These fats, particularly AA and DHA, are vital for neural development and visual acuity. Infants fed formula containing only linoleic and alpha-linolenic acid, the precursors for AA and DHA, are able to synthesize only a limited amount of long-chain fatty acids. When compared with breast-fed infants, formula-fed infants had less mature neurophysiologic maturation and brain function (Khedr, Farghaly, Amry Sel, & Osman, 2004).

Research Studies by Formula Companies

A study sponsored by Ross Products Division, Abbott Labs, makers of Similac, Neosure, and Isomil infant formulas, found that the addition of DHA and AA to infant formula increased DHA and AA plasma levels to those commonly seen in breast-fed infants without improvement in measures of visual acuity or other neurodevelopment tests (Auestad et al., 2001). A study sponsored by Mead Johnson Nutritionals, makers of Enfamil Lipil, found that when infants received a continuous supply of DHA and AA throughout the first year of life they had improved visual acuity at 1 year of age (Morale et al., 2005). Compared with women in other countries where greater intakes of fish are consumed, the DHA levels in the milk of mothers from the United States are much lower and do not meet the WHO recommendations.

Iron

Iron deficiency anemia is the most common childhood nutritional deficiency worldwide, with consequences of delays in motor and cognitive development caused by irreversible brain injury. Developmental deficits occur when iron deficiency becomes severe and chronic enough to result in anemia. Although iron supplementation increases iron stores, poor developmental outcomes may persist with lower scores on mental and motor tests and functional impairment in school-aged children. A high prevalence of nutritional iron deficiency anemia was first noted in the United States in infants in the 1930s and has decreased dramatically since the 1960s when it was acknowledged as a public health problem. Interventions, including an increase in breast-feeding, the start of the Special Supplemental Nutrition Program for Women, Infants, and Children (**WIC**) in 1972, and education of physicians and the public, resulted in a dramatic decrease in iron deficiency anemia across all socioeconomic groups in the United States. The intervention was so successful that in the 1980s it was suggested that routine screening of all infants be replaced by selective screening of high-risk patients.

It now appears that the prevalence of iron deficiency anemia is increasing in 1- to 3-year-olds (Kazal, 2002). Data from the 2001 Pediatric Nutrition Surveillance System indicated that 16.6% of 6- to 11-month-old infants and 15.3% of 12- to 17-month old children were anemic. The subjects in this national sample were largely from low-income populations, in which 82% were enrolled in WIC (Altucher, Rasmussen, Barden, & Habicht, 2005). It is not unusual for children ages 1 to 3 years to have low intakes of iron. Most 12-month-olds receive 100% of the daily requirement for iron, but this declines to less than recommended intake by 18 months, likely due to cessation of breast-feeding and switching from iron-fortified infant formula to cow's milk and reduced intake of iron-fortified cereals (Kazal, 2002). Juice intake can decrease a child's appetite for other, more nutritional solid foods, further contributing to iron deficiency.

Healthy, normal-birth-weight, full-term infants receive adequate iron from human milk for approximately the first 6 to 9 months of life. Reserves at birth are a critical factor for anemia. Total body iron is fairly stable in infants from birth through age 4 months as stored iron is gradually used to support growth. Between 4 and 12 months there is a significant increase in iron requirements as body size increases. These needs cannot be met through the iron available in human milk. The concentration of iron in human milk is 0.2 to 0.4 mg/L and remains stable throughout lactation. Although the absolute amount of iron in human milk is low, efficiency of iron absorption from human milk is quite high, at about 50%. Once iron stores are depleted, iron-related physiologic functions may become compromised with both cognitive and motor deficits even in the absence of anemia. After age 2 years when growth velocity decreases, iron stores start to accumulate and the risk for deficiency decreases (AAP, 2008).

The risk for anemia is much greater in low-birth-weight infants. In a study of low-birth-weight infants born in Honduras, infants with birth weights less than 3,000 g were at risk for anemia at 6 months even when iron-fortified complementary foods were introduced between ages 4 and 6 months (Dewey, Peerson, & Brown, 1998). It is recommended that low-birth-weight breast-fed infants receive iron drops beginning at age 2 to 3 months.

Fomon (2001) stated that infants who are exclusively or predominantly breast-fed are at risk of becoming iron deficient by 8 to 9 months of age. Whereas Fomon recommended beginning iron supplementation of breast-fed infants at an early age to prevent depletion of body stores, the AAP notes that iron deficiency is rare in breast-fed infants due to increased absorption and the absence of microscopic blood loss in the intestinal tract that may occur with whole cow's milk. Supplementation of healthy breast-fed infants with iron to prevent deficiency is controversial. Unnecessary supplementation can increase the prevalence of gastrointestinal infection, sepsis, and cancer because iron is essential for the growth of microorganisms and malignant cells. Gastrointestinal effects such as nausea, vomiting, constipation, and abdominal pain have been reported by individuals on iron supplementation. Routine iron supplementation of breast-fed infants with normal hemoglobin levels resulted in increased diarrhea and poor linear growth, possibly due to the pro-oxidant effect of iron on the intestinal mucosa. Reduction in zinc absorption leading to poor growth can occur from excessive iron intake (Dewey, Domellof, et al., 2002).

Iron deficiency anemia: The most common childhood nutritional deficiency resulting in motor and cognitive developmental deficits.

WIC: The Special Supplemental Nutrition Program for Women, Infants, and Children that serves to safeguard the health of low-income women, infants, and children up to age 5 who are at nutritional risk by providing nutritious foods to supplement diets, information on healthy eating, and referrals to health care.

Ermis and colleagues (2002) found that supplementation of breast-fed infants from ages 5 to 9 months with iron at a dose of 2 mg/kg every other day prevented iron deficiency and iron-deficiency anemia. Every-other-day dosing improved compliance and reduced unpleasant side effects.

Domellof, Lonnerdal, Abrams, and Hernall (2002) found that regulation of iron absorption in breast-fed infants undergoes developmental changes from ages 6 to 9 months that enhances the ability of the infant to adapt to a low-iron diet. Unlike iron absorption in adults that increases in states of iron depletion, iron absorption in infants was found to be directly related to dietary intake rather than to iron status. Iron status as measured by serum ferritin was improved in infants given iron supplementation, but there was a significant inverse relationship between dietary iron provided and absorption of iron from human milk. Unsupplemented infants absorbed 37% of the iron in human milk, compared with only 17% absorption in breast-fed infants supplemented with 1 mg/kg/day. Supplemental iron drops had a greater effect on decreasing iron absorption from human milk than iron in complementary foods. Domellof et al. concluded that breast-feeding with the addition of complementary foods containing adequate iron likely provides sufficient iron for some, but not all, healthy 9-month-old infants, possibly due to up-regulation of iron in response to low dietary intake, thus avoiding iron deficiency.

Iron absorption from foods varies greatly from less than 1% to 50% of available iron. About 4% of the iron in fortified infant formula is absorbed versus 50% of the iron in human milk. The AAP estimates that for infants consuming iron-fortified formula there is an 8% risk of iron deficiency and a less than 1% risk of iron deficiency anemia. Infants drinking cow's milk have a 30% to 40% risk of iron deficiency by ages 9 to 12 months. Exclusively breast-fed infants have a 20% risk of iron deficiency by 9 to 12 months of age. Formula-fed infants should not be switched to whole cow's milk until after 1 year of age, and there is no medical indication for low-iron formulas. The AAP has recommended that the manufacture of low-iron formulas be discontinued because there is no scientific evidence to support the claim that iron-fortified formulas increase gastrointestinal distress in infants.

The main sources of iron from complementary foods in the infant diet are iron-fortified cereal and meats. Absorption of iron from infant cereal is only about 4%. The form of iron used in dry infant cereals is an insoluble iron salt or metallic iron powder that is used to reduce oxidative rancidity, and these forms have low bioavailability. Meat is a much better source of iron because the iron is in the heme form, with an absorption efficiency of 10% to 20%. Non-heme iron from plant foods and fortified products is less well absorbed. Plant-based foods have a high phytic acid, polyphenol, and/or dietary fiber content that can inhibit absorption of micronutrients. Ascorbic acid counteracts the effects of phytate on iron absorption by preventing it from binding with available iron.

Zinc

The AI for zinc for infants from birth to age 6 months reflects the usual zinc intake of infants fed human milk exclusively. Human milk alone is inadequate to meet infants' needs for zinc after 6 months of age (IOM, 2001). **Zinc deficiency** is prevalent in undernourished children and is linked to reduced activity and play with subsequent poor developmental outcomes. Zinc deficiency is associated with poor growth as well as diarrheal disease. It is estimated that 12- to 24-month-olds meet only 50% to 60% of the DRI/RDA for zinc (Krebs, 2000). Meeks Gardner et al. (2005) found that when poor, undernourished Jamaican children aged 9 to 30 months were supplemented with 10 mg zinc daily and also participated in a weekly program to improve mother-child interactions, the developmental quotient and hand/eye coordination improved. Diarrheal morbidity was reduced, but there were no improvements in the children's growth.

Zinc deficiency: Prevalent in undernourished children and associated with poor growth, poor developmental outcomes, and diarrheal disease.

Zinc concentration in human milk is low, but bioavailability is high. Neonatal stores are likely sufficient to maintain zinc homeostasis until 6 months of age. The young infant has a relatively high zinc requirement to support the rapid growth of early infancy. Zinc concentration in human milk decreases throughout lactation, but as the infant's growth rate declines with increasing age so does the requirement for zinc (Lawrence, 1999). The concentration of zinc in human milk decreases rapidly from 4 mg/L at 2 weeks to 2 mg/L at 2 months and to 1.2 mg/L at 6 months (Krebs, Reidinger, Robertson, & Hambridge, 1994). Despite an increased intake in volume over the first 6 months, this steep decline in zinc concentration in human milk results in a decline in zinc intake. Zinc concentration in human milk of well-nourished mothers is resistant to changes in the maternal diet. Although zinc supplementation is associated with improved growth, exclusively breast-fed infants grow well without additional zinc. Dewey, Peerson, and Brown (1998) found that when breast-fed children received complementary foods fortified with zinc to double their average zinc intake, there was no significant increase in weight or length.

Zinc absorption is greater from a diet high in animal protein, and the best source of zinc is red meat. Plant-based foods containing phytic acid bind with zinc in the intestines and reduce absorption. Vegetarians who rely on a plant-based diet may need to increase their zinc intake by 50% due to decreased bioavailability of zinc from phytic acid.

Vitamin D

Rickets was almost universally seen in African-American infants living in the northern United States at the turn of the 20th century. With the discovery of vitamin D and a public health campaign to fortify infant foods and supplement breast-fed infants with cod liver oil, rickets was nearly eradicated (Rajakumar & Thomas, 2005). Once again, nutritional rickets is a public health concern. Breast-fed infants are at risk for vitamin D deficiency due to limited amounts of vitamin D in breast milk and the current trend to limit sun exposure (Fomon, 2001). Vitamin D–deficiency rickets can cause significant morbidity, including delays in growth and motor development, failure to thrive, short stature, tetany, seizures, and skeletal deformities. A review of published reports from 1986 to 2001 found 166 cases of rickets in children in North Carolina, Texas, Georgia, and the mid-Atlantic region (Weisberg, Scablon, Li, & Cogswell, 2004). Most cases (83%) were in African-American children, and 96% were breast-fed. Only 5% of the breast-fed infants received vitamin D supplementation, and most were weaned from the breast to a diet low in vitamin D and calcium.

Rickets: Vitamin D deficiency resulting in growth deficits, developmental delay, failure to thrive, short stature, tetany, seizures, and skeletal deformities.

Dark-skinned infants who are exclusively breast-fed are at particular risk. From 1990 to 1999 in North Carolina 30 cases of nutritional rickets were seen in African-American children who were breast-feeding without supplemental vitamin D, even though infants living in sunny southern states were believed to be at low risk (Kreiter et al., 2000). Vitamin D–deficiency rickets is common in infants in Pakistan, Saudi Arabia, and the United Arab Emirates, where breast-feeding women have limited sun exposure and a diet low in vitamin D. Infants are not routinely supplemented with vitamin D while breast-feeding, and many mothers avoid consumption of fortified dairy products. Despite abundant sunshine, only rural women who spent more time working outdoors had adequate serum levels of vitamin D (Dawodu, Adarwal, Hossain, Kochiyil, & Zayed, 2003).

Revised guidelines from the AAP for vitamin D are based on new evidence from clinical trials demonstrating the importance of vitamin D in maintaining innate immunity and prevention of diseases, including diabetes and cancer. The recommended daily intake of vitamin D is 400 IU per day for all infants, children, and adolescents beginning in the first few days of life (Wagner, Greer, & the Section on Breastfeeding and Committee on Nutrition, 2008). This recommendation replaces earlier recommendations that all infants, including those exclusively breast-fed, require a minimum intake of 200 IU of vitamin D per day beginning the first 2 months of life to prevent vitamin D–deficiency rickets (Gartner, Greer, & the Section on Breastfeeding and Committee on Nutrition, 2003). Vitamin D drops are available to provide the recommended 400 IU per day for all infants. Supplementation with a multivitamin is not necessary or recommended.

Vitamin D synthesis occurs in the skin from exposure to ultraviolet B light from sunlight. Dietary sources include fish liver oils, fatty fish, and foods fortified with vitamin D, particularly cow's milk, infant formula, and breakfast cereals. Sunlight exposure may not be sufficient at higher latitudes during winter months or with sunscreen use. Individuals with dark skin pigmentation have limited vitamin D synthesis with sunlight exposure. Human milk typically contains 25 IU/L of vitamin D, which is not enough to meet the recommended requirement. Maternal vitamin D status has a direct effect on the vitamin D content in human milk. Traditionally, sunlight exposure provided adequate vitamin D for both mothers and breast-feeding infants. For instance, in light-skinned individuals, 10 to 15 minutes of total body peak sunlight exposure endogenously produces and releases into circulation 20,000 IU of vitamin D. The daily recommended intake for vitamin D for lactating women is 400 IU, an amount unlikely to provide for optimal vitamin D levels in human milk. Wagner, Hulsey, Fanning, Ebeling, and Hollis (2006) found that by supplementing lactating mothers with 6,400 IU/day of vitamin D they were able to increase maternal vitamin D levels sufficiently to increase the amount of vitamin D in human milk from 82 to 873 IU/L and to significantly improve circulating vitamin D in both the mother and the breast-fed infant.

Supplemental Nutrients

Human milk continues to provide many nutrients in the second half of the first year of life during the period of **complementary feeding**. Human milk intake of infants aged 9 to 11 months meets the estimated needs for vitamin C, folate, vitamin B$_{12}$, selenium, and iodine. After the age of 6 months complementary foods are needed to provide 12% of vitamin A; 25% to 50% of copper; 50% to 75% of thiamin, niacin, and manganese; and up to 98% of iron and zinc (Gibson & Holtz, 2000).

Complementary feeding: The period that begins with the introduction of the first nonmilk food and ends with the cessation of breast- or formula-feeding.

Despite the fact that most young children receive adequate vitamins and minerals from their diet, many families supplement their child's diet with additional vitamins and minerals. Eichenberger Gilmore, Hong, Broffitt, & Levy (2005) studied trends in children younger than 2 years in Iowa and found that by 24 months 31.7% used some type of supplement. In the first 6 months of life, 3.5% to 6.3% of non–breast-fed infants received supplements, compared with 18.3% to 29.2% of breast-fed infants. After 6 months of age use of multiple vitamin supplements and multiple vitamins with minerals increased with age. Diet alone provided AI of most vitamins and minerals, and with additional supplementation intake of vitamin A exceeded the recommended upper limit. Hypervitaminosis A is a concern because reports associate excessive vitamin A intake with decreased bone mineral density and increased risk of fracture. The long-term adverse effects of high intakes of vitamin A during early life are not clear.

Vegetarianism

A vegetarian diet during infancy and childhood can be adequate in all essential nutrients, with normal growth and nutritional status expected unless the diet is severely restricted. A breast-fed infant of a well-nourished vegetarian mother receives adequate nutrition, particularly if the mother pays close attention to her own intake of iron, vitamin B$_{12}$, and vitamin D. Women who consume 3 or more servings of dairy products receive sufficient amounts of vitamins D and B$_{12}$ from their diet. Women following a vegan diet need to supplement with foods fortified with vitamin B$_{12}$, such as nutritional yeast or soy milk. Vegan infants who are not breast-fed need to receive soy infant formula until 1 year of age. Soy milk, rice milk, and homemade formulas do not provide adequate nutrition for infants younger than 1 year and should not be used to replace breast milk or commercial infant formula (American Dietetic Association, 2003).

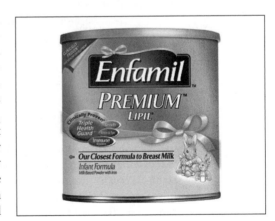

A variety of protein-rich vegetarian foods are available for the older infant and toddler, including tofu, legumes, soy or dairy yogurt and cheese, eggs, and cottage cheese. These foods can be easily pureed or mashed for increased acceptance when the child is first introduced to complementary foods. Later, soft cooked beans, bean spreads, or nut butters on toast, chunks of tofu, or cheese and soy burgers can be offered as finger foods. Fat is an important source of energy and should not be restricted in children younger than 2 years. Vegan infants need a supplementary source of vitamin B$_{12}$ when they are weaned from breast milk or infant formula. Read more about vegetarianism in Chapter 7.

Complementary Feeding

Transitioning from All Milk to Family Foods

Complementary feeding is defined as the period extending from the first introduction of nonmilk feeds to the cessation of breast- or formula-feeding (Weaver, 2000). Any food that provides energy and displaces breast milk is considered a complementary food. A gradual progression from an exclusive milk diet to a variety of complementary foods allows the infant's gastrointestinal function to accommodate new types of foods, including starch, sucrose, and fiber. In many other mammals there are abrupt and well-defined changes in the intestinal mucosa and enzyme activity as weaning occurs. However, in humans these changes are less obvious and more gradual. Human milk contains many bioactive substances, including digestive enzymes, such as bile salt-stimulated lipase, amylase, and protease, that may be involved in the digestion of complementary foods.

The timing of complementary feeding varies according to cultural practices and the personal beliefs of the mother as well as guidance she receives from her pediatrician. In some instances pediatricians may suggest adding cereal to the infant's diet before age 4 months if a mother is concerned about the baby's sleeping patterns or growth. Child nutrition experts agree that there is no reason to introduce complementary foods before 4 months of age. At least 60 countries have policies in place to recommend the introduction of complementary foods after 6 months of age. Earlier introduction of complementary foods can affect immune function and immunotolerance, development of chronic disease, and risk of atopy.

At birth the gut of a full-term infant may be anatomically and functionally mature, but subtle immaturities in luminal digestion, mucosal absorption, and protective function could predispose the infant to gastrointestinal and systemic disease during the first 6 months of life. It is not known exactly when the period of immature immune function ends and when it is safe to feed foreign proteins. Early introduction can cause protein-induced enteropathies, leading to mucosal inflammation, villous atrophy, diarrhea, and failure to thrive (Muraro et al., 2004). The question of when the normal-term infant is developmentally ready to discontinue **exclusive breast-feeding** and begin the intake of solid and semisolid complementary foods is an important one. There probably is not a single optimal age for introduction of complementary foods but rather optimal ages that are determined by factors such as infant birth weight, maternal nutrition while breast-feeding, and environmental conditions.

Exclusive breast-feeding:
When an infant receives only breast milk and no other foods or drinks for the first 6 months.

Feeding Guidelines

From 1979 until 2001 the WHO recommended that normal full-term infants be exclusively breast-fed for 4 to 6 months. Later, it was found that discontinuing exclusive breast-feeding before 6 months increased infant morbidity and mortality, and the WHO recommendations were revised to encourage exclusive breast-feeding for at least 6 months. Early introduction of complementary foods and exposure to pathogens in food could result in symptomatic infection and illness in the infant and reduced sucking at the breast, followed by a decrease in the amount of milk and immune substances consumed as well as decreased maternal milk production from reduced demand. Exclusive breast-feeding for 6 months results in greater immunologic protection and limits exposure to pathogens at an early age, when the immune system is immature. Energy and nutrients that are valuable for normal growth and development can be used for their intended purpose rather than diverted for immunologic function.

Malnutrition is the leading cause of death worldwide in children younger than 1 year. Inappropriate feeding practices include early cessation of exclusive breast-feeding, introducing complementary foods too early or too late, and providing nutritionally inadequate or unsafe foods. Malnourished children who survive are frequently sick and may suffer lifelong consequences. Overweight and obesity are increasing at alarming rates throughout the world and are associated with poor feeding practices that often begin in early childhood. Global strategies for infant and young child feeding can impact social and economic development.

The WHO feeding guidelines (WHO, 2003) are for generally healthy breast-fed infants. These guidelines primarily target low-income countries where most children are breast-fed and safe low-cost alternatives to breast milk are not readily available. No information is included for feeding premature infants or children with infections or other acute or chronic diseases that could affect nutritional status. No information is provided on feeding non–breast-fed infants. An important goal of the WHO is to improve complementary feeding practices in terms of timeliness, quality, quantity, and safety to ensure adequate global nutrition. It is difficult to make recommendations regarding the optimal age for introduction of complementary foods. Ideally, recommendations for the appropriate time to introduce complementary foods and the optimal duration of breast-feeding consider infant outcomes, such as growth, behavioral development, micronutrient status, and the risks of infection, allergy, and impaired intestinal function, as well as those of the mother, such as general health and nutritional status and return to fertility.

The AAP states that there is no evidence of harm when safe, nutritious, complementary foods are introduced after 4 months when the infant is developmentally ready. The AAP Section on Breastfeeding (2005) recommends that complementary foods rich in iron be introduced gradually around 6 months of age, but due to the unique needs of individual infants the need to introduce complementary foods could occur as early as 4 months or as late as 8 months of age. Exclusive breast-feeding in the first 6 months is defined by the AAP as consumption of human milk with no supplementation of any type (no water, no juice, no nonhuman milk, and no foods) except for vitamins, minerals, and medications. During the first 6 months, water, juice, or other liquids are unnecessary, even in hot climates, and can introduce contaminants or allergens. Exclusive breast-feeding provides protection from many acute and chronic diseases. Breast-feeding is also more likely to continue for at least the first year of life when infants are exclusively breast-fed for the first 6 months. For optimal health benefits, breast-feeding should continue for 12 months or longer. The recommendations of the WHO are to breast-feed for at least 2 years, and the AAP states that there is no upper limit to the duration of breast-feeding and no evidence of psychological or developmental harm from breast-feeding into the third year of life or longer (AAP, Section on Breastfeeding, 2005). Indeed, in late infancy, breast milk provides significant amounts of energy and micronutrients and is a key source of PUFAs crucial for brain development and neurologic function (Villalpando, 2000).

A partnership of the Agricultural Research Service (ARS) at the U.S. Department of Agriculture– Children's Nutrition Research Center at the Baylor College of Medicine in Houston, Texas, and the American Dietetic Association, funded by Gerber Food Products Company, developed the "Start Healthy Feeding Guidelines for Children Ages 0–24 Months." The expert panel realized that guidance was needed to help parents through the transition period from an all-milk diet to the first introduction of solid foods by adding variety and texture throughout the weaning process and to establish healthy eating patterns. These new guidelines are an effort to address the growing problem of childhood obesity and inappropriate food choices at an early age. They are intended to complement and expand on already existing guidelines from the AAP, CDC, and other expert groups. These evidence-based guidelines answer the important questions "when, what, and how" complementary foods should be introduced (Butte, Cobb, et al., 2004). Where scientific evidence was limited or unavailable, expert opinion was referenced. For instance, there is only limited evidence to suggest any order for introduction of textures, and expert opinion suggests a general progression based on the child's readiness for and acceptance of different food textures.

Complementary Foods and Growth

Introducing complementary foods to the exclusively breast-fed infant before the age of 6 months does not increase total calorie intake or improve growth. A breast-fed infant who receives complementary foods at 4 months decreases his or her intake of human milk to maintain the same level of calories. Complementary foods displace human milk, and the infant receives fewer immune factors and is at greater risk for infection. No significant improvement in weight or length was observed by Dewey (2001) in infants up to 12 months of age when they received complementary foods at 4 months compared with infants who received exclusive human milk until 6 months.

Despite recommendations to exclusively breast-feed for the first 6 months of life, this practice may be uncommon. Carruth, Skinner, Houck, and Moran (2000) found that in a study of 94 mothers, 60 added solid food by 4 months and 8 were feeding cereal in a bottle. The median age for introduction of cereal was 4 months and for juice 4½ months. Thirteen mothers introduced cereal, juice, or fruit as early as 2 months. In looking at the growth of the children who had early solids, there was no association between the age of introduction of complementary foods and change in weight or length from 2 to 8 months or from 12 to 24 months. These results were similar to the WHO data (WHO Working Group, 2002) showing only minor differences in growth among infants receiving complementary foods at different ages. The WHO data were based on a unique longitudinal seven-country study of predominantly breast-fed infants. They found little evidence of risk or benefit related to growth based on timing of introduction or types or frequency of complementary foods in healthy infants living in environments without major economic restraints and with low rates of illness.

The amount of energy and nutrients needed from complementary foods depends on the amount of breast milk or formula the infant is consuming. Although it is possible for an infant to receive adequate nutrition for the first year solely from iron-fortified formula, all infants need complementary foods for exposure to novel tastes and textures and to develop appropriate feeding skills. A variety of flavors and foods is important in the first 2 years of life and may increase the likelihood that children will try new foods.

Meal Patterns and Nutrient Intakes

During infancy and early childhood, lifelong patterns of eating are formed that can influence later eating habits and overall health. As the child makes the transition from an all-milk diet to sharing foods from the family table, meeting nutritional guidelines may become more problematic for families. Families strive to follow nutrition recommendations to provide the best for their children, particularly in the year after birth when the infant is eating mostly jarred baby foods. As the infant matures and begins to incorporate more of the family foods into his or her diet, less than optimal nutrition becomes evident. Transitioning from baby food to table food has been associated with a decreased intake of vitamin A, iron, and folate at meals as baby-food fruits, vegetables, and meats are not replaced with equivalent table foods.

> **● Learning Point** Breast-feeding exposes the infant to a variety of flavors from the very beginning through mother's milk. Repeated exposures to a new food may be necessary before it is accepted.

Children imitate what others around them are eating, and if no one else eats fruits or vegetables, the young child will quickly abandon these foods. When other family members drink sweetened carbonated beverages and eat high-calorie, low-nutrient-dense foods, such as french fries, doughnuts, and potato chips, the young child will happily join in. As rates of obesity, excess weight, and type 2 diabetes are increasing in children, it is evident that the influence of early diet needs to be addressed. At a surprisingly young age many infants and toddlers do not receive a variety of fruits and vegetables and instead are consuming high-calorie, high-fat, salty snacks and sweetened drinks. It is the parent's responsibility to offer nutritious foods to infants and toddlers. Although a preference for sweet foods is innate, repeated exposure at an early age and observing other family members eating these foods increases the likelihood that young children will develop preference for these foods. The disappearance of the family meal and the increase in the number of meals eaten outside the home and from fast-food establishments has concerned experts as the prevalence of snacking and the quantity and quality of foods consumed by children and adolescents in recent years has changed.

Feeding Skills and Neuromuscular Development

Reflexes

A normal progression of sucking and feeding reflexes is necessary for the child to advance from a milk-only diet to consumption of foods from the family diet. Swallowing is present in early fetal life at the end of the first trimester. The fetus has ample opportunities to practice by swallowing amniotic fluid even before the development of the sucking reflex, which appears by the middle of the second trimester. The sucking reflex is quite strong in the newborn and can be easily elicited by stroking the infant's lips, cheeks, or inside the

> **● Learning Point** Food-related behaviors are established early in life, and how and what an infant or toddler eats in the first years of life can influence later food choices.

mouth. By about 3 months of age sucking becomes less automatic and more voluntary. The gag reflex is present in the third trimester and is stimulated by contact of the posterior two-thirds of the tongue. This reflex gradually diminishes to one-fourth of the posterior tongue by 6 months of age. The rooting reflex, which assists the infant to locate the breast and nipple by turning the head side to side and opening the mouth wide when the skin surrounding the mouth is stroked, disappears by 3 months of age.

Advanced Motor Skills

Infants need new oral motor skills to transition from a full liquid milk-based diet to a more solid diet of complementary foods. Disappearance of the rooting and sucking reflexes and the accompanying changes in anatomy help prepare the infant for this transition. Phasic biting, resulting in the rhythmic opening and closing of the jaw when the gums are stimulated, disappears between 3 and 4 months of age. Between 6 and 9 months it becomes possible for the infant to receive a bolus of food without reflexively pushing it out of the mouth. By 12 months of age rotary chewing is well established, along with sustained controlled biting that permits the infant to consume a variety of foods (Kleinman, 2000c).

During the first 2 years of life there is increasing head and torso control that permits a child to achieve developmental milestones required for proper self-feeding abilities. Finger coordination to permit self-finger feeding usually is adequate by 6 to 7 months of age. The infant must be able to sufficiently stabilize the head and balance the trunk before he or she can sit without support and use arm and hand movements for self-feeding. Carruth, Ziegler, Gordon, and Hendricks (2004) found that one-third of 4- to 6-month-old infants and 99% of 9- to 11-month-olds can sit without support. Stability of the trunk is crucial in the process of progressing to complementary foods, and by 6 months most infants have achieved greater strength in the trunk, shoulder, and neck muscles. There is a wide range of ages when feeding skills emerge, and it is crucial that caregivers allow ample opportunities for appropriate exploratory activities. Offering the child a variety of nutritious foods and allowing them to self-feed when they have sufficiently developed this skill is appropriate and will not jeopardize adequate nutrient intake.

Beginning at 6 months most infants are ready for pureed, mashed, and semisolid foods. By 7 months soft foods that can be pressed down by the infant's tongue can be introduced, and at 9 months the infant can handle foods that can be compressed by the gums. Teeth are not necessary for chewing of soft, lumpy foods. The ability to handle advanced textures increases day by day, and children require multiple opportunities to practice new feeding skills. By 8 months they can progress to finger foods they can pick up and feed themselves. By 12 months of age most children can transition to the same diet as the rest of the family, keeping in mind the need for calorically and nutrient-dense foods because of the smaller portion size. Infants possessing self-feeding skills are reported to have higher energy and nutrient intakes (Carruth, Ziegler, Gordon, & Hendricks, 2004). Foods that are a choking risk that can lodge in the trachea, such as grapes, nuts, hard raw vegetables and fruits, and popcorn, should be avoided. Introduction to a cup usually occurs after 6 months, and by 12 months most infants are drinking from a "sippy cup."

Chewing Ability

Advances in gross motor skills parallel advances in dentition as the first primary teeth erupt at 7 to 8 months and continue throughout the first 2 years, with approximately 15 teeth erupting by 19 to 24 months of age. Carruth, Ziegler, Gordon, and Hendricks (2004) found that the ability to consume foods that required chewing increases with age. Nutrient intakes of energy, fat, protein, vitamin B_6, vitamin B_{12}, folate, zinc, thiamin, niacin, and magnesium were greater for infants under 1 year of age who were able to eat foods that required chewing. Individual differences in the age of eruption of teeth can influence the ability to chew certain foods, especially meat and fibrous vegetables.

Feeding difficulties, particularly difficulty with chewing tough or fibrous foods, in Japanese children are thought to be caused by inappropriate transition from a milk-based diet to a diet of family foods. Sakashita, Inoue, and Kamegai (2004) found that at 2 years of age many preschool children swallowed without chewing or were unable to chew and swallow certain foods and that many kindergarten children did not chew properly, retained food in the side of their mouth, or frequently spit food out (Sakashita, Inoue, & Kamegai, 2004). A transitional diet containing very soft and pureed foods for an extended period has been suspected of preventing children from developing a proper masticatory system and chewing and swallowing ability. Leafy vegetables were usually offered early as a weaning food but were not well accepted because the fiber makes it difficult to chew. Meats were often introduced later than recommended, possibly due to parental concerns related to food allergies (Sakashita, Inoue, & Tatsuki, 2003). In Japan, foods were specially cooked and fed to children with a spoon, inhibiting the proper development of the masticatory system and mature chewing and swallowing behavior.

Determinants of Food Acceptance

Sakashita, Inoue, and Kamegai (2004) found that acceptance of new foods was greatest in children who were offered food prepared from the family table and was lowest in children fed jarred baby food. Offering infants foods prepared from the family table promotes feeding progress by giving the infant an opportunity to experience a variety of food textures from an early age. Infants first offered lumpy solid foods between ages 6 and 9 months had fewer feeding difficulties and improved acceptance than infants not introduced to these foods until after age 10 months. Observing other family members eating at the family table and having the opportunity to try new foods is also an important component of transitioning an infant to family

foods. Sakashita, Inoue, and Kamegai (2004) found that first-born children experience more feeding difficulties than second- or third-born children. This may be a result of limited opportunities to observe other family members eating and to learn feeding behavior from older siblings.

The number of accepted foods increases rapidly from 6 months to 1 year and continues to increase throughout the first 2 years. Foods requiring significant chewing before swallowing, such as leafy vegetables and sliced meat, may be poorly accepted. Processed sliced deli meats are often more readily accepted when offered. Because chewing ability affects ability to swallow and therefore food acceptance, breast-fed infants who have more opportunity to develop the masticatory system have a higher rate of food acceptance than bottle-fed infants. Exposure to food flavors through mother's milk also prepares the infant for a variety of flavors. Breast-feeding seems to facilitate increased acceptance of different foods due to the greater variation in breast milk flavors compared with infant formula.

Other causes of food refusal include dislike of the taste or smell and an unfamiliar appearance. Often, a child's food preferences reflect those of other family members. Early food experiences can be imprinted on the memory, and when children refuse to eat vegetables at an early age, these food preferences may remain throughout the childhood and adolescent years with significant health consequences. Child-feeding practices contribute to the development of food intake controls and energy balance and can affect childhood obesity. Obese individuals tend to prefer fatty foods to fruits and vegetables and dislike tough or fibrous texture. Exposure to fruits and vegetables in infancy and early childhood should be encouraged to reduce risk factors for obesity and obesity-related diseases.

Caregiver Behaviors

Although early childhood malnutrition can be attributable to poverty and lack of resources, family and caregiver characteristics, such as education and household management or coping skills of the mother, can determine normal growth and development. Lack of knowledge regarding appropriate foods and feeding practices can contribute to malnutrition to a greater degree than lack of food. Not only is providing the appropriate combination of complementary foods to meet the child's nutritional needs important, feeding practices such as frequency of feeds and feeding style need to be considered. Caregiving behaviors that have been identified as promoting normal growth and development are (1) active or interactive feeding, (2) selecting foods appropriate to the child's motor skills and taste preferences, (3) feeding in response to the child's hunger cues, (4) feeding in a nondistracting safe environment, and (5) talking and playing with the child in the context of the meal. This type of responsive parenting has been described as sensitive and supportive caregiving associated with good growth and development.

Feeding interactions should include the caregiver observing the infant's intake and nonverbal cues and responding accordingly (Pelto, 2000). If children refuse many foods, parents should be encouraged to be creative and experiment with different food combinations, tastes, and textures. Parents should be taught to encourage children to eat, but never to force, because this can lead to food aversion and behavioral problems.

Effect of Feeding Mode in Infancy

In early infancy parents choose whether the child will be breast-fed or bottle fed and whether human milk or formula will be consumed. They may also control the timing of the feedings and the volume consumed, although this is less likely when the infant is breast-fed. When a mother breast-feeds and her infant's sucking slows or stops, the mother assumes the child is satisfied and is finished eating. The amount of milk consumed is primarily under the infant's control. Breast-fed infants are able to adjust the amount of milk consumed to maintain a constant energy intake. Formula-feeding mothers may rely on visual cues of formula remaining in the bottle and encourage the infant to continue feeding after he or she has exhibited signs of satiety.

Taveras et al. (2004) found that the longer a mother breast-fed, the less likely she was to restrict her child's intake at 1 year. Compared with mothers who formula fed, mothers who exclusively breast-fed for 6 months were less likely to restrict their child's intake. Breast-feeding for at least 12 months was associated with lower levels of controlling feedings and resulted in improved intake by toddlers (Orlet Fisher, Birch, Smiciklas-Wright, & Picciano, 2000). Breast-feeding may protect against obesity by allowing the infant to naturally regulate energy intake based on hunger cues and by preventing parents from overriding these cues by controlling the feeding. Mothers who breast-feed may be more responsive to their infants' signals regarding the timing and volume of feedings.

Feeding Relationship

As the child transitions to a variety of family foods, the need to be independent and autonomous will be evident in the feeding relationship as the child assumes more control of his or her eating. The feeding relationship reflects the overall parent-child relationship, and feeding struggles may be indicative of other difficulties involving parent-child interactions. Feeding is a major area of frequent daily exchanges between the parent and the child, reflecting the characteristics of both the parent and the child that can either support or hinder the child's development. Feeding involves more than providing the correct mix of calories and vitamins to ensure adequate nutrition. The feeding relationship itself is crucial for the child's growth and development (Slaughter & Bryant, 2004). Feeding is a blend of nutrition, parenting, and human development and provides an opportunity for parents to be present and to provide love, support, and attention that can affect the child's physical, social, and emotional health.

As infants progress from a milk-based diet to sharing family foods, they develop unique likes and dislikes regarding the foods they are offered and will communicate these preferences to their parents. How the parents respond to this assertiveness can impact the child's developing sense of self and autonomy. The ability to refuse food and have this be accepted by the parents is paramount to future interactions between the child and the parents and provides a base for all future social interactions. It is important for the child's development to be able to say "no" and still be unconditionally loved and supported. If the parent withholds love from the child or forces or pressures the child to eat, the child feels helpless and abandoned. Furthermore, the child learns that he or she does not have the ability to say "no" and be respected, which can have far-reaching effects. By allowing a child to refuse to eat a certain food or to not eat at all because he or she is not hungry, parents are giving the child permission to express his or her needs without fear of repercussions.

High levels of maternal control over when and what children eat are associated with increased adiposity and an increased desire to consume restricted foods. Maternal restrictive feeding practices have been found to increase the child's preference for the restricted food and to promote overeating when the restricted foods are available and are counterproductive in preventing obesity (Birch, Orlet Fisher, & Krahnstoever Davison, 2003). In place of restricting desirable foods, parents should be taught skills that help children learn how to consume appropriate portion sizes, to like healthy foods, and to recognize hunger and satiety cues to determine when and how much to eat.

Portion Size

Children demonstrate an innate ability for self—regulation of energy intake. They can compensate for changes in energy density by adjusting the quantity of food they consume. Parents and caregivers potentially interfere with this natural hunger-driven mechanism by coercing children to eat when they are not hungry or by directing them to "finish their plate" or to "take one more bite" when they have demonstrated signs of satiety. Over-restriction of intake to prevent overeating in infants and toddlers can have negative consequences by preventing the natural development of feeding self-regulation. **Table 2.1** indicates food types and corresponding development infants usually demonstrate; some variances should be expected.

TABLE 2.1 Infant Feeding by Age and Development

Age	Development	What to Feed
Birth to 6 mo	Baby can suck and swallow. Baby should be held for feeding.	Breast milk is best. Use formula if not breast-feeding. No water or juice.
6–8 mo	Baby can sit with support and control head movement. Spoon feeding begins. *No honey entire first year.*	Breast-fed infants: begin puree meats first and then eggs, puree fruits and vegetables, and infant cereal. Formula-fed infants: begin infant cereals and then pureed fruits, vegetables, and meats and eggs. Wait 3–5 days between new foods. Watch for signs of food allergies such as rash, vomiting, or diarrhea.
7–9 mo	Baby can chew, grasp, and hold items. Finger feeding begins. Introduce a cup with water, juice, breast milk, or formula. Baby can eat with a spoon and will feed self more often. Expect baby to eat with hands and make a mess.	Try well-cooked carrots, sliced bananas, unsweetened dry cereals, graham crackers, soft cheeses, pancake bits, and well-cooked pasta. Offer new tastes and textures such as plain yogurt, cottage cheese, tofu, and refried beans. Offer soft foods from the family meal. Limit juice to 4 oz/day. Offer fewer pureed foods and more foods from the family meal. Always try to eat together as a family. Parents should set a good example by eating fruits and vegetables. Avoid dangerous foods that are a choking hazard: raw vegetables,

Age	Development	What to Feed
		nuts, seeds, whole grapes or cherry tomatoes, hot dogs, po corn, and spoonfuls of peanut butter.
9–12 mo 1 year and beyond	Encourage self-feeding. Continue breast-feeding. Wean from bottle. Begin offering whole cow's milk in cup. No low-fat or skim milk until 2 years of age.	Infant should eat three meals and two to three snacks each day. Feeding should be a happy time for the entire family. Let infant decide when enough is enough. Never force infant to eat or drink. No sweetened drinks or soda. Avoid sweets. Offer fruit for dessert.

The presence of self-regulation of dietary intake in infants and toddlers was confirmed by analysis of the relationship between portion size, number of eating occasions, number of unique foods, and energy density (Fox, Devaney, Reidy, Razafindrakoto, & Ziegler, 2006). Children who ate less often during the day consumed larger portions, and children who ate more often ate smaller portions. For infants, energy density was negatively associated with portion size. As the energy density increased, portion size decreased, and as energy density decreased, portion size increased. The number of different foods consumed by 6- to 11-month-olds was also positively associated with portion size, indicating that infants with a more varied diet consume larger portions.

Children under 2 years of age typically eat 7 times a day, although the number of meals and snacks reported ranges from 3 to 15. It is appropriate for infants and toddlers to consume many small meals and snacks because of their small stomachs and high energy demands. Snacks often provide about 25% of toddlers' energy intake (Skinner, Ziegler, Pac, & Devaney, 2004a). The breakfast, lunch, dinner, and snacks pattern emerges at ages 7 to 8 months and is well established by 9 to 11 months.

Issues to Debate

1. Discuss the nutritional impact of commercial formula on infants.
2. Should more be done to promote breast-feeding?
3. Should there be more food labeling because of the potential for infant food allergies?
4. What are some cultural aspects that affect the transitioning from an all-milk infant diet to a diet of family foods?

Case Studies

(Answers to all case studies are in the Instructor's Manual available at jbpub.com.)

Normal Infant Nutrition Case Study

Caleb was born by standard vaginal delivery to a healthy 30-year-old mother. Caleb's mother decided while she was pregnant to exclusively breast-feed him for the first 6 months of life because she was familiar with the advantages associated with exclusive breast-feeding, such as reduction of illness and allergies, enhanced intelligence, convenience of feedings, and cost savings. Caleb weighed 7 pounds at birth (25th percentile) and gained weight appropriately for the first 6 months of life. At his 6-month checkup he weighed 18 pounds and was at the 50th to 75th percentile for weight.

Continues

Caleb's mother chose to introduce pureed foods she prepared herself when Caleb was 6 months old. At this time he exhibited an interest in what his parents were eating and had developed good head and neck control. She prepared sweet potatoes, carrots, squash, and peas and pureed them in a food processor until they were a smooth consistency. She froze them in single-serving portions in an ice cube tray.

She introduced one food at a time and waited 3 to 5 days between foods while observing Caleb for signs of food allergy. Gradually, she added more foods to his diet, including chicken, turkey, beef, cereal, pears, peaches, and bananas. When Caleb was 7 months old he was offered a sippy cup with water at meals.

Caleb was developing fine motor control and was able to grasp foods and attempt self-feeding. His mother offered him small pieces of toast, Cheerios, cut-up fresh melon, soft-cooked carrots, French toast, and pieces of cheese and turkey. He also began to eat cottage cheese and yogurt and a greater variety of foods from the family meal. Caleb continued to breast-feed, but the number of feedings per day began to decrease as he increased his intake of complementary foods. Caleb was breast-fed without any supplemental formula until he was 13 months old, when he was offered whole cow's milk by cup. By 1 year of age he had gradually transitioned from an all-milk diet in the first 6 months to a mixed diet of breast milk and pureed foods and finally to a diet of family foods including a variety of fruits and vegetables, grains, meats, and dairy.

What did Caleb's mother do correctly?

References

Altucher, K., Rasmussen, K., Barden, E., & Habicht, J. (2005). Predictors of improvement in hemoglobin concentration among toddlers enrolled in the Massachusetts WIC program. *Journal of the American Dietetic Association, 105,* 709–715.

American Academy of Pediatrics (AAP). (2008). *Pediatric Nutrition Handbook* (6th ed.). Elk Grove Village, IL: American Academy of Pediatrics.

American Academy of Pediatrics (AAP), Committee on Nutrition. (2000). Hypoallergenic infant formulas. *Pediatrics, 106,* 346–349.

American Academy of Pediatrics (AAP), Committee on Nutrition. (2003). Prevention of pediatric overweight and obesity. *Pediatrics, 112,* 424–430.

American Academy of Pediatrics (AAP), Section on Breastfeeding. (2005). Breastfeeding and the use of human milk. *Pediatrics, 115,* 496–506.

American Dietetic Association. (2003). Position of the American Dietetic Association and Dietitians of Canada: Vegetarian diets. *Journal of the American Dietetic Association, 103,* 748–765.

Auestad, N., Halter, R., Hall, R., Blatter, M., Bogle, M., Burks, W., et al. (2001). Growth and development in term infants fed long-chain polyunsaturated fatty acids: A double-masked, randomized, parallel, prospective, multivariate study. *Pediatrics, 108,* 372–381.

Baker, R. D. (2002). Infant formula safety. *Pediatrics, 110,* 833–835.

Bergmann, K. E., Bergmann, R. L., Kries, R. von, Böhm, O., Richter, R., Dudenhausen, J. W., et al. (2003). Early determinants of childhood overweight and adiposity in a birth cohort study: Role of breast-feeding. *International Journal of Obesity, 27,* 162–172.

Birch, L., Orlet Fisher, J., & Krahnstoever Davison, K. (2003). Learning to overeat: Maternal use of restrictive feeding practices promotes girls' eating in the absence of hunger. *American Journal of Clinical Nutrition, 78,* 215–220.

Bogen, D. L., Hanusa, B. H., & Whitaker, R. C. (2004). The effect of breast-feeding with and without formula use on the risk of obesity at 4 years of age. *Obesity Research, 12,* 1527–1535.

Briefel, R., Reidy, K., Karwe, V., Jankowski, L., & Hendricks, K. (2004b). Toddlers' transition to table foods: Impact on nutrient intakes and food patterns. *Journal of the American Dietetic Association, 104,* S38–S44.

Butte, N., Cobb, K., Dwyer, J., Graney, L., Heird, W., & Rickard, K. (2004). The Start Healthy Feeding Guidelines for infants and toddlers. *Journal of the American Dietetic Association, 104,* 442–454.

Butte, N., Wong, W., Hopkinson, J., Heinz, C., Mehta, N., & Smith, E. O. (2000). Energy requirements derived from total energy expenditure and energy deposition during the first 2 y of life. *American Journal of Clinical Nutrition, 72,* 1558–1569.

Butte, N., Wong, W., Hopkinson, J., Smith, E. O., & Ellis, K. (2000). Infant feeding mode affects early growth and body composition. *Pediatrics, 106,* 1355–1366.

Canadian Paediatric Society. (2003). Dietary manipulations for infantile colic. *Paediatrics & Child Health, 8,* 449–452.

Carruth, B. R., Skinner, J., Houck, K., & Moran, J. D. (2000). Addition of supplementary foods and infant growth. *Journal of the American College of Nutrition, 19,* 405–412.

Carruth, B. R., Ziegler, P., Gordon, A., & Hendricks, K. (2004). Developmental milestones and self-feeding behaviors in infants and toddlers. *Journal of the American Dietetic Association, 104,* S51–S56.

Centers for Disease Control. (2002). *Enterobacter sakazakii* infections associated with the use of powdered infant formula—Tennessee. *Morbidity and Mortality Weekly Report, 51,* 297–300.

Clifford, T., Campbell, K., Speechley, K., & Gorodzinsky, F. (2002). Infant colic: Empirical evidence of the absence of an association with source of early infant nutrition. *Archives of Pediatric and Adolescent Medicine, 156,* 1123–1128.

Dawodu, A., Adarwal, M., Hossain, M., Kochiyil, J., & Zayed, R. (2003). Hypovitaminosis D and vitamin D deficiency in exclusively breastfeeding infants and their mothers in summer: A justification for vitamin D supplementation of breastfeeding infants. *Journal of Pediatrics, 142,* 169–173.

de Onis, G., Garza, C., Onyango, A. W., & Borghi, E. (2007). Comparison of the WHO Child Growth Standards and the CDC 2000 Growth Charts. *Journal of Nutrition, 137,* 144–148.

Devaney, B., Kalb, L., Briefel, R., Zavitsky-Novak, T., Clusen, N., & Ziegler, P. (2004a). Feeding Infants and Toddlers Study: Overview of the study design. *Journal of the American Dietetic Association, 104,* S8–S13.

Devaney, B., Ziegler, P., Pac, S., Karwe, V., & Barr, S. (2004b). Nutrient intakes of infants and toddlers. *Journal of the American Dietetic Association, 104,* S14–S21.

Dewey, K. G. (2000a). Complementary feeding and breastfeeding. *Pediatrics, 106,* 1301–1302.

Dewey, K. G. (2000b). Protein and amino acids. *Pediatrics, 106,* 1292.

Dewey, K. G. (2001). Nutrition, growth, and complementary feeding of the breastfed infant. *Pediatric Clinics of North America, 48,* 87–104.

Dewey, K. G., Beaton, G., Fjeld, C., Lonnerdal, B., & Reeds, P. (1996). Protein requirements of infants and children. *European Journal of Clinical Nutrition, 50,* S119–S150.

Dewey, K. G., Cohen, R. J., Rivera, L. L., Canahuati, J., & Brown, K. H. (1996). Do exclusively breast-fed infants require extra protein? *Pediatric Research, 39,* 303–307.

Dewey, K. G., Domellof, M., Cohen, R., Rivera, L. L., Hernell, O., & Lonnerdal, B. (2002). Iron supplementation affects growth and morbidity of breast-fed infants: Results of a randomized trial in Sweden and Honduras. *Journal of Nutrition, 132,* 3249–3255.

Dewey, K. G., Peerson, J. M., & Brown, K. H. (1998). Effects of age of introduction of complementary foods on iron status of breastfed infants in Honduras. *American Journal of Clinical Nutrition, 67,* 878–884.

Dietz, W. H. (2001). Breastfeeding may help prevent childhood overweight. *Journal of the American Medical Association, 285,* 2506–2507.

Domellof, M., Lonnerdal, B., Abrams, S., & Hernall, O. (2002). Iron absorption in breast-fed infants: Effects of age, iron status, iron supplements, and complementary foods. *American Journal of Clinical Nutrition, 76,* 198–204.

DuPont, C. (2003). Protein requirements during the first year of life. *American Journal of Clinical Nutrition, 77*(Suppl.), 1544S–1549S.

Eichenberger Gilmore, J., Hong, L., Broffitt, B., & Levy, S. (2005). Longitudinal patterns of vitamin and mineral supplement use in young white children. *Journal of the American Dietetic Association, 105,* 763–772.

Ermis, B., Demirel, F., Demircan, N., & Gurel, A. (2002). Effects of three different iron supplementations in term healthy infants after 5 months of life. *Journal of Tropical Pediatrics, 48,* 280–284.

European Food Safety Authority. (2004). January 8, 2005 Retrieved from http://www.efsa.europa.eu/EFSA/efsa_locale-1178620753812_1178620781033.htm

FDA Talk Paper. (2002). FDA warns about possible *Enterobacter sakazakii* infections in hospitalized newborns fed powdered infant formulas. Retrieved January 7, 2005. Retrieved from http://www.fda.gov/Food/FoodSafety/Product-SpecificInformation/InfantFormula/AlertsSafetyInformation/default.htm

Fomon, S. (2001). Feeding normal infants: Rationale for recommendations. *Journal of the American Dietetic Association, 101,* 1002–1005.

Fox, M. K., Devaney, B., Reidy, K., Razafindrakoto, C., & Ziegler, P. (2006). Relationship between portion size and energy intake among infants and toddlers: Evidence of self-regulation. *Journal of the American Dietetic Association, 106,* S77–S83.

Fox, M. K., Pac, S., Devaney, B., & Jankowski, L. (2004). Feeding infants and toddlers study: What foods are infants and toddlers eating? *Journal of the American Dietetic Association, 104,* S22–S30.

Fox, M. K., Reidy, K., Karwe, V., & Ziegler, P. (2006b). Average portions of foods commonly eaten by infants and toddlers in the United States. *Journal of the American Dietetic Association, 106,* S66–S76.

Fox, M. K., Reidy, K., Novak, T., & Ziegler, P. (2006c). Sources of energy and nutrients in the diets of infants and toddlers. *Journal of the American Dietetic Association, 106,* S28–S42.

Gartner, L., Greer, F., and the Section on Breastfeeding and Committee on Nutrition. (2003). Prevention of rickets and vitamin D deficiency: New guidelines for vitamin D intake. *Pediatrics, 111,* 908–910.

Gibson, R., & Holtz, C. (2000). The adequacy of micro-nutrients in complementary foods. *Pediatrics, 106,* 1298–1300.

Gillman, M. W., Rifas-Shiman, S. L., Camargo, C. A., Berkey, C. S., Frazier, A. L., Rockett, H. R. H., et al. (2001). Risk of overweight among adolescents who were breastfed as infants. *Journal of the American Medical Association, 285,* 2461–2467.

Greer, F., Shannon, M., the Committee of Nutrition, & the Committee on Environmental Health. (2005). Infant methemoglobinemia: The role of dietary nitrate in food and water. *Pediatrics, 116,* 784–786.

Hediger, M., Overpeck, M., Kuczmarski, R., & Ruan, W. J. (2001). Association between infant breastfeeding and overweight in young children. *Journal of the American Medical Association, 285,* 2453–2460.

Heine, R., Hill, D., & Hosking, C. (2004). Primary prevention of atopic dermatitis in breastfed infants: What is the evidence? *Journal of Pediatrics, 44,* 564–567.

Hill, D., Roy, N., Heine, R., Hosking, C., Francis, D., Brown, J., et al. (2005). Effect of a low-allergen maternal diet on colic among breastfed infants: A randomized, controlled trial. *Pediatrics, 116,* e709–e715.

Institute of Medicine (IOM). (2001). *Dietary Reference Intake for Vitamin A, Vitamin K, Arsenic, Boron, Chromium, Copper, Iodine, Iron, Manganese, Molybdenum, Nickel, Silicon, Vanadium, and Zinc.* Washington, DC: National Academy Press.

Institute of Medicine (IOM). (2002). *Dietary Reference Intake for Energy, Carbohydrate, Fiber, Fat, Fatty Acids, Cholesterol, Protein, and Amino Acids. Part I.* Prepublication copy. Washington, DC: National Academy Press.

Institute of Medicine (IOM). (2005). Report brief. *WIC Food Packages: Time for a Change.* October 4, 2007. Retrieved from www.iom.edu/report.asp?id=26667

Joppu, U., Kalliomaki, M., & Isolauri, E. (2000). Maternal diet rich in saturated fat during breastfeeding is associated with atopic sensitization of the infant. *European Journal of Clinical Nutrition, 54,* 702–705.

Kalliomaki, M., Salminen, S., Arvilommi, H., Kero, P., Koskinene, P., & Isolauri, E. (2001). Probiotics in primary prevention of atopic disease; a randomised placebo-controlled trial. *Lancet, 357,* 1076–1079.

Kattelmann, K. K., Ho, M., & Specker, B. L. (2001). Effect of timing of introduction of complementary foods on iron and zinc status of formula fed infants at 12, 24, and 36 months of age. *Journal of the American Dietetic Association, 101,* 443–447.

Kazal, L. (2002). Prevention of iron deficiency in infants and toddlers. *American Family Physician, 66,* 1217–1224.

Khedr, E. M., Farghaly, W. M., Amry Sel, D., & Osman, A. A. (2004). Neural maturation of breastfed and formula-fed infants. *Acta Paediatrics, 93,* 734–738.

Kill, I., Wickman, M., Lilja, G., Nordvall, S. L., & Pershagen, G. (2002). Breast feeding and allergic diseases in infants—a prospective birth cohort study. *Archives of Diseases in Children, 87,* 478–481.

Kleinman, R. (2000a). American Academy of Pediatrics recommendations for complementary feeding. *Pediatrics, 106,* 1274.

Kleinman, R. (2000b). Complementary feeding and later health. *Pediatrics, 106,* 1287–1288.

Kleinman, R. (2000c). Complementary feeding and neuromuscular development. *Pediatrics, 106,* 1279.

Koletzko, B. (2000). Complementary foods and the development of food allergy. *Pediatrics, 106,* 1285.

Kramer, M., Guo, T., Platt, R., Shapiro, S., Collet, J. P., Chlamers, B., et al. (2002). Breastfeeding and infant growth: Biology or bias? *Pediatrics, 110,* 343–347.

Krebs, N. (2000). Dietary zinc and iron sources, physical growth and cognitive development of breastfed infants. *Journal of Nutrition, 130,* 358S–360S.

Krebs, N. F., Reidinger, C. J., Robertson, A. D., & Hambridge, K. M. (1994). Growth and intakes of energy and zinc in infants fed human milk. *Journal of Pediatrics, 124,* 32–39.

Kreiter, S., Schwartz, R., Kirkman, H., Charlton, P., Calikoglu, A., & Davenport, M. (2000). Nutritional rickets in African-American breast-fed infants. *Journal of Pediatrics, 137,* 153–157.

Kries, R. von, Koletzko, B., Sauerwald, T., Mutius, E. von, Barnert, K., Grunert, V., et al. (1999). Breast feeding and obesity: Cross sectional study. *British Medical Journal, 319,* 147–150.

Lack, G., Fox, D., Northstone, K., & Golding, J. (2003). Factors associated with the development of peanut allergy in childhood. *New England Journal of Medicine, 348,* 977–985.

Lawrence, R. (1999). *Breastfeeding: A Guide for the Medical Profession* (5th ed.). St. Louis: Mosby.

Lucas, A., & St. James-Robert, I. (1998). Crying, fussing and colic behavior in breast and bottle-fed infants. *Early Human Development, 53,* 9–18.

Lust, K., Brown, J., & Thomas, W. (1996). Maternal intake of cruciferous vegetables and other foods and colic symptoms in exclusively breastfed infants. *Journal of the American Dietetic Association, 96,* 47–48.

Martorell, R., Stein, A. D., & Schroeder, D. G. (2001). Early nutrition and later adiposity. *Journal of Nutrition, 131,* 874S–880S.

Meeks Gardner, J. M., Powell, C. A., Baker-Henningham, H., Walker, S. P., Cole, T. J., & Grantham-McGregor, S. M. (2005). Zinc supplementation and psychosocial stimulation: Effects on the development of undernourished Jamaican children. *American Journal of Clinical Nutrition, 82,* 399–405.

Michaelsen, K. F. (2000). Cow's milk in complementary feeding. *Pediatrics, 106,* 1302–1303.

Morale, S., Hoffman, D., Castañeda, Y., Wheaton, D., Burns, R., & Birch, E. (2005). Duration of long-chain polyunsaturated fatty acids availability in the diet and visual acuity. *Early Human Development, 81,* 197–203.

Motarjemi, Y. (2000). Research priorities on safety of complementary feeding. *Pediatrics, 106,* 1304–1305.

Muraro, A., Dreborg, S., Halken, S., Høst, A., Niggemann, B., Aalberse, R., et al. (2004). Dietary prevention of allergic diseases in infants and small children. Part III. Critical review of published peer-reviewed observational and interventional studies and final recommendations. *Pediatric Allergy and Immunology, 15,* 291–307.

National Center for Health Statistics. (2000). Vital and health statistics of the Centers for Disease Control and Prevention. *Advance Data,* 314.

National WIC Association Position Paper. (2004). *Breastfeeding Promotion and Support in the WIC Program.* Washington, DC: Author.

Norris, J., Barriga, K., Hoffenber, E., Taki, I., Miao, D., Haas, J., et al. (2005a). Risk of celiac disease autoimmunity and timing of gluten introduction in the diet of infants at increased risk of disease. *Journal of the American Medical Association, 293,* 2343–2351.

Norris, J., Barriga, K., Klingensmith, G., Hoffman, M., Eisenbarth, G., Erlich, H., et al. (2005b). Timing of initial cereal exposure in infancy and risk of islet autoimmunity. *Journal of the American Medical Association, 290,* 1713–1720.

Nowak-Wegrzyn, A. (2003). Future approaches to food allergy. *Pediatrics, 111,* 1672–1680.

Odijk, J. van, Hulthen, L., Ahlstedt, S., & Borres, M. P. (2004). Introduction of food during the infant's first year: A study with emphasis on introduction of gluten and of egg, fish, and peanut in allergy-risk families. *Acta Paediatrics, 93,* 464–470.

Orlet Fisher, J., Birch, L., Smiciklas-Wright, H., & Picciano, M. F. (2000). Breast-feeding through the first year predicts maternal control in feeding and subsequent toddler energy intakes. *Journal of the American Dietetic Association, 100,* 641–646.

Owen, C. G., Martin, R. M., Whincup, P. H., Davey Smith, G., & Cook, D. G. (2005). Effect of infant feeding on the risk of obesity across the life course: A quantitative review of the published evidence. *Pediatrics, 115,* 1367–1377.

Pelto, G. (2000). Improving complementary feeding practices and responsive parenting as a primary component of interventions to prevent malnutrition in infancy and early childhood. *Pediatrics, 106,* 1300–1301.

Ponce-Rivera, L. N. M., Blanco-Montero, A., Reyes-Vazquez, H., Lopez-Enriquez, C., & Fuentes-Lugo, D. (2008). Assessment of differences between the new World Health Organization Child–Growth Standards and the Centers for Disease Control and Prevention 2000 Growth Charts in Latin American children: Which reference should we use? *Pediatrics, 121,* S114.

Ponza, M., Devaney, B., Ziegler, P., Reidy, K., & Squatrito, C. (2004). Nutrient intakes and food choices of infants and toddlers participating in WIC. *Journal of the American Dietetic Association, 104,* S71–S79.

Rajakumar, K., & Thomas, S. (2005). Reemerging nutritional rickets: A historical perspective. *Archives of Pediatric and Adolescent Medicine, 159,* 335–341.

Ryan, A. S., Wenjun, Z., & Acosta, A. (2002). Breastfeeding continues to increase into the new millennium. *Pediatrics, 110,* 1103–1109.

Saarinen, K. M., Pelkonen, A. S., Makela, M. G., & Savilahti, E. (2005). Clinical course and prognosis of cow's milk allergy are dependent on milk-specific IgE status. *Journal of Allergy and Clinical Immunology, 116,* 869–875.

Sakashita, R., Inoue, N., & Kamegai, T. (2004). From milk to solids: A reference standard for the transitional eating process in infants and preschool children in Japan. *European Journal of Clinical Nutrition, 58,* 643–653.

Sakashita, R., Inoue, N., & Tatsuki, T. (2003). Selection of reference foods for a scale of standards for use in assessing the transitional process from milk to solid foods in infants and pre-school children. *European Journal of Clinical Nutrition, 57,* 803–809.

Savino, F., Costamagna, M., Prino, A., Oggero, R., & Silvestro, L. (2002). Leptin levels in breast-fed and formula-fed infants. *Acta Paediatrics, 91,* 897–902.

Schach, B., & Haight, M. (2002). Colic and food allergy in the breast-fed infant: Is it possible for an exclusively breastfed infant to suffer from food allergy? *Journal of Human Lactation, 18,* 50–52.

Schmitz, J. (2000). Complementary feeding and enteropathies. *Pediatrics, 106,* 1286.

Sicherer, S. (2003). Clinical aspects of gastrointestinal food allergy in childhood. *Pediatrics, 111,* 1609–1616.

Skinner, J., Ziegler, P., Pac, S., & Devaney, B. (2004). Meal and snack patterns of infants and toddlers. *Journal of the American Dietetic Association, 104,* S65–S70.

Skinner, J., Ziegler, P., & Ponza, M. (2004). Transitions in infants' and toddlers' beverage patterns. *Journal of the American Dietetic Association, 104,* S45–S50.

Slaughter, C., & Bryant, A. H. (2004). Hungry for love: The feeding relationship in the psychological development of young children. *Permanente Journal, 8,* 23–29.

Stang, J. (2006). Improving the eating patterns of infants and toddlers. *Journal of the American Dietetic Association, 106,* S7–S9.

Stettler, N., Stallings, V. A., Troxel, A., Zhou, J., Schinnar, R., Nelson, S. E., et al. (2005). Weight gain in the first week of life and overweight in adulthood. *Circulation, 111,* 1897–1903.

Stettler, N., Zemel, B. S., Kumanyika, S., & Stallings, V. A. (2002). Infant weight gain and childhood overweight status in a multicenter, cohort study. *Pediatrics, 109,* 194–199.

Taveras, E., Scanlon, K., Birch, L., Rifas-Shiman, S., Rich-Edwards, J., & Gillman, M. (2004). Association of breastfeeding with maternal control of infant feeding at age 1 year. *Pediatrics, 114,* e577–e583.

Upham, J., & Holt, P. (2005). Environment and development of atopy. *Current Opinion in Allergy and Clinical Immunology, 5,* 167–172.

Vadas, P., Wai, Y., Burks, W., & Perelman, B. (2001). Detection of peanut allergens in breast milk of lactating women. *Journal of the American Medical Association, 285,* 1746–1748.

vanDijk, C. E. & Innis, S. M. (2009). Growth-curve standards and the assessment of early excess weight gain in infancy. *Pediatrics, 123,* 102–108.

Villalpando, S. (2000). Feeding mode, infections, and anthropometric status in early childhood. *Pediatrics, 106,* 1282–1283.

Wagner, C. L., Greer, F. R., & the Section on Breastfeeding and Committee on Nutrition. (2008). Prevention of rickets and vitamin D deficiency in infants, children, and adolescents. *Pediatrics, 122,* 1142–1152.

Wagner, C. L., Hulsey, T. C., Fanning, D., Ebeling, M., & Hollis, B. W. (2006). High-dose vitamin D3 supplementation in a cohort of breastfeeding mothers and their infants; a 6-month follow-up pilot study. *Breastfeeding Medicine, 1,* 59–70.

Weaver, L. (2000). Gastrointestinal digestive and absorptive function. *Pediatrics, 106,* 1280–1281.

Weisberg, P., Scablon, K., Li, R., & Cogswell, M. (2004). Nutritional rickets among children in the United States: Review of cases reported between 1986 and 2003. *American Journal of Clinical Nutrition, 80*(Suppl.), 1697S–16705S.

Wharton, B. (2000). Patterns of complementary feeding (weaning) in countries of the European Union: Topics for research. *Pediatrics, 106,* 1273–1274.

WHO Working Group on the Growth Reference Protocol and the WHO Task Force on Methods for the Natural Regulation of Fertility. (2002). Growth of healthy infants and the timing, type and frequency of complementary foods. *American Journal of Clinical Nutrition, 76,* 620–627.

Wood, R. A. (2003). The natural history of food allergy. *Pediatrics, 111,* 1631–1637.

World Health Organization (WHO). (2003). *Global Strategy for Infant and Young Child Feeding* [pamphlet]. Geneva: Author.

Zeiger, R. (2003). Food allergen avoidance in the prevention of food allergy in infants and children. *Pediatrics, 11,* 1662–1671.

Zutavern, A., Mutius, E. von, Harris, J., Mills, P., Moffatt, S., White, C., et al. (2004). The introduction of solids in relation to asthma and eczema. *Archives of Diseases in Children, 89,* 303–308.

Normal Nutrition for Toddler Through School-Aged Children and the Role of Parents in Promoting Healthy Nutrition in Early Childhood

Jennifer Sabo, RD, LDN, CNSD

CHAPTER OUTLINE

Reader Objectives

After studying this chapter and reflecting on the contents, you should be able to

1. Understand the different nutritional factors that may affect growth and development in a toddler.
2. Understand the use of vitamins and minerals in a toddler and how to provide them naturally.
3. Identify the differences in portion sizes that are appropriate for toddlers versus adults.
4. Understand the importance of "mealtime" with toddlers.
5. Identify reasons for excess weight gain in toddlers and how this can be prevented.

After infancy, nutrition continues to be vital to the growth and **development** of children. As the child becomes less dependent on breast milk and/or formula, a more comprehensive form of nutrition becomes essential to provide an appropriate variety of foods. Doing so will ensure that the growing child is obtaining the necessary macro- and micronutrients for growth. This goal is made difficult by the emerging independence of the child. Strategies designed to incorporate, understand, and compensate for particular behaviors centered on mealtime and eating may be just as vital as providing healthy choices.

Development: A process in which something passes by degrees to a different, more advanced stage.

Growth Expectations

Growth is measured and plotted on standard Centers for Disease Control and Prevention (CDC) growth charts based on age and sex. Head circumference and weight for height are measured and plotted until 36 months of age. After age 2 body mass index (BMI) is used to assess appropriate weight for height (National Institutes of Health, n.d.). The use of BMI after the age of 2 is appropriate because of a correlation between height and adiposity before age 12 (Freedman et al., 2004).

Growth rates may vary considerably for each individual child. This is thought to be associated with a variety of factors, including parents' growth history and patterns. It is essential for clinicians to note that approximately 25% of normal infants and toddlers in the first 2 years of life drop to a lower growth percentile and subsequently remain on this new growth track (Krugman & Dubowitz, 2003). **Tables 3.1 and 3.2** demonstrate average weight and height growth, respectively, for the 1st through 10th years of life. It is helpful for health care professionals to be aware of these growth trends to assess each child's growth.

TABLE 3.1	Weight Growth	
Age (yr)	**Average Daily Growth (g/day)**	
1–3	4–10	
4–6	5–8	
7–10	5–12	

Based on growth velocity of the 50th percentile weight for age and height for age from the National Center for Health Statistics growth charts (2000).

TABLE 3.2	Height Growth	
Age (yr)	**Average Daily Growth (g/day)**	
1–3	0.7–1.1	
4–6	0.5–0.8	
7–10	0.4–0.6	

Based on growth velocity of the 50th percentile weight for age and height for age from the National Center for Health Statistics growth charts (2000).

Energy and Nutrient Needs

As growth rates differ for each child, so do their energy needs. The energy requirements of toddlers and children vary greatly based on differences in both growth rate and level of activity (Zlotkin, 1996). As shown in Tables 3.1 and 3.2, the growth rate for ages 1 to 3 years and 7 to 10 years are more rapid, thus necessitating greater energy needs. The chronologic age and the current stage of development of the child also relate to and influence energy needs. Current energy need recommendations from the Food and Agriculture Organization, World Health Organization, and United Nations University Expert Con-

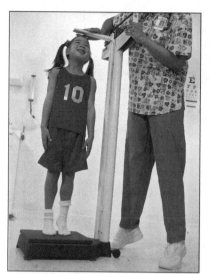

sultation (1985) for growing children ages 1 to 10 years are based
on the actual observed intakes of healthy children and can aid clinicians in establishing norms.

   Current weight and height, as well as trends in growth velocity, can also be used to assess a particular child's needs. It is essential to note that throughout childhood there appears to be no difference
in energy requirements between boys and girls. A study by Butte et
al. (2000) used the total energy expenditure and energy deposition data of a group
of healthy children to demonstrate that current recommendations for energy intake in the first 2 years of life may exceed modern energy expenditures and perhaps need to be revised.

Protein

Protein is the primary factor in many body tissues.
Proteins build, maintain,
and restore tissues in the
body, such as muscles and
organs. As a child grows and
develops, protein is a cru-

cial nutrient needed to provide optimal growth. Current recommendations
state that protein intake should comprise approximately 10% to 20% of the child's
daily energy intake. This recommendation is designed to ensure that enough
energy is provided to the body from all nutrients so that protein is spared for
growth and development of tissues. **Table 3.3** provides the current dietary reference intake for protein for growing toddlers and children (Institute of Medicine [IOM], Food and Nutrition Board, 2000–2005).

TABLE 3.3	Protein Requirements

Age (yr)	Dietary Reference Intake for Protein (g/kg/day)
1–3	0.87
4–8	0.76

Based on growth velocity of the 50th percentile weight for age and height for age from the National Center for
Health Statistics growth charts (2000).

Fat

Until age 3, dietary fat plays a role in brain development. Fat makes up approximately 60% of the central and peripheral nervous systems that essentially control, regulate, and integrate every body system;
thus it is essential that growing toddlers obtain adequate fat from their diet. Furthermore, the fat content of the diet is known to be the crucial element in providing sati-
ety. Therefore, low-fat meals or snacks for children can lead to hunger
and subsequent overeating between meals. After infancy most children are able to meet their daily calorie and nutrient requirements
for growth with a diet consisting of 30% of total calories from fat
(American Academy of Pediatrics [AAP], Committee on Nutrition,
1992; Butte, 2000). If excess weight gain is a concern, often only mi-

nor changes in dietary choices are needed to help keep fat intake at or below 30% of daily calories to promote optimal growth (Fisher, Van Horn, & McGill, 1997).

It should be noted that all fats are not equal in their benefits to one's health. Most fat intake should be derived from poly- and monounsaturated fat, such as fish, most nuts, and vegetable oils (American Heart Association [AHA], n.d.). These fats help to keep total cholesterol low and "good" cholesterol, or **high-density lipoproteins**, high. Foods high in saturated fat, such as butter, cheese, and beef, should be offered in moderation, because these can contribute to high total cholesterol and high **low-density lipoproteins**. Although hypercholesterolemia has not traditionally been a concern for this age group, recent trends in obesity coincide with a rise in cholesterol levels, therefore mandating that clinicians become more cognizant of fat intake.

Vitamins and Minerals

Calcium

Calcium is the principal mineral required by the body for the process of bone mineralization. Toddlers and young children have an increased need for calcium to promote the rapid bone growth and skeletal development that takes place during these early years of life. Despite the essential nature of this mineral, studies demonstrate that only about 50% of children aged 1 to 5 years meet the Dietary Reference Intake (DRI) for calcium (Dennison, 1996). **Table 3.4** provides the current DRI for calcium in growing children (IOM, 2000–2005).

> **High-density lipoprotein:** A blood constituent involved in the transport of cholesterol and associated with a decreased risk of heart attack.
>
> **Low-density lipoprotein:** A lipoprotein that transports cholesterol in the blood, composed of a moderate amount of protein and a large amount of cholesterol. High levels are associated with increased risk of heart disease.

TABLE 3.4	Calcium Requirements	
Age (yr)	**Dietary Reference Intake for Calcium (mg/day)**	
1–3	500	
4–8	800	
9–13	1,300	

Based on current Dietary Reference Intake for calcium (IOM, 2000–2005).

Storey, Forchee, and Anderson (2004) demonstrated that soft drink and juice consumption begin to increase at 4 to 8 years of age, often replacing milk at meals and snacks. This study found that intake of milk and milk products decreased more significantly with age for girls as compared with boys. These authors suggest discouraging and/or restricting juice and soft drink intake to avoid the displacement of milk with these largely unhealthy beverages (Storey, Forchee, & Anderson, 2004).

If it is determined that the recommended daily calcium intake is not being met, by using diet histories and food frequencies, health professionals should consider recommendation of a daily calcium supplement. Many studies have shown that males demonstrate a superior result in building peak bone mass with calcium supplementation (Carter et al., 2001). It is essential to recognize that milk and milk products contain additional necessary nutrients for health, including protein and vitamin D, which continues to make these the superior means of meeting calcium needs. Thus, health care professionals should continue to find means of increasing intake of milk and milk products (Storey, Forchee, & Anderson, 2004). Because vitamin D is needed for the best utilization of calcium, many calcium supplements are now including vitamin D to aid in the efficiency of the product. As demonstrated by Johnston et al. (1992), daily calcium supplementation lasting longer than 12 months may result in great gains in bone mass as compared with control groups.

Recent studies indicate that calcium intake of about 800 mg/day is associated with adequate bone mineralization in preadolescent children (AAP, 1999). The importance of providing adequate calcium to growing children is becoming more apparent. Storey, Forchee, and Anderson (2004) found that adequate calcium intake in preadolescent and adolescent girls is necessary to help decrease the incidence of osteoporosis in adulthood. Therefore, good prevention efforts for osteoporosis should focus on "young people in their growing years" (Carter et al., 2001).

Dairy products are typically the main source of calcium in the diet, including milk, yogurt, cheese, and ice cream. However, more recently and perhaps reflecting trends of inadequate calcium intake, many

TABLE 3.5	Easy Ways to Increase Calcium in the Diet

Drink milk. Two 8-ounce glasses of milk each day can provide over 600 mg of calcium. Lactose-reduced milk is a good source of calcium if regular milk is not tolerated.

Use heated milk in place of hot water to make hot cereals, such as oatmeal or hot chocolate.

Add cheese to sandwiches, casseroles, meat loaf, salads, and snacks.

Add broccoli and cheese to a baked potato.

Choose desserts made with milk such as pudding, custard, frozen yogurt, and ice cream.

Substitute milk and yogurt in recipes instead of cream or sour cream.

Add dried powdered milk or evaporated milk when preparing soups, mashed potatoes, sauces, and hot cereals.

Drink a glass of calcium-fortified juice, such as orange juice.

Add almonds to muffin and bread recipes.

Remember to read labels for percentage of calcium. If it has greater than 30% of your calcium requirement for the day, then it would be a high-calcium choice. Many foods are fortified with calcium, such as orange juice, rice, cereals, waffles, and pasta.

Choosing one high-calcium food at each meal will help you to meet your goal every day!

Note: Low-fat products contain the same amount of calcium as whole milk products.

foods are being fortified with calcium, such as waffles, juice, and cereals. Calcium is often represented as a percent daily value on food labels, using 1,000 mg/day as 100% daily value (AAP, 1999). **Table 3.5** provides ways to increase calcium in a child's diet.

CRITICAL **Thinking**

Though controversial, flavored milk can be a good source of calcium and may increase calcium intake in young children. It may be helpful to choose lower-fat milk and add flavoring with sugar-free syrups as a way to keep fat and added sugar intake low for toddlers over age 2 but still give them the benefits of calcium.

Vitamin D

Vitamin D is available to humans through the photochemical action of sunlight or ultraviolet light on 7-dehydrocholesterol in skin and through dietary sources such as fish oils, fatty fish, and foods fortified with vitamin D, including cow's milk and infant or supplemental formulas (Holick, Shils, Olsen, Shike, & Ross, 1999). The amount of vitamin D synthesized through sunlight exposure is affected by time spent outside, the amount of skin exposed, air pollution, cloud cover, time of day, latitude, time of year, and skin pigmentation (Tomashek et al., 2001).

Specker and colleagues (1985) estimated that white infants require approximately 30 minutes of sunlight per week to obtain adequate vitamin D if wearing only a diaper but require 2 hours per week if fully clothed without a hat. The melanin in our skin decreases the amount of vitamin D synthesized from sunlight. Therefore, children with darker skin need to spend more time outside than those with lighter skin to obtain sufficient vitamin D (Weisberg, Scanlon, Li, & Cogswell, 2004).

Adequate vitamin D intake is important for optimal calcium absorption. Dietary products such as yogurts and orange juice are now fortified with vitamin D. As toddlers are advanced off of infant formula and onto table foods, parents should be educated to offer a diet adequate in both nutrients (Weisberg et al., 2004). National data as to the prevalence of hypovitaminosis D among children are not yet available (Weisberg et al., 2004). More extensive study is needed to determine the extent of vitamin D deficiency in the United States.

Iron

Daily requirements for iron intake are based on age and iron stores. During periods of rapid growth the body's need for iron increases, as shown in **Table 3.6** (IOM, 2000–2005).

Iron can be classified as being derived from heme or nonheme sources. Heme sources include animal meats and products, such as beef and chicken, whereas nonheme sources include fortified grains, fruits, and vegetables (IOM, 2000–2005). Although iron can be obtained from either source, absorption of this essential nutrient is found to be higher from heme sources than from nonheme. Of note, consuming foods with vitamin C while eating an iron-containing food can promote better absorption of iron into the body. Conversely, taking antacids during the meal may inhibit iron absorption. **Table 3.7** provides ways to increase iron in the diet.

Iron deficiency **anemia** is the most common nutritional deficiency in the world and remains relatively common among at-risk groups in the United States (Schneider et al., 2005). Risk factors for iron deficiency include low household income, lack of consistent medical care, poor diet quality, and parents with minimal education. Identification of deficiency is crucial, because side effects for infants and children with iron deficiency may include impaired neurodevelopment, leading to decreased attention span and lower scores on standardized tests (Grantham-McGregor & Ani, 2001).

Iron deficiency often occurs secondary to insufficient dietary iron intake. It should also be noted that increased calcium intake may lead to anemia. This is due to calcium and iron competing for absorption at the same receptor sites within the body. Therefore, drinking large amounts of high-calcium milk is a common cause of iron deficiency in children. Refusal of meats is also a common cause of low iron intake in developing children. The increased availability of iron-fortified foods and formulas has helped to decrease the incidence of iron deficiency.

An objective of *Healthy People 2010* is to reduce iron deficiency in 1- to 2-year-olds by 5% and in 3- to 4-year-olds by 1% (U.S. Department of Health and Human Services, 2000). The goal to reduce anemia and iron deficiency in high-risk populations, such as toddlers, has been addressed through programs such as the Special Supplemental Nutrition Program for Women, Infants, and Children (WIC) of the U.S. Department of Agriculture by enrolling families at the highest risk for anemia and iron deficiency and providing them with vouchers for iron-fortified formulas and cereals. WIC also screens children for low hemoglobin with the goal of identifying at-risk children, educating families, and reducing the incidence of anemia (Schneider et al., 2005).

Vitamin Supplements

After infancy, supplemental vitamin use decreases, but it is still relatively common. Typically, a general multivitamin is not routinely recommended for toddlers and young children unless the diet history demonstrates the child's intake to be inadequate.

Supplementation is recommended for children without the means to eat a balanced diet and for those with chronic medical conditions or treatments who may lose necessary vitamins—for example, children

TABLE 3.6	Iron Requirements
Age (yr)	Dietary Reference Intake for Iron (mg/day)
1–3	7
4–8	10
9–13	8

Based on current Dietary Reference Intake for iron (IOM, 2000–2005).

TABLE 3.7 Increasing Iron in the Diet

Include a protein source at meals, such as fish, beef, or poultry.

Look for iron enriched or fortified grains, such as cereals, breads, and pasta.

Offer oatmeal or cream of wheat at breakfast.

Add foods high in vitamin C to the meal, including citrus fruit, melon, and dark green leafy vegetables, for improved iron absorption.

Add pureed meats to pasta sauce or casseroles for toddlers with difficulty advancing to chewing meats.

Encourage children with advanced chewing skills to eat the skin of the baked potato for added dietary iron.

Anemia: A quantitative deficiency of hemoglobin, often accompanied by a reduced number of red blood cells and causing pallor, weakness, and breathlessness. May be related to inadequate dietary consumption of iron or blood loss.

with dialysis, cystic fibrosis, gastrointestinal conditions, or food allergies. Megadoses of vitamins and minerals should be discouraged unless prescribed by a doctor for a specific medical condition.

Many everyday foods are fortified with multiple vitamins and minerals; therefore, vitamin and mineral deficiencies are rare in the United States (Dietz & Stern, 1999). Consuming the recommended daily servings of the many food groups typically provides adequate nutrients. A diet evaluation by a health care professional is recommended for children whose parents are questioning the child's need for multivitamin intake. Many pediatricians believe minimal risk is involved if a child is given the daily standard multiple vitamin. However, although vitamin and mineral toxicities are rare, possible excess intakes of some nutrients due to supplements and high intake of fortified foods should be considered (Briefel, Hanson, Fox, Novak, & Ziegler, 2006).

> **● Learning Point**   Many vitamins often look and taste like candy; special care should be taken to keep them out of reach of children, and under no circumstances should they be referred to as a treat by parents or caregivers.

If a child has an inadequate diet, providing a daily vitamin addresses the problem only in the short term. Working on improving the diet is the best way to ensure a child is receiving optimal nutrition. Health care professionals should stress the importance of whole foods rather than individual nutrients (Fox, Reidy, Novak, & Ziegler, 2006) to ensure the diet is complete with all nutrients, including fiber.

Fluoride

Fluoride has been demonstrated to promote tooth formation and also to inhibit the progression of dental caries (IOM, 2000–2005). However, children who begin to use fluoride toothpaste before age 2 are at higher risk for enamel **fluorosis**. This is due to a poorly controlled swallowing reflex, thereby leading to increased ingestion of fluoride. To avoid excess ingestion, child-strength toothpaste (which contains a decreased quantity of fluoride) may be used in children aged 2 to 6 years. After age 6 regular fluoridated toothpaste is approved for children (CDC, 2001).

> **Fluorosis:** An abnormal condition caused by excessive intake of fluorides, characterized in children by discoloration and pitting (mottling) of the teeth.

Deficiencies in fluoride are not common but may occur in children who live in areas with nonfluoridated water or who receive nonfluoridated bottled water. Fluoride supplementation may be prescribed by a health care professional for infants over age 6 months who are at risk for dental caries and primarily drink water with minimal fluoride content (CDC, 2001).

Water

Water helps the body to maintain homeostasis, allows for the transport of nutrients into cells, and also functions in the removal of the waste products of metabolism (IOM, 2000–2005). Therefore, water is a very important, though often overlooked, component of the daily diet. All beverages contain water, as do high-moisture foods, such as fruit, soups, and ice cream. Water can be offered to the growing child for hydration, but care should be taken not to replace adequate milk or formula intake to prevent displacing vital nutrients in the diet.

Whole Milk

The use of whole milk should typically stop after age 2, unless otherwise directed by a health care professional. To promote adherence, families should take care to drink skim or 1% milk together.

Foods at 1 Year

After 1 year of age toddlers begin to eat more like their caregivers. An important aspect of feeding toddlers is the knowledge that portion sizes should be kept appropriate for their age. Toddlers often eat 6 small meals each day versus 3 larger meals. Dietz and Stern (1999) suggested that toddler serving sizes be one-fourth to one-half that of adults. Some examples follow:

- Grains: bread, one-fourth to one-half slice; cereal, rice, or pasta, cooked, 4 tablespoons; dry cereal, ¼ cup

- Cooked vegetables: 1 tablespoon per year of age
- Fruit: cooked or canned, ½ cup; fresh, one-half piece; 100% juice, ¼ to ½ cup
- Dairy: milk, ½ cup; cheese, ½ ounce; yogurt, ⅓ cup
- Protein: chicken, turkey, beef, or fish, 1 ounce; ground meat, 2 tablespoons

Mealtime with Toddlers

As toddlers continue to advance in their feeding skills, it is crucial to provide a healthy feeding and eating environment. Structure at meals can have a significant influence on a child's eating patterns (Patrick & Nicklas, 2005). Suggestions to provide such a structured environment include the complete absence of television and other distractions of a similar ilk. As often as possible the family should sit at the dining room or kitchen table together and enjoy the meal as a unit. In addition to providing structure and promoting family bonding, eating together as a family has been shown to be associated with increased intakes of fruits and vegetables at a meal (Patrick & Nicklas, 2005).

As with most behaviors, the child's stage of development can influence food choices. A toddler may prefer finger foods that encourage them to demonstrate their new independence. **Table 3.8** provides examples of finger foods that are typically safe to offer. To avoid conflict at meals, parents should be educated that the child may also decide mealtime is over before a large amount of food is consumed because of their comparatively small stomach size. The AHA recommends that infants and young children should not be forced to finish a meal, because calorie intake is likely to vary at each mealtime (AHA, n.d.). In fact, Fisher et al. found that children forced to eat everything on their plates became less sensitive to their body's signs of satiety (Fisher & Birch, 1999).

TABLE 3.8	Finger Foods

Foods should be easily dissolved.

Serve cheese sticks, rice puffs, wagon wheels, cheese puffs, meat sticks, soft vegetable pieces, peeled apple or pear sticks, and soft fruit pieces.

Note: Types of foods offered must match developmental abilities.

Introducing New Foods

As toddlers and young children develop new feeding skills, there is potential for greater dietary variety. To the frustration of many caregivers, children often initially refuse a new food simply because it is unfamiliar. However, multiple exposures to a new food have been found to ultimately achieve food acceptance. It has been found that up to 10 exposures to the new food promote clear changes in acceptance of the food (Sullivan & Birch, 1993). However, Carruth et al. (1998) found that most caregivers tried a new food an average of 2.5 times before deciding the child disliked that particular food, falling well below the recommended number of experiences needed to truly determine an actual dislike for the food. This demonstrates that parents and caregivers can greatly benefit from consistent education regarding presentation of new foods.

It is important to introduce one food at a time to avoid confusion or overwhelming the child. Consistency with each new food, offering it at least once per day, helps the child to develop a familiarity. Offering vegetables more frequently throughout the day has been shown to help increase a child's daily intake (Dennison, Rockwell, & Baker, 1998). Similar-appearing foods may be more readily received once one type of food has previously been accepted. Conversely, limited exposure to a variety of foods could lead to rejection of other products that have a similar visual appearance to the initially rejected food (Carruth et al., 1998). Many parents state their child does not like vegetables, but vegetables are rarely available in the home for the child to become familiar with. Therefore, not only exposure but also the opportunity to taste a food increases food acceptance (Birch & Fisher, 1998).

Caregivers should be educated on providing a variety of healthful new foods to their child. Foods without overall nutritional value should not be introduced merely to provide calories (AHA, n.d.). **Table 3.9** provides tips on promoting increased fruit and vegetable intake.

TABLE 3.9	How To Promote Increased Fruit and Vegetable Intake

Add fruit purees into mixes, such as pancakes, waffles, and muffins.

Apples, pears, bananas, and blueberries are great fruits to try. Using purees avoids the child finding chunks of the fruit, which may prevent the child from eating the food. Sometimes starting with a very small amount of fruit and increasing the amount as the child becomes familiar with the flavor is the best way for more sensitive children.

Pureed fruits can also be mixed into yogurt, milk shakes, and pudding to add flavor.

Adding dried fruits to cereal or trail mixes is a good way to increase fruit intake. Serving sizes are smaller for dried fruit, so the child does not have to eat as much. Note: This should be used for children over age 3 to prevent a choking risk.

Mix vegetable purees into soups and sauces, such as spaghetti sauce or chicken noodle soup. Carrots, green beans, and sweet potatoes are good vegetables to start out with. You can also mix these purees into homemade meat loaf, meatballs, or hamburgers.

Bring the child along to the store to select a new fruit or vegetable he or she would like to try. Have the child help prepare the new food. If the child feels more involved with the selection of the food, he or she is more likely to try it.

Planning Children's Meals

When planning meals for the growing toddler or child it is important to keep in mind the different food groups and nutrient needs. It can be difficult to meet daily recommendations for fruit and vegetable intake if one offers these foods only at the three main meals. Low intake of fruits and vegetables is correlated with suboptimal intake of many nutrients, including fiber and vitamins A and C, and also appears

to be linked with higher fat intakes (Dennison et al., 1998). Fruits and vegetables are a good choice at snack time, thereby helping to meet optimal intake.

It is important to plan balanced meals, demonstrating healthy eating early while the child is developing feeding behaviors. Starting a heart-healthy diet before reaching adulthood can help to reduce the prevalence of obesity (Fisher, Van Horn, & McGill, 1997).

It is essential for health care providers to be aware that preparing and providing healthy meals can be expensive. The high cost of fruits and vegetables is often reported as the main reason a parent or caregiver does not frequently purchase these foods (Dennison et al., 1998). Parents should be educated on creative ways to provide fruits and vegetables. For example, shopping for produce at local farmers' markets can be more affordable. Furthermore, canned fruits and vegetables are often less expensive and remain an excellent source of nutrients. It is important, however, to let caregivers know to purchase fruit canned in its own juice and vegetables without added salt or sugar to avoid providing extra sugar or sodium to the child.

Children tend to eat more of foods they are familiar with, so it is important for healthy foods to always be available in the home. Patrick and Nicklas (2005, p. 84) reported that "children are more likely to eat foods that are available and easily accessible." This should always be considered when planning and shopping for a meal.

Hunger and Behavior

Children gain knowledge of dietary behaviors from watching others (Hayman, 2003; Patrick & Nicklas, 2005). As children age they begin to spend more time outside of the home, learning new feeding behaviors from those around them. By age 3 or 4 eating becomes influenced by environmental cues more than the previous "deprivation-driven response" during infancy (Patrick & Nicklas, 2005).

However, regardless of behaviors developed the child should not control meal planning. Satter suggested caregivers develop a "division of labor" between caregivers and the child. In this model the caregiver's role is to provide healthy foods that are accessible. It is the child's responsibility to decide when to eat and how much food they will eat at a particular meal (Satter, 1986, 1996).

Food behaviors can also be related to the availability of certain foods and how easy they are to consume for the developing child. Baranowski, Cullen, and Baranowski (1999) found that children tend to choose foods more often that are in an accessible location and also of an appropriate size for their developmental capacity. Fruits and vegetables that are cut into sticks or bite-size pieces are more likely to be chosen than whole fruits and vegetables simply because the child is able to handle them independently.

Growing toddlers and children should typically not be restricted at meals. Restriction of foods that are high in fat and sugar often lead to the child "fixating on the forbidden food" and consuming more of these foods outside of the home or when full (Fisher & Birch, 2000). If seconds are requested it is beneficial to develop a habit of offering an additional serving of vegetables or fruits, though not forcing the child to take what or *only* what is offered.

Picky Eating

Picky eating is common in toddlers and may continue throughout childhood. Often, picky eating may represent an attempt at acquiring independence rather than a declaration of actual likes and dislikes. A caregiver may try to accommodate a picky eater or to develop techniques that may help increase amount and quality of foods eaten. However, using rewards, prodding, or punishment to encourage eating may only enforce the "picky eater phenomenon" (Pelcaht & Pliner, 1986). Caregivers should continue to provide healthy food options and not make special foods or entire meals for the picky child.

Working with a child who is exhibiting picky behaviors can certainly be challenging. Parents and caregivers may need information and strategies from their health care professional to increase the number of foods acceptable to their toddlers and children and to develop a sound eating plan (Carruth et al., 1998).

Grazing

Growing toddlers and children may not be hungry on a schedule, and they often do not want to stop for a meal or snack that may interrupt their playtime. If a child asks for food or liquids more frequently than every 2 to 3 hours, it is important to encourage him or her to wait until the next meal or snack time to eat.

Grazing may produce a constant feeling of fullness and cause the child to avoid eating an appropriate amount at mealtime and therefore not expand the stomach size. Constant snacking and early satiety may result in the child not receiving adequate calories each day, ultimately leading to failure to thrive (Krugman & Dubowitz, 2003). A child who sits at a table away from distractions while eating will better understand the difference between mealtime and playtime.

Failure to Thrive

Failure to thrive is defined by "inadequate physical growth diagnosed by observation of growth over time using a standard growth chart" (Krugman & Dubowitz, 2003, p. 879). This failure to maintain adequate growth can be caused by a multitude of factors. Most often, failure to thrive is classified as organic (inability to meet calorie needs due to medical conditions, malabsorption, or increased metabolism with specific disease states) or inorganic (food shortage, incorrect mixing of formula, or neglect) (Krugman & Dubowitz, 2003).

Health care professionals should be aware of any factors that may contribute to poor growth. Taking a full diet history, including formula-mixing techniques, can help assess if adequate calories are in fact being provided to the child. If all possible inorganic etiologies are ruled out, then a medical workup for organic failure to thrive should be undertaken. Read more about failure to thrive in Chapter 5.

Lactose Intolerance

According to Vesa, Marteau, and Korpela (2000, p. 165S), lactose is the "most important source of energy during the first year of human life." Intolerance is uncommon in healthy infants but can present as a result of a gastrointestinal illness, ultimately resolving with improvement of the illness. Symptoms of intolerance are similar to other gastrointestinal dysfunctions (Vesa et al., 2000), causing stomach pain, flatulence, and loose stools.

Hypolactasia can present early in childhood in African-American and Asian children but seems to appear in late childhood or adolescence for white children (Scrimshaw & Murray, 1988). Many lactose maldigesters are able to tolerate small amounts of lactose without discomfort (Vesa et al., 2000). For example, children with lactose intolerance can often drink a small amount of regular milk. Alternatives such as solid cheeses that are low in lactose and yogurt may be better tolerated.

More recently, lactose-free and low-lactose milks and ice creams are readily available. Soy milk may also be a good substitute, but caregivers should be educated that whatever the variety of substituted milk, it must be fortified with calcium and vitamin D. Careful diagnosis is important to prevent unnecessary diet restrictions that may lead to deficiencies in the essential nutrients provided by dairy products (Vesa et al., 2000). Families should be instructed on ways to meet nutrient needs if a dairy restriction is ultimately recommended.

Television Watching and Media Influence on Food Cravings

Many children spend more time watching television than interacting with their families, creating a change in key influences. More than 50% of food advertisements on television target children (Story & French, 2004). Messages often show "junk" foods as fun, exciting, and glamorous. Young people often have difficulty discriminating between education provided in television programs and information in commercials, therefore misinterpreting advertising as life-style instruction. Furthermore, because commercials are brief and to the point, they target the child's short attention span, conveying an efficient and powerful message.

It is suggested that television viewing contributes to obesity by one or more of three mechanisms: displacement of physical activity, an increase in calorie consumption while watching or as a direct result of the effects of advertising, and/or reducing resting metabolism (Robinson, 2001).

The AAP Committee on Nutrition (2001) proposes that children should spend no more than 2 hours per day watching television or using other electronic forms of entertainment. (Note: The AAP recommends no television watching at all for children under age 2.) Making sure that meals and snacks are not eaten while watching television may help to reduce daily television viewing. Saelens et al. (2002) found that the frequency of meals eaten while watching television was the most important predictor of long-term increase in television viewing time among children. Creating rules about eating meals in front of the television was found to decrease the probability of the child watching television for more than 2 hours per day (Saelens et al., 2002).

Simply restricting meals while watching television may not be an entirely adequate strategy for decreasing overall inactivity. The relationships among the family environment, television viewing, and low level of activity are complex. Restricting television viewing during mealtimes may be effective, but focusing on increasing physical activity is also a component not to be overlooked (Waller, Du, & Popkin, 2003; Salmon, Timperio, Telford, Carver, & Crawford, 2005).

A study by Burdette and Whitaker (2005) on preschool children found that television viewing and outdoor play minutes were not correlated to one another or to the child's BMI. However, in an article by Gortmaker, Must, and Sobol (1996), a dose-dependent relationship between television viewing and obesity was demonstrated. Given the conflicting evidence, more research is needed regarding any possible real-world correlation between daily television viewing, activity, and excessive weight gain.

Learning Through Participation

As children grow and mature, involving them in the preparation of the meal may help to increase variety in the diet. A child will often taste what he or she has participated in preparing. Time spent in the kitchen can also be used to talk about the different colors of fruit and vegetables, to help the child understand the healthy reasons behind eating a wider variety of foods, and to promote family bonding. Furthermore, offering a choice of fruits or vegetables at a meal may help the child feel a modicum of control and inclusion. Such a practice may also promote better intake of the chosen food during the meal.

Interestingly, many studies have shown that it can be beneficial to allow children to be involved in portioning foods onto their own plate at meals. Orlet Fisher, Rolls, and Birch (2003) showed that allowing children to serve themselves at meals may decrease the incidence of exposure to excessive portion sizes.

Choking Prevention

Having an adult always present whenever a child is eating constitutes the ultimate in safe eating practices. Because many children do not develop the skill of chewing with a grinding motion until about 4 years of age (Dietz & Stern, 1999), foods with a firmer texture that need adequate chewing may not be appropriate for young children. To prevent choking, foods should be cut into small, bite-size pieces and children should remain sitting at all times while eating. Choking is more likely to occur if the child is running or falling with food in the mouth. The child should be encouraged to take small bites and avoid stuffing his or her mouth full of food. **Table 3.10** lists foods that may present a choking risk.

Snacks

Snacking among children is an important source of energy (Jahns, Siega-Riz, & Popkin, 2001). Toddlers and children have a comparatively small stomach size and cannot consume large amounts at meals; therefore, snacks provide needed servings of healthy foods. However, Jahns et al. (2001) found that children obtain an inordinate percentage of their daily calories from snacks, so much so that at times children may snack to such an extent that they are not hungry at mealtime. In contrast, many children continue to eat normal-sized meals and simply consume excess calories during the day, leading to increased weight gain.

Instead of skipping snacks, caregivers should provide healthy snack choices. Nutritious snacks include, but are not limited to, cheese slices, carrot sticks, orange slices, yogurt, apple pieces, and peanut butter on wheat crackers. Snacks should be easy to prepare and on hand to reduce the need for quick, often unhealthy, snack choices.

Caregivers should be aware of what and how much their child is eating while watching television. Sometimes television viewing may condition a child who is not hungry to snack (Epstein, Coleman, & Myers, 1996). As stated previously, it can be helpful to prohibit meals or snacks in front of the television.

Dental Health

It is beneficial to start tooth care at a young age. Introducing a toothbrush during the toddler years can initiate a good oral hygiene routine that continues through life (Mahan & Escott-Stump, 2000). Children often snack on sugary, sticky foods that may stay in the teeth and provide an ideal environment for growth

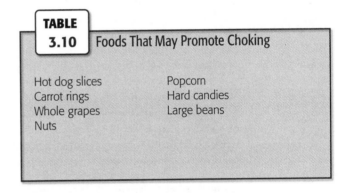

CRITICAL Thinking

Evidence suggests that more young girls are becoming concerned with gaining weight because of the influence of caregivers and the media. Can you give some examples of this? What can be done to prevent this?

TABLE 3.10 Foods That May Promote Choking

Hot dog slices	Popcorn
Carrot rings	Hard candies
Whole grapes	Large beans
Nuts	

of the bacteria that cause dental caries. Also, the continued exposure of the teeth to the sugary drinks, such as juice, contributes to dental caries in children (AAP, Committee on Nutrition, 2001). Teaching young children to brush their teeth after meals and snacks can help to reduce the incidence of cavities.

Role Models

Children learn by observing the behaviors of others and then incorporating and imitating these practices. Parents modeling healthy behaviors, accessibility to sedentary pursuits at home, sibling influences, and family television viewing habits may be important determinants of a child's activity level and healthy behaviors (Rachlin, Logue, Gibbon, & Frankel, 1986). Food choices and dietary quality in the early years of life are usually influenced by parents or other primary caregivers.

As children mature they tend to eat more meals outside the home. Therefore, it is essential to model good habits while the child is at a young, impressionable age. Modeling food behaviors is one of the most effective ways to promote increased consumption of healthy foods (Dennison et al., 1998). Parents who do not eat fruits and vegetables tend to raise children who refuse these foods as well.

Negative thoughts regarding food can also begin at a young age. Preadolescent girls are becoming more at risk for picking up dieting habits from female caregivers. Girls who diet by adolescence tend to have mothers who are often overtly encouraging or unconsciously demonstrating the means to diet through their own restrictive habits (Birch & Fisher, 2000).

Breakfast

As children enter school there is often less time in the morning for simple things, such as eating a healthy breakfast. It is important to develop the habit of including breakfast in the daily morning routine. Eating breakfast has been shown to increase energy and concentration at school. It also allows for a balanced metabolism, aiding in the child's ability to maintain a healthy weight. Studies have shown that skipping breakfast is related to increased BMI and risk of obesity (Cho, Dietrich, Brown, Clark, & Block, 2003).

Breakfast is an excellent time to consume a needed serving of fruit, whole grains, dairy, or protein. Many schools have a breakfast program, but it is important to be aware of what foods are being offered and how much the child is consuming during this time. At breakfast, schools provide 25% or more of the daily recommended levels of key nutrients that children need (School Breakfast Program Food and Research Action Center, n.d.), but the menus are often not controlled to avoid excess. The child is usually able to make his or her own food choices, so education concerning appropriate portion sizes and healthy choices can be helpful.

Nutrition at School

Many schools participate in the government-funded National School Lunch Program. Regulations create a standard for school lunches in order to provide one-third of the Recommended Daily Allowance (RDA) for protein, vitamins A and C, calcium, iron, and calories (U.S. Department of Agriculture, 2005). Meals must meet nutritional requirements, but individual schools are able to decide what foods to serve and how to prepare them.

The program guarantees that every child will meet at least 33% of his or her daily needs each day. It is true that many children rely on this program for needed nutrition. However, to meet the required 33% of calories, at times meal options do not contain particularly healthy choices. Less than nutritious options such as nachos, giant hoagies, and hot dogs are common at many schools. Also, many children receive a large portion of their daily calories from snacks, which often leads to excess daily calories when combined with school lunches and fast food consumption. Lunch is often provided at a discount or may be free to students, making it unrealistic to expect these children to pack lunches containing healthier options. Therefore, it seems reasonable for schools to become more adept at offering well-balanced meals.

Peer influence also plays a role in lunchtime nutrition. Food choices are often affected by what friends at school are eating. Children may be encouraged to try a new food if others around them are eating it. In contrast, such influence may also contribute to requesting more "junk" foods that other children bring to school.

Parents and children may benefit from education on choosing healthier options at school. If available, reviewing the monthly menu with the child can prompt discussion on which foods are the healthiest choices.

Physical Activity

Physical activity is an important part of a healthy life-style. It promotes muscle building, increased metabolism, and disease prevention. Among children, overweight, obesity, and low levels of physical activity have been shown to be associated with increased risk of disease later in life (Baranowski, 1992). Exercise is also a vital aspect of achieving maximal peak bone mass (AAP, 1999).

With age and increased independence, physical activity often decreases. The CDC demonstrated that 61% of 9- to 13-year-olds do not participate in organized after-school activities and 23% did not participate in any physical activity during their free time (CDC, 2003). Something as simple as parental encouragement may be all some children need to become more active. Studies have shown that parents who are supportive of their children's participation in physical activities are more likely to have an active child (Sallis, Prochaska, & Taylor, 2000).

Sedentary activities such as watching television and playing video games have become the preferred after-school pastime. Parents, caregivers, health educators, and teachers should promote enjoyable alternatives to sedentary behaviors to increase children's participation in physical activity and prevent unhealthy weight gain (Salmon et al., 2005). If the safety of the neighborhood is poor, then caregivers should work to create indoor activities that keep the child active and away from sedentary pursuits.

The bottom line is that physical activity should be a part of everyday life. If children are cared for outside of the home after school, parents may need to discuss with day-care providers or other caregivers the stated preference that their child be active and not spend the afternoon involved in sedentary activities. Being active as a family can help everyone to stay healthy and provides an excellent means of spending quality time together.

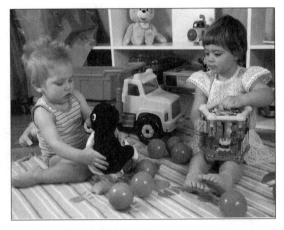

Excessive Weight Gain

Obesity prevention programs focused on diet and exercise are becoming more and more available to young children. However, Etelson et al. (2003) reported that participation in obesity prevention programs and life-style changes are dependent on the parents' ability to recognize that their child is overweight. In their study it was determined that no parents of children above the 75th percentile for BMI/age were able to correctly estimate how overweight their children were. These parents universally believed their children were less overweight than actually recorded. Therefore, if a parent perceives a child to be at low risk for being overweight, the intervention is likely to be delayed. Read more about childhood obesity in Chapter 7.

Obesity is becoming a more common problem with young children. Fifteen percent of children aged 6 to 11 years are estimated to be overweight in the United States (Ogden, Flegal, Carroll, & Johnson, 2002). Inactivity and larger portion sizes are contributors to this multifaceted and increasingly severe prob-

Juice Consumption

In the past fruit juice was consistently recommended by pediatricians as a good source of vitamin C for children and also an additional source of hydration (AAP, Committee on Nutrition, 2001). Juices high in vitamin C have been shown to aid in the body's absorption of iron. However, the high carbohydrate content of juice often leads to malabsorption of vitamin C in children.

Continues

> Over time juice has become the preferred beverage among many children. Children aged 1 to 12 years make up about 18% of the total population but are responsible for almost one-third of the average daily intake of juice and juice drinks (AAP, Committee on Nutrition, 2001).
>
> In toddlers and children juice intake often inappropriately replaces formula, milk, and water intake and is also used as a replacement for whole fruit and vegetable servings. Fruit juice accounts for about 33% of all fruit and vegetable intake among preschoolers and 50% of fruit intake by children aged 2 to 18 (Dennison, 1996). When replacing formula and milk, the child often does not receive optimal calories and nutrients needed for growth. Excessive juice consumption has been shown to contribute to inorganic failure to thrive and decreased stature in some children. Juice provides empty carbohydrate calories and decreases the child's appetite at mealtime, causing overall decreased calorie intake (Smith & Lifshitz, 1994; Dennison, 1996). Conversely, it has also been shown to be associated with high caloric intake and obesity in some studies when consumed frequently throughout the day (Dennison, 1996).
>
> Only pasteurized 100% fruit juice is recommended for growing children and is the specific type of juice provided by WIC. Juice should be watered down for the child and should not be available to be sipped throughout the day. Juice should be limited to no more than 4 to 6 ounces per day for children aged 1 to 6 years (AAP, Committee on Nutrition, 2001).
>
> The IOM has recommended a change in the WIC package to decrease the juice content. Also, the AAP's Top Ten Resolutions for 2005 stated that their number 2 priority is to get the message out that juice is not a healthy choice for children.

lem. Studies demonstrate that increased size of food portions offered can stimulate a young child's food intake, causing excess calorie consumption at meals (Orlet Fisher et al., 2003).

Supplements for Increased Calories

Children who are not able to consume adequate calories each day may need a high-calorie nutritional supplement. There are multiple supplements available designed specifically for growing children. Pediasure®, Nutren Jr®, Resource Just for Kids®, and Carnation Instant Breakfast Junior® are just a few supplements available for children ages 1 through 10 years. These supplements are often packaged in child-friendly containers and come in a variety of popular flavors. After age 10 most adult supplements, such as Ensure®, Boost®, and Nutren 1.0®, are acceptable. It is essential to note that supplements should be used under the care of a health care professional.

Summary

It is undeniable that to provide essential nutrients for optimal growth and development, toddlers and young children must consume a wide variety of foods. A varied diet, coupled with physical fitness, is an excellent beginning for these young lives.

Growing toddlers and children rely on caregivers to provide them with adequate nutrition and guide them in the development of proper mealtime behaviors, ultimately resulting in healthy life-styles into the adult years and beyond. However, outside influences, including the media and the food and beverage industries, make this challenge ever more difficult. Health care professionals must provide support for each family, with the goal of fostering understanding regarding the importance of good nutrition and consistent physical activity, and they must help parents acquire the necessary parenting skills to put their beliefs into practice when raising their young children.

Case Studies

(Answers to all case studies are in the Instructor's Manual available at jbpub.com.)

Case Study 1

Anna is a 2½-year-old girl. Her mother considers her a picky eater. She loves milk, and sometimes will only drink at a meal and pick at the other foods. Her favorite foods are oatmeal, yogurt, dried cereal, macaroni and cheese, and pasta with tomato sauce. Her mom is concerned that she is not getting enough nutrients. Her growth has started to slowly fall off her normal curve, and she also seems pale and more tired during the day.

Questions: What are some nutritional concerns you may have for Anna? What suggestions could you make to her mother?

Case Study 2

Mark is a 5-year-old boy who loves snack foods. He doesn't really like to sit down for a meal. His mom leaves the snacks out so while he is playing he can grab a bite or two and then continue to play. He carries his sippy cup of juice around with him too in case he gets thirsty. He has not been growing well, but his mom says that once he grows out of this phase, he will catch up.

Questions: Why might Mark's growth be inadequate? What changes to Mark's current eating habits would you recommend?

Case Study 3

Tony is an 11-year-old boy whose favorite activity is his PlayStation system. He loves to come home from school and start playing right away. He usually grabs a large bag of potato chips and a soda from the fridge and snacks while he plays. He takes a break for dinner, but then he heads right back to the game. Tony has always plotted around the 50th percentile for weight and height for age, but lately he has been gaining weight and is now greater than the 95th percentile for weight. His father is not concerned, reporting that he was the same way at his age but "thinned out" as he got older.

Questions: Should Tony's weight gain be a concern, despite his family history? What recommendations could be made to the family?

Websites

For Families and Professionals
Bright Futures www.brightfutures.org
Ellyn Satter Associates www.ellynsatter.com
Food for Tots www.foodfortots.com
Kids Health http://websrv01.kidshealth.org/parent
Nutrition for Kids www.nutritionforkids.com
Tiny Tummies www.tinytummies.com

For Professionals
Pediatric Basics: Journal of Pediatric (Early Childhood) Nutrition and Development http://www.gerber.com/Pledge/Taking-Action.aspx
Zero to Three: a resource organization for the first 3 years of life www.zerotothree.org

For Parents, Professionals, and Children
Celebrate Healthy Eating www.celebratehealthyeating.org
Small Step www.smallstep.gov

References

American Academy of Pediatrics (AAP). (1999). Calcium requirements of infants, children, and adolescents. *Pediatrics, 104,* 1152–1157.

American Academy of Pediatrics (AAP). (2001). Children, adolescents, and television. *Pediatrics, 107,* 423–426.

American Academy of Pediatrics (AAP), Committee on Nutrition. (1988). *Cholesterol in Childhood.* Elk Grove, IL: Author. Retrieved October 11, 2007, from http://pediatrics.aappublications.org/cgi/content/abstract/118/1/201

American Academy of Pediatrics (AAP), Committee on Nutrition. (1992). Statement on Cholesterol. *Pediatrics, 90,* 469–473.

American Academy of Pediatrics (AAP), Committee on Nutrition. (2001). The use and misuse of fruit juice in pediatrics. *Pediatrics, 107,* 1210–1213.

American Heart Association (AHA). (n.d.). *AHA scientific position. Dietary guidelines for healthy children.* Retrieved February 10, 2007, from http://www.americanheart.org

Baranowski, T. (1992). Assessment, prevalence, and cardiovascular benefits of physical activity and fitness in youth. *Medicine and Science in Sports and Exercise, 24,* S237–S247.

Baranowski, T., Cullen, K. W., & Baranowski, J. (1999). Psychosocial correlates of dietary intake: Advancing dietary intervention. *Annual Review of Nutrition, 9,* 17–40.

Birch, L. L., & Fisher, J. O. (1998). Development of eating behaviors among children and adolescents. *Pediatrics, 101,* 539–549.

Birch, L. L., & Fisher, J. O. (2000). Mothers' child-feeding practices influence daughters' eating and weight. *American Journal of Clinical Nutrition, 71,* 1054–1061.

Briefel, R., Hanson, C., Fox, M. K., Novak, T., & Ziegler, P. (2006). Feeding infants and toddlers study: Do vitamin and mineral supplements contribute to nutrient adequacy or excess among US infants and toddlers? *Journal of the American Dietetic Association, 1*(Suppl.), S52–S65.

Burdette, H. L., & Whitaker, R. C. (2005). A national study of neighborhood safety, outdoor play, television viewing, and obesity in preschool children. *Pediatrics, 116,* 657–662.

Butte, N. (2000). Fat intake of children in relation to energy requirements. American *Journal of Clinical Nutrition, 72*(Suppl.), 1246S–1252S.

Butte, N. F., Wong, W. W., Hopkinson, J. M., Heinz, C. J., Mehta, N. R., & O'Brian Smith, E. (2000). Energy requirements derived from total energy expenditure and energy deposition during the first 2 y of life. *American Journal of Clinical Nutrition, 72,* 1558–1569.

Carruth, B. R., Skinner, J., Houck, K., Moran, J., Coletta, F., & Ott, D. (1998). The phenomenon of "picky eater": A behavioral marker in eating patterns of toddlers. *Journal of the American College of Nutrition, 17,* 180–186.

Carter, L. M., Whiting, S. J., Drinkwater, D. T., Zello, G. A., Faulkner, R. A., & Baily, D. A. (2001). Self-reported calcium intake and bone mineral content in children and adolescents. *Journal of the American College of Nutrition, 20,* 502–509.

Centers for Disease Control and Prevention (CDC). (2001). Recommendations for using fluoride to prevent and control dental caries in the United States. *Morbidity and Mortality Weekly Report, 50*(RR-14), 26–27.

Centers for Disease Control and Prevention (CDC). (2003). Physical activity levels among children aged 9–13 years: United States, 2002. *Morbidity and Mortality Weekly Report, 52,* 785–788.

Cho, S., Dietrich, M., Brown, C. J., Clark, C. A., & Block, G. (2003). The effect of breakfast type on total daily energy intake and body mass index: Results from the Third National Health and Nutrition Examination Survey (NHANES III). *Journal of the American College of Nutrition, 22,* 296–302.

Dennison, B. A. (1996). Fruit juice consumption by infants and children: A review. *Journal of the American College of Nutrition, 15*(Suppl. 5), 4S–11S.

Dennison, B. A. (2004). Prevention of childhood overweight: The Role Child Care Settings. Presented at the Site Specific Approaches: Prevention or Management of Pediatric Obesity Workshop, July 14–15.

Dennison, B. A., Rockwell, H. L., & Baker, S. L. (1998). Fruit and vegetable intake in young children. *Journal of the American College of Nutrition, 17,* 371–378.

Dietz, W. H., & Stern, L. (1999). *American Academy of Pediatrics: Guide to Your Child's Nutrition* (pp. 41–60). New York: Random House.

Epstein, L. H., Coleman, K. J., & Myers, M. D. (1996). Exercise in treating obesity in children and adolescents. *Medicine and Science in Sports and Exercise, 28,* 428–435.

Etelson, D., Brand, D. A., Patrick, P. A., & Shirali, A. (2003). Childhood obesity: Do parents recognize this health risk? *Obesity Research, 11,* 1362–1368.

Fisher, J. O., & Birch, L. L. (1999). Restricting access to palatable foods affects children's behavioral response, food selection, and intake. *American Journal of Clinical Nutrition, 69,* 1264–1272.

Fisher, J. O., & Birch, L. L. (2000). Parent's restrictive feeding practices are associated with young girls' negative self-evaluation of eating. *Journal of the American Dietetic Association, 100,* 1341–1346.

Fisher, E. A., Van Horn, L., & McGill, H. C. (1997). Nutrition and children: A statement for healthcare professionals from the Nutrition Committee, American Heart Association. *Circulation, 95,* 2332–2333.

Food and Agricultural Organization, World Health Organization, and United Nations University Expert Consultation. (1985). Energy and protein requirements. *World Health Organization Technical Report Series, 724,* 1–206.

Fox, M. K., Reidy, K., Novak, T., & Ziegler, P. (2006). Sources of energy and nutrients in the diets of infants and toddlers. *Journal of the American Dietetic Association, 1*(Suppl.), S28–S42.

Freedman, D. S., Thornton, J. C., Mei, Z., Wang, J., Dietz, W. H., Pierson, R. N., et al. (2004). Height and adiposity among children. *Obesity Research, 12,* 846–853.

Gortmaker, S. L., Must, A., & Sobol, A. M. (1996). Television viewing as a cause of increasing obesity among children in the United States. *Archives of Pediatric and Adolescent Medicine, 150,* 356–362.

Grantham-McGregor, S., & Ani, C. (2001). A review of studies on the effect of iron deficiency on cognitive development in children. *Journal of Nutrition, 131,* 649S–668S.

Hayman, L. L. (2003). The Dietary Intervention Study in Children (DISC): Progress and prospects for primary prevention. *Progress in Cardiovascular Nursing, 18,* 4–5.

Holick, M. F., Shils, M. E., Olsen, J., Shike, M., & Ross, C.A. (Eds.). (1999). *Modern Nutrition in Health and Disease* (9th ed.). Baltimore, MD: Williams & Wilkins.

Institute of Medicine (IOM), Food and Nutrition Board. (2000–2005). *Dietary Reference Intakes.* Retrieved February 10, 2007, from http://www.nal.usda.gov/fnic/etext/000105.html

Jahns, L., Siega-Riz, A. M., & Popkin, B. M. (2001). The increasing prevalence of snacking among U.S. children from 1977 to 1996. *Journal of Pediatrics, 138,* 493–498.

Johnston, C. C., Miller, J. Z., Slemenda, C. W., Reister, T. K., Hui, S., Christian, J. C., et al. (1992). Calcium supplementation and increases in bone mineral density in children. *New England Journal of Medicine, 327,* 82–87.

Kaiser, L. (2004). *What Are Infants and Toddlers Eating? Maternal and Infant Briefs: Jan/Feb Edition.* Retrieved February 10, 2007, from http://nutrition.ucdavis.edu/briefs/ (See Jan/Feb 2004)

Krugman, S., & Dubowitz, H. (2003). Failure to thrive. *American Family Physician, 68,* 879–884.

Mahan, L. K., & Escott-Stump, S. (2000). *Krause's Food, Nutrition, and Diet Therapy* (10th ed.). Philadelphia: W. B. Saunders.

National Center for Health Statistics, in collaboration with the National Center for Chronic Disease Prevention and Health Promotion. (2000). *CDC Growth Charts.* Retrieved February 1, 2007, from http://www.cdc.gov/growthcharts

National Institutes of Health. (n.d.). *BMI Chart.* Retrieved October 11, 2007, from www.nhlbi.nih.gov/guidelines/obesity/bmi_tbl.pdf

Ogden, C. L., Flegal, K. M., Carroll, M. D., & Johnson, C. L. (2002). Prevalence and trends in overweight among US children and adolescents, 1999–2000. *Journal of the American Medical Association, 288,* 1728–1732.

Orlet Fisher, J., Rolls, B. J., & Birch, L. L. (2003). Children's bite size and intake of an entrée are greater with large portions than with age-appropriate or self-selected portions. *American Journal of Clinical Nutrition, 77,* 1164–1170.

Patrick, H., & Nicklas, T. A. (2005). A review of family and social determinants of children's eating patterns and diet quality. *Journal of the American College of Nutrition, 24,* 83–92.

Pelcaht, M. L., & Pliner, P. (1986). Antecedents and correlates of feeding problems in young children. *Journal of Nutrition Education, 18,* 23–29.

Rachlin, H., Logue, A. W., Gibbon, J., & Frankel, M. (1986). Cognition and behavior in studies of choice. *Psychology Review, 93,* 33–45.

Robinson, T. N. (2001). Television viewing and childhood obesity. *Pediatric Clinics of North America, 48,* 1017–1025.

Saelens, B. E., Sallis, J. F., Nader, P. R., Broyles, S. L., Berry, C. C., & Taras, H. L. (2002). Home environment influences on children's television watching from early to middle childhood. *Journal of Developmental and Behavioral Pediatrics, 23,* 127–132.

Sallis, J. F., Prochaska, J. J., & Taylor, W. C. (2000). A review of correlates of physical activity of children and adolescents. *Medicine and Science in Sports and Exercise, 32,* 963–975.

Salmon, J. O., Timperio, A., Telford, A., Carver, A., & Crawford, D. (2005). Association of family environment with children's television viewing and with low level of physical activity. *Obesity Research, 13,* 1939–1951.

Satter, E. M. (1986). The feeding relationship. *Journal of the American Dietetic Association, 86,* 352–356.

Satter, E. M. (1996). Internal regulation and the evolution of normal growth as the basis for prevention of obesity in children. *Journal of the American Dietetic Association, 96,* 860–864.

Schneider, J. M., Fujii, M. L., Lamp, C. L., Lonnerdal, B., Dewey, K. G., & Zidenberg-Cherr, S. (2005). Anemia, iron deficiency, and iron deficiency anemia in 12–36-mo-old children from low-income families. *American Journal of Clinical Nutrition, 82,* 1269–1275.

School Breakfast Program and Food and Research Action Center. (n.d.). *Child Nutrition Fact Sheet.* Retrieved January 15, 2007, from www.frac.org/pdf/cnsbp.PDF

Scrimshaw, N. S., & Murray, E. B. (1988). Prevalence of lactose maldigestion. *American Journal of Clinical Nutrition, 48*(Suppl.), 1086–1098.

Smith, M. M., & Lifshitz, F. (1994). Excess fruit juice consumption as a contributing factor in nonorganic failure to thrive. *Pediatrics, 93,* 438–443.

Specker, B. L., Valanis, B., Hertzberg, V., Edwards, N., & Tsang, R. (1985). Sunshine exposure and serum 25-hydroxy-vitamin D concentrations in exclusively breast-fed infants. *Journal of Pediatrics, 107,* 372–376.

Storey, M. L., Forchee, R.A., & Anderson, P. A. (2004). Associations of adequate intake of calcium with diet, beverage consumption, and demographic characteristics among children and adolescents. *Journal of the American College of Nutrition, 23,* 18–33.

Story, M., & French, S. (2004). Food advertising and marketing directed at children and adolescents in the US. *International Journal of Behavioral Nutrition and Physical Activity, 1,* 1–17.

Sullivan, S. A., & Birch, L. L. (1993). Infant dietary experience and acceptance of solid foods. *Pediatrics, 93,* 271–278.

Tomashek, K. M., Nesby, S., Scanlon, K. S., Cogswell, M. E., Powell, K. E., Parashar, U. D., et al. (2001). Nutritional rickets in Georgia. *Pediatrics, 107,* e45.

U.S. Department of Agriculture. (2005). *Nutrition Program Facts. National School Lunch Program.* Retrieved February 10, 2007, from www.fns.usda.gov/cnd/Lunch/AboutLunch/NSLP FactSheet.pdf

U.S. Department of Agriculture, Food and Nutrition Service. (n.d.). *Women, Infants, and Children (WIC).* Retrieved February 2, 2007, from www.fns.usda.gov/wic/aboutwic/default.htm

U.S. Department of Health and Human Services. (2000). *Tracking Healthy People 2010.* Retrieved February 21, 2007, from http://www.healthypeople.gov/0

Vesa, T. H., Marteau, P., & Korpela, R. (2000). Lactose intolerance. *Journal of the American College of Nutrition, 19,* 165S–175S.

Waller, C. E., Du, S., & Popkin, B. M. (2003). Patterns of overweight, inactivity, and snacking in Chinese children. *Obesity Research, 11,* 957–961.

Weisberg, P., Scanlon, K. S., Li, R., & Cogswell, M. E. (2004). Nutritional rickets among children in the United States: Review of cases reported between 1986 and 2003. *American Journal of Clinical Nutrition, 80*(Suppl.), 1697S–1705S.

Zlotkin, S. H. (1996). A review of the Canadian nutrition recommendations update: Dietary fat and children. *Journal of Nutrition, 126*(Suppl.), 1022S–1027S.

Normal Adolescent Nutrition

CHAPTER

4

Pamela S. Hinton, PhD

CHAPTER OUTLINE

Growth and Development

Physical Growth • Hormonal Mediators of the Adolescent Growth Spurt • Assessment of Growth and Development

Cognitive and Psychosocial Development During Adolescence

Cognitive and Affective Development • Psychosocial Development

Nutrient Requirements and Temporal Consumption Trends

Macronutrients • Minerals • Vitamins

Dietary Patterns

Serving Size • Food Groups • Skipping Breakfast • Added Sugars • Fast Food Consumption • Sociodemographic Moderators of Dietary Intake • School Food Environment

Health Status of U.S. Adolescents

Excessive Weight and Obesity • Metabolic Syndrome • Iron Deficiency • Tobacco Use and Nutritional Status • Adolescent Pregnancy

● ● ● ● ● **Reader Objectives**

After studying this chapter and reflecting on the contents, you should be able to

1. Understand nutritional regulation of the hormones that moderate growth and sexual maturation.
2. Describe gender differences in growth and development and in nutrient requirements.
3. Appreciate how psychosocial development during adolescence affects health-related behaviors, including dietary patterns.
4. Identify and describe sociodemographic factors affecting dietary patterns.
5. Describe trends in chronic disease incidence among adolescents.

Adolescence is a period of rapid linear growth, altered body composition, reproductive maturation, and psychosocial development. Nutrient requirements are increased to meet the demands of growth and development. There are significant gender differences in the timing and rate of peak linear growth, puberty, and sexual development, resulting in divergent nutrient needs. Normal growth and development are influenced by nutritional status because the hormones responsible for linear growth, alteration in body composition, and sexual development are nutritionally regulated. Food intake during adolescence is influenced by psychosocial factors; peers and popular culture, including the mass media and advertising, significantly affect dietary patterns.

Growth and Development

Physical Growth

Peak Height Velocity

The adolescent growth spurt takes 2 to 4 years to complete and is generally longer in boys than in girls. The average height velocity is 5 to 6 cm/yr during adolescence; peak height velocity is 8 to 10 cm/yr. Girls, on average, begin their pubertal growth spurt at age 9 years (Veldhuis et al., 2005) and achieve their maximal rate of linear growth (i.e., peak height velocity) at an average chronologic age of 11.5 years, corresponding to Tanner breast stages 2 and 3. The onset of the pubertal growth spurt occurs at age 11 years in boys, and peak height velocity occurs at age 13.5 years, normally Tanner genital stages 3 and 4. The onset of the adolescent growth spurt is more closely associated with bone age than with chronologic age. Boys, because their peak height velocity is greater than that of girls, 9.5 cm/yr versus 8.3 cm/yr, and because peak height velocity occurs later in boys than in girls, are on average 13 cm taller than girls. Interindividual variation in the onset and rate of pubertal growth and development is significant because of interaction between a child's genetic potential and his or her environment.

Body Composition

Normative body composition data from prospective population-based samples are lacking in adolescent populations, especially ethnicity- and gender-specific data. During adolescence girls gain fat mass at an average rate of 1.14 kg/yr. In contrast, boys do not experience a significant increase in absolute fat mass. Boys also gain fat-free mass at a greater rate and for a longer period of time than girls; as a result, boys are relatively leaner than girls after puberty. At ages 8 to 10 boys, on average, have 15% body fat and 24 kg fat-free mass. At the end of puberty, ages 18 to 20 years, young men have 13% body fat and 60 kg fat-free mass. In contrast, girls have 20% body fat and 24 kg fat-free mass at ages 8 to 10 years. By ages 18 to 20 years, young women have 26% body fat and 44 kg fat-free mass (Guo, Chunlea, Roche, & Siervogel, 1997).

Bone Growth and Mineralization

In the immature skeleton the ends of the long bones (**epiphyses**) are separated from the shafts of the long bones (**diaphyses**) by the growth plate. After puberty the growth plate becomes mineralized and the epiphyses fuse. Thus the mature skeleton is incapable of additional growth in height or length.

Epiphyses:
Ends of long bones.

Diaphyses:
Shafts of long bones.

Bone mass doubles between the onset of puberty and young adulthood. Bone growth is greatest approximately 6 months after peak height velocity (Whiting et al., 2004); approximately 25% of peak adult bone mass is acquired during the 2 years of peak adolescent skeletal growth. Growth of the skeleton occurs via modeling, which changes

CRITICAL Thinking

After reading the statement "Thus the mature skeleton is incapable of additional growth in height or length," how do you think nutrition in childhood affects skeletal growth?

● **Learning Point** There are ethnic differences in BMD; African-American teenagers have higher BMD than white teenagers.

Periosteal apposition: Deposition of bone on the outer surface.

Endosteal resorption: Removal of bone from the inner surface.

both the size and shape of the bones. Bones increase in length by ossification of the growth plates and in diameter by **periosteal apposition** and **endosteal resorption**. When the growth plates fuse after puberty, bone mass density (BMD) is 90% to 95% of peak BMD (Riggs, Khosla, & Melton, 2002). Boys are, on average, 10% taller and have 25% greater peak bone mass than girls because of their later pubertal onset and longer growth spurt (Riggs et al., 2002).

Calcium Absorption and Retention

The maximal rate of calcium accretion in the skeleton occurs at ages 11 to 14 years in girls and 16 to 18 years in boys. During the 2 years of peak bone growth, boys gain approximately 400 g of bone mineral, and girls deposit approximately 325 g. Fractional calcium absorption is increased to approximately 40% during peak bone mineral deposition (Molgaard, Thomsen, & Michaelsen, 1999). In adolescents there is a linear relationship between dietary calcium intake and calcium retention. During adulthood, fractional absorption decreases with increasing dietary calcium. In contrast, increasing calcium consumption to 47.4 mmol/day did not reduce fractional calcium absorption compared with 21.2 mmol/day in adolescent girls (Wastney et al., 2000; Weaver, 2000). Because the additional calcium suppressed bone resorption, calcium retention was significantly increased by the higher calcium intake (Weaver, 2000). In a calcium balance study of adolescent girls, African-Americans were found to have increased calcium retention, bone formation relative to bone resorption, fractional calcium absorption, and decreased urinary excretion compared with whites (Bryant et al., 2003).

Bone Turnover Markers

Biochemical markers of bone formation and resorption also are increased during puberty and generally parallel the rate of linear growth (Federico, Baroncelli, Vanacore, Fiore, & Saggese, 2003). Bone turnover during puberty is up to 10-fold higher than during adulthood (Eastell, 2005). The rate of remodeling is increased, linear growth occurs at the epiphyseal growth plates, and there is modeling of bone, which changes the shape of the bones by periosteal or endosteal apposition. Longitudinal studies demonstrate that bone turnover markers are greatest early in puberty, whereas maximal mineral deposition occurs late in puberty when bone turnover markers in serum are decreasing (Eastell, 2005). Mechanical stress on the skeleton is critical to all these processes; the growing skeleton is more sensitive to loading than the mature skeleton. Thus, physical activity during adolescence is necessary to maximize peak bone mass.

Peak Bone Mass and Prevention of Osteoporosis

Loss of bone mass during adulthood is inevitable; thus, prevention of osteoporosis depends, in part, on maximizing peak bone mass during young adulthood. Because a large fraction of adult bone mass is acquired during adolescence, it is important to optimize skeletal growth during this stage in the life cycle. Strategies to maximize peak bone mass include ensuring adequate nutrition, engaging in regular weight-bearing exercise, and maintaining normal endocrine function to retain calcium and stimulate bone growth (Weaver, 2000).

Fracture Risks

Although 75% to 85% of the variance in bone strength can be attributed to bone mass, the fragility of a bone also is determined by the shape of the bone, remodeling rates, and chemical properties of the bone. Most fractures occur later in life; thus, fracture risk depends not only on bone mass but on bone geometry, bone turnover, and risk of falling. Furthermore, the rate of bone loss during adulthood is accelerated by poor nutrient intake and lack of regular weight-bearing exercise. Therefore, acquisition of peak bone mass during adolescence does not guarantee that an individual will be protected against fractures during late adulthood (Schonau, 2004).

Hormonal Mediators of the Adolescent Growth Spurt

Pattern of Hormone Secretion

Normal physical growth and development during puberty depends on the integration of the growth hormone (GH) insulin-like growth factor (IGF) and gonadotropin axes. Nutritional and metabolic signals, in part, control these hormonal systems by acting on the hypothalamus and pituitary gland. During childhood, the activity of the hypothalamic–pituitary–gonadal axis is suppressed by the central nervous system. Animal data suggest that in females gamma-aminobutyric acid is responsible for the juvenile pause; in males **neuropeptide Y** prevents the onset of puberty. At puberty, excitatory neurotransmitters stimulate the release of gonadotropin-releasing hormone in the hypothalamus. As a result, the pulse amplitude of the **gonadotropins,** luteinizing hormone (LH) and follicle-stimulating hormone (FSH), increases and the nocturnal rise in LH secretion is amplified. Pulse frequency, however, is unchanged during puberty. This nocturnal rhythm is specific to puberty and disappears in adulthood. Increased circulating concentrations of LH and FSH stimulate development of the gonads and production of sex steroid hormones. Androgens are synthesized in the Leydig cells of the testes, to a lesser degree the ovaries, and are secreted in response to LH. Testosterone stimulates sperm protein synthesis and development of secondary sex characteristics. FSH stimulates release of estrogens from the ovaries. Progesterones are synthesized in the **corpus luteum** and secreted in response to LH. Estrogen and progesterone control the menstrual cycle and the development of the female secondary sex characteristics.

An increase in spontaneous GH secretion precedes the onset of puberty. GH peak amplitude per pulse is elevated, and integrated 24-hour GH secretion (Styne, 2003) is increased 1.5- to 3-fold (Leung, Johannsson, Leong, & Ho, 2004). GH release stimulated by insulin, arginine, and other secretagogues is also elevated during puberty. Serum levels of IGF-I increase in parallel with increased GH secretion and are elevated 3-fold above prepubertal levels (Leung et al., 2004). Because the secretion of the acid-labile subunit and IGF binding protein 3 (IGFBP-3) do not match the increased production of IGF-I, free IGF-I concentrations are also elevated. GH deficiency diseases illustrate the importance of the somatotropic axis in pubertal growth. Children with GH deficiency are of short stature and have reduced growth velocity and delayed pubertal onset. Thus, normal function of the GH–IGF axis is needed for onset and maintenance of puberty and male sexual development.

Leptin, a peptide hormone secreted by adipocytes, plays a role in pubertal development, although its role in the onset of puberty is not clear. Leptin levels parallel the changes observed in fat mass during puberty, suggesting that leptin does not initiate puberty. However, administration of recombinant human leptin to post-menarcheal women with hypothalamic amenorrhea increases secretion of LH, FSH, and estradiol and stimulates follicular development independent of changes in body weight (Welt et al., 2004). In addition, individuals who are deficient in leptin or who have leptin receptor defects fail to go through puberty. Boys have lower serum leptin concentrations than girls, and this gender difference increases throughout puberty. The lower leptin concentrations in males compared with females at a given body mass index (BMI) may be due to the suppressive effects of androgens on leptin expression (Federico et al., 2003).

Neuropeptide Y: A 36–amino acid peptide neurotransmitter found in the brain and autonomic nervous system; it augments the vasoconstrictor effects of noradrenergic neurons.

Gonadotropin: Hormones secreted by the pituitary gland that affect the function of the male or female gonads.

Corpus luteum: A yellow glandular mass in the ovary formed by an ovarian follicle that has matured and released its egg; secretes progesterone.

Sex Hormones

The sex steroids, estrogen and testosterone, increase spontaneous and stimulated GH secretion. Estrogen appears to be primarily responsible for increased GH secretion associated with the pubertal growth spurt. The effects of testosterone are likely mediated through conversion to estradiol by the enzyme aromatase. Sex steroids also modulate IGF-I bioactivity via regulation of IGFBPs and proteases. IGF-I enhances gonadotropin-releasing hormone secretion in some species and augments the effects of LH and FSH on sex steroid production in the ovaries and testes both in vitro and in vivo (Veldhuis et al., 2005).

Assessment of Growth and Development

Growth

Serial measurements of height and weight plotted on height for age, weight for age, and weight for height growth charts from the National Center for Health Statistics (2000) are used to evaluate growth statistics (see Appendix 1). Height growth potential is calculated from parental height. Skeletal age is assessed using radiography of the left hand and wrist. An open epiphysis indicates skeletal immaturity and poten-

Lordosis: An abnormal forward curvature of the lumbar spine.

tial for additional growth. Stature of pregnant adolescents should be assessed using a knee height measuring device to determine the length of the lower leg. Vertebral compression during pregnancy due to changes in posture (increased **lordosis**) and gestational weight gain makes stature an invalid measure of growth.

Height and weight are used to calculate BMI (kg/m^2); BMI for age growth charts also are available. Excessive weight in adolescents is defined as BMI greater than or equal to the 95th percentile; adolescents with the 85th percentile less than or equal to BMI less than or equal to the 95th percentile are classified as "at risk for overweight." Underweight is defined as BMI less than the 5th percentile.

Reproductive Development

Reproductive development is assessed using Tanner stages that characterize pubic hair and breast (female) and genital (male) maturation. Progression from Tanner stages 2 to 5 typically takes 2.5 to 5 years. In girls, Tanner staging of breasts and pubic hair usually occurs in parallel; for boys, genital staging precedes pubic hair staging. Menarche typically occurs at Tanner stage 4. Pubertal onset, including age at menarche, is in part genetically determined. The normal age of pubertal onset is ages 8 to 16 years in girls and ages 9 to 17 years in boys.

Cognitive and Psychosocial Development During Adolescence

Cognitive and Affective Development

The brain develops during puberty; in particular, areas involved in regulation of behavior and emotion and in perception and evaluation of risk and reward undergo considerable change (Steinberg, 2005). Cognitive development during adolescence results in increased self-awareness, self-direction, and self-regulation. However, the changes in arousal and motivation that take place during puberty occur before acquisition of the ability to regulate affect (Steinberg, 2005). The limbic areas of the brain associated with emotion increase in volume during puberty. The cortical gray area is reduced in volume, and there is lo-

calized synaptic pruning that increases the efficiency of information processing. Frontal brain activity, which is responsible for abstract thought, planning, and attention, is increased (Waylen & Wolke, 2004). There is increased connectivity among brain regions via myelination of nerve fibers; in particular, increased connections between the cortex and the limbic systems augment the ability to evaluate and make decisions regarding risk and reward.

During early adolescence, teenagers improve their deductive reasoning, information processing, and specialized knowledge. The capacity for abstract, multidimensional, planned, and hypothetical thought increases into middle adolescence. Although adults and adolescents have similar reasoning capacities, adolescents and adults differ in social and emotional factors, leading to divergent behaviors with age. For example, adolescents are more susceptible to peer influences than adults, and their reasoning about real-life situations or personal choices is not as sound as their reasoning about hypothetical or ethical questions.

Age and life experience are associated with most aspects of cognitive development during adolescence; however, maturation in arousal, motivation, and emotion are more closely linked with the onset of puberty. Emotional intensity and reactivity and reward-seeking and risk-taking behaviors also are influenced by puberty and not by chronologic age. Vulnerability to social status appears to increase at pubertal onset, coinciding with increased risk-taking behaviors. Cognitive development enhances the ability to regulate affect; conversely, emotion alters decision-making thought processes and behavior. Because teenagers are more likely to engage in high-risk behaviors (e.g., drug use and unprotected sex), it previously was thought that their ability to accurately evaluate risk was lacking. However, there is evidence that adolescents are able to understand risk but make poor decisions regardless. Thus, decision-making behaviors that affect health, including diet and exercise, are highly influenced by emotion and social influences, despite understanding of associated risks and benefits.

Psychosocial Development

Adolescence is the transition from childhood to adulthood, requiring maturation of psychosocial functioning. During the teenage years, individuals move from same- to mixed-sex peer groups, develop romantic relationships, and transfer relational dependence and modeling of behaviors from parents to peers (Waylen & Wolke, 2004). Adolescence is also a time of increased independence with regard to academic performance and economic self-sufficiency. In the United States and other Western societies, physical maturity precedes achievement of these developmental tasks; this period of prolonged adolescence has been termed the "maturity gap." The length of the maturity gap differs significantly between genders and among individuals; the maturity gap is larger for boys than for girls.

The cognitive and affective development that occurs during adolescence changes a teenager's self-concept and self-esteem. Adolescents are concerned with the identity they project to others (Waylen & Wolke, 2004). The discrepancy between an adolescent's self-identity and the expectations of others may be problematic. Rapid pubertal development or pubertal onset that deviates from one's peers also may result in maladaptive behaviors. In females early maturation is associated with increased affective disorders, delinquency and drop-out rates, and pregnancy. In boys early physical maturation has mostly positive consequences—namely, increased social status and high self-esteem. In contrast, males with late pubertal onset are more likely to engage in status-seeking antisocial behaviors. Thus, biological and social factors interact to affect behaviors, including those with long-term effects on health.

Drug use is one maladaptive coping mechanism that adolescents may adopt to deal with stress. Puberty is associated with the onset of mental health disorders in girls; in particular, the incidence of anxiety and depressive disorders, eating disorders, and smoking is increased in female adolescents. Among U.S. girls participating in the National Longitudinal Study of Adolescent Health (Harris, Gordon-Larsen, Chantala, & Udry, 2006), 10% to 15% reported feelings of depression and 13% to 33% had suicidal thoughts. In contrast, boys were less likely to feel depressed (6% to 9%) or to report suicidal ideation (8% to 14%). Girls also are more likely to attempt suicide (Grunbaum et al., 2002). This gender difference may be attributed to hormonal changes and to the female ruminative response style.

In the Youth Risk Behavior Surveillance nearly one-half of high school students reported that they used alcohol, 30% said they binge drink, and approximately one-fourth reported current marijuana use (Grunbaum et al., 2002). The prevalence of cocaine, inhalant, heroin, and methamphetamine use is lower; lifetime rates of use range from 3% to 15% (Grunbaum et al., 2002). Five percent of high school students reported using illegal steroids during their lifetime (Grunbaum et al., 2002). Among girls, 13% to 33% reported that they binge drink, 7% to 21% used marijuana, and 2% to 8% used hard drugs (Harris et al., 2006). Adolescent boys were more likely than girls to binge drink (17% to 32%), use marijuana (14% to 28%), or use hard drugs (3% to 8%) (Grunbaum et al., 2002; Harris et al., 2006). In a national sample of U.S. youth, 49.3% had consumed at least one drink in the previous month. On average, adolescents aged 15 to 21 years consumed 14.3 drinks per month (Snyder, Milici, Slater, Sun, & Strizhakova, 2006).

Alcohol use, smoking, marijuana use, and truancy are co-occurring behaviors; teens who use marijuana are more likely to also use tobacco than nonusers (Weden & Zabin, 2005). Regular or excessive alcohol consumption is positively associated with marijuana use (Boys et al., 2003; Rey, Martin, & Krabman, 2004). These behaviors are less likely to persist into adulthood if the onset occurs during adolescence, if the frequency of the behaviors is occasional, and if the behaviors occur within the peer group (Waylen & Wolke, 2004).

Tobacco use, poor diet/inactivity, alcohol abuse, and illicit drug use are among the leading modifiable causes of death in the United States (McGinnis, 1993; Mokdad et al., 2000). Unfortunately, the prevalence of these risk factors is high among adolescents.

Tobacco use, particularly cigarette smoking, also is common among adolescents. In 2004 about 12% of middle school students and 28% of high school students reported smoking at least one cigarette in the past 30 days (Centers for Disease Control and Prevention [CDC], 2005). Each day approximately 4,000 children and adolescents younger than 18 years of age smoke their first tobacco cigarette. One-half of these teens become regular smokers (U.S. Department of Health and Human Services, Office of Applied Studies, 2003). Teenagers perceive increased social status from cigarette smoking. Girls often smoke cigarettes to control their body weight. Adolescents also believe cigarette smoking is harmless during the first few years of smoking (Waylen & Wolke, 2004). Advertising increases risk of cigarette smoking by glamorizing smoking and by fostering brand recognition and desirability (CDC, 2005).

Nutrient Requirements and Temporal Consumption Trends

Absolute nutrient requirements are increased in adolescence compared with childhood due to increased growth and body size. Adolescent boys have greater requirements for most nutrients compared with girls due to differences in growth and development. The exception is iron; postmenarcheal adolescent girls need more iron than boys due to menstrual blood losses (Institute of Medicine [IOM], Food and Nutrition Board, 2001).

Macronutrients

Average daily energy consumption, as assessed in the National Health and Nutrition Examination Survey (NHANES) I (1971–1974) and III (1988–1994), has remained relatively constant, except in the case of adolescent girls, whose energy intake increased from 1,735 to 1,996 kcal/day (Troiano, Briefel, Carroll, & Bialostosky, 2000; Briefel & Johnson, 2004). The proportion of energy derived from fat and saturated fat decreased over time but remained above the recommendations in the Dietary Guidelines at 33.5% for total fat and 12.5% for saturated fat (Troiano et al., 2000). In children over 6 years of age, 10% to 18% of saturated fat and 5% to 10% of total fat was consumed in 2% fat and whole-milk products.

Minerals

Calcium

The Food and Nutrition Board of the IOM established the adequate intake (AI) for calcium based on maximal calcium retention using data from epidemiologic studies, randomized controlled trials, and balance studies (IOM, Food and Nutrition Board, 1997). Calcium balance studies in adolescents determined that retention increased with dietary intake up to 1,300 mg/day. Recent longitudinal data of bone mineral deposition suggest that calcium requirements may be higher—1,500 mg for girls and 1,700

CRITICAL **Thinking**

Milk consumption declined 36% among teenaged girls from the late 1970s to the mid-1990s. Teenaged girls may avoid dairy products because they believe dairy products promote weight gain. Lactose intolerance is another reason that teenagers, especially nonwhites, do not consume dairy products. Consumption of soft drinks has been associated with reduced bone mineral deposition in adolescent girls with average calcium intakes less than 900 mg/day but not in boys, whose calcium intakes averaged more than 1,000 mg (Whiting et al., 2004). Noncaffeinated carbonated soft drinks do not increase urinary calcium losses (Heaney & Rafferty, 2001). Because soft drinks often replace milk, reduced calcium consumption likely explains the relationship between soft drinks and bone mineral. What effects will this have in the aging process?

mg for boys—during peak calcium accretion (Whiting et al., 2004). Dairy foods supply 75% of the calcium in the American diet (Weaver, 2000). Some vegetables contain calcium, but the bioavailability is poor: 5 servings of broccoli and 15 servings of spinach provide as much absorbable calcium as 1 cup of milk (Weaver, 2000).

Adolescent boys aged 9 to 13 years consume, on average, 79% of the AI for calcium (1,022 mg/day) and girls, 65% of the AI for calcium (842 mg/day) (Storey, Forshee, & Anderson, 2004). Older adolescent boys aged 14 to 18 years consume 1,156 mg calcium per day (89% of AI per day). However, calcium consumption is reduced among older adolescent girls aged 14 to 18 years; average daily calcium intake among these girls is only 750 mg/day, or 57% of the AI (Storey et al., 2004). There also are significant ethnic differences in calcium consumption; African-American and Hispanic-American teenagers have lower daily calcium intakes than whites (Storey et al., 2004).

Iron

Iron requirements increase during adolescence to meet the demands of growth and inevitable losses. Iron is lost from the gastrointestinal tract, skin, and urine and from menstrual blood in females. The requirements for absorbed iron for adolescent boys and girls are estimated to be 1.47 and 1.15 mg/day, respectively (Fomon et al., 2003). The mean iron intake of adolescent boys aged 14 to 16 years is approximately 15 mg/day (Egan, Tao, Pennington, & Bolger, 2002). Thus, most boys probably meet the absorbed iron requirement. In contrast, female adolescents average a daily intake of 11 mg (Egan et al., 2002) and thus are at risk for iron deficiency.

Sodium

Average daily sodium consumption increased by approximately 1,000 mg for adolescent boys and girls between NHANES I (1971–1974) and NHANES III (1988–1994) with data released in 1999–2000. The average daily sodium intake for teenaged boys was about 4,000 mg, and for girls, 3,000 mg.

Vitamins

Vitamin D

The AI for vitamin D is 5 µg (200 IU) per day for individuals aged 1 to 50 years (IOM, Food and Nutrition Board, 1997). Synthesis of vitamin D in the skin is adequate to meet the requirement with sufficient exposure to ultraviolet light. Skin vitamin D synthesis is reduced by use of sunscreen and by dark skin pigmentation. Recently, there have been increased reports of vitamin D insufficiency and deficiency, including reports

> ### CRITICAL **Thinking**
>
> Individuals who live at northern latitudes above the 35th parallel do not receive enough ultraviolet radiation to support adequate synthesis of vitamin D; between November and March vitamin D synthesis is dramatically reduced in the northern hemisphere (C. Moore et al., 2005). What effect does global warming have on this issue?

of rickets among African-American children and vitamin D deficiency in adolescents. Individuals with darkly pigmented skin have reduced ability to synthesize vitamin D and therefore are at greater risk for insufficiency when dietary intakes are marginal.

Dietary intake of vitamin D among adolescents varies by ethnicity; non–Hispanic-American whites had the highest intakes of vitamin D, and African-Americans the lowest (C. Moore, Murphy, & Holick, 2005). As a group, adolescent boys are more likely to have adequate vitamin D intakes than girls and older males. However, there are significant ethnic differences; approximately 75% of non–Hispanic-American whites meet or exceed the AI, compared with 45% of non–Hispanic African-Americans and 58% of Mexican-Americans (C. Moore et al., 2005). Approximately one-half of adolescent girls meet or exceed the AI for vitamin D; only 38% of non–Hispanic African-Americans met the AI, compared with 59% of whites and 60% of Mexican-Americans (C. Moore et al., 2005).

Fortified foods, mainly fortified milk, are the primary dietary sources of vitamin D. Because the prevalence of lactose intolerance is higher among African-Americans (75%) than among Hispanic-Americans (53%) and whites (6% to 22%), avoidance of dairy products may explain the reduced vitamin D intakes among African-American adolescents (Jackson & Savaiano, 2001). In 2003 the U.S. Food and Drug Administration approved vitamin D fortification of calcium-fortified juices and juice drinks. African-Americans and Mexican-Americans who avoid dairy products may benefit from these fortified products; for example, 8 ounces of fortified orange juice provides up to 2.5 µg (100 IU) of vitamin D.

The current recommended intakes for vitamin D are probably too low, based on optimal calcium absorption. Without ultraviolet synthesis of vitamin D, 20 to 25 µg (800 to 1,000 IU) of dietary vitamin D

Parathyroid hormone:
Peptide hormone secreted by the parathyroid gland; it increases blood calcium by acting on the bone, intestine, and kidneys.

a day is needed to maintain serum vitamin D concentrations within the desired range (Dawson-Hughes, 2004). During peak pubertal growth, low serum concentrations of 25-hydroxyvitamin D increase serum **parathyroid hormone**, 1,25-dihydroxyvitamin D, and, consequently, fractional calcium absorption (Abrams et al., 2005). In contrast to the relationship observed in adults, 25-hydroxyvitamin D was not correlated with fractional calcium absorption in adolescents. These findings suggest that adolescents adapt to suboptimal vitamin D status better than adults. Possible mechanisms include enhanced responsiveness of calcium absorption to 1,25-dihydroxyvitamin D, increased conversion of 25-hydroxy to 1,25-dihydroxyvitamin D, or increased vitamin D–independent calcium absorption (Abrams et al., 2005).

Dietary Patterns

Serving Size

Average serving sizes for foods eaten at home and away from home have increased during the past 30 years. The average serving sizes for foods frequently consumed by adolescents—salty snacks, French fries, ready-to-eat cereals, and soft drinks—have significantly increased. The volume of soft drinks consumed per occasion increased more than 50% among female adolescents. Foods with low nutrient density, such as soft drinks, candy, desserts, salty snacks, and added sugar and fats, account for 30% of daily energy intake in children aged 8 to 18 years (Briefel & Johnson, 2004). Consumption of these low-nutrient-density foods is associated with higher energy intakes and lower consumption of vitamin A, folate, calcium, magnesium, iron, and zinc.

Food Groups

Adolescents do not consume the recommended number of servings of fruits, vegetables, and dairy products, and they consume excessive amounts of added sugar (Xie, Gilliland, Li, & Rockett, 2003), fat, and saturated fat (Briefel & Johnson, 2004). In a study of 18,000 adolescents who participated in the National Longitudinal Study of Adolescent Health, many did not eat the minimum recommended number of servings of vegetables (71%), fruits (55%), and dairy products (47%) (Videon & Manning, 2003). Teenagers who did not consume milk had inadequate intakes of vitamin A, folate, calcium, phosphorous, and magnesium (Briefel & Johnson, 2004).

Skipping Breakfast

One-fifth of adolescents report skipping breakfast (Videon & Manning, 2003). Children who skip breakfast have lower daily intakes of vitamins A, E, D, and B_6; calcium; phosphorous; and magnesium compared with breakfast eaters (Nicklas, Bao, Webber, & Berenson, 1993). Eating breakfast is associated with increased school attendance and academic performance (Pollitt, 1995).

Added Sugars

Adolescents have the highest intake of added sugars than any other age group; approximately 40% of added sugars are consumed in carbonated soft drinks (Briefel & Johnson, 2004). Soft drinks supply approximately 8% of total energy intake among adolescents. Overweight adolescents derive more of their daily energy intake from soft drinks than normal-weight teens (Troiano et al., 2000). Teenagers consume more carbonated soft drinks than they do fruit juices, fruit-ades, or milk. Consumption of soda and fruit drinks among adolescent girls doubled and milk consumption decreased between NHANES I (1971–1974) and NHANES III (1988–1994). Based on the U.S. Department of Agriculture (USDA) Continuing Survey of Food Intakes by Individuals for adolescents aged 12 to 17 years, consumption of sweetened breakfast cereals is positively associated with dietary intakes of calcium, folate, and iron, and sweetened dairy products increase calcium intakes. However, consumption of other foods and beverages that are high in sugar was associated with poor diet quality, including reduced intakes of calcium, iron, and folate (Frary, Johnson, & Wang, 2004). Displacement of milk by high-sugar beverages reduces consumption of protein, calcium, and vitamins B_2, B_{12}, and D (St. Onge, Keller, & Heymsfield, 2003).

Fast Food Consumption

Most adolescents frequently eat meals and snacks away from home. In one study 26% of all meals and snacks were consumed away from home, accounting for 32% of total energy (Lin, Guthrie, & Frazao, 1999). In another survey 75% of adolescents reported eating at a fast-food restaurant in the previous week (French, Story, Neumark-Sztainer, Fulkerson, & Hannan, 2001). Teens who ate at a fast-food restaurant at least 3 times in the past week had energy intakes about 40% higher than adolescents who did not eat fast food. Frequency of fast food consumption is also inversely related to daily servings of vegetables, fruit, and dairy products (French, Story, Neumark-Sztainer, et al., 2001). Adolescents who described themselves as overweight were more likely to have poor dietary consumption patterns (Videon & Manning, 2003) but did not differ in frequency of fast food consumption compared with normal-weight teens (French, Story, Neumark-Sztainer, et al., 2001). Adolescent boys are more likely than girls to eat away from home (Briefel & Johnson, 2004). Teenagers who were employed ate fast food more frequently than those who did not work (French et al., 2001).

Sociodemographic Moderators of Dietary Intake

Gender, ethnicity, parental income, and education affect diet quality in adolescents. Non–Hispanic-American whites have the lowest intakes of fruit; African-Americans and Asian-Americans have significantly higher consumption of vegetables (Xie et al., 2003). Degree of acculturation affects nutrient intake among Hispanic-American youths. Adolescents whose families were less acculturated had lower intakes of energy, protein, sodium, and percentage of energy from fat and saturated fat and greater intakes of folate compared with acculturated families (Mazur, Marquis, & Jensen, 2003). Higher parental education level was associated with better diet quality, and the presence of a parent at the evening meal was positively associated with consumption of fruits, vegetables, and dairy products. Another study of 3,200 adolescents reported higher intakes of polyunsaturated fat, protein, calcium, and folate in teenagers from families with higher incomes and lower intakes of total fat, saturated fat, and cholesterol with higher parental education (Xie et al., 2003). Snacking is more common among families with higher incomes, and income modifies the selection of snack foods. Family income at or below 130% of the poverty line reported higher intakes of fried potatoes, potato chips, whole milk, and fruit drinks and ades than those with incomes at or above 300% of the poverty line (Briefel & Johnson, 2004).

As children make the transition from dependence on their parents to autonomy, normative family development includes increased frequency and intensity of parent-child conflicts. During this time peer influence on values and behavior becomes stronger as peers replace parents as the primary source of social support. Teenagers may use diet as a means of expressing their self-identity and autonomy. Peers may exert either positive or negative influences on food intake.

Advertising and marketing of foods and beverages influences the food preferences, purchase requests, purchase, and consumption of children and youth (IOM, Food and Nutrition Board, 2006). Television is the primary source of advertising, but other forms of marketing such as radio, print, billboards, and the Internet also are used to influence purchases by adolescents. Most products marketed to children and teenagers are high in energy, sugars, fat, and salt and low in micronutrients. Children are more vulnerable to advertising than teenagers because they are not able to differentiate between informative and commercial programming. There is strong evidence that advertising influences food preferences, purchase requests, and short-term food consumption of children 2 to 11 years of age. There are insufficient data to determine the effect of advertising on teenagers. However, television advertising is positively correlated with body fat in children and adolescents (IOM, Food and Nutrition Board, 2006). Televi-

Effect of Advertising

Advertising influences the consumption of alcoholic beverages by adolescents. One study showed that exposure to alcohol advertising on television, radio, magazines, and billboards increased alcohol consumption in a dose-dependent manner in individuals aged 15 to 20 years. Each additional advertisement seen increased the number of drinks consumed by 1% (Snyder et al., 2006).

sion and video viewing are associated with reduced consumption of fruits and vegetables in adolescents (Boynton-Jarrett et al., 2003).

School Food Environment

The recent increase in excessive weight and obesity in adolescents has brought the food environment in schools under increasing scrutiny. Most schools have "competitive" foods for sale in addition to the USDA National School Breakfast and Lunch Programs that provide free and reduced-cost meals to students from low-income families. The USDA meals programs are subject to federal regulations, including nutrient standards (USDA, 2005). Despite these regulations, the meals offered by these programs have been reported to exceed the USDA's recommendations for fat (38% versus < 30% of total energy), saturated fat (15% versus < 10% of total energy), and sodium (~1,500 mg per meal versus < 2,400 mg/day).

Competitive foods include those that are sold a la carte, in vending machines, from school stores, or as school fundraisers. The only federal regulation regarding competitive foods is restriction of the sale of "foods of minimal nutritional value" (e.g., carbonated beverages, water ices, chewing gum, and some candy) in the lunch rooms during meals (French, 2005). Fruits, fruit juices, and vegetables are rarely offered for sale in school stores or in vending machines (St. Onge et al., 2003). Concern about the increasing incidence of excessive weight in children has caused some states and local school districts to regulate competitive foods through legislation and policy. Sales of a la carte foods and vending machine purchases are significant in middle and high schools, and many of the available selections are high in fat and/or added sugar (Kann, Grunbaum, McKenna, Wechsler, & Galuska, 2005). The School Health Profiles assessment of schools from 27 states and 11 large urban school districts found that nearly 90% of districts offered competitive foods. The most prevalent types of less nutritious foods were chocolate candy (65% of schools); other candy (68%); salty snacks, not low in fat (75%); and soft drinks, sports drinks, or fruit drinks. Low-fat salty snacks (80%) and 100% fruit juice (84%) were the most common choices with higher nutritional value; fruits and vegetables were offered by 45% of schools surveyed (Kann et al., 2005). In a survey of public high schools in Pennsylvania the top-selling items were pizza, hamburgers, and sandwiches; baked goods not low in fat; French-fried potatoes; salty snacks not low in fat; carbonated beverages, sports drinks, and fruit drinks; and bottled water (Probart et al., 2005).

Availability of competitive foods reduces diet quality (French & Stables, 2003). Interventions in the school food environment designed to promote consumption of fruits and vegetables significantly increase fruit intake with a negligible effect on vegetable consumption (French & Stables, 2003). Increased availability of fruit and fruit juices effectively increases intake. Reducing the cost of healthful food items offered in school snack bars and vending machines increases the purchases of these items. Alternatively, increasing the cost of higher-fat "junk" foods reduces purchase and consumption of these foods (French, 2005). Other innovative strategies include school gardening programs, use of produce from local farmers' markets in school salad bars, and free fruit and vegetables.

Health Status of U.S. Adolescents

Excessive Weight and Obesity

The prevalence of excessive weight (i.e., ≥ 95th percentile for BMI on 2000 CDC growth charts) among adolescents increased from 6.1% in NHANES I (1974–1976) to 15.5% in NHANES III (1988–1994). The increase in excessive weight was greatest in African-American and Mexican-American teens; the prevalence of excessive weight approaches 25% in these ethnic groups (Moore, 2004). Adolescents from lower income households are twice as likely to be overweight or obese compared with those from higher income families.

The increase in excessive weight and obesity in adolescents has been attributed to a dietary shift away from fruits and vegetables toward fats and simple carbohydrates and to decreased energy expenditure in physical activity. Among children aged 12 to 19 years, only 50% report regular vigorous physical activity and 25% do not get any vigorous exercise (T. Moore, 2004). The time spent in sedentary activities also is increasing among adolescents. In 1997 parents reported that their children (aged 2 to 17 years) watched an average of 2.1 hours of television per day; by 2000 the average time spent watching television increased to 2.45 hours per day, and a total of 382 minutes were spent watching television, playing video games, using a computer, talking on the telephone, or reading (Ford, Mokdad, & Ajani, 2004).

Excess adiposity during adolescence increases the risk of adult obesity and chronic diseases. In the National Longitudinal Study of Adolescent Health of 9,795 adolescents, baseline prevalence of obesity was 12.5%, and only 1.6% of adolescents who were obese between ages 13 and 20 years were not obese 5 years later (Ford, Mokdad, & Ajani, 2004). Non–Hispanic African-American females were more likely to become and remain obese than non–Hispanic-American whites; Asian women were less likely to become and remain obese (Ford, Mokdad, & Ajani, 2004). The risk of hypertension is increased 10-fold, dyslipidemias 3- to 8-fold, and diabetes mellitus 2-fold by excess adiposity. Surprisingly, only 39.6% of adolescents aged 12 to 15 years and 51.6% of older teens aged 16 to 19 years were ever informed of their overweight status by a physician or health care provider (Ogden, 2005). Read more about childhood obesity in Chapter 7.

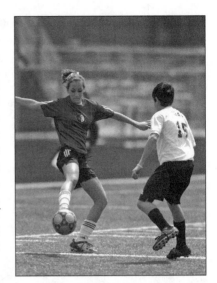

Metabolic Syndrome

The comorbidities of diabetes, hypertension, and hyperlipidemia in patients with cardiovascular disease have been described as the metabolic syndrome. Using the guidelines from NHANES III, the metabolic syndrome is defined as having 3 or more of the following risk factors: abdominal obesity (i.e., waist circumference 90th percentile for age and gender), triglycerides at least 110 mg/dL, fasting glucose at least 110 mg/dL, systolic or diastolic blood pressure at least in the 90th percentile (age, height, gender specific), and no more than 40 mg/dL high-density lipoprotein for males and no more than 50 mg/dL for females.

Data from NHANES III of 1,366 adolescents aged 12 to 17 years found the prevalence of the metabolic syndrome to be 6.3% among boys and 4.1% among girls. Abdominal obesity, assessed by waist circumference, was identified in 17.9%, hypertriglyceridemia was present in 21.0%, 18.0% had low high-density lipoprotein, and 7.1% had hypertension. Furthermore, the prevalence of elevated C-reactive protein was nearly 4 times greater in adolescents with the metabolic syndrome compared with those without it (Ford, Ajani, Mokdad, & National Health and National Examination, 2005). Using slightly different criteria for the metabolic syndrome (i.e., waist circumference < 75th percentile and high-density lipoprotein < 45 mg/dL for adolescent boys), the prevalence of the metabolic syndrome was 9.2% in 1,960 adolescents aged 12 to 19 years and was comparable among boys and girls (de Ferranti et al., 2004).

There were small changes in risk factors for the metabolic syndrome in children and adolescents between NHANES III and NHANES (1988–1994): Waist circumference increased by 2.0 cm in children aged 2 to 17 years, systolic blood pressure increased 2.2 mm Hg in children aged 8 to 17 years, and triglycerides decreased by 8.8 mg/dL and glucose by 2.5 mg/dL in teens aged 12 to 17 years. Total cholesterol, high-density lipoprotein and low-density lipoprotein cholesterol, and glycosylated hemoglobin were unchanged (Ford, Mokdad, & Ajani, 2004).

Cultural Diversity: Among overweight children the metabolic syndrome was nearly 3 times as common, with a prevalence of 31.2%. Non–Hispanic African-Americans (2.5%) were less likely to have the metabolic syndrome than non–Hispanic-American whites (10.9%) and Mexican-Americans (12.9%) (de Ferranti et al., 2004).

Iron Deficiency

Approximately 9% of girls aged 12 to 15 years and 16% of adolescent girls aged 16 to 19 years are iron deficient (Looker, 2002). Iron deficiency anemia affects 2% of girls aged 12 to 19 years. The prevalence of iron deficiency among males 12–15 years is 5%. Iron deficiency causes reduced exercise capacity, immune function, and cognitive performance. Adolescent girls who were iron deficient scored lower in verbal learning and memory (Ford, Mokdad, & Ajani, 2004) and in math (Halterman, Kaczorowski, Aligne, Auinger, & Szilagyi, 2001) compared with those with normal iron status. Iron deficiency also may contribute to attention deficit hyperactivity disorder. Children with attention deficit hyperactivity disorder have significantly lower concentrations of ferritin than control subjects (Konofal, Lecendreux, Arnulf, & Mouren, 2004).

Tobacco Use and Nutritional Status

Although the prevalence of smoking among adults in the United States has decreased in the 40 years after the Surgeon General's report describing the adverse consequences of cigarette smoking, more adolescents are smoking now than in the past. In 2004, 30% of adolescents smoked. In addition, children are starting to smoke at a younger age. Rates of regular tobacco use increase significantly at age 11 years (DuRant & Smith, 1999; Winkleby, Robinson, Sundquist, & Kraemer, 1999). Non–Hispanic-American white adolescents are more likely to smoke cigarettes than African-American, Mexican-American, and Native American teens (CDC, Division of Adolescent and School Health and Office on Smoking and Health, 1999). Most adolescents smoke to control their weight, and some substitute smoking a cigarette for eating (Dowdell & Santucci, 2004).

Adult smokers have significantly higher intakes of energy, total fat, saturated fat, cholesterol, and alcohol and lower intakes of polyunsaturated fat, fiber, vitamin C, vitamin E, and beta-carotene than nonsmokers (Dallongeville, Marécaux, Fruchart, & Amouyel, 1998). Similarly, adolescent smokers consume less fiber and fewer vitamins and minerals than nonsmokers (Hampl & Betts, 1999). The more a teenager smokes, the less likely he or she is to exercise at least 3 times per week and consume at least 1 serving per day of vegetables or dairy products (Wilson et al., 2005). Adolescents who smoke consume more alcohol than nonsmokers (Crawley & While, 1996). For some teens who smoke, their poor diet may reflect the poor diet quality of their parents, who also smoke. Nonsmoking children of parents who smoke had lower intakes of folate and vitamins C and E than children whose parents do not smoke (Crawley & While, 1996). Among young women, passive and active smokers had lower intakes of folate and concentration of folate in serum compared with nonsmokers and values reported in the 1999–2000 NHANES (Ortega et al., 2004).

Data from NHANES III show that environmental tobacco smoke exposure and active cigarette smoking increase the risk of the metabolic syndrome among adolescents. Teens exposed to environmental tobacco smoke were 4.7 times as likely to develop the metabolic syndrome compared with nonexposed adolescents; the odds ratio for active smokers was 6.1 (Weitzman et al., 2005). Among overweight adolescents 19.6% of those exposed to environmental tobacco smoke and 23.6% of smokers had the metabolic syndrome, compared with 5.6% of nonexposed teens (Weitzman et al., 2005). Unfortunately, 43% of children in the United States live in a household with at least one smoker. Alcohol and marijuana users eat more snack foods and less fruit, vegetables, and milk than nonusers (Farrow, Rees, & Worthington-Roberts, 1987).

Adolescent Pregnancy

There are approximately 0.9 million adolescent pregnancies in the United States per year; more than 40% of adolescent girls have been pregnant at least once before 20 years of age (Kirby, Coyle, & Gould, 2001). About 51% of these pregnancies end in live births. Pregnant adolescents are more likely to have nutritional and medical complications than adult women; the risk is greatest for the youngest teenagers. Teenagers are twice as likely to deliver a low-birth-weight infant, and the rate of neonatal death is increased nearly 3-fold compared with adult women. Premature delivery is more common in teenagers. Inadequate and excessive maternal weight gain (Howie, Parker, & Schoendorf, 2003), pregnancy-induced hypertension, and anemia are common nutrition-related problems among pregnant adolescents (Klein, 2005). Low prepregnancy body weight and **gynecologic age,** parity, and poor nutritional status negatively affect pregnancy outcome (Klein, 2005). Smoking tobacco or marijuana, behaviors that are relatively common among adolescents, reduces birth weight (Fergusson & Woodward, 2000).

> ● **Learning Point** An increase in leptin during gestation may mediate the increased maternal adiposity and fetal growth restriction in growing adolescents (Scholl, Stein, & Smith, 2000). Leptin also may mediate the increased postpartum weight retention observed in growing adolescents compared with nongrowing teens (Scholl et al., 2000).

Gynecologic age: Years since menarche.

To optimize infant birth weight the IOM (1990) recommended that pregnant adolescents gain weight at the upper end of the recommended rates for each prepregnancy BMI category. However, the recommendation for greater weight gain in adolescents is controversial because it may increase the risk of maternal obesity (McAnarney & Stevens-Simon, 1993). Early and continuous weight gain is also important (American Dietetic Association, 1994). Inadequate weight gain in the first 24 weeks of pregnancy increases the risk of having an infant that is small for gestational age; low rates of weight gain late in gestation increase the risk of premature delivery (Hediger, Scholl, Belsky, Ances, & Salmon, 1989).

In addition to gestational weight gain, maternal growth is an important determinant of birth weight. Among teens who are still growing, gestational weight gain is positively associated with increased maternal subcutaneous adiposity and not with birth weight (Scholl, Hediger, Schall, Khoo, & Fischer, 1994). Growing adolescents give birth to infants that weigh 150 to 200 g less than the infants of nongrowing teens or adult women. Reduced placental perfusion and transfer of micronutrients to the fetus explain, at least in part, the lower birth weight.

Nutrition is one of the most important modifiable factors that alters pregnancy outcome. Adolescents may improve their diet quality during pregnancy, but total energy and iron intake are often inadequate (American Dietetic Association, 1994). Suboptimal intakes of magnesium, zinc, folate, and vitamin B_6 have also been reported among pregnant adolescents (Pope, Skinner, & Carruth, 1992). Calcium, vitamin B_6, vitamin C, and folate supplements are recommended for teens at risk for poor dietary intakes (American Dietetic Association, 1994). Food cravings and aversions to previously preferred foods are common among adolescents. Cravings for sweet foods increase the consumption of sugar, and craving salty snacks is associated with increased consumption of sodium and fat (Pope et al., 1992).

Issues to Debate

1. If girls experience peer pressure to eat like other teens, including boys, what might be the result?
2. Discuss how psychosocial development during adolescence affects health-related behaviors, including dietary patterns.
3. What are the sociodemographic factors affecting dietary patterns? How do they affect a pregnant teen?
4. What are the dietary implications for chronic disease incidence among adolescents?

References

Abrams, S. A., Griffin, I. J., Hawthorne, K. M., Gunn, S. K., Gundberg, C. M., & Carpenter, T. O. (2005). Relationships among vitamin D levels, parathyroid hormone, and calcium absorption in young adolescents. *Journal of Clinical Endocrinology and Metabolism, 90,* 5576–5581.

American Dietetic Association. (1994). Position of the American Dietetic Association: Nutrition care for pregnant adolescents. *Journal of the American Dietetic Association, 94,* 449–450.

American Psychiatric Association. (2000). *Diagnostic and Statistical Manual of Mental Disorders* (4th ed.). Washington, DC: Author.

Bonny, A. E., Ziegler, J., Harvey, R., Debanne, S. M., Secic, M., & Cromer, B. (2006). Weight gain in obese and non-obese adolescent girls initiating depot medroxyprogesterone, oral contraceptive pills, or no hormonal con-tra-ceptive method. *Archives of Pediatric and Adolescent Medicine, 160,* 40–45.

Boynton-Jarrett, R., Thomas, T. N., Peterson, K. E., Wiecha, J., Sobol, A. M., & Gortmaker, S. L. (2003). Impact of television viewing patterns on fruit and vegetable consumption among adolescents. *Pediatrics, 112,* 1321–1326.

Boys, A., Farrell, M., Taylor, C., Marsden, J., Goodman, R., Brugha, T., et al. (2003). Psychiatric morbidity and substance use in young people aged 13–15 years: Results from the Child and Adolescent Survey of Mental Health. *British Journal of Psychiatry, 182,* 509–517.

Briefel, R. R., & Johnson, C. L. (2004). Secular trends in dietary intake in the United States. *Annual Review of Nutrition, 24,* 401–431.

Bryant, R. J., Wastney, M. E., Martin, B. R., Wood, O., McCabe, G. P., Morshidi, M., et al. (2003). Racial differences in bone turnover and calcium metabolism in adolescent females. *Journal of Clinical Endocrinology and Metabolism, 88,* 1043–1047.

Centers for Disease Control and Prevention. (2005). Tobacco use, access, and exposure to tobacco in media among middle and high school students—United States, 2004. *Morbidity and Mortality Weekly Report, 54,* 297–301.

Centers for Disease Control and Prevention, Division of Adolescent and School Health and Office on Smoking and Health. (1999). Cigarette smoking among high school students—11 states, 1991–1997. *Journal of School Health, 69(8),* 303–306.

Crawley, H. F., & While, D. (1996). Parental smoking and the nutrient intake and food choice of British teenagers aged 16–17 years. *Journal of Epidemiology and Community Health, 50,* 306–312.

Dallongeville, J., Marécaux, N., Fruchart, J. C., & Amouyel, P. (1998). Cigarette smoking is associated with unhealthy patterns of nutrient intake: A meta-analysis. *Journal of Nutrition, 128,* 1450–1457.

Dawson-Hughes, B. (2004). Racial/ethnic considerations in making recommendations for vitamin D for adult and elderly men and women. *American Journal of Clinical Nutrition, 80,* 1763S–1766S.

de Ferranti, S. D., Gauvreau, K., Ludwig, D. S., Neufeld, E. J., Newburger, J. W., & Rifai, N. (2004). Prevalence of the metabolic syndrome in American adolescents: Findings from the Third National Health and Nutrition Examination Survey. *Circulation, 110,* 2494–2497.

Dowdell, E. B., & Santucci, M. E. (2004). Health risk behavior assessment: Nutrition, weight, and tobacco use in one urban seventh-grade class. *Public Health Nursing, 21,* 128–136.

DuRant, R. H., & Smith, J. A. (1999). Adolescent tobacco use and cessation. *Primary Care, 26,* 553–575.

Eastell, R. (2005). Role of oestrogen in the regulation of bone turnover at the menarche. *Journal of Endocrinology, 185,* 223–234.

Egan, S. K., Tao, S. S. H., Pennington, J. A. H., & Bolger, P. M. (2002). US Food and Drug Administration's Total Diet Study: Intake of nutritional and toxic elements, 1991–96. *Food Additives and Contaminants, 19,* 103–125.

Farrow, J. A., Rees, J. M., & Worthington-Roberts, B. S. (1987). Health, developmental, and nutritional status of adolescent alcohol and marijuana abusers. *Pediatrics, 79,* 218–223.

Federico, G., Baroncelli, G.I., Vanacore, T., Flore, L. & Saggese, G. (2003). Pubertal changes in biochemical markers of growth. *Hormone Research, 60 (Suppl 1),* 46-51.

Fergusson, D. M., & Woodward, L. J. (2000). Educational, psychosocial, and sexual outcomes of girls with conduct problems in early adolescence. *Journal of Child Psychology and Psychiatry, 41,* 779–792.

Fomon, S. J., Drulis, J. M., Nelson, S. E., Serfass, R. E., Woodhead, J. C., & Ziegler, E. E. (2003). Inevitable iron loss by human adolescents, with calculations of the requirement for absorbed iron. *Journal of Nutrition, 133,* 167–172.

Ford, E. S., Ajani, U. A., Mokdad, A. H., & National Health and National Examination. (2005). The metabolic syndrome and concentrations of C-reactive protein among U.S. youth. *Diabetes Care, 28,* 878–881.

Ford, E. S., Mokdad, A. H., & Ajani, U. A. (2004). Trends in risk factors for cardiovascular disease among children and adolescents in the United States. *Pediatrics, 114,* 1534–1544.

Frary, C. D., Johnson, R. K., & Wang, M. Q. (2004). Children and adolescents' choices of foods and beverages high in added sugars are associated with intakes of key nutrients and food groups. *Journal of Adolescent Health, 34,* 56–63.

French, S. A. (2005). Public health strategies for dietary change: Schools and workplaces. *Journal of Nutrition, 135,* 910–912.

French, S. A., & Stables, G. (2003). Environmental interventions to promote vegetable and fruit consumption among youth in school settings. *Preventive Medicine, 37,* 593–610.

French, S. A., Story, M., Fulkerson, J. A., & Gerlack, A. F. (2003). Food environment in secondary schools: À la carte, vending machines, and food policies and practices. *American Journal of Public Health, 93,* 1161–1167.

French, S. A., Story, M., Neumark-Sztainer, D., Fulkerson, J. A., & Hannan, P. (2001). Fast food restaurant use among adolescents: Associations with nutrient intake, food choices and behavioral and psychosocial variables. *International Journal of Obesity and Related Metabolic Disorders, 25,* 1823–1833.

Fujiwara, S., Kasagi, F., Yamada, M., & Kodama, K. (1997). Risk factors for hip fracture in a Japanese cohort. *Journal of Bone and Mineral Research, 12,* 998–1004.

Grunbaum, J. A., Kann, L., Kinchen, S. A., Williams, B., Ross, J. G., Lowry, R. & Kolbe, L. (2002). Youth risk behavior surveillance. *The Journal of School Health, 72,* 313-328.

Guo, S. S., Chunlea, W. C., Roche, A. F., & Siervogel, R. M. (1997). Age- and maturity-related changes in body composition during adolescence into adulthood: The Fels Longitudinal Study. *International Journal of Obesity and Related Metabolic Disorders, 21,* 1167–1175.

Halterman, J. S., Kaczorowski, J. M., Aligne, C. A., Auinger, P., & Szilagyi, P. G. (2001). Iron deficiency and cognitive achievement among school-aged children and adolescents in the United States. *Pediatrics, 107,* 1381–1386.

Hampl, J. S., & Betts, N. M. (1999). Cigarette use during adolescence: Effects on nutritional status. *Nutrition Reviews, 57,* 215–221.

Harris, K. M., Gordon-Larsen, P., Chantala, K., & Udry, J. R. (2006). Longitudinal trends in race/ethnic disparities in leading health indicators from adolescence to young adulthood. *Archives of Pediatric and Adolescent Medicine, 160,* 74–81.

Heaney, R. P., & Rafferty, K. (2001). Carbonated beverages and urinary calcium excretion. *American Journal of Clinical Nutrition, 74,* 343–347.

Hediger, M. L., Scholl, T. O., Belsky, D. H., Ances, I. G., & Salmon, R. W. (1989). Patterns of weight gain in adolescent pregnancy: Effects on birth weight and preterm delivery. *Obstetrics and Gynecology, 74,* 6–12.

Howie, L. D., Parker, J. D., & Schoendorf, K. C. (2003). Excessive maternal weight gain patterns in adolescents. *Journal of the American Dietetic Association, 103,* 1653–1657.

Institute of Medicine (IOM). (1990). *Nutrition During Pregnancy. Part I: Weight Gain. Part II: Supplements.* Washington, DC: National Academy Press.

Institute of Medicine (IOM), Food and Nutrition Board. (1997). *Dietary Reference Intakes for Calcium, Magnesium, Phosphorous, Vitamin D.* Washington, DC: National Academy of Sciences.

Institute of Medicine (IOM), Food and Nutrition Board. (2001). *Dietary Reference Intakes for Vitamin A, Vitamin K, Arsenic, Boron, Chromium, Copper, Iodine, Iron, Manganese, Nickel, Silicon, Vanadium, and Zinc.* Washington, DC: National Academy Press.

Institute of Medicine (IOM), Food and Nutrition Board. (2006). *Food Marketing to Children and Youth: Threat or Opportunity.* Washington, DC: National Academy Press.

Jackson, K. A., & Savaiano, D. A. (2001). Lactose maldigestion, calcium intake and osteoporosis in African-, Asian-, and Hispanic-Americans. *Journal of the American College of Nutrition, 20,* 198S–207S.

Kann, L., Grunbaum, J., McKenna, M. L., Wechsler, H., & Galuska, D. A. (2005). Competitive foods and beverages available for purchase in secondary schools—selected sites, United States, 2004. *Morbidity and Mortality Weekly Report, 54,* 917–921.

Kirby, D., Coyle, K., & Gould, J. B. (2001). Manifestations of poverty and birthrates among young teenagers in California zip code areas. *Family Planning Perspectives, 33*, 63–69.

Klein, J. D. (2005). Adolescent pregnancy: Current trends and issues. *Pediatrics, 116*, 281–286.

Konofal, E., Lecendreux, M., Arnulf, I., & Mouren, M. C. (2004). Iron deficiency in children with attention-deficit/hyperactivity disorder. *Archives of Pediatric and Adolescent Medicine, 158*, 1113–1115.

Leung, K. C., Johannsson, G., Leong, G. M., & Ho, K. K. (2004). Estrogen regulation of growth hormone action. *Endocrine Reviews, 25*, 693–721.

Lin B-H., Guthrie, J., & Frazao, E. (1999). Nutrient contribution of food away from home. In Frazao, E. (Ed.), *America's Eating Habits: Changes and Consequences*. USDA, ERS Agriculture Information Bulletin 750.

Looker, A. C. (2002). Iron deficiency—United States, 1999–2000. *Mortality and Morbidity Weekly Report, 51*, 897–899.

Mazur, R. E., Marquis, G. S., & Jensen, H. H. (2003). Diet and food insufficiency among Hispanic-American youths: Acculturation and socioeconomic factors in the third National Health and Nutrition Examination Survey. *American Journal of Clinical Nutrition, 78*, 1120–1127.

McAnarney, E. R., & Stevens-Simon, C. (1993). First, do no harm. Low birth weight and adolescent obesity. *American Journal of Diseases of Children, 147*, 983–985.

McGinnis, J. M. (1993). Actual causes of death in the United States. *Journal of the American Medical Association, 270*, 2207–2212.

Mokdad, A. H., Serdula, M. K., Dietz, W. H., Bowman, B. A., Marks, J. S., & Koplan, J. P. (2000). The continuing epidemic of obesity in the United States. *Journal of the American Medical Association, 284*, 1650–1651.

Molgaard, C., Thomsen, B. L., & Michaelsen, K. F. (1999). Whole body bone mineral accretion in healthy children and adolescents. *Archives of Disease in Childhood, 81*, 10–15.

Moore, C. E., Murphy, M. M., & Holick, M. F. (2005). Vitamin D intakes by children and adults in the United States differ among ethnic groups. *Journal of Nutrition, 135*, 2478–2485.

Moore, T. R. (2004). Adolescent and adult obesity in women: A tidal wave just beginning. *Clinical Obstetrics and Gynecology, 47*, 884–889.

National Center for Health Statistics. (2000). *CDC Growth Charts: United States*. U.S. Department of Health and Human Services, Centers for Disease Control and Prevention.

Nicklas, T. A., Bao, W., Webber, L. S., & Berenson, G. S. (1993). Breakfast consumption affects adequacy of total daily intake in children. *Journal of the American Dietetic Association, 93*, 886–891.

Ogden, C. (2005). Children and teens told by doctors that they are overweight—United States, 1999–2002. *Mortality and Morbidity Weekly Report, 54*, 848–849.

Ortega, R. M., Requejo, A. M., López-Sobaler, A. M., Navia, B., Mena, M. C., Basabe, B., et al. (2004). Smoking and passive smoking as conditioners of folate status in young women. *Journal of the American College of Nutrition, 23*, 365–371.

Pollitt, E. (1995). Does breakfast make a difference in school? *Journal of the American Dietetic Association, 95*, 1134–1139.

Pope, J. F., Skinner, J. D., & Carruth, B. R. (1992). Cravings and aversions of pregnant adolescents. *Journal of the American Dietetic Association, 92*, 1479–1482.

Probart, C., McDonnell, E., Weirich, J. E., Hartman, T., Bailey-Davis, L., & Prabhakher, V. (2005). Competitive foods available in Pennsylvania public high schools. *Journal of the American Dietetic Association, 105*, 1243–1249.

Rey, J. M., Martin, A., & Krabman, P. (2004). Is the party over? Cannabis and juvenile psychiatric disorder: The past 10 years. *Journal of the American Academy of Child and Adolescent Psychiatry, 43*, 1194–1205.

Riggs, B. L., Khosla, S., & Melton, L. J. 3rd. (2002). Sex steroids and the construction and conservation of the adult skeleton. *Endocrine Reviews, 23*, 279–302.

Roy, D. K., O'Neill, T. W., Finn, J. D., Lunt, M., Silman, A. J., Felsenberg, D., et al. (2003). Determinants of incident vertebral fracture in men and women: Results from the European Prospective Osteoporosis Study (EPOS). *Osteoporosis International, 14*, 19–26.

Scholl, T. O., Hediger, M. L., Schall, J. L., Khoo, C. S., & Fischer, R. L. (1994). Maternal growth during pregnancy and the competition for nutrients. *American Journal of Clinical Nutrition, 60*, 183–188.

Scholl, T. O., Stein, T. P., & Smith, W. K. (2000). Leptin and maternal growth during adolescent pregnancy. *American Journal of Clinical Nutrition, 72*, 1542–1547.

Schonau, E. (2004). The peak bone mass concept: Is it still relevant? *Pediatric Nephrology, 19*, 825–831.

Snyder, L. B., Milici, F. F., Slater, M., Sun, H., & Strizhakova, Y. (2006). Effects of alcohol advertising exposure on drinking among youth. *Archives of Pediatric and Adolescent Medicine, 160*, 18–24.

Steinberg, L. (2005). Cognitive and affective development in adolescence. *Trends in Cognitive Science, 9*, 69–74.

St. Onge, M. P., Keller, K. L., & Heymsfield, S. B. (2003). Changes in childhood food consumption patterns: A cause for concern in light of increasing body weights. *American Journal of Clinical Nutrition, 78*, 1068–1073.

Storey, M. L., Forshee, R. A., & Anderson, P. A. (2004). Associations of adequate intake of calcium with diet, beverage consumption, and demographic characteristics among children and adolescents. *Journal of the American College of Nutrition, 23*, 18–33.

Styne, D. M. (2003). The regulation of pubertal growth. *Hormone Research, 60*, 22–26.

Troiano, R. P., Briefel, R. R., Carroll, M. D., & Bialostosky, K. (2000). Energy and fat intakes of children and adolescents in the United States: Data from the national health and nutrition examination surveys. *American Journal of Clinical Nutrition, 72*, 1343S–1353S.

U.S. Department of Agriculture (USDA). (2005). *National School Lunch Program: Nutrition program facts*. Retrieved October 11, 2007, from www.fns.usda.gov/cnd/Lunch/AboutLunch/NSLPFactsheet.pdf

U.S. Department of Health and Human Services, Office of Applied Studies. (2003). *Results from the 2002 National Survey on Drug Use and Health: National findings*. Retrieved October 11, 2007, from http://oassamhsagov/nhsda/

Veldhuis, J. D., Roemmich, J. N., Richmond, E. J., Rogol, A. D., Lovejoy, J. C., Sheffield-Moore, M., et al. (2005). Endocrine control of body composition in infancy, childhood, and puberty. *Endocrine Reviews, 26*, 114–146.

Videon, T. M., & Manning, C. K. (2003). Influences on adolescent eating patterns: The importance of family meals. *Journal of Adolescent Health, 32*, 365–373.

Wastney, M. E., Martin, B. R., Peacock, M., Smith, D., Jiang, X. Y., Jackman, L. A., et al. (2000). Changes in calcium kinetics in adolescent girls induced by high calcium intake. *Journal of Clinical Endocrinology and Metabolism, 85,* 4470–4475.

Waylen, A., & Wolke, D. (2004). Sex 'n' drugs 'n' rock 'n' roll: The meaning and social consequences of pubertal timing. *European Journal of Endocrinology, 151,* S151–S159.

Weaver, C. M. (2000). The growing years and prevention of osteoporosis in later life. *Proceedings of the Nutrition Society, 59,* 303–306.

Weden, M. M., & Zabin, L. S. (2005). Gender and ethnic differences in the co-occurrence of adolescent risk behaviors. *Ethnic Health, 10,* 213–234.

Weitzman, M., Cook, S., Auinfer, P., Florin, T. A., Daniels, S., Nguyen, M., et al. (2005). Tobacco smoke exposure is associated with the metabolic syndrome in adolescents. *Circulation, 112,* 862–869.

Welt, C. K., Chan, J. L., Bullen, J., Murphy, R., Smith, P., DePaoli, A. M., et al. (2004). Recombinant human leptin in women with hypothalamic amenorrhea. *New England Journal of Medicine, 351,* 987–997.

Whiting, S. J., Vatanparast, H., Baxter-Jones, A., Faulkner, R. A., Mirwald, R., & Bailey, D. A. (2004). Factors that affect bone mineral accrual in the adolescent growth spurt. *Journal of Nutrition, 134,* 696S–700S.

Wilson, D. B., Smith, B. N., Speizer, I. S., Bean, M. K., Mitchell, K. S., Uguy, L. S., et al. (2005). Differences in food intake and exercise by smoking status in adolescents. *Preventive Medicine, 40,* 872–879.

Winkleby, M. A., Robinson, T. N., Sundquist, J., & Kraemer, H. C. (1999). Ethnic variation in cardiovascular disease risk factors among children and young adults: Findings from the Third National Health and Nutrition Examination Survey, 1988–1994. *Journal of the American Medical Association, 281,* 1006–1013.

Xie, B., Gilliland, F. D., Li, Y. F., & Rockett, H. R. (2003). Effects of ethnicity, family income, and education on dietary intake among adolescents. *Preventive Medicine, 36,* 30–40.

Special Topics in Prenatal and Infant Nutrition: Failure to Thrive

Claire Blais, RD, LDN, CNSD

Special Section: Genetics and Inborn Errors of Metabolism
Laura Harkness, PhD, RD; Sara Snow, MS, RD

CHAPTER OUTLINE

Reader Objectives

After studying this chapter and reflecting on the contents, you should be able to

1. Identify and classify failure to thrive.
2. Evaluate the diet of the patient with failure to thrive and describe techniques to treat failure to thrive in the outpatient and inpatient settings.
3. Discuss medical nutrition therapy for inborn errors of metabolism.

The American Academy of Pediatrics (AAP) uses two criteria for diagnosing failure to thrive (FTT). The first of these is when weight (or weight for height) falls to less than two standard deviations below the mean (z-score less than –2.0) for sex- and age-matched peers (Kleinman, 2004). The second relates to weight for age having declined across more than two major percentile lines after having achieved a previously stable growth pattern. The latter definition highlights the importance of clinical judgment when diagnosing a child with failure to thrive. Up to 39% of infants cross two major percentile lines before stabilizing into a growth pattern (Mei, Grummer-Strawn, Thompson, & Dietz, 2004), so it is prudent not to use weight for age as a single measure for identifying failure to thrive.

> ### CRITICAL **Thinking**
>
> **Clair Blais, RN, LDN, CNDS**
>
> Critical Thinking About Clinical Judgment: Never let definitions outweigh your clinical judgment. These classifications are meant to help guide your practice, not replace it. If you have a child who was born at low birth weight and is plotting consistently below the third percentile on the weight for age chart, would you classify her with failure to thrive? Some previously accepted definitions would say yes—weight for age below the third percentile classifies as failure to thrive. But use your judgment; perhaps this patient is just following her own growth curve. Someone has to be in the bottom 3%!

z-score: A numeric value assigned to the standard deviation from the mean of a data set. A z-score of 1.0 equates to one standard deviation above the mean.

A **z-score** is defined as the standard deviation from the mean. For example, in the National Center for Health Statistics (NCHS) growth charts the mean weight for age is defined by the 50th percentile. The fifth percentile expresses 1.75 standard deviations below the mean, or a z-score of 21.75. Categorizing growth according to z-scores is the most accurate technique for classifying growth failure. It is more precise than defining an infant's growth as "at or near" a percentile or "just below" a percentile (Kleinman, 2004). Nonetheless, this technique is less practical in the acute care setting, and growth charts tend to be the established norm.

It is important to distinguish children who are constitutionally small from those who are truly failing to thrive. Bone age can be useful in differentiating genetic short stature from abnormal growth (Corrales & Utter, 2004). If the bone age is less than the chronologic age, there exists potential for more growth, and the child is likely failing to thrive. If the bone age is consistent with the chronologic age, then the child is likely exhibiting genetic short stature.

Classification of Failure to Thrive

In 1972 Waterlow established criteria for comparing weight and height of a malnourished child with standards for age- and sex-matched peers. He described a weight-for-height deficit as wasting, indicating acute malnutrition, and a height-for-age deficit as stunting, indicating chronic malnutrition. No one method of classifying failure to thrive is infallible (Raynor & Rudolf, 2000), providing further evidence for the need to exercise clinical judgment when making the diagnosis of failure to thrive. The **Waterlow criteria** are still widely accepted today as among the primary classifications of pediatric malnutrition (Waterlow, 1972). The growth charts found in Appendix 1 can also be used to assess failure to thrive, which is summarized in **Table 5.1**.

Waterlow criteria: A set of calculations used to classify the severity of malnutrition in children.

The three factors that lead to energy imbalance in the failure-to-thrive population are inadequate energy intake, inefficient energy utilization, and increased energy expenditure **(Table 5.2)**. Failure to thrive can be characterized by the presence of one or more of the above conditions.

The Cultural Diversity of Poverty

Poverty is the most omnipresent of the social risk factors for failure to thrive. One study documented that 13% of its patients with poor growth were homeless, which makes access to the medical care needed to prevent and correct malnutrition difficult (Frank & Zeisel, 1988). It becomes crucial to proper treatment of your patients that you consider their socioeconomic status in designing an individualized care plan.

TABLE 5.1 NCHS Growth Charts and Failure to Thrive

Failure to thrive is defined as malnutrition resulting in inadequate physical growth as determined by failure to meet the norms established by the National Center for Health Statistics (NCHS):

* Growth below the 5th percentile, or a change in growth that has crossed two major growth percentiles (i.e., from above the 75th percentile to below the 25th) in a short time are generally accepted criteria for a diagnosis of failure to thrive.

* Growth parameters for premature infants should be corrected for gestational age until the age of 24 months for head circumference, age 24 months for weight, and age 24 months for height.

Source: PHN Guideline: Failure to Thrive. Available at: www.ok.gov/health/documentsa/Failure%20to%20thrive. Retrieved 06/04/09.

TABLE 5.2 Energy Imbalance

Inadequate Energy Intake
    Anorexia
    Inappropriate formula preparation
    Poor nutritional quality of breast milk
    Poor nutritional quality of food offered
    Poor oral feeding (including dysphagia, uncoordinated suck/swallow)
Inefficient Energy Utilization
    Frequent emesis
Gastroesophageal Reflux
    Malabsorption/maldigestion (cystic fibrosis, inflammatory bowel disease, short gut syndrome, pancreatitis)
Increased Energy Expenditure
    Bronchopulmonary dysplasia
Cancer
Congential Heart Disease
Cystic Fibrosis

Source: PHN Guideline: Failure to Thrive. Available at: www.ok.gov/health/documentsa/Failure%20to%20thrive. Retrieved 06/04/09.

There are a variety of causes for the three factors, which are broken up into two classes: organic and nonorganic. **Organic failure to thrive (OFTT)** is lack of growth associated with an identifiable disease or disorder. Almost all chronic illnesses in childhood can result in poor weight gain related to any of the factors described in Table 5.2. **Nonorganic failure to thrive (NOFTT)** is present in most of all diagnosed cases of failure to thrive (Kleinman, 2004). Children have nonorganic failure to thrive when their lack of growth cannot be attributed to an identifiable disease. The cause of nonorganic failure to thrive is psychosocial in origin. Risk factors for the development of nonorganic failure to thrive can be found in **Table 5.3.**

Organic failure to thrive: Lack of growth associated with an identifiable disease.

Nonorganic failure to thrive: Lack of growth that cannot be attributed to an identifiable disease or condition.

TABLE 5.3	Risk Factors for the Development of OFTT and NOFTT

Risk Factors for OFTT	Risk Factors for NOFTT
Bronchopulmonary dysplasia	Poverty
Cleft palate	Abuse
Cystic fibrosis	Maternal/paternal deficits in appropriate
Developmental delay	feeding practices
Fetal alcohol syndrome	Feeding difficulties
HIV/AIDS	Factors leading to poor bonding
Intrauterine growth restriction	Unwanted pregnancy
Prematurity	Mother of young age ($<$ 17 yr)
Low birth weight	Depression
Very low birth weight	Psychopathology (including Munchausen
Extremely low birth weight	syndrome by proxy
Short gut syndrome	

Source: PHN Guideline: Failure to Thrive. Available at: www.ok.gov/health/documentsa/Failure%20to%20thrive. Retrieved 06/04/09.

The development of failure to thrive is multifactorial and complex. It would be errant to assume that all cases of failure to thrive have a mutually exclusive presentation. In fact, many children present with features of both organic and nonorganic failure to thrive (Corrales & Utter, 2004).

Assessment of the Patient with Failure to Thrive

Assessment of the patient with failure to thrive should include a thorough medical, social, and nutritional evaluation. The medical evaluation should include a complete history and physical, paying careful attention to pre- and perinatal history, clinical examination, and family history, especially that of older siblings (Kleinman, 2004). The medical evaluation should also assess for lead toxicity, anemia, and zinc deficiency. A low serum alkaline phosphatase may indicate zinc deficiency. During the clinical examination the physician should observe for signs of neglect, which may include poor general hygiene, poor oral health, or diaper rash (Kleinman, 2004).

Given that the vast majority of cases of failure to thrive present with some form of inadequate caloric intake, nutritional rehabilitation should be attempted before extensive laboratory workup is commenced. A social evaluation should be conducted to assess the family dynamics and economic situation (Kleinman, 2004). During all evaluations careful attention should be paid to caregiver-child interaction, including eye contact, physical proximity, and verbalization.

The assessment performed by the nutrition professional is most essential. A thorough assessment of intake and output is necessary to evaluate truly the child's nutriture. If the infant is breast-feeding, the registered dietitian should ask if the child feeds at both breasts at each feeding, how long the child sucks at each breast, and how many times daily the child feeds. If the infant is formula feeding, careful attention must be paid to formula preparation. The most common error in formula feeding is improper dilution of the formula (Kleinman, 2004). The dietitian should determine how the formula is prepared, how much the child feeds, and how often. It is important here to be specific. Many parents are tempted to say, "2 to 3 ounces every 3 to 4 hours." This could be as little as 12 ounces of formula or as much as 24 ounces of formula. Asking a parent to keep a detailed 3- to 5-day food record is the most accurate method of determining energy intake, but a 24-hour recall can be very effective when this is not possible (Kleinman, 2004).

For the child who is also taking solid foods, it is important to ask what types and textures are being offered, how long the child takes to eat, what the portion size is and how much the child actually eats of it, and the timing of meals and snacks. The dietitian should also inquire into food allergies or intolerances, including the child's reaction to the food item. If possible, a direct observation of the feeding would be helpful. An in-home evaluation is ideal, but often an office or hospital setting must suffice. In addition to evaluating intake, the dietitian should also garner an understanding of the child's output. Number and consistency of stools and number of wet diapers (or strict measurement of urine output in the acute care setting) can be helpful in determining the child's absorptive capacity. The dietitian should also ask about spits or emesis and, if at all possible, try to quantify the frequency and volume of such spits and emesis.

It is important to inquire about the child's activity level as well, because fidgety or very active children can be difficult to feed and could also be burning off more calories than they are consuming. It is also the responsibility of the dietitian to plot the growth curves carefully, correcting for prematurity where necessary. For a child who was born premature, the weight should be corrected until the child is 24 months old, the length until the child is 40 months old, and the head circumference until the child is 18 months old (Kleinman, 2004).

The nutrition evaluation should also include an assessment of kilocalorie and protein needs for catch-up growth. The equation for catch-up growth is as follows:

$$\frac{(\text{Ideal Body Weight for Height} \times \text{RDA for Weight Age})}{\text{Current Weight}}$$

where Ideal Body Weight for Height is the weight at the 50th percentile for the current height, RDA is the Recommended Daily Allowance, and Weight Age is the age at which the current weight is at the 50th percentile (Corrales & Utter, 2004; Kleinman, 2004). This equation can be used for both kilocalorie needs and protein needs. For example, an 8-month-old male who weighs 7 kg and is 78 cm long has a weight age of 4.5 months and an ideal body weight for length of 8 kg. You would then multiply 8 kg by 108 kcal/kg and divide by 7 kg. The result is 123 kcal/kg. If the RDA for weight age is equal to the RDA for current age, then it is generally acceptable to use 120 kcal/kg as the standard reference for this value. For example, a 5-month-old female who weighs 5 kg and measures 59 cm long has a weight age of 2.5 months and an ideal body weight for length of 5.7 kg. The RDA for her weight age is the same as the RDA for her chronologic age, so we would multiply 5.7 kg by 120 kcal/kg and divide by 5 kg to get 134 kcal/kg.

Calculation of needs for catch-up growth is always an estimate. It is important to exercise clinical judgment. If a child's catch-up needs calculate out to be substantially more than his or her current level of intake, it is best to make small increases in the level of intake, following weight gain and adjusting as needed. Efforts to promote catch-up should continue until the child regains his or her previously established growth percentiles (Kleinman, 2004). The best measure of whether a child is meeting his or her needs for growth is by following the child's weight gain after interventions (Corrales & Utter, 2004). If the child is gaining weight at or above the expected rate for age, then the child is receiving adequate kilocalories. See **Table 5.4** for expected rates of weight gain by age.

Nutritional Interventions

Weight gain or loss in the hospital may not be reproducible in the home environment, and it may not distinguish between organic and nonorganic failure to thrive, so it is best to avoid hospitalization if possible (Kleinman, 2004). Many failure-to-thrive cases are initially treated in the outpatient setting, with behavioral and nutritional interventions.

Regardless of the cause of the failure to thrive, the primary intervention is to increase intake of kilocalories. This presents a unique challenge for the breast-fed infant, because breast milk is only 20 kcal/oz. What will inevitably take place is that the mother will pump her breast milk, add infant formula powder or other modular kilocalorie supplements to the breast milk to fortify it, and feed this to the infant by bottle. In a case where malnutrition is present, the benefits of direct nursing are outweighed

<table>
<tr><td colspan="2">**TABLE 5.4** Expected Rates of Growth by Age</td></tr>
</table>

Age	Expected growth (g/day)
Preterm infant	15–30
0–3 months	20–30
3–7 months	15–21
7–12 months	10–13
1–7 years	5–8

Source: PHN Guideline: Failure to Thrive. Available at: www.ok.gov/health/documentsa/Failure%20to%20thrive. Retrieved 06/04/09.

by the infant's need for adequate kilocalories. In the formula-fed infant the first intervention is to concentrate the formula to a higher caloric density. This can be done by concentration up to 24 kcal/oz and by modular kilocalorie supplements as needed up to 30 kcal/oz. The modular kilocalorie supplements typically used are in the form of fat or glucose polymers. It is not generally recognized as safe to concentrate beyond 24 kcal/oz strictly from powder, because the potential renal solute load becomes too high for the infant and vomiting and dehydration could occur (Corrales & Utter, 2004).

For the child who is taking additional solid foods, adding kilocalories to food without adding volume becomes imperative to maximize their intake. Parents should be taught label reading to offer their infants younger than 12 months old high-kilocalorie baby foods. These foods can also be fortified with small amounts of infant cereal, glucose polymer modular supplements, corn oil, or margarine. Children over 1 year of age can be offered drinks with added powdered skim milk, instant breakfast powder, glucose polymer modular supplements, table sugar, or corn oil. Cheese, gravy, margarine, peanut butter, and cream cheese can be added to solid foods, in addition to the supplements listed above for beverage addition. Juice should be limited to 4 ounces daily or eliminated completely from the diet (Corrales & Utter, 2004).

It is important to teach caregivers to develop a standard mealtime routine with their children. Some suggestions for what to tell caregivers are as follows (University of Iowa, 2002):

- Set definitive meal and snack times, and limit their duration to 30 minutes or less.
- Do not allow eating between scheduled meals and snacks, regardless of how much was eaten at the previous feeding.
- Always feed your child at the table in a high chair or a booster seat.
- Praise the positive behaviors.
- Ignore the negative behaviors.
- Allow your child to get messy while eating.
- Model good eating behavior.

Another less common approach to treatment includes the use of appetite stimulants. Homnick and coworkers (2004) found the use of appetite stimulants such as cyproheptadine to be effective in promoting weight gain among individuals aged 5 and older with organic failure to thrive; however, the AAP and U.S. Food and Drug Administration (FDA) believe the costs outweigh the benefits of the use of this appetite stimulant in infants with failure to thrive (Kleinman, 2004).

Occasionally, when behavioral management fails and the child continues to fail to take adequate amounts of nutrition by mouth, a nasogastric feeding tube must be placed. It is up to the health care team to determine how much of the child's nutrition will be administered through the tube at this point, but it generally depends on how much the child can reliably take by mouth. In most cases 75% to 77% of the child's nutritional needs should be provided through nasogastric feedings. For infants under age 1 year, standard infant formulas can be given. It is best to start with the standard dilution of 20 kcal/oz and advance by 2 kcal/oz daily as tolerated by the infant until the goal concentration is met. The same rules for concentrating infant formula and breast milk for oral feedings apply to tube feedings as well. For children over 1 year of age, a standard 30 kcal/oz pediatric formula can be used, provided there is no cow's milk protein allergy present. If the child is allergic, there are a variety of hydrolyzed protein and hypoallergenic formulas available on the market. Full-strength feedings should be initiated at a low rate and advanced slowly as tolerated, monitoring for vomiting, diarrhea, or abdominal distension. If it becomes evident that the child will need aggressive nutrition supplementation for a period of several weeks to months, it would be wise to consider more permanent enteral access, typically in the form of a gastrostomy tube.

The prognosis of children with failure to thrive depends largely on the severity of the illness and the risk factors present. Evidence from studies on the effects on cognitive development in children with a history of failure to thrive in infancy has shown an adverse effect on intellectual outcomes in older childhood (Corbett & Drewett, 2004). A multidisciplinary team (a registered dietitian, a speech-language pathologist, and an occupational therapist, at a minimum) approach to the treatment of the patient with failure to thrive is the most effective method of intervention in these patients. In many cases prognosis can be excellent if the diagnosis is made early enough and intervention is commenced immediately (Corrales & Utter, 2004).

Summary

Individualized medical nutrition therapy must be initiated immediately upon diagnosis of an inborn error of metabolism. Nutrition therapy is necessary to prevent further adverse health outcomes and to optimize growth and development. Medical nutrition therapy must be continuously monitored to ensure that the individual needs of each patient are being met and that blood levels of key substances are being monitored. In addition, for some inborn errors of metabolism, consumption of foods may cause physical distress such as gastrointestinal (GI) pain, and the individual may be reluctant to eat foods or may develop anorexia. In planning nutrition support, a formal dietary prescription must be carefully written, including all macronutrients and key micronutrients as well as fluid. A plan for monitoring the nutrition support must also be enacted to ensure that both physical and biochemical status are monitored regularly. Last, compliance with the medical nutrition therapy is a very challenging area and must be constantly supported to enable parents and patients to maintain their diet.

"Failure to thrive" is a term used to describe children whose growth is significantly below that of their peers. This term has been used for centuries but remains controversial (Kleinman, 2004). There exists no one agreed-on definition for failure to thrive but rather several clinically acceptable diagnostic criteria. This section touched on some of these diagnostic criteria as well as accepted methods for classifying malnutrition in the pediatric population. It reviewed necessary components of the medical and nutritional evaluation of the patient with failure to thrive and described several techniques found to be effective in treatment of failure to thrive. Because there are so many factors that can contribute to the development of failure to thrive, outcomes are variable. Continued education and heightened awareness of clinicians is necessary to prevent and treat failure to thrive in at-risk populations.

Case Studies

(Answers to all case studies are in the Instructor's Manual available at jbpub.com.)

Case Study: Failure to Thrive

MN is a 2-year, 2-month-old boy admitted to the hospital with failure to thrive. As the clinical dietitian you are consulted to evaluate this patient on his first day of admission. In your chart review you determine that he was a full-term infant and was strictly breast-fed until he was 6 months old; he then began to take rice cereal and eventually strained fruits and vegetables were added to his diet. During your interview mom reports that MN is difficult to feed. He throws food on the floor, plays with it, pushes the spoon away, laughs at his older brothers (ages 4 and 7), and generally does not seem interested in eating. It takes him over an hour to eat each meal and snack, and it is not a pleasant experience for the patient or his mother.

Continues

Birth Wt: 7 lb, 2 oz
Birth Length: 20.5″
12-month check-up: 19 lb, 6 oz
Current Wt: 9.86 kg
Current Length: 90.5 cm
Labs: unremarkable, albumin WNL
Meds: none
24-hr Recall
Breakfast: 6–8 oz orange juice, ½ cup toasted oat o-shaped cereal, ½ banana, sliced. MN mostly throws the cereal on the floor and mashes the banana into his hair.
Morning snack: 4–6 oz apple juice, 2–3 wheat crackers, 1 string cheese.
Lunch: 8 oz whole milk, 1 cup spaghetti with tomato sauce. MN very much enjoys the milk, but most of the spaghetti ends up on his clothes and in the high chair.
Afternoon snack: 4 oz water, ½ cup cooked carrot coins.
Dinner: 8 oz whole milk, 1 to 2 chicken nuggets, a few bites of corn.
Dessert: 8 oz whole milk, a few bites of chocolate brownie.

Questions

1. Other than the information provided above, what other questions would you ask the mother?
2. What other services do you believe should be consulted for this patient while in the hospital?
3. Plot MN's weights on a NCHS growth chart. Describe his weight trend.
4. Estimate MN's calorie and protein needs.
5. What suggestions can you give to MN's mother?

SPECIAL SECTION: GENETICS AND INBORN ERRORS OF METABOLISM
Laura Harkness, PhD, RD, and Sara Snow, MS, RD

Autosomal recessive: Both parents must be carriers of a gene on one of the autosomal (non-sex) chromosomes for a child to inherit the disease. If both parents are carriers, there is a 25% chance that the child will inherit the disease and a 50% chance the child will be a carrier.

The inheritance of a genetic disease is determined by whether the gene is dominant or recessive as well as the type of chromosome that carries the gene (autosomal or sex chromosome). **Autosomal recessive** describes a form of inheritance of genetic traits located on the autosomes (the non-sex chromosomes 1–22). Sex-linked diseases are inherited through the X chromosome (because diseases cannot be inherited through the Y chromosome).

A recessive gene is an allele that causes a phenotype (a detectable or visible characteristic) that is seen only on a homozygous genotype (one with two copies of the same allele). Each of us has two copies of every gene on an autosomal chromosome, one from the mother and one from the father.

For a child to inherit a recessive disease, both parents must carry at least one gene for the disease and the child must inherit two abnormal alleles; in other words, the individual is homozygous for the trait. If only one gene is inherited, the child will not have the disease but will be a carrier and can pass the gene on to future generations.

If both parents are carriers (heterozygous for the trait), there is a 25% chance a child will inherit two abnormal genes and inherit the disease and a 50% chance a child will inherit one abnormal gene and be a carrier for the disease. If only one parent is a carrier, the trait will occur only if the other parent is also a carrier of the trait.

Inborn errors of metabolism: Traits arising from a variation in the structure of enzymes or protein molecules.

The number and complexity of **inborn errors of metabolism** present a notable challenge to health care providers. More than 300 genetic disorders are associated with adverse production, either deficiency, excess, or altered metabolism, of normally occurring cellular compounds (Burton, 1998). Because early diagnosis and treatment are vitally important to prevent poor outcomes in infants born with inherited metabolic disorders, newborn screening programs are common nationwide to diagnose many of these genetic disorders. In many cases early treatment has been shown to be effective in reducing long-term risks in such disorders as phenylketonuria (PKU), maple syrup urine disease (MSUD), isovaleric academia, and galactosemia. For some inborn errors of metabolism, medical nutrition therapy is the primary treatment modality and will prevent manifestation of toxic substances. Unfortunately, diagnosis of genetic disorders often takes place after irreversible damage has occurred. Early diagnosis and appropriate medical nutrition therapy are paramount to optimal patient outcome.

For nutritional management of inborn errors of metabolism, use of restricted diets and medical nutritional foods are principal components of disease treatment. Medical nutrition therapy must be maximized to maintain normal growth and development. Frequently, energy needs are higher in individuals with inborn errors of metabolism, because protein, carbohydrate, or fat is restricted. Children can require supplemental feedings in the form of enteral or parenteral support to promote growth and to prevent protein catabolism. For inborn errors of metabolism of essential amino acids, it is not possible to completely eliminate the amino acids from the diet for a long period of time without causing adverse outcomes, so careful and continuous monitoring of biochemical measures is crucial. In addition, identifying and managing all key metabolic pathways and compounds that are affected by the inborn error are essential for adequate medical nutritional therapy. The adverse consequences that can result from inborn errors of metabolism include accumulation of toxic substances both locally and remotely, loss of production of key intermediates and products, increased production of intermediates or products that are normally produced in small amounts, lack of substrates for formation of biological compounds, and loss of normal feedback compounds that normally inhibit or stimulate other pathways (Elsas & Acosta, 2006). Therefore, the purpose of this section is to review the more prevalent inborn errors of metabolism and to discuss key aspects of medical nutrition therapy management.

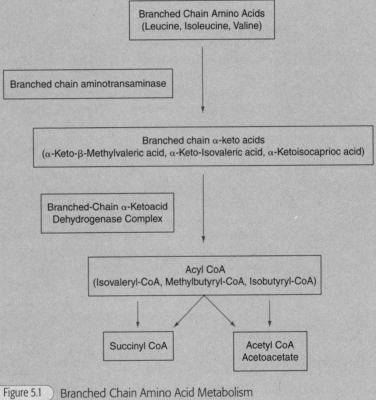

Very low birth weight (VLBW): Birth weight of less than 1,500 g.

Extremely low birth weight: Birth weight of less than 1,000 g.

Small for gestational age (SGA): Birth weight plots below the 10th percentile (see Appendix 1).

Intrauterine growth restriction: When an infant has not achieved his or her full in utero growth potential.

Prematurity: Less than 37 weeks gestation at birth.

Figure 5.1 Branched Chain Amino Acid Metabolism

Branched Chain Amino Acids and Inborn Errors of Metabolism

The **branched chain amino acids** (BCAAs) (leucine, valine, and isoleucine) constitute most of the essential amino acids in healthy individuals, accounting for 40% of essential amino acids. The primary role of BCAAs is incorporation into body proteins. In newborns 75% of BCAAs are used for the synthesis of protein. BCAAs are an important source of nitrogen for the synthesis of nonessential amino acids. Those not used in protein metabolism are catabolized to provide intermediates (acetyl-coenzyme A [CoA], succinyl-CoA, and acetoacetate) for energy metabolism. The BCAAs share common first steps in catabolism with tricarboxylic acid cycle intermediates. This irreversible oxidative decarboxylation of the keto acids yields intermediates for energy metabolism **(Figure 5.1)**.

Branched chain amino acids: Leucine, isoleucine, and valine; present in and help maintain skeletal muscle tissue; important in gluconeogenesis.

Maple Syrup Urine Disease (Branched Chain Alpha-Ketoaciduria)

Maple syrup urine disease is a defect in the metabolism of the BCAAs (isoleucine, leucine, and valine). This autosomal recessive disorder is caused by a deficiency of branched chain α-ketoacid dehydrogenase, which is needed for the oxidative decarboxylation of the keto acids that are produced from the BCAAs. The result is accumulation of the BCAAs in the plasma (Harris et al., 1990).

> **Maple syrup urine disease (MSUD):** An autosomal recessive disorder characterized by a defect in the metabolism of the branched chain amino acids isoleucine, leucine, and valine caused by a deficiency of branched chain α-ketoacid dehydrogenase resulting in the accumulation of the branched chain amino acids in the plasma.

MSUD is rare in the general population (1/100,000 to 1/300,000 births) but has a high incidence (1/200 to 1/700 births) in the Mennonite population. In 1954 Menkes and colleagues at Boston Children's Hospital first described MSUD. Menkes, Hurst, and Craig (1954) documented the deaths of four children from the same family. All the children displayed severe ketoacidosis in the first week of life, and their urine had a strong smell of maple syrup.

Nutrition Therapy for MSUD

Long-term nutrition therapy is required to provide appropriate dietary BCAA intake to support optimal growth and development while maintaining plasma concentrations of BCAA at nontoxic levels. Timely initiation of nutrition therapy is key to preventing impaired physical and mental development. The aim of the therapeutic regime in MSUD is to keep the concentration of toxic metabolites within individual tolerance limits. BCAAs are essential amino acids and therefore cannot be eliminated from the diet. BCAA requirement in patients with MSUD is mainly determined using indirect markers such as growth and elimination of symptoms. Direct measurement of BCAA requirements in patients with MSUD has been done using indicator amino acid oxidation technique (Riazi et al., 2004). Total mean BCAA requirement was found to be 45 mg/kg/day with an upper limit of 62 mg/kg/day (Raizi et al., 2004). Nutritionally complete protein substitutes, free from leucine, isoleucine, and valine, are used to provide protein and calories for patients with MSUD (Hallam, Lilburn, & Lee, 2005).

The long-term restriction of BCAA intake in diets has proven effective in controlling plasma BCAA levels and mitigating some of the neurologic manifestations. Individualized nutrition therapy must be carefully planned to provide for adequate growth and development while maintaining BCAA concentrations at nontoxic levels. Nutrition therapy that is frequently modified is necessary using laboratory analysis of plasma BCAA concentrations. Long-term plasma leucine levels are associated with impaired cognitive outcome in patients with classic MSUD. To achieve the best possible intellectual outcome for affected individuals, the target range for plasma leucine should not exceed 200 mmol/L in children (Hoffman, Helbling, Schadewaldt, & Wendel, 2006). All patients with MSUD should be evaluated for thiamin responsiveness, because some forms of MSUD respond to thiamin therapy. Thiamin-responsive MSUD is due to a reduced affinity of the mutant branched chain alpha-keto acid dehydrogenase for thiamin pyrophosphate (Chuang, Ku, & Cox, 1982). For these patients, 100 to 500 mg of oral thiamin should be provided for up to 3 months (Fernhoff, 1985).

Figure 5.2   Phenylalanine Conversion to Tyrosine

Aromatic Amino Acids and Inborn Errors of Metabolism

Phenylalanine Metabolism

Phenylalanine is an essential amino acid used for tissue protein synthesis and hydroxylation reactions that result in the formation of tyrosine. The reaction requires phenylalanine hydroxylase, tetrahydrobiopterin, and dihydropteridine reductase (Scriver, Kaufman, Eisensmith, & Woo, 2001) **(Figure 5.2)**. Hyperphenylalaninemia is caused by a defect in phenylalanine hydroxylase activity. If phenylalanine hydroxylase or its cofactor tetrahydrobiopterin is absent or deficient, phenylalanine accumulates in body fluids and the central nervous system and tyrosine becomes an essential amino acid (Behrman, Kleigman, & Arvin, 1996; Scriver et al., 2001).

Hyperphenylalaninemia primarily affects the brain tissue. The high concentration of phenylalanine interferes with the transport of the amino acids tyrosine and tryptophan into the brain (Behrman et al., 1996). Tyrosine is needed to provide energy and to synthesize protein, catecholamines, melanin, and thyroid hormones (Elsas & Acosta, 2006). Excess phenylalanine in the blood results in the accumulation of phenyl ketones that are excreted in the urine—thus the term **phenylketonuria**.

Phenylketonuria: A form of hyperphenylalaninemia caused by the complete or near complete deficiency of the liver enzyme phenylalanine hydroxylase resulting in an accumulation of phenylalanine in body fluids and the central nervous system.

Phenylketonuria

Phenylketonuria (PKU), first described in 1933, is a form of hyperphenylalaninemia, defined as plasma phenylalanine value above 120 mM (2 mg/dL) (Scriver et al., 2001). It is an autosomal recessive disorder caused by the complete or near complete deficiency of the liver enzyme phenylalanine hydroxylase. The most severe form is classic PKU. The observation that phenylpyruvic acid was excreted in the urine of patients with mental defects was the first identification of a specific chemical deficiency in a central nervous system disorder (Udenfriend, 1961). Untreated, PKU can result in severe to profound mental retardation and behavioral difficulties. The severity of the disease can vary with each affected person. Mild and moderate PKU are less severe forms and carry less risk for brain damage; however, most patients with the disorder need to follow a lifelong restricted diet.

At least 200 different mutations that cause the "PKU phenotype" have been identified. They involve deletions in coding frames, missense mutations, and intron splice mutations (Scriver et al., 2001). PKU is an autosomal recessive disorder (both parents must have and pass on the gene). A rare disorder, PKU occurs in approximately 1 in 13,500 to 19,000 newborns. The incidence of non-PKU hyperphenylalaninemia is 1 in 48,000. PKU is more common in whites and Native Americans and occurs less often in African-Americans, Hispanics, and Asians (National Institutes of Health [NIH], Consensus Development Panel, 2006). It is also common in those of Irish descent (Acosta & Yannicelli, 2001; Elsas & Acosta, 2006).

Clinical Symptoms and Diagnosis of PKU

The infant with PKU is normal at birth. Mental retardation can develop over time and may not be evident for the first few months. Left untreated, mental retardation can become severe. On physical examination, infants with PKU are lighter in complexion than their siblings and have blue eyes and fair skin because phenylalanine cannot be converted to melanin. Some appear with seborrheic or eczematoid rash that disappears as the child gets older. A musty odor caused by phenylacetic acid may be present in the child's breath, skin, and/or urine. Most infants with PKU are hypertonic with hyperactive deep tendon reflexes. Twenty-five percent of children have seizures, with more than 50% exhibiting electroencephalographic abnormalities. Other common findings include microencephaly, prominent maxilla with widely spread teeth, enamel hyperplasia, and growth retardation (Behrman et al., 1996).

Newborn screening and subsequent dietary treatment of PKU have significantly reduced the incidence of severe mental retardation (MacCready, 1974; Luder & Greene, 1989; Koch et al., 2003). Screening for PKU was initiated in the early 1960s after the Guthrie bacterial inhibition assay was developed (Guthrie, 1961; Guthrie & Susi, 1963). All states require that newborns be screened for PKU. Blood is routinely collected from the infant's heel within the first 24 to 48 hours of life after protein ingestion (Behrman et al., 1996). Criteria for a positive PKU screen can vary state to state, and decision-making policies, funding, and availability of follow-up services can also vary. Because of this, not all newborns and families have the same level of care for PKU (NIH, 2006). In addition to newborn testing, prenatal screening can be done using chorionic villus sampling, DNA analysis, or enzyme assay (Scriver et al., 2001). Early screening coupled with early dietary treatment has led to major improvements in the intellectual and behavioral outcomes for persons with PKU (Fishler, Azen, Henderson, Friedman, & Koch, 1987; Fishler, Azen, Friedman, & Koch, 1989).

Medical Nutrition Therapy for PKU

Treatment of PKU involves the immediate and lifelong avoidance of excess dietary phenylalanine. It was once thought that the diet could be discontinued in adolescence, but today it is recommended the diet be followed for life (Scriver et al., 2001; Elsas & Acosta, 2006). The diet provides supplemental tyrosine and small amounts of phenylalanine for essential functions. Frequent laboratory testing and growth records are used to determine phenylalanine and tyrosine requirements. Requirements differ for each person depending on the extent of phenylalanine hydroxylase deficiency, age, health status, and, for pregnant women, the stage of pregnancy. The diet consists of phenylalanine-free medical foods that supply protein and essential nutrients and measured amounts of low-protein foods and free foods (foods with little or no phenylalanine). High-protein foods such as meat, fish, poultry, eggs, dairy products, nuts, dried beans, and peas are not allowed. Foods without PHE, such as sugar, oil, and pure starch, are added as needed to meet energy needs. Although expensive, low-protein specialty products such as bread, pasta, and baking mixes are available and can help to provide variety. A diet that is too low in phenylalanine may cause a phenylalanine deficiency, which could cause harm; thus, small, measured amounts of low-protein foods such as cereals, fruits, and vegetables are allowed (Acosta & Yannicelli, 2001; NIH, 2006). The amount of protein may be greater than the Dietary Reference Intake when an elemental formula is the primary source of protein equivalent (Acosta, Yannicelli, Singh, et al., 2003). Aspartame products should not be used because they contain 56% phenylalanine. Baby formulas and breast milk contain phenylalanine, so infants must be fed phenylalanine-free formula; however, some infants can tolerate a measured amount of breast milk depending on the level of enzyme deficiency (Acosta & Yannicelli, 2001; Elsas & Acosta, 2006).

The strict limitations of the diet make compliance difficult and lead to noncompliance in 80% of patients (Walter et al., 2002). In addition, nutrient deficiencies, such as vitamin B_{12}, are associated with protein restriction (Hanley, Feigenbaum, Clarke, Schoonheyt, & Austin, 1996; Robinson et al., 2000). As a result, researchers have been investigating alternatives to traditional diet therapy. The transport of phenylalanine across the blood-brain barrier has been shown to be completely inhibited by dietary supplementation of large neutral amino acids in adults who have been unable to follow the PKU diet (Pietz et al., 1999; Weglage et al., 2001; Moats, Moseley, Koch, & Nelson, 2003). Treatment using tetrahydrobiopterin, a cofactor of phenylalanine hydroxylase, has been shown to decrease blood phenylalanine in tetrahydrobiopterin-sensitive PKU, although more research needs to be done to find the optimal dose (Trefz, Scheible, Frauendienst-Egger, Korall, & Blau, 2005).

Disorders of Carbohydrate Metabolism

Galactosemia

Most cases of **galactosemia** are categorized as classic, or type I, galactosemia and are caused by mutations in the GALT gene. This gene produces the enzyme galactose-1-phosphate uridyl-transferase, which is important in processing galactose. Mutations in the GALT gene cause two forms of type I galactosemia, classic and Duarte variant. Individuals with the classic type of galactosemia lack nearly all the enzyme activity necessary to metabolize galactose. Individuals with the Duarte variant have approximately 5% to 20% of the enzyme activity necessary to metabolize galactose and often do not have signs or symptoms of galactosemia (Podskarbi et al., 1996). Classic galactosemia is an inherited disorder that occurs in approximately 1 in 30,000 live births. The incidence of the Duarte variant, a mild type of galactosemia, is more common. This variant affects an estimated 1 in 16,000 live births (Tyfield et al., 1999).

Galactosemia: An inborn error of metabolism caused by a deficiency of galactosyl-1-phosphate uridyl-transferase, which inhibits glycogen breakdown and glucose synthesis, causing severe hypoglycemia after the ingestion of glucose.

Clinical Symptoms and Diagnosis of Galactosemia

Vomiting, liver enlargement, and jaundice are often the earliest signs of the disease, but bacterial infections (often severe), irritability, failure to gain weight, and diarrhea may also occur (Bosch, 2006). If unrecognized in the newborn period, the disease may produce liver, brain, eye, and kidney damage; thus, galactosemia should be considered in any jaundiced infant (Bosch, 2006). Galactosemia is diagnosed by measuring levels of galactose-1-phosphate uridyl-transferase. In patients with galactosemia there is no enzyme activity. If infants are fed galactose-containing feedings, there will be large amounts of galactose excreted in urine (Bosch, 2006).

Medical Nutrition Therapy for Galactosemia

Nutrition therapy is to provide a galactose-free diet by using galactose-free foods. For infants with galactosemia, feeding special galactose- and lactose-free formula is required. Infants cannot be fed breast milk. With early therapy any liver damage that occurred in the first few days of life will nearly completely heal. Careful lifelong monitoring of dietary therapy must be maintained, including elimination of both lactose and galactose from the diet. Galactose is found mainly in milk and dairy products as part of lactose, but it is also contained in galactoproteins and galactolipids in others foods. The use of galactose-restricted diets must include attention to galactose contributions from all food sources, including bound galactose found in meat, dairy, and cereals as well as free galactose in peas, lentils, some legumes, organ meats, cereals, and some fruits and vegetables (Gropper, Weese, West, & Gross, 2000; Weese, Gosnell, West, & Gropper, 2003).

Careful monitoring of growth in children with galactosemia is important, because altered growth has been found with decreased height, less fat mass, and less lean body mass (Panis, Forgot, Nieman, Van Kroonenburgh, & Rubio-Gozalbo, 2005). Long-term complications usually develop in patients with galactosemia, despite a restricted diet. Complications, including mental retardation, motor abnormalities, hypergonadotropic hypogonadism, and speech disorders, are common (Bosch, 2006).

Issues to Debate

1. When is it appropriate to feed an infant nasogastrically? Moreover, when does it become imperative?
2. At what point should permanent enteral access be considered in a failure-to-thrive infant or toddler?

Websites

Failure to Thrive

American Academy of Pediatrics (AAP) www.aap.org
American Dietetic Association (ADA) www.eatright.org

Genetic and Inborn Errors of Metabolism

Medline Plus http://www.nlm.nih.gov/medlineplus/ency/article/002438.htm
Medline Plus http://www.nlm.nih.gov/medlineplus/ency/article/001166.htm
Maple Syrup Urine Disease www.nlm.nih.gov/medlineplus/ency/article/000373.htm

References

Failure to Thrive

Corbett, S. S., & Drewett, R. F. (2004). To what extent is failure to thrive in infancy associated with poorer cognitive development? A review and meta-analysis. *Journal of Child Psychology and Psychiatry, 45,* 741–754.

Corrales, K. M., & Utter, S. L. (2004). Failure to thrive. In P. Q. Samour, K. K. Helm, & C. E. Lang (Eds.), *Handbook of Pediatric Nutrition* (2nd ed., pp. 395–412). Sudbury, MA: Jones and Bartlett.

Feldman, R., Keren, M., Gross-Rozval, O., & Tyano, S. (2004). Mother-touch patterns in infant feeding disorders: Relation to maternal, child, and environmental factors. *Journal of the American Academy of Child and Adolescent Psychiatry, 43,* 1089–1097.

Fomon, S. J., Haschke, F., Zeigler, E. E., & Nelson, S. E. (1982). Body composition of reference children from birth to age 10 years. *American Journal of Clinical Nutrition, 35,* 1169–1175.

Frank, D. A., & Zeisel, S. H. (1988). Failure to thrive. *Pediatric Clinics of North America, 35,* 1187–1207.

Homnick, D. N., Homnick, B. D., Reeves, A. J., Marks, J. H., Pimentel, R. S., & Bonnema, S. K. (2004). Cyproheptadine is an effective appetite stimulant in cystic fibrosis. *Pediatric Pulmonology, 38,* 129–134.

Kleinman, R. E. (2004). Failure to thrive (pediatric undernutrition). In American Academy of Pediatrics and R. E.

Kleinman (Eds.), *Pediatric Nutrition Handbook* (5th ed., pp. 443–458). Elk Grove, IL: American Academy of Pediatrics.

Mei, Z., Grummer-Strawn, L. M., Thompson, D., & Dietz, W. H. (2004). Shifts in percentiles of growth during early childhood: Analysis of longitudinal data from the California Child Health and Development Study. *Pediatrics, 113,* e717–e727.

Raynor, P., & Rudolf, M. C. (2000). Anthropometric indices of failure to thrive. *Archives of Disease in Childhood, 82,* 374–375.

Waterlow, C. (1972). Classification and definition of protein-calorie malnutrition. *British Medical Journal, 3,* 577–579.

University of Iowa. (2002). "Mealtime routine" suggestions. Adapted from Intensive Course in Pediatric Nutrition, University of Iowa, Iowa City, May 7–10, 2002.

Genetics and Inborn Errors of Metabolism

Acosta, P. (1995). Nutrition support of maternal phenylketonuria. *Seminars in Perinatology, 19,* 182–190.

Acosta, P., Matalon, K., Castiglioni, L., Rohr, F. J., Wenz, E., Austin, V., et al. (2001). Intake of major nutrients by women in the Maternal Phenylketonuria (MPKU) Study and effects on plasma phenylalanine concentrations. American *Journal of Clinical Nutrition, 73,* 792–796.

Acosta, P., & Yannicelli, S. (2001). *The Ross Metabolic Formula System: Nutrition Support Protocols* (4th ed.). Columbus, OH: Abbott Laboratories.

Behrman, R. E., Kleigman, R. M., & Arvin, A. A. (1996). *Nelson Textbook of Pediatrics* (15th ed.) Philadelphia: W. B. Saunders.

Behrman, R. E., Kleigman, R. M., & Arvin, A. A. (2004). *Nelson Textbook of Pediatrics* (17th ed.). Philadelphia: W. B. Saunders.

Bosch, A. M. (2006). Classical galactosaemia revisited. *Journal of Inherited Metabolic Disease,* July 11 [epub]. Retrieved October 29, 2007, from http://www.springerlink.com/content/102938/

Burton, B. K. (1998). Inborn errors of metabolism in infancy: A guide to diagnosis. *Pediatrics, 102,* 69–78.

Chuang, D. T., Ku, L. S., & Cox, R. P. (1982). Thiamin-responsive maple-syrup-urine disease: Decreased affinity of the mutant branched-chain alpha-keto acid dehydrogenase for alpha-ketoisovalerate and thiamin pyrophosphate. *Proceedings of the National Academies of Science, 79,* 3300–3304.

Elsas, L. J., & Acosta, P. B. (2006). Inherited metabolic disease: Amino acids, organic acids, and galactose. In M. E. Shils, M. Shike, A. C. Ross, B. Caballero, & R. J. Cousins (Eds.), *Modern Nutrition in Health and Disease* (9th ed., pp. 909–959). Baltimore: Williams & Wilkins.

Fisch, R. O., Chang, P. N., Weisberg, S., Gulberg, P., Guttler, F., & Tsai, M. Y. (1995). Phenylketonuria patients decades after diet discontinuation. *Journal of Inherited Metabolic Disease, 18,* 347–353.

Fishler, K., Azen, C. G., Friedman, E. G., & Koch, R. (1989). School achievement in treated PKU children. *Journal of Mental Deficiency Research, 33,* 493–498.

Fishler, K., Azen, C. G., Henderson, R., Friedman, E. G., & Koch, R. (1987). Psychoeducational findings among children treated for phenylketonuria. *Journal of Mental Deficiency Research, 92,* 65–73.

Gropper, S. S., Weese, S. J. O., West, P. A., & Gross, K. C. (2000). Free galactose content of fresh fruits and strained fruits and vegetable baby foods: More foods to consider for the galactose-restricted diet. *Journal of the American Dietetic Association, 100,* 573–575.

Guthrie, R. (1961). Blood screening for phenylketonuria. *Journal of the American Medical Association, 178,* 863.

Guthrie, R., & Susi, A. (1963). A simple phenylalanine method for detecting phenylketonuria in large populations of newborn infants. *Pediatrics, 32,* 338–343.

Hallam, P., Lilburn, M., & Lee, P. J. (2005). A new protein substitute for adolescents and adults with maple syrup urine disease (MSUD). *Journal of Inherited Metabolic Disease, 28,* 665–672.

Hanley, W. B., Feigenbaum, A. S., Clarke, J. T., Schoonheyt, W. E., & Austin, V. J. (1996). Vitamin B12 deficiency in adolescents and young adults with phenylketonuria. *European Journal of Pediatrics, 155,* 145S–147S.

Harris, R. A., Zhang, B., Goodwin, G. W., Kuntz, M. J., Shimomura, Y., Rougraff, P., et al. (1990). Regulation of the branched-chain alpha-ketoacid dehydrogenase and elucidation of a molecular basis for maple syrup urine disease. *Advances in Enzyme Regulation, 30,* 245–263.

Hoffman, B., Helbling, C., Schadewaldt, P., & Wendel, U. (2006). Impact of longitudinal plasma leucine levels on the intellectual outcome in patients with classic MSUD. *Pediatric Research, 59,* 17–20.

Luder, A. S., & Greene, C. L. (1989). Maternal phenylketonuria and hyperphenylalanemia: implications for medical practice in the United States. *American Journal of Obsetrics and Gynocology, 161,* 1102–1105.

Koch, R., Moseley, K. D., Yano, S., Nelson, M. Jr., & Moats, R. A. Large neutral amino acid therapy and phenylketonuria: a promising approach to treatment. *Molecular Genetics and Metabolism, 79,* 110–113.

Moats, R. A., Moseley, K. D., Koch, R., & Nelson, M. (2003). Brain phenylalanine concentrations in phenylketonuria: Research and treatment of adults. *Pediatrics, 112,* 1575–1579.

National Institutes of Health (NIH), Consensus Development Panel. (2006). National Institutes of Health Consensus Development Conference statement: Phenylketonuria: screening and management, October 16–18, 2000. *Pediatrics, 105,* 972–982.

Panis, B., Forgot, P. P., Nieman, F. H., Van Kroonenburgh, M. J., & Rubio-Gozalbo, M. E. (2005). Body composition in children with galactosemia. *Journal of Inherited Metabolic Disease, 28,* 931–937.

Pietz, J., Kreis, R., Rupp, A., Mayatepek, E., Rating, D., Boesch, C., et al. (1999). Large neutral amino acids block phenylalanine transport into brain tissue in patients with phenylketonuria. *Journal of Clinical Investigation, 103,* 1169–1178.

Podskarbi, T., Kohlmetz, T., Gathof, B. S., Kleinlein, B., Bieger, W. P., Gresser, U., et al. (1996). Molecular characterization of Duarte-1 and Duarte-2 variants of galactose-1-phosphate uridyltransferase. *Journal of Inherited Metabolic Disease, 19,* 638–644.

Riazi, R., Rafii, M., Clarke, J. T. R., Wykes, L. J., Ball, R. O., & Pencharz, P. B. (2004). Total branched chain amino acids requirements in patients with maple syrup urine disease by use of indicator amino acid oxidation with L-$[1-_{13}C]$ phenylalanine. *American Journal of Physiology, Endocrinology and Metabolism, 287,* E142–E149.

Scriver, C. R., Kaufman, S., Eisensmith, R., & Woo, S. L. C. (2001). The hyperphenylalaninemias. In C. R. Scriver, A. L. Beaudet, W. S. Sly, & D. Valle (Eds.), *The Metabolic and Molecular Basis of Inherited Disease* (8th ed.). New York: McGraw-Hill.

Trefz, F. K., Scheible, D., Frauendienst-Egger, G., Korall, H., & Blau, N. (2005). Long-term treatment of patients with mild and classical phenylketonuria by tetrahydrobiopterin. *Molecular Genetics and Metabolism, 86,* 75S–80S.

Udenfriend, S. (1961). Phenylketonuria. *American Journal of Clinical Nutrition, 9,* 691–694.

Waterlow, C. (1972). Classification and definition of protein-calorie malnutrition. *British Medical Journal, 3,* 577–579.

Weese, S. J., Gosnell, K., West, P., & Gropper, S. S. (2003). Galactose content of baby food meats: Considerations for infants with galactosemia. *Journal of the American Dietetic Association, 103,* 373–375.

Special Topics in Toddler and Preschool Nutrition: Vitamins and Minerals in Childhood

Aaron Owens, MS, RD

CHAPTER OUTLINE

Vitamins

Water-Soluble Vitamins • Fat-Soluble Vitamins • Multiple Vitamin Supplementation

Minerals

Calcium • Iron • Magnesium • Potassium • Phosphorus • Copper • Zinc • Selenium • Iodine • Chromium

Reader Objectives

After studying this chapter and reflecting on the contents, you should be able to

1. Recognize the overall purposes of vitamin and mineral functions in growth and development.
2. Review the specific contributions of the major vitamins in growth and development.
3. Review the specific contributions of the major minerals in growth and development.

Vitamins and minerals are nutrients that are essential to life because of their involvement in cellular metabolism, maintenance, and growth throughout the life cycle. Vitamins and minerals are often called micronutrients because in comparison with the four major nutrients—carbohydrate, protein, fat, and water—they are needed in relatively small amounts. Changing life-styles and dietary patterns over the past two decades have conspired to increase a number of micronutrient imbalances in diets of children. Poor dietary patterns, such as skipping meals, a preference for low-nutrient-dense foods in place of nourishing ones, and frequent snacking, can contribute to suboptimal nutrition status during childhood (Kim, Kim, & Keen, 2005). The Commission on the Nutrition Challenges of the 21st Century (2000) stated that although protein-energy malnutrition remains a concern for many of the world's children, micronutrient malnutrition is recognized increasingly as a more widespread problem (Tanner & Finn-Stevenson, 2002).

Malnutrition permeates all aspects of health—growth, cognition, and motor and social development. Micronutrient deficiencies, such as iron deficiency anemia, have been shown to positively correlate with decreased school performance. Lack of adequate micronutrients, especially zinc, selenium, iron, and the antioxidant vitamins, can also lead to clinically significant immune deficiency and infections in children. More than 50% of deaths of children in developing countries are a result of infections related to malnutrition. Irreversible and lifelong sequelae may prevent children from reaching their fullest potential (Neuman, Gewa, & Bwibo, 2004). Therefore, it is important that healthy dietary patterns are established during childhood.

Vitamins

Vitamins are organic compounds that occur naturally in plants and animals and are distinct from carbohydrates, fats, and proteins. Vitamins are also typically found naturally in foods in minute amounts and are not synthesized by the body in adequate amounts to meet physiologic needs. Vitamin needs are often dependent on energy intake or other nutrient levels. Therefore, inadequate consumption of vitamins results in a specific deficiency syndrome. Vitamin functions are determined by their chemical and associated physical properties and serve essential roles in numerous metabolic processes. Few, however, show close chemical or functional similarities. By and large, vitamins function as coenzymes, which are fundamental parts of enzymes.

Vitamins are usually classified into two groups, based on their solubility. Some are soluble in nonpolar solvents (i.e., vitamins A, D, E, and K), whereas others are soluble in polar solvents (i.e., vitamin C, thiamin, riboflavin, niacin, vitamin B_6, biotin, pantothenic acid, folate, and vitamin B_{12}). The **fat-soluble vitamins** tend to be absorbed and transported with dietary lipids, whereas the **water-soluble vitamins** are absorbed by passive and active processes. Vitamins remain in the body for varying amounts of time. Utilization of water-soluble vitamins begins the minute they are absorbed through the digestive system, and they remain in the body for 2 to 4 days. Water-soluble vitamins are not stored and are quickly excreted in the urine either intact or as water-soluble metabolites. Thus, water-soluble vitamins must be replenished regularly, and toxicities are virtually unknown. Fat-soluble vitamins stay in the body for longer periods of time and are usually stored in lipid tissue of organs, especially the liver. In general, the fat-soluble vitamins are excreted with the feces via enterohepatic circulation. Toxicity is probable with some but only when taken in very large doses (Mahan & Escott-Stump, 2000).

Vitamins: Organic compounds that occur naturally in plants and animals and are not synthesized by the body in adequate amounts to meet physiologic needs.

Fat-soluble vitamins (e.g., A, D, E, and K): Soluble in polar solvents, absorbed and transported with dietary lipids, and excreted in the feces.

Water-soluble vitamins (e.g., vitamin C, thiamin, riboflavin, niacin, vitamin B_6, biotin, pantothenic acid, folate, and vitamin B_{12}): Soluble in nonpolar solvents, absorbed by passive and active processes, and excreted in the urine.

Water-Soluble Vitamins

Vitamin B

Although each B vitamin has its own unique biological role and individual properties, as a group these nutrients are often thought of as a single entity because of their commonality. B vitamins work together in the body by maintaining healthy nerves, skin, hair, eyes, liver, and mouth and by preserving good muscle tone in the gastrointestinal tract. B vitamins are used as coenzymes in almost all parts of the body and also provide energy, because they are necessary for metabolism of carbohydrate, fat, and protein. Emotional stress, surgery, illness, pregnancy, and breast-feeding all increase B vitamin requirements. Deficiency in a single B vitamin is rare; rather, people tend to have multiple deficiencies, making subtle deficiency symptoms more difficult to diagnose yet more likely to be present. Because of competition for absorption in the intestines, high doses of a single B vitamin should be avoided. When considering supplementation, the ratio of B vitamins is most beneficial when 1:1. In general, no toxicity of B vitamins has been reported.

Vitamin B₁ (Thiamin)

Thiamin was the first B vitamin to be discovered, in the 1920s, and it plays an essential role in metabolism of carbohydrates, a major source of energy in our cells. As daily intake of complex and simple carbohydrates increases, the need for thiamin increases as extra carbohydrates use more thiamin. The cells of the brain and central nervous system are the first to show signs of thiamin deficiency due to extreme sensitivity to carbohydrate metabolism. During periods of physical and emotional stress, including times of fever, muscular activity, overactive thyroid, pregnancy, and lactation, thiamin requirements increase. Thiamin is also involved in converting fatty acids into steroid hormones, such as cortisone and progesterone, necessary for proper growth and maintenance of healthy skin. Thiamin may play a role in resistance to disease (Libermann & Branning, 1997).

Classic thiamin deficiency results in **beriberi,** a disease that affects the gastrointestinal tract, cardiovascular system, and peripheral nervous system and is usually confined to alcoholics. Advanced symptoms of deficiency are indigestion, constipation, headaches, insomnia, and heavy weak legs, followed by cramping or numb feet. Thiamin deficiency can also produce ventricular dilatation and dysfunction resulting in a damaged, enlarged, or irregularly beating heart (Prabhu & Dalvi, 2000). Subclinical deficiency symptoms are fatigue, apathy, mental confusion, inability to concentrate, poor memory, insomnia, anorexia, weight loss, decreased strength, emotional instability, depression, and irrational fears. Such symptoms have been reported in children with B-cell leukemia/lymphoma being treated with chemotherapy and total parenteral nutrition. In this group, profound lethargy developed because of severe lactic acidosis caused by an impairment of pyruvate dehydrogenase complex. This was due to a lack of its necessary cofactor, thiamin, in the total parenteral nutrition. Treatment with added thiamin resulted in an improved clinical and laboratory status (Svahn et al., 2003).

Beriberi: Classic thiamin deficiency disease that affects the gastrointestinal tract, cardiovascular system, and peripheral nervous system and is usually confined to alcoholics.

Significant food sources include organ meats, pork, dried beans, peas, soybeans, peanuts, whole grains, wheat germ, rice bran, egg yolk, poultry, and fish. Foods with anti-thiamin activity include blueberries, red chicory, black currants, Brussels sprouts, red cabbage, and raw seafood. Ascorbic acid has been shown to protect against thiamin destruction in some of these foods.

Vitamin B₂ (Riboflavin)

Riboflavin plays an important role in the oxidation of amino acids, synthesis of fatty acids, and oxidation of glucose and thyroid hormone metabolism, processes that influence metabolism and energy production. An increased need for riboflavin is associated with tissue damage, including from burns, surgery, injuries, fever, and malignancies. The blood, too, requires riboflavin, a deficiency of which can lead to vitamin B₂ anemia. There is reasonably good evidence that poor riboflavin status interferes with iron handling and contributes to the etiology of anemia when iron intakes are low. Correcting a riboflavin deficiency in children improves the hematologic response of iron supplements. Riboflavin is also found in the pigment of the retina, enabling eyes to adapt to light, with photophobia resulting in times of vitamin B_2 deficiency. Current interest is focused on the role that riboflavin plays in determining circulating concentrations of homocysteine, a risk factor for cardiovascular disease.

Biochemical signs of depletion arise within only a few days of dietary deprivation. Riboflavin deficiency among Western children seems to be largely confined to adolescents, primarily girls, despite the diversity of riboflavin-rich foods available. Classic deficiency symptoms are cheilosis (tiny lesions and cracks in the corners of the mouth); an inflamed purple tongue; tearing, burning, and itching of the eyes; flaking of the skin; and behavior changes. Riboflavin deficiency may exert some of its effects by reducing the metabolism of other B vitamins, notably folate and vitamin B_6. Some children may be marginally deficient as a result of taking antibiotics because antibiotics interfere with absorption and utilization of riboflavin. Phototherapy used to treat hyperbilirubinemia in neonates is also associated with transient deterioration in riboflavin status, although no functional deficits have been described. Riboflavin deficiency has also been implicated as a risk factor for cancer, although this has not been satisfactorily established.

Riboflavin is unique among the water-soluble vitamins in that milk and dairy products make the greatest contribution to its intake in Western diets. Meat and fish are also good sources of riboflavin, and certain fruits and vegetables, especially dark-green leafy vegetables, contain reasonably high concentrations. Breast milk concentrations of riboflavin are fairly sensitive to maternal riboflavin intake and can be moderately increased by riboflavin supplementation of the mother when natural intake is low. Even in well-nourished communities, concentrations of riboflavin in breast milk are considerably lower than in cow's milk. Infants receiving banked breast milk through nasogastric tubing may be at risk of developing transient riboflavin deficiency because of losses in the milk during collection, storage, and administration.

Intakes of riboflavin in excess of tissue requirements are excreted in the urine as riboflavin or other metabolites. Some urinary metabolites reflect bacterial activity in the gastrointestinal tract as well. Urinary excretion, however, is not a sensitive marker of very low riboflavin intakes (Powers, 2003).

Vitamin B_3 (Niacin)

There are two forms of niacin, nicotinic acid and niacinamide, which our bodies make from tryptophan. Nicotinic acid and niacinamide have identical vitamin activities but have very different pharmacologic activities. Niacin is a coenzyme in many important biochemical reactions involved in maintaining healthy skin, properly functioning gastrointestinal tract and central nervous system, and metabolism of lipids (Hendler & Rorvik, 2001). Because of niacin's role in the metabolism of fats, much of its use involves the treatment of elevated cholesterol. There is strong evidence that the onset of atherosclerosis occurs in childhood. Identifying and treating children and adolescents at risk for hypercholesterolemia should lead to a decrease in adult atherosclerotic disease. Studies show that niacin is effective in decreasing triglycerides in the blood. Long-term studies, however, are needed to determine if delivery of niacin truly provides long-term benefits for those children with hypercholesterolemia (Kronn, Sapru, & Satou, 2000).

Niacin deficiency can occur under certain conditions, which include malabsorption syndromes, cirrhosis, and the provision of total parenteral nutrition with inadequate niacin supplementation. The well-known disorder of niacin deficiency is **pellagra**. Pellagra is a nutritional wasting disease attributable to a combined deficiency of the essential amino acid tryptophan and niacin (nicotinic acid). It is characterized clinically by four classic stages, often referred to as the four Ds: dermatitis, diarrhea, dementia, and death. Before the development of these symptoms, other nonspecific symptoms develop gradually and mostly affect dermatologic, neuropsychological, and gastrointestinal systems. Easily observable deficiency generally occurs only in severely malnourished people. A review of literature reveals several case reports describing pellagra in patients with anorexia nervosa, with the most common features being cutaneous manifestations such as erythema on sun-exposed areas, glossitis, and stomatitis. Pellagra may be diagnosed if cutaneous symptoms resolve within 24 to 48 hours of oral niacin administration (Prousky, 2003). Although pellagra was commonly found in the United States through the 1930s, the disorder is rare today in industrialized countries. This is in large part due to the enrichment of refined flours with niacin (Hendler & Rorvik, 2001).

Pellagra: A nutritional wasting disease attributable to a combined deficiency of the essential amino acid tryptophan and niacin (nicotinic acid).

Niacin is found naturally in meat, poultry, fish, legumes, and yeast. Consumption of corn-rich diets has resulted in niacin deficiency in certain populations. The reason for this is that niacin contained in corn exists in bound forms, which exhibits little or no nutritional availability. Soaking corn in a lime solution, which releases the niacin, has prevented such a deficiency in parts of the world where corn-based diets are prevalent.

Flushing is the adverse reaction first observed after intake of a large dose of nicotinic acid because it causes vasodilatation of cutaneous blood vessels. Other adverse reactions of nicotinic acid include dizziness, shortness of breath, sweating, nausea, vomiting, insomnia, abdominal pain, and tachycardia. Excessive intake of niacin can also exacerbate gastric ulcers. With liver disorders, high-dose therapeutic supplementation needs to be monitored because of potential increased liver function tests (Hendler & Rorvik, 2001).

Vitamin B_6 (Pyridoxine)

Pyridoxine is one of the most essential and widely used vitamins in the body and participates as a coenzyme in more than 60 enzymatic reactions involved in the metabolism of amino acids and essential fatty acids. Vitamin B_6 is needed for proper growth and maintenance of almost all of our body structures and functions. One of the many systems dependent on vitamin B_6 is the nervous system. Pyridoxine is necessary for the production of serotonin and other neurotransmitters in the brain. Infants fed formulas low in vitamin B_6 have been reported to suffer from epileptic-like convulsions, weight loss, nervous irritability, and stomach disorders (Libermann & Branning, 1997). Pyridoxine-dependent epilepsy usually presents in the neonatal period or even in utero, is resistant to antiepileptic medications, and is treatable with lifelong administration of pyridoxine. The seizures are typically generalized as tonic-clonic, although myoclonic seizures or infantile spasms have been described (Yoshii, Takeoka, Kelly, & Krishnamoorthy, 2005).

Deficiency can cause anemia and depression of immune system responses. Symptoms of vitamin B_6 deficiency are dermatitis of the nose, eyes, and mouth; acne; cheilosis; stomatitis; and glossitis. Deficiency symptoms also include alteration of the nervous system, depression, confusion, dizziness, insomnia, irritability, nervousness, and convulsions.

All foods contain small amounts of vitamin B_6, but foods with the highest concentration are eggs, fish, spinach, carrots, peas, meat, chicken, brewer's yeast, walnuts, sunflower seeds, and wheat germ. The amount

of vitamin B_6 in foods does not necessarily represent the amount that is bioavailable or active in the tissues after ingestion. Studies have shown that bioavailability is quite limited (Libermann & Branning, 1997).

Vitamin B_6 is relatively nontoxic, but some problems with the nervous system have been reported when consumed in huge doses of 2,000 to 6,000 mg/day, with reversal of side effects when dosage is discontinued. Inconclusive studies have suggested that social isolation, verbal delays, and self-stimulating behaviors of autistic children have been shown to improve when they are given high doses of vitamin B^6 along with magnesium (Libermann & Branning, 1997; Samour & King, 2005). The use of megavitamin intervention began in the 1950s with the treatment of schizophrenic patients. A number of studies attempted to assess the effects of vitamin B_6 magnesium (Yoshii et al., 2005). It is thought that total vitamin B_6 is abnormally high in children with autism due to impaired conversion of pyridoxine to pyridoxal-5-phosphate. This may explain the published benefits of high-dose vitamin B_6 supplementation (Adams, George, & Audhya, 2006). Because of the small number of studies, the methodologic quality of studies, and small sample sizes, no recommendation can be advanced regarding the use of high doses of vitamin B_6 as a treatment for autism.

Vitamin B_{12} (Cobalamin)

Recent data indicate that cobalamin status undergoes marked changes during childhood, particularly during the first year. During the first year of life vitamin B_{12} uptake may be limited because of low vitamin B_{12} content in breast milk and immature intrinsic factor system, but the estimated vitamin B_{12} stores in the neonatal liver are assumed to be sufficient for normal growth. Serum cobalamin has been shown to be lower during the first 6 months of life, with total homocysteine and methylmalonic acid particularly high, suggesting impaired cobalamin function. Children have the ability to produce vitamin B_{12} in the intestines, but it is not definite how much can be absorbed by the body. Older children with an omnivorous diet are thought to ensure meeting the daily dietary requirement for vitamin B_{12}.

Cobalamin is a coenzyme in a methyl transfer reaction that converts homocysteine to methionine, which is later converted to L-methylmalonyl-coenzyme A to succinyl-coenzyme A. This explains why increased total homocysteine and methylmalonic acid in the blood are indicative of impaired cobalamin status, which may occur even in the presence of normal serum cobalamin concentrations. The reported occurrence of low serum cobalamin and increased methylmalonic acid in a significant portion of healthy infants, as demonstrated by newborn screening tests, may be more prevalent than once recognized. The increased metabolite concentrations in infants may be a harmless phenomenon related to developmental, physiologic, or nutritional factors or may reflect the common occurrences of impaired cobalamin function in infants. Because impaired cobalamin function may have long-term effects related to psychomotor development, intervention studies with cobalamin supplementation in pregnancy and infancy may be warranted (Monsen, Refsum, Markestad, & Ueland, 2003).

Some causes of deficiency are various forms of intestinal malabsorption, inborn errors of cobalamin metabolism, exposure to nitrous oxide, infants born to vitamin B_{12}–deficient mothers, and children adhering to strict vegetarian diets (Korenke, Hunneman, Eber, & Hanefeld, 2004; Kim et al., 2005). Vitamin B_{12} is absorbed from the terminal ileum, which is the commonly affected segment of gut in Crohn's disease. Its absorption may be compromised in these children secondary to inflammatory lesions, ileal bacterial overgrowth, and surgical resection. Prolonged depletion of vitamin B_{12} is one of the major causes of megaloblastic anemia and ultimately leads to neuropathy (Ahmed & Jenkins, 2004). An example of such a disorder characterized by megaloblastic anemia due to malabsorption of cobalamin is Imerslund-Grasbeck disease (Eitenschenck, Armari-Alla, Plantaz, Pagnier, & Ducros, 2005). Cobalamin deficiency is prevalent in vegetarian teens and has been associated with increased risk of osteoporosis. In adolescents, signs of impaired cobalamin status, as judged by elevated concentrations of methylmalonic acid, have been associated with low bone mineral density. This is especially true in adolescents fed a macrobiotic diet during the first years of life, when cobalamin deficiency is more prominent (Dhonukshe-Rutten, van Dusseldorp, Schneede, de Groot, & van Staveren, 2005). Childhood pernicious anemia is exceedingly rare; etiology is varied and may result despite adequate dietary intake.

Deficiency in infancy presents as failure to thrive, developmental delay, progressive neurologic disorders, or hematologic changes. Symptoms may be evident as early as 3 to 4 months of age but are often nonspecific and difficult to diagnose. Because the age at onset and the duration of neurologic symptoms may contribute to the development of long-term symptoms, early diagnosis and treatment are important for vitamin B_{12}–deficient children (Monsen et al., 2003; Korenke et al., 2004).

The amount of vitamin B_{12} in food sources is small, with good sources including beef, herring, mackerel, egg yolk, milk, cheese, clams, sardines, salmon, crab meat, and oysters. Vegetarian teens should be counseled on the need to identify and regularly consume dietary sources of vitamin B_{12}, especially breast-feeding teen girls. Infants of vegan mothers should also receive vitamin B_{12} supplements starting at birth while breast-feeding if the mother's diet is not supplemented.

Folic Acid (Folate)

One of the most important roles of folate is that it works closely with vitamin B_{12} in metabolism of amino acids, synthesis of proteins, and production of genetic material such as RNA and DNA. Abnormal metabolism of homocysteine and methylmalonic acid, which is directly related to folate metabolism, has been associated with neurologic disorders, such as autism (Miller, 2003; Muntjewerff et al., 2003). The observed imbalance of folate metabolism in autistic children is complex and not easily explained by one single pathway or isolated genetic or nutritional deficiency (James et al., 2004).

The greatest attention received by folic acid is secondary to its ability to prevent **neural tube defects.** The neural tube is the structure of the embryo that gives rise to the brain, spinal cord, and other parts of the central nervous system. Neural tube defects occur in 1 to 2 per 1,000 births and are the most significant fetal anomalies leading to long-term morbidity. Evidence from a number of studies demonstrated that periconceptional use of vitamin supplements containing folic acid reduces the risk of neural tube defects by at least 60% (Lumley, Watson, Watson, & Bower, 2000; Persad, Van den Hof, Dube, & Zimmer, 2002). Although the mechanism of action of this nutrient in influencing the risk of neural tube defects is poorly understood, the evidence of the benefit of folic acid has led many health organizations to recommend periconceptional supplementation at a level of 400 mg/day. Because of the concern that public education campaigns alone cannot achieve optimal periconceptional intake of folic acid, food fortification has been proposed as a strategy to supplement all women of childbearing age. The fortification of grain products with folic acid has been controversial because of the potential to mask vitamin B_{12} deficiency. A study in Newfoundland implemented the food fortification strategy with a marked decrease (78%) in the rate of neural tube defects. No evidence of adverse effect of folic acid fortification on the detection of vitamin B_{12} deficiency was identified (Liu et al., 2004).

Because of folic acid's vital role in healthy cell division, replication, and tissue growth, deficiency of this nutrient is associated with dysplasia, an abnormal growth of tissues that is considered precancerous. Acute lymphoblastic leukemia is the most common childhood cancer in developed countries. Little is known about its causes, although its diagnosis at an early age has focused interest on maternal and perinatal factors. The second most common pediatric tumor is neuroblastoma, an embryonic tumor that is also the most prevalent extracranial solid tumor in children. Results of previous studies suggested a protective effect of maternal folate supplementation during pregnancy against acute lymphoblastic leukemia and neuroblastoma tumors. Other studies of genes and environment interaction in acute lymphoblastic leukemia and other cancers provided contradictory results, perhaps because of varying definitions of folate exposure (French et al., 2003; Milne et al., 2006). Further investigation into the interaction of folate intake and the role of metabolism in the formation and prevention of embryonically determined cancers is needed.

Like vitamin B_{12}, folic acid is needed for formation of red blood cells. Without adequate amounts of folic acid, specific types of anemia result, characterized by oversized red blood cells. Symptoms of deficiency are irritability, weakness, sleep difficulty, and pallor. When testing for anemia it is imperative to use diagnostic tests to distinguish vitamin B_{12} anemia from folic acid anemia. If folic acid is supplemented when a child is deficient in vitamin B_{12}, severe vitamin B_{12} deficiency will develop, because the body needs vitamin B_{12} to use folic acid. The reverse, severe folic acid deficiency, occurs if vitamin B_{12} is given to a child deficient in folic acid (Libermann & Branning, 1997).

Cerebral folate deficiency is defined by low active folate metabolites in the presence of normal folate metabolism. Cerebral folate deficiency could result from either disturbed folate transport or increased folate turnover in the central nervous system. Typical features begin to manifest from age 4 months, starting with irritability, sleep disturbances, psychomotor retardation, cerebellar ataxia, spastic paraplegic, and epilepsy. Children often show signs of decelerated head growth from ages 4 to 6 months. Visual disturbances begin around age 3 years, and progressive hearing loss starts at age 6 years. Cerebral folate deficiency has been treated with carefully titrated doses of folinic acid to prevent over- or under-dosage of folinic acid. Various conditions such as Rett syndrome, Aicardi-Goutieres syndrome, and Kearns-Sayre syndrome may also be related to cerebral folate deficiency (Ramaekers & Blau, 2004).

Food sources include beef, lamb, pork, chicken liver, deep-green leafy vegetables, asparagus, broccoli, whole wheat, and brewer's yeast. Twenty-five percent to 50% of folic acid in food is bioavailable.

Vitamin C (Ascorbic Acid)

The usefulness of vitamin C in the diet stems from its role as an antioxidant, preventing free radical damage and other antioxidant vitamins from being oxidized and thus keeping them potent. It is also essential for growth and repair of tissues in all parts of the body, such as formation of collagen, bone, and cartilage. The skin may also be protected from free radical damage associated with ultraviolet light with adequate intake of vitamin C. Synthesis of hormones in the adrenal glands requires vitamin C, with vast amounts of this micronutrient depleted during times of stress such as surgery, illness, and infection. Studies have shown that ascorbic acid may help prevent increased blood pressure, atherosclerosis, and decreased serum cholesterol. Vitamin C also plays a role in the bioavailability of other micronutrients, such as converting folic acid to its active form and increasing the body's ability to absorb iron from non-heme sources.

Both cross-sectional and follow-up studies have shown an association between decreased intake of vitamin C–containing fruits during the winter and an increased risk of wheezing symptoms in children. Asthma has been associated with oxidant and antioxidant imbalance. Patients with asthma have been shown to have decreased plasma concentrations of vitamin C and increased oxidative stress. Protective effects of citrus fruit consumption do not seem to follow a dose-related response, with positive effects shown with as little as fruit once a week. Results, however, of various experimental studies regarding the effect of vitamin C supplementation on lung function and bronchial responsiveness are conflicting (Forastiere et al., 2000).

Vitamin C deficiency in the United States is rare, with the classic disease being **scurvy.** Symptoms are often subtle and difficult to diagnose, with early signs being listlessness, weakness, irritability, vague muscle and joint pain, and weight loss. Late symptoms of deficiency include bleeding gums, gingivitis, loosening of teeth, and fatigue. Unlike most other animals, humans are incapable of producing vitamin C in their bodies and depend on the daily food supply. The level at which tissue saturation occurs is approximately 1,500 mg/day. Concentrated food sources include broccoli, Brussels sprouts, black currants, collards, guava, horseradish, kale, turnip greens, parsley, and sweet peppers. Interestingly enough, citrus fruits are not the most concentrated sources of vitamin C. The bioflavonoids in the skin are responsible for increased vitamin C absorption from citrus fruits. Few people realize that an orange loses 30% of its vitamin C concentration after being squeezed, with nonfortified commercial juice almost having no natural vitamin C left. No proven toxicity has been identified. However, there is a potential for formation of kidney stones, intestinal gas, and loose stools when extremely large doses are consumed (Libermann & Branning, 1997).

Scurvy: Classic vitamin C deficiency in which symptoms are often subtle and difficult to diagnose, with early signs being listlessness, weakness, irritability, vague muscle and joint pain, and weight loss.

Fat-Soluble Vitamins

Vitamin A

Vitamin A has essential roles in the proper function of the eye, growth and maintenance of epithelial tissue, protection from cardiovascular disease and cancer, immune system function, and reproduction. Vitamin A is especially useful in the prevention of both infectious and noninfectious diseases of the respiratory system.

Each function of vitamin A can be satisfied by ingesting the compounds that form vitamin A, which are retinoids (preformed vitamin A) and carotenoids (precursors to vitamin A that the body converts into active vitamin A). Over 400 carotenoids exist, such as beta-carotene, lutein, canthaxanthin, zeaxanthin, lycopene, alpha-carotene, and cryptoxanthin. Although not all have vitamin A activity, many have powerful antioxidant properties. All forms of active vitamin A, both fat and water soluble, are stored in the liver, where they can be mobilized for distribution to peripheral tissues. Because active vitamin A

Vitamin A Research

Chronic infection and illness can decrease the body's level of vitamin A, thereby weakening the mucous membranes and making them more susceptible to viral infection. Randomized controlled trials have shown inconsistent responses of childhood pneumonia with the use of vitamin A as an adjunct to the standard treatment of pneumonia (Huiming, Chaomin, & Meng, 2005; Rodriguez et al., 2005). There is growing evidence that vitamin A and beta-carotene provide some protection against various forms of cancer.

Beta-carotene may also offer hope to children infected with HIV in developing countries where the infection has a devastating impact on children. Poor nutrition and HIV-related adverse health outcomes contribute to a vicious cycle that may be slowed down by using nutritional interventions, including supplemental vitamin A. Periodic supplementation with vitamin A starting at age 6 months has been shown to be beneficial in reducing both mortality and morbidity among HIV-infected children (Fawzi, Msamanga, Spiegelman, & Hunter, 2005).

Vitamin A has been proposed as a nutrient for which infants at risk for chronic pulmonary insufficiency may have special requirements. There is suggestive evidence that high doses when given intramuscularly may reduce the incidence of death from chronic lung disease. Exogenous steroid therapy, which is often used to improve pulmonary compliance in ventilated premature infants, may compromise vitamin A status and induce restricted somatic and bone mineral growth (Atkinson, 2001). Further studies are needed to verify the role that vitamin A may play in preventing severe chronic lung disease in premature infants.

and beta-carotene have slightly different functions in the body, a combination should be consumed. Palmitate, a synthetic form of vitamin A, is water miscible and appropriate for children experiencing fat malabsorption. Chain-shortened and oxidized forms of vitamin A are excreted in the urine with intact forms excreted in the bile and lost with the feces (Mahan & Escott-Stump, 2000).

An estimated 250 million children globally are at risk for vitamin A deficiency. Traditionally recognized symptoms of deficiency are night blindness, skin disorders, suboptimal growth, and reproductive failure. In 1991 nearly 14 million preschool children, most from South Asia, had clinical eye disease (xerophthalmia) due to vitamin A deficiency. Xerophthalmia involves atrophy of the periocular glands, hyperkeratosis of the conjunctiva, and finally involvement of the cornea, leading to softening of keratomalacia and blindness. Although the condition is rare in the United States, where it is usually associated with malabsorption, it is more common in developing countries, where it is a major source of blindness among children. Two-thirds of new patients die within months of going blind, due to enhanced susceptibility to infections. Even subclinical vitamin A deficiency increases child morbidity and mortality (Mahan & Escott-Stump, 2000).

Measles is also a major cause of childhood morbidity and mortality, with vitamin A deficiency recognized as a risk factor for severe measles infections. The World Health Organization recommends administration of an oral dose of vitamin A (200,000 IU for children or 100,000 IU for infants) each day for 2 days to children with measles when they live in areas where vitamin A deficiency may be present. Comparing several studies showed no evidence that vitamin A in a single dose was associated with a reduced risk of mortality among children with measles (Huiming et al., 2005).

Vitamin A deficiency produces characteristic changes in skin texture. These involve follicular hyperkeratosis in which blockage of the hair follicles with plugs of keratin causes "goose flesh" or "toad skin." The skin becomes dry, scaly, and rough. At first the forearms and thighs are involved, but in advanced stages the whole body is affected. Subsequently, deficiency leads to failures in systemic functions characterized by anemia and impaired immunocompetence. A deficiency also leads to the keratinization of the mucous membranes that line the respiratory tract, alimentary canal, urinary tract, skin, and epithelium of the eye. These changes hinder the roles that these membranes play in protecting the body against infections. Clinically, these conditions are manifest as poor growth, blindness, periosteal overgrowth of the cranium, or increased susceptibility to infections. Primary deficiencies result from inadequate intakes of preformed vitamin A and provitamin A carotenoids. Secondary deficiencies can result from malabsorption due to insufficient dietary fat, biliary or pancreatic insufficiency, liver disease, protein-energy malnutrition, or zinc deficiency.

Acute vitamin A deficiency is treated with large oral doses of vitamin A. When it is part of concomitant protein-energy malnutrition, correction of this condition is needed to realize benefits of vitamin A treatment. The signs and symptoms of vitamin A deficiency respond to vitamin A supplementation in the same order as they appear: Night blindness resolves quickly, whereas the skin abnormalities may take several weeks to resolve. Treatment with single doses of 200,000 IU of vitamin A has reduced child mortality by 35% to 70%. This approach is very costly, which has stimulated interest in increasing vitamin A content of local food systems as a more sustainable approach to preventing the deficiency (Mahan & Escott-Stump, 2000).

Active vitamin A is found only in food sources with preformed vitamin A present in foods of animal origin, either in storage areas such as the liver or associated with the fat of milk and eggs. Very high concentrations occur in fish liver oil from cod, halibut, salmon, and shark. Provitamin A carotenoids are found in dark leafy, green, and yellow-orange vegetables and fruit; deeper colors are associated with higher carotenoid levels. In much of the world carotenoids supply most of the dietary vitamin A.

Persistent large doses of vitamin A, which overcome the capacity of the liver to store the vitamin, can produce intoxication. Hypervitaminosis A can be induced by single doses of retinal greater than 330,000 IU in children, potentially resulting in liver disease. Vitamin A toxicity is characterized by changes in the skin and mucous membranes. Early signs of toxicity include fatigue, nausea, vomiting, muscular incoordination, and dryness of the lips. Dryness of the nasal mucosa and eyes, erythema, scaling and peeling of the skin, hair loss, and nail fragility follow. Chronic hypervitaminosis can result from chronic intakes, usually from misuse of supplements, greater than at least 10 times the Recommended Dietary Allowance of 14,000 IU for an infant (Mahan & Escott-Stump, 2000). Reversal of symptoms occurs when supplementation is discontinued. In contrast, beta-carotene, a naturally occurring pigment, can be given for long periods of time virtually without risk of toxicity. Carotenemia, a harmless condition, is a sign that the body converted as much beta-carotene to active vitamin A as it could, leaving the excess as an orange-yellow pigment in the skin (Libermann & Branning, 1997).

Vitamin D

Vitamin D is not truly a vitamin and can be described as a steroid hormone because it does not need to be supplied from a source outside the body. Now recognized as the "sunshine vitamin," it is a hormone produced in the body by the photoconversion of 7-dehydrocholesterol in the skin. With adequate exposure to solar ultraviolet B radiation (290 to 320 nm), no dietary supplement is needed (Mughal, 2002). There are two forms of vitamin D: vitamin D_2 (ergocalciferol) and vitamin D_3 (cholecalciferol), which is the preferred form because of its natural occurrence in the body. Both vitamins D_2 and D_3 become active hormone vitamin D after passing through the liver and kidneys. The bioactive form of vitamin D is produced not only in the kidneys but also in the placenta during pregnancy. In the active form it is considered to be a hormone because of its roles in calcium and phosphorous homeostasis, cell differentiation, and bone formation and maintenance. As compared with the knowledge of vitamin D in calcium homeostasis and skeletal growth, very little is known about its role in the central nervous system. Vitamin D may also have anticancer properties and play a role in treatment of immunologic disorders, mood behavior, and improvement in muscle strength (Libermann & Branning, 1997; Chaudhuri, 2005).

Life-style, skin pigmentation, clothing, degree of air pollution, and geographic latitude affect the degree of exposure to the sun and therefore the amount of vitamin D internally produced by the body. It is also speculated that iron deficiency may affect vitamin D handling in the skin, gut, or its intermediary metabolism (Wharton & Bishop, 2003). It is difficult to determine amount of sun exposure needed; however, modest exposure to sunlight is sufficient for most children to produce their own vitamin D. Light

Vitamin D Research

It has been previously hypothesized that vitamin D deficiency in early life may be a risk factor for various neurologic and psychiatric diseases, including multiple sclerosis (MS), which is a demyelinating disease of the central nervous system that runs a chronic course and disables young people. The suggestion that vitamin D may have a protective effect on MS is not new. In areas of high latitudes where MS is common, ultraviolet radiation is too low to produce sufficient vitamin D in the fair-skinned population throughout the year. Vitamin D supplementation may significantly reduce the incidence of MS. The protective roles of sunlight exposure in early life and cutaneous vitamin D synthesis on the lifetime risk of developing MS is probably not without genetic predisposition because the population prevalence of MS does not parallel the prevalence of rickets. Although subclinical vitamin D deficiency is more common in dark-skinned races, MS is more common in fair-skinned races of European descent. Low vitamin D, however, appears to be an important modifiable external risk factor for MS (Chaudhuri, 2005).

sun exposure to the hands and face for 20 to 30 minutes two to three times per week has been shown to release approximately 50,000 IU into circulation within 24 hours of exposure (Hollis & Wagner, 2004). Most vitamin D in older children and adolescents is supplied by sunlight exposure. Ethnic populations living in geographic areas with high levels of solar exposure throughout the year have darkly pigmented skin, a feature associated with a reduced rate of cutaneous vitamin D. It is also questionable whether any vitamin D is synthesized during the winter months and whether the body's stores of this vitamin are able to meet the daily requirements during this period because the half-life of 25-hydroxyvitamin D is only 19 days (Mughal, 2002; Chaudhuri, 2005). In general, dermatologists discourage unprotected exposure to sun due to the increased risk of skin cancer and premature aging.

The incidence of vitamin D deficiency, also known as **nutritional rickets,** was thought to have vanished, but it is reappearing. Concerns about vitamin D resurfaced because of the promotion of exclusive breast-feeding for long periods without vitamin D supplementation, particularly for infants whose mothers are vitamin D deficient; reduced opportunities for production of the vitamin within the skin because of cultural practices and fear of skin cancer; and the high prevalence of rickets in groups in more temperate regions (Gartner, Greer, & Section on Breastfeeding and Committee on Nutrition, 2003; Pawley & Bishop, 2004). Rickets has been reported in children with chronic problems of lipid malabsorption and in those receiving long-term anticonvulsant therapies. Rickets can also be secondary to disorders of the gut, pancreas, liver, kidney, or metabolism; however, it is most likely due to nutrient deprivation not only of vitamin D but also of calcium and phosphorus (Wharton & Bishop, 2003).

Nutritional rickets: Vitamin D deficiency that was thought to have vanished but is reappearing.

Clinical features of rickets vary in severity and age at onset, with symptoms present for months before diagnosis. Juvenile deficiency affects ossification at the growth plates, resulting in deformity and impaired linear growth of long bones (Pawley & Bishop, 2004). A state of deficiency occurs months before structural abnormalities of the weight-bearing bones and is associated with bone pain, muscular tenderness, and hypocalcemic tetany. Soft, pliable, rachitic bones cannot withstand ordinary stresses, resulting in the appearance of bowlegs, knock-knees, pigeon breast, and frontal bossing of the skull. Improvement in clinical symptoms, such as aches and pains, occurs within 2 weeks of supplementation. Full correction of bowlegs and knock-knees can take up to 2 years. Adolescents are usually left with residual skeletal deformities that require surgical correction (Mughal, 2002).

Regular sources of dietary vitamin D are recommended for those otherwise at risk for deficiency. The National Academy of Sciences recommends the regular intake of a multiple vitamin with 200 IU vitamin D per day for all infants who are breast-fed unless weaned to 500 mL/day of formula, for all non–breast-feeding infants with less than 500 mL/day formula or milk, and for children not regularly exposed to sunlight and not ingesting 500 mL of fortified milk. It is generally accepted that nutritional rickets can be prevented by dietary supplementation of 400 IU/day. In the past human milk was thought to be an adequate source of vitamin D for neonates and growing infants (Hollis & Wagner, 2004). However, it has been determined that human milk typically contains 25 IU/L or less of vitamin D. Thus the recommended intake cannot be met with expressed breast milk as a sole source (Gartner et al., 2003). More data are needed to support adequacy of present recommendations and possibly even higher recommendations for vitamin D daily intake.

Vitamin D deficiency has also been associated with **osteopenia** in adults with cystic fibrosis, and cystic fibrosis is also potentially related to a childhood deficiency. Studies have shown, however, that most children with cystic fibrosis had normal 25-hydroxyvitamin D levels. Interpretation is difficult due to a lack of knowledge of optimal levels of 25-hydroxyvitamin D required for healthy bone accretion. Lower levels in adolescents may be a precursor to low levels in adulthood and do not seem to be simply related to poor compliance with supplementation. This may, however, reflect normal physiology (Chavasse, Francis, Balfour-Lynn, Rosenthal, & Bush, 2004).

Osteopenia: Bone mineral density that is lower than normal peak bone mineral density but not low enough to be classified as osteoporosis; often present in preterm infants, resulting in fractures.

Excessive intake of vitamin D can produce intoxication characterized by hypercalcemia and hyperphosphatemia and, ultimately, calcinosis of the kidney, lungs, heart, and even the tympanic membrane of the ear, which can result in deafness. Infants given excessive amounts of vitamin D may have gastrointestinal upsets, bone fragility, poor appetite, and retarded growth.

Nutritional hypervitaminosis results from pharmacologic doses of vitamin D consumed over a long period of time and is defined by a large increase in circulating 25-hydroxyvitamin D concentration. The tolerable upper level has been established at 1,000 IU day for infants and 2,000 IU day for children. The amount consumed to cause toxicity is thought to be 20,000 IU/day. Hypervitaminosis of vitamin D is a serious, albeit very rare, condition, with mild cases being treatable (Hollis & Wagner, 2004). Evidence exists that synthetic active forms of vitamin D, available by prescription, may be better in individuals with malabsorption because smaller doses can be used and thus decrease the risk of toxicity. Currently available solitary vitamin D preparations (containing up to 800 IU) are too concentrated for use in children when the recommendation is filled by standard multiple vitamin preparation (1 mL = 400 IU) (Gartner et al., 2003).

Calcium and magnesium, as well as other vitamins and minerals, should be taken with vitamin D because these nutrients all work together in the body to form and maintain bone mass. Vitamin D_3 occurs naturally in animal products, the richest sources being fish liver oils and eggs. However, approximately 98% of all fluid milk sold in the United States is fortified with vitamin D_2 (usually at the level of 400 IU per quart), as is most dried whole milk and evaporated milk, as well as some margarines, butter, soy milk, certain cereals, and infant formulas. A typical American diet does not supply the recommended 200 to 400 IU/day, thus requiring supplementation or fortification (Mughal, 2002; Samour & King, 2005). In many European countries, supplemented foodstuffs with vitamin D are limited; therefore, solar exposure is responsible for providing most of the body's vitamin D.

Vitamin E

Vitamin E is now recognized as having a fundamental role in the normal metabolism of all cells as a powerful antioxidant and anticarcinogen. Benefits may be due to its ability to protect vitamin A and C from oxidation, thus keeping them potent. In addition, vitamin E helps to increase the body's level of superoxide dismutase, an enzyme that is a powerful free radical scavenger. The antioxidant function of vitamin E can be affected by the nutritional status of a child with respect to one or more other nutrients that, collectively, protect against the potentially damaging effects of oxidative degradation. Therefore, deficiency can affect several different organ systems. The absorption of vitamin E is highly variable, with efficiencies in the range of 20% to 70% (Mahan & Escott-Stump, 2000). Vitamin E actually consists of eight substances, with alpha, beta, delta, and gamma tocopherols being the most active forms. The naturally occurring form is D-alpha-tocopherol, which appears to be the most absorbable.

Deficiencies of vitamin E in childhood present in a variety of ways. Children with progressive neuromuscular diseases are reported to have vitamin E deficiency, which may take 5 to 10 years to develop. Deficiency is manifested clinically as abnormal reflexes, impaired ability to walk, changes in balance and coordination, muscle weakness, and visual disturbances, which are improved after vitamin E supplementation. Additional deficiency symptoms include anemia caused by premature aging and death of red blood cells. These symptoms generally appear only when severe fat malabsorption results due to disorders of the pancreas, celiac disease, and cystic fibrosis. The limited transplacental movement of vitamin E results in newborn infants having low tissue concentrations of vitamin E. Premature infants may therefore be at increased risk of vitamin E deficiency because they typically have limited lipid absorptive capacity for some time (Mahan & Escott-Stump, 2000). Premature infants may also suffer from disorders of the retina, which can lead to blindness, as a result of vitamin E deficiency.

Vitamin E is synthesized only by plants and therefore is found primarily in plant products, the richest sources being oils such as cottonseed, corn, soybean, and safflower, and wheat germ having the highest concentration. Smaller amounts may be found in whole grains, green leafy vegetables, nuts, and

Vitamin E Research

A variety of studies have provided inconclusive, but promising, results identifying additional roles vitamin E may play in childhood. The results of a study in China ($n = 120$) suggest that chronic childhood constipation causes oxidative stress, in which levels of vitamin C and E are both decreased (Wang, Wang, Zhou, & Zhou, 2004). Because of its antioxidant capability, vitamin E also helps protect the body from mercury, lead, carbon tetrachloride, benzene, ozone, and nitrous oxide exposure that bring about harm through their ability to act as free radicals. The use of vitamin E during cancer treatment to enhance the ability of radiation treatment to shrink cancer cells has been considered. Vitamin E may also play a role in wound healing and reduction of scar formation (Libermann & Branning, 1997).

legumes. Animal tissues tend to contain low amounts of vitamin E, mainly found in fatty tissues and tissues of animals fed large amounts of the vitamin.

Vitamin E is one of the least toxic of the vitamins. Humans appear to be able to tolerate relatively high intakes, at least 100 times the nutritional requirement. At very high doses, however, vitamin E can antagonize the utilization of other fat-soluble vitamins (Mahan & Escott-Stump, 2000). Many supplements contain only alpha-tocopherols. However, it is recommended that a mixture of tocopherols be provided because this is how they exist in foods. For children experiencing fat malabsorption, vitamin E succinate is an alternative, synthetic, oil-free powder that is water miscible and well tolerated. With very high doses of more than 1,200 IU/day some adverse effects result, such as nausea, flatulence, diarrhea, heart palpitations, and fainting, which are reversible upon decrease in dose. To avoid adverse side effects, the recommendation is to begin with the provisional low dose and increase gradually (Libermann & Branning, 1997).

Vitamin K

Vitamin K is a general term used to describe a group of similar compounds. Vitamin K_1 is found in food, vitamin K_2 is made by intestinal bacteria, and vitamin K_3 is a synthetic form only available by prescription. For this reason vitamin K is not strictly considered a vitamin, with its most important function being the role it plays in production of coagulation factors in the body. Vitamin K is required to make prothrombin, which is converted to thrombin, which converts fibrinogen to fibrin and creates a blood clot. Newborn infants, particularly those who are premature or exclusively breast-fed, are susceptible to hypoprothrombinemia during the first few days of life as a result of poor placental transfer of vitamin K and failure to establish a vitamin K–producing intestinal microflora. This is associated with hemorrhagic disease of the newborn, which is treated prophylactically by administering vitamin K intramuscularly on delivery, which has been a standard of care since 1961 (American Academy of Pediatrics Committee on Fetus and Newborn, 2003; Samour & King, 2005).

Vitamin K is also essential for development of normal bone density during childhood and is thought to be important in preventing the development of osteoporosis in later life. There has been relatively little research emphasis on the effect of vitamin K on bone health during childhood. Better vitamin K status is associated with lower levels of markers of bone resorption and bone formation, suggesting a lower rate of bone turnover. There is a need for randomized supplementation trials to better understand the role of vitamin K on bone acquisition in growing children (Cashman, 2005). A marked reduction in bone mineral density has also been observed in children on long-term use of warfarin, a vitamin K antagonist. The etiology for reduced bone density is likely to be multifactorial; however, screening children on long-term warfarin for reduced bone density should be considered (Barnes et al., 2005).

Because vitamin K is easily obtained from the diet and synthesized in the body, deficiencies are rare and usually occur only with lipid malabsorption, destruction of intestinal flora as with chronic antibiotic therapy, and liver disease in which supplementation is recommended. The predominant sign of vitamin K deficiency is hemorrhage, which in severe cases can cause a fatal anemia. The underlying condition is hypoprothrombinemia, which manifests as prolonged clotting time (Mahan & Escott-Stump, 2000).

Vitamin K is found in large amounts in green leafy vegetables, especially broccoli, cabbage, turnip greens, and dark lettuces. Breast milk tends to be low in vitamin K content, providing insufficient amounts of the vitamin for infants less than 6 months of age. An important source of vitamin K is a result of microbiologic synthesis in the gut, which is affected by long-term antibiotic treatment by altering the gut flora (Samour & King, 2005). The synthetic form, vitamin K_3, is known to potentially result in toxicity when consumed in large doses. Major symptoms of overdose include hemolytic anemia, in which red blood cells die more quickly than the body can replace them.

Multiple Vitamin Supplementation

Multiple vitamin supplementation is a common practice in the United States, with approximately 54% of preschool children taking a supplement, typically a multiple vitamin and mineral preparation with iron. Use of supplementation generally decreases in older children and adolescents. Children taking supplements do not necessarily represent those who need them the most. Higher rates of use are found in families of higher socioeconomic status and education levels. Supplements may be taken inappropriately when the marginal or deficient nutrient is not supplied. For example, a child may be taking a children's vitamin but may actually need extra calcium, not always provided in a supplement. Except for fluoride supplementation in nonfluoridated areas, the American Academy of Pediatrics (AAP) does not recommend routine supplementation for normal healthy children. The American Medical Association and the American Dietetic Association recommend that nutrients for a healthy child come from food, not supplements. Dietary evaluation determines the need for supplementation. The AAP identifies six groups of children or adolescents at nutrition risk who might benefit from supplementation: (1) those with anorexia, poor appetites, and fad dieting; (2) those with chronic disease states such as cystic fibrosis or irritable bowel syndrome; (3) those from deprived families involving abuse or neglect; (4) those who use diet to manage obesity; (5) those who have an inadequate consumption of dairy products; and (6) those who have limited sun exposure or no consumption of vitamin D–fortified milk. Children with food allergies, those who omit entire food groups, and those with limited food acceptances may also be likely candidates for supplementation. Megadose levels of nutrients should be discouraged and parents counseled regarding dangers of toxicity, especially with fat-soluble vitamins. The Dietary Reference Intakes include the tolerable upper limit levels, which can be used to detect excess levels of vitamins and minerals from supplemental sources. Because many children's vitamins look and taste like candy, parents should be educated to keep them out of reach of children. Megavitamin therapy has been promoted, despite the lack of controlled studies, for many disorders, such as attention deficit hyperactivity disorder (ADHD), autism, and various behavioral problems.

> **● Learning Point** Except for fluoride supplementation in nonfluoridated areas, the AAP does not recommend routine supplementation for normal healthy children. The American Medical Association and the American Dietetic Association recommend that nutrients for a healthy child come from food, not supplements. Dietary evaluation determines the need for supplementation.

Minerals

Minerals are inorganic elements not produced by plants and animals and are primarily stored in bone and muscle tissues. Like vitamins, many minerals function as coenzymes enabling chemical reactions to occur throughout the body. Minerals belong to two groups: **macrominerals**, which are needed in large amounts (calcium, magnesium, and phosphorus), and microminerals or **trace minerals**, which are needed in much smaller amounts (zinc, iron, and potassium). Currently, nine trace minerals are considered to have a nutrient requirement: iron, zinc, copper, selenium, iodine, manganese, molybdenum, chromium, and cobalt. Notable differences between trace elements are the availability of biomarkers such as tissue concentration, mineral homeostasis and metabolism, body stores, functional indices, and response to increased intake.

> **Minerals:** Inorganic elements not produced by plants and animals and primarily stored in bone and muscle tissues.
>
> **Macrominerals:** Needed in large amounts (calcium, magnesium, and phosphorus).
>
> **Trace minerals:** Needed in much smaller amounts (iron, zinc, copper, selenium, iodine, manganese, molybdenum, chromium, and cobalt).

Calcium

Calcium is an essential mineral with a wide range of biological roles. Apart from being a major constituent of bones and teeth, calcium is crucial for muscle contraction and relaxation, transmission of nerve impulses, the beating of the heart, blood coagulation, glandular secretion, and the maintenance of immune function. Calcium is also used to activate enzymes involved in fat and protein digestion and production of energy. Calcium also aids in the absorption of many nutrients, especially vitamin B_{12}. Studies have also shown potential anticarcinogenic, antihypertensive, and hypocholesterolemia activity (Hendler & Rorvik, 2001).

Bodies contain approximately 2½ pounds of calcium, 99% of which is stored in the bones and teeth, with the remaining 1% (13 ounces) distributed throughout the body in the bloodstream and fluids surrounding our cells. Calcium is primarily found in bone and teeth in the form of the calcium phosphate compound hydroxyapatite (Hendler & Rorvik, 2001). The skeleton functions as a bank from which the body can draw the calcium it needs for various purposes. Therefore, identifying skeletal growth is a dynamic process. Approximately 100 mg of calcium per day is retained as bone during the preschool years. This triples and quadruples for adolescents during peak growth. Normally, sufficient calcium absorption from diet, blood, and bone calcium levels remains in balance and fluctuates only slightly. From the body's point of view, however, it is more important to maintain enough calcium in the blood to keep the heart beating regularly than it is to keep the bones strong. Because the body gives top priority to the maintenance of normal calcium levels in the blood, blood tests are an ineffective means of determining calcium levels in either the bone or diet. The concentration of calcium in the blood may be perfectly normal, whereas bone mineral density is suboptimal. If a child's diet is deficient in calcium, the body will always choose to maintain plasma calcium concentration by drawing it out of the bone, often resulting in osteopenia (Libermann & Branning, 1997; Samour & King, 2005).

Optimal dietary calcium and possibly vitamin D intake throughout childhood and adolescence may enhance bone mineral accrual and are central to osteoporosis prevention. During adolescence, children often receive less calcium because of rapid growth, dieting, and substitution of carbonated beverages for milk. From early childhood to late adolescence it has been reported that milk intake decreases by 25%. Mean calcium intake from ages 5 to 9 is positively related to bone mineral density at 9 years of age and is weakly related to bone mineral content after control for pubertal development and height at age 9. Adolescence is a critical period for optimal calcium retention to achieve peak bone mass, especially for females at risk for osteoporosis in later years. During this period of rapid bone mineral acquisition, adolescent girls' calcium intakes are reported to be 30% to 40% below the 1,300 mg/day recommendation (Fisher, Mitchell, Smiciklas-Wright, Mannino, & Birch, 2004; Samour & King, 2005), placing these adolescents at risk for calcium deficiency. Studies have also shown that gender, life-style factors, and socioeconomic status are significant predictors of calcium and vitamin D intake (Salamoun et al., 2005). Children who are vegetarians and do not consume fortified foods may also be at risk for not consuming the recommended calcium requirement. These findings have important implications regarding the institution of public health strategies to promote skeletal health during a critical time for bone mass accrual.

Bone health is now recognized to contribute to overall lifetime management of children and adolescents with disabling conditions, including physical and intellectual disability, and with many chronic disease processes. Increased skeletal fragility in the disabled child is well recognized. Strategies to address bone health, including public and medical education concerning consumption of calcium, appropriate selection of vitamin D preparations, and possible use of newer drugs, such as bisphosphonates, are changing the outlook for this large group (Zacharin, 2004).

Nutrition and oral health are also closely related. Micronutrients such as calcium, vitamin D for mineralization, and fluoride for enamel formation are critical to developing and maintaining oral structures. Because of individual variability, children receiving less than the recommended allowance of calcium may not necessarily be at risk.

Clinical signs of calcium depletion from bone gradually develop and are not usually apparent until the symptoms of osteopenia begin to appear. Even x-rays are incapable of picking up bone loss until 30% to 40% of bone has disappeared. Calcium-deficient diets, over long periods of time, result in bones that become porous, brittle, and weak. Children may easily suffer fractures from normal activity such as sneezing, bending over, or receiving a hug. The spinal vertebrae have also been reported to compress or fracture. Inconclusive studies have linked diets high in protein and fat with loss of calcium from the bone. Medications, such as antibiotics, anticonvulsants, and laxatives, can also affect absorption and utilization of calcium (Libermann & Branning, 1997).

Needs are determined by growth velocity, rate of absorption, and phosphorus and vitamin D status. The absorption efficiency of calcium varies throughout the life cycle. It is highest during infancy, when it is about 60%, with a decrease to approximately 28% in prepubescent children. During early puberty, at the time of the growth spurt, it increases to about 34% and then again drops to 25% two years later; it remains at this level for several years. The efficiency of absorption from a calcium supplement is greatest when taken in doses of 500 mg or lower (Hendler & Rorvik, 2001). Genetics and life-style also affect bone mineral density and possible calcium requirements. When assessing calcium status, vitamin D intake should be considered because of its major role in calcium metabolism. Concomitant use of vitamin D and calcium may increase absorption of calcium. The ratio of calcium to phosphorus has also been advised by researchers to be at least 1:1 to improve calcium absorption (Hambridge, 2003). Concomitant use of iron and calcium may inhibit the absorption of iron. Similarly, concomitant use of fluoride, magnesium, phosphorus, or zinc and calcium may decrease the absorption of these minerals (Hendler & Rorvik, 2001).

Food sources include dairy, canned salmon or sardines including the bones, green leafy vegetables, clams, oysters, shrimp, broccoli, soybeans, and soy products. Although unfortified plant foods have less calcium than milk, their increased absorption rate makes them good sources of this nutrient overall. Vitamin D–fortified milk is a primary source of this nutrient. It has been estimated that humans actually absorb as little as 20% to 40% of the calcium in food. This may be a result of the presence of oxalic acid, a substance that has been shown to bind with calcium, preventing its absorption in the colon. Limited known toxic effects have been reported, such as the rare development of kidney stones as a result of extremely large doses (Libermann & Branning, 1997).

Iron

Iron is an essential trace mineral that is involved in the entire process of respiration due to its role in the synthesis of hemoglobin, which carries oxygen in the blood. In addition to its fundamental roles in energy production, iron is involved in DNA synthesis and may also play roles in normal brain development and in immune function. Iron is also involved in the synthesis of collagen, serotonin, dopamine, and norepinephrine.

Iron, in the form of ferritin, is the most notable example of a mineral that is stored by the body. Ferritin provides a generous form of bioavailable iron that is released as required when intake is less adequate. Serum ferritin is highly correlated with total body iron stores, making it the most sensitive index of iron status among healthy children. Requirements are determined by rate of growth, iron stores, increased blood volume, and rate of absorption from food sources. Menstrual loss and rapid growth increases the need in adolescent girls. Reliable biomarkers of the total quantity of dietary iron are unavailable because of the wide variation in bioavailability and especially due to the large difference in absorption of heme iron versus inorganic iron. In contrast, a range of biomarkers is available that in combination allows for reliable assessment of iron status, therefore identifying the adequacy of iron intake, especially in noninfected, nonstressed individuals. Biomarkers can distinguish three generally accepted levels of iron deficiency and are also useful in the evaluation of iron overload. The three levels of iron deficiency are depleted iron stores, early functional iron deficiency, and iron deficiency anemia (Pollitt, 2001; Hambridge, 2003).

Iron deficiency is the most common nutritional disorder in the world, with approximately 25% of the world's population being deficient. Iron deficiency anemia is most common in children between ages 1 and 3 years, with a prevalence of approximately 9%. Over the past two decades there has been an overall decrease in prevalence of iron deficiency anemia. Factors that have influenced this are prolonged use of iron-fortified infant formulas, increased breast-feeding, iron intake in the form of food sources, and the Special Supplemental Nutrition Program for Women, Infants, and Children. The AAP recommends universal or selective screening for infants between 9 and 12 months of age, followed by a second screening 6 months later. Universal screening up to age 2 years for communities with significant levels of iron deficiency or infants whose diets put them at risk is also recommended. Selective screening may be based on risk factors such as prematurity, low birth weight, and dietary intake. Routine screening is not recommended for children over 2 years of age except when risk factors such as poor diet, poverty, or special needs are present (Samour & King, 2005).

Iron deficiency: The most common nutritional disorder in the world, with approximately 25% of the world's population being deficient.

The relationship between iron deficiency and cognition has been debated for many years. Much of the research has been focused on the idea that even in the early stages of iron deficiency, iron dependent neurotransmitters can be altered, which in turn can impair learning ability and behaviors. It is plausible that some cerebral changes occur soon after the reserve of iron is depleted and there is a decreased activity in nutrient-dependent enzymes. This could be followed by constraint in motor development and physical activity secondary to a drop in the oxygen supply to muscle fibers. Iron deficiency during infancy may have long-term consequences, as demonstrated by impaired cognitive development and impaired learning ability. Anemic children have been reported to be at risk of delayed acquisition of developmentally appropriate emotional regulation (Pollitt, 2001). It is not certain, however, whether iron status is the major factor contributing to poor school performance of children with general lack of nutrition, such as that which often occurs in rural areas. For these children, cumulative overall nutrient intake may affect school performance more significantly than their iron intake. Despite the improving trends, iron deficiency is especially common among children from low-income families, with many of these children having the more severe form of the disorder, iron deficiency anemia (Kim et al., 2005).

Rapid growth during the first year of life requires an adequate supply of iron for synthesis of blood, muscle, and other tissues. Preterm infants have an increased requirement for dietary iron to facilitate appropriate growth. Most health authorities recommend exclusively breast-feeding for 4 to 6 months, a practice thought to prevent development of iron deficiency anemia in term healthy infants. Iron in human milk, however, is low, but it is thought that the high bioavailability partly compensates for decreased concentration. Iron absorption is regulated by recent dietary iron intake, independent of the size of iron stores and the rate of erythropoiesis. Observational studies suggest that dietary regulation of iron absorption is immature in an infant less than 6 months of age and is subject to developmental changes between 6 and 9 months of age. Changes in the regulation of iron absorption between 6 and 9 months of age enhance the infant's ability to adapt to a low-iron diet and provide a mechanism by which some, but not all, infants avoid iron deficiency despite low iron intake in late infancy. This adaptation may not be sufficient to prevent iron deficiency in exclusively breast-fed infants, especially those who were born prematurely. To prevent this, iron supplements are often recommended for breast-fed infants after 4 to 6 months if not consuming adequate amounts of iron-rich complementary foods. Iron supplementation is also often recommended for older breast-feeding infants who are not consuming iron-rich infant cereals. Little, however, is known about factors affecting iron absorption from human milk or supplements (Domellof, Lonnerdal, Abrams, & Hernell, 2002).

Different stages of iron deficiency involve different systemic changes, which in turn affect different psychobiological domains. During early iron deficiency the supply of iron to the bone marrow is marginal, not causing measurable decline in hemoglobin. Iron deficiency anemia is associated with variation in red blood cell width. Hemoglobin and hematocrit are the main biological screening tests because of the simplicity of measurements. Low values occur only during later stages of deficiency and result in impairment of normal physiology (Hambridge, 2003). Acute blood loss, acute and chronic infection, micronutrient deficiency (vitamin B_{12} or folate), and defects in red blood cell production (sickle cell or thalassemia) may also cause low values. An advantageous side effect of correcting low iron levels with iron supplements has been shown to be improved appetite (Pawley & Bishop, 2004).

Iron absorption from food depends on iron status of the individual (those with low iron stores have increased absorption rate) and increased absorption rate from heme iron versus non-heme sources. It is uncertain if excessive dietary iron levels result in abnormally high ferritin levels. A typical American mixed diet contains approximately 6 mg iron per 1,000 calories. Adolescents dieting to lose weight will likely have minimal iron intake, especially if animal protein is limited. The best dietary sources of iron are green vegetables, legumes, and meat. Much of the iron ingested in the American diet in the form of bread and cereals is not well absorbed. Although iron is clearly essential for a wide range of vital biological processes, it is also a potentially toxic substance. Iron overload disorders, which can lead to cirrhosis, coronary heart disease, and congestive heart failure, are also a public health concern (Hendler & Rorvik, 2001).

Magnesium

Magnesium is an essential mineral involved with over 300 metabolic reactions. It is necessary for every major biological process, including the production of cellular energy and the synthesis of nucleic acids and proteins. It is also important for the electrical stability of cells, the maintenance of membrane integrity, muscle contraction, nerve conduction, and regulation of vascular tone. About 50% to 60% of the body's magnesium content is in the bone, whereas a mere 1% is found extracellularly. Magnesium is the second most abundant intracellular cation, with potassium being the most abundant. There is much about the pharmacokinetics of magnesium that is not known.

Magnesium deficiency is associated with the pathogenesis of numerous serious disorders, notably ischemic heart disease, congestive heart failure, sudden cardiac death, diabetes, and hypertension. Treatment with supplemental magnesium is often helpful in these conditions. It may help prevent or reduce the incidence of cerebral palsy (CP) and mental retardation in pre-term infants. Symptoms and signs of magnesium deficiency include anorexia, nausea and vomiting, diarrhea, generalized muscle spasticity, confusion, seizures, and cardiac arrhythmias. Magnesium deficiency may be found in diabetes mellitus, malabsorption syndromes, and hyperthyroidism. Long-term use of diuretics may also result in magnesium deficiency. Magnesium deficiency itself is an important cause of hypokalemia (Hendler & Rorvik, 2001).

Magnesium is associated with a low risk of adverse effects that are most often related to the rate of administration and the dose given. The most common adverse reaction from the use of magnesium supplements is diarrhea. Other gastrointestinal symptoms that may occur with the use of magnesium supplements are nausea and abdominal cramping. Magnesium, which is excreted by the kidney, is contraindicated in patients with renal failure. Those with renal failure may develop hypermagnesemia with use of magnesium supplements. Magnesium seems to have a wide therapeutic window in which doses expected to produce clinical benefits should not result in significant adverse effects. There is currently very little information to guide physicians regarding the frequency with which magnesium boluses may be administered (Scarfone, 1999).

Foods rich in magnesium include unpolished grains, nuts, and green leafy vegetables, which are particularly good sources because of their chlorophyll content. Refined and processed foods are generally poor sources of magnesium. The efficiency of absorption of magnesium is inversely proportional to the amount of magnesium ingested.

Potassium

Potassium is an essential micromineral that is important in the transmission of nerve impulses; contraction of the cardiac, smooth, and skeletal muscles; production of energy; and synthesis of nucleic acids. Its antihypertensive properties were first identified in 1928. Evidence suggests that high intakes of potassium also protect against strokes and cardiovascular disease (Hendler & Rorvik, 2001).

The major cause of potassium depletion is excessive losses through the alimentary tract and kidneys. Depletion typically occurs as a result of chronic diuretic use, from severe diarrhea, or in children receiving long-term total parenteral nutrition inadequately supplemented with potassium. The effects of potassium depletion on the rapidly growing infant have not been well studied. Chronic hypokalemia has been associated with renal hypertrophy, interstitial disease, and hypertension in adults. Additional symptoms of depletion include metabolic alkalosis, anorexia, fatigue, and cardiac arrhythmias (Hendler & Rorvik, 2001). Animal studies, including in young rats, have shown significant growth retardation and increased renin-angiotensin system activity. Potassium-depleted kidneys also showed early fibrosis. Systolic blood pressure was also elevated in potassium-depleted rats, which persisted even after the serum potassium was normalized (Ray, Suga, Liu, Huang, & Johnson, 2001).

Foods that are rich in potassium include fresh fruits and vegetables. Therefore, children following vegetarian diets tend to have higher intakes of potassium. The efficiency of absorption of supplementary potassium is significant at approximately 90% via the gastrointestinal tract. Dietary potassium is absorbed at a similar rate. The most common adverse effects of potassium supplementation include nausea, vomiting, abdominal discomfort, and diarrhea. Oral potassium supplements rarely result in hypokalemia when normal renal function is present.

Phosphorus

Phosphorus is an essential macromineral that plays a pivotal role in the structure and function of the body. Phosphorus is essential for the process of bone mineralization and makes up the structure of the bone. Phosphorus in the form of phospholipids makes up the structure of cellular membranes. Phosphorus also makes up the structure of nucleic acids and nucleotides, including adenosine triphosphate. During the last trimester of pregnancy, the human fetus accrues about 80% of the calcium, phosphorus, and magnesium present at term. Therefore, infants born prematurely require higher intakes of these minerals per kilogram of body weight than do term infants. Providing adequate amounts of these nutrients, particularly phosphorus, to very-low-birth-weight infants during the first few weeks of life is not always possible. As a result, osteopenia is frequent in these infants, with fractures developing in some. Preterm human milk is low in phosphorus and has been associated with impaired bone mineralization and rickets. The addition of human milk fortifiers has improved bone mineralization (Kleinman and American Academy of Pediatrics Committee on Nutrition, 2004).

Phosphorus deficiency states are usually a result of malabsorption syndromes and diseases causing renal tubular losses of phosphorus. In addition, those with malnutrition and critically ill patients, such as those being treated for diabetic ketoacidosis, are at risk for phosphorus deficiency and phosphorus imbalance. The so-called refeeding syndrome can cause hypophosphatemia, which may be life threatening. Phosphorus deficiency can result in anorexia, impaired growth, osteomalacia, skeletal demineralization, proximal muscle atrophy, cardiac arrhythmias, respiratory insufficiency, susceptibility to infectious rickets, nervous system disorders, and even death.

Phosphorus supplements, in the form of phosphate salts, are not widely used in the United States to treat phosphorus deficiency. The one exception is calcium phosphate, which is mainly used as a delivery form of calcium. The most common adverse reaction to use of sodium or potassium phosphate is diarrhea. The salts are less likely to cause diarrhea when they are used by phosphorus-deficient individuals than when used by those with normal phosphorus status. Those with renal failure may develop hyperphosphatemia, which can result in ectopic calcification (Hendler & Rorvik, 2001).

Phosphorus, mainly in the form of phosphates, is widely distributed in the food supply, and phosphorus intake from the normal diet is usually sufficient to meet the body's needs. Milk and milk products are particularly good sources of phosphorus.

Copper

Copper essentiality was first demonstrated in the late 1920s when malnourished children with anemia were nonresponsive to iron supplementation. Anemia, neutropenia, and osteopenia are found with frank copper deficiency. Twenty years later the essentiality of copper (Cu) for fetal development was reestablished when it was shown that deficits of this nutrient during pregnancy can result in gross structural malformations in the fetus and persistent neurologic and immunologic abnormalities. Copper is required for normal infant development, red and white blood cell maturation, iron transport, bone strength, cholesterol metabolism, myocardial contractility, brain development, and immune function. Premature and small-for-gestational-age infants who are born with low Cu stores can exhibit signs of Cu deficiency, including neutropenia, normocytic hypochromic anemia, osteopenia, pathologic bone fractures, depigmentation of the skin and hair, and distended blood vessels. During the past decade there has been increasing interest in the concept that marginal deficits of this element can contribute to the development and progression of a number of disease states, including cardiovascular disease and diabetes.

Several human disorders with genetic mutations in Cu transporters have further defined the role of Cu in human health. Infants with **Menkes disease,** an X-linked genetic disorder, have a gene mutation that is responsible for Cu deficiency. Symptoms are characterized by hypothermia; neuronal degeneration; mental retardation; abnormalities in hair, skin, and connective tissue; bone fractures; and widespread vascular abnormalities, with death typically occurring by age 4 years. Some of the above symptoms are likely secondary to excessive iron accumulation and subsequent oxidative stress (Uriu-Adams & Keen, 2005).

Plasma copper and ceruloplasmin levels are the most frequently used biomarkers of copper status and are depressed in Cu deficiency states. Levels plateau when copper intake reaches an adequate level, and these biomarkers do not reflect the magnitude of copper intake beyond this point (Hambridge, 2003). Low intakes of Cu in the diet can result in marginal Cu deficiency in young children. Although the mean dietary intake of Cu in most countries is close to the Recommended Dietary Allowance, a substantial percentage of individuals have intakes less than the recommendation, fueling the concern that marginal Cu deficiency may be a common public health concern. Moreover, high dietary intakes of iron or zinc can adversely affect Cu status. For example, infants consuming infant formula with a high level of iron absorb less Cu than those consuming formulas with a low level of iron. Manifestations of mild copper deficiency may include abnormal glucose intolerance, hypercholesterolemia, myocardial disease, arterial disease, cardiac arrhythmias, loss of pigmentation, and neurologic symptoms.

Although copper is clearly essential for a wide range of biochemical processes, which are necessary for the maintenance of good health, it is also a potentially toxic substance. There are a number of case reports of acute Cu toxicity in the literature. Typically, these case reports represent instances when the acute toxicity is due to ingestion of beverages (including water) that have been contaminated with Cu. Acute Cu toxicity can result in a number of pathologies and, in severe cases, death. **Wilson disease** is an inherited disorder of copper metabolism characterized by a failure of the liver to excrete copper, leading to its accumulation in the liver, brain, cornea, and kidney, with resulting chronic degenerative changes. Cu toxicity, typically due to genetic disorders, can also be a significant health concern (Uriu-Adams & Keen, 2005).

The richest food sources of copper include nuts, seeds, legumes, liver, kidneys, and shellfish. Absorption efficiency appears to depend on the level of dietary copper intake, with a range of approximately 15% to 97%. As dietary copper increases, the fractional absorption of copper decreases. Excessive intake of non-heme iron, zinc, and vitamin C may decrease copper status (Hendler & Rorvik, 2001).

Menkes disease: X-linked genetic disorder that is responsible for Cu deficiency. Symptoms are characterized by hypothermia; neuronal degeneration; mental retardation; abnormalities in hair, skin, and connective tissue; bone fractures; and widespread vascular abnormalities, with death typically occurring by age 4.

Wilson disease: An inherited disorder of copper metabolism characterized by a failure of the liver to excrete copper, leading to its accumulation in the liver, brain, cornea, and kidney, with resulting chronic degenerative changes.

Zinc

Zinc is an essential nutrient that because of its fundamental role in many aspects of cellular metabolism is critical for normal immune function and physical growth. Zinc is critically involved in several biological mechanisms related to growth, including protein synthesis, gene expression, and hormonal regulation. Zinc is a trace mineral that is involved with RNA and DNA synthesis and is critical to cellular growth, differentiation, and metabolism. The body also appears to have the ability, though much more modest, to store zinc. As the global public health importance of zinc deficiency has attracted increasing attention during the past decade, so have the limitations of current biomarkers. Plasma zinc is currently the most widely used and accepted biomarker despite poor sensitivity and imperfect specificity. Investigators often use indirect measures of zinc status because only a small percentage of the body's zinc is in plasma. Most of the body's zinc is located in muscle, bone, and the liver, where it turns over slowly (Black, 2003; Hambridge, 2003).

Animal studies have shown that zinc deficiency probably begins to affect the growth process before birth (Merialdi et al., 2004). Zinc deficiency may be particularly relevant to early development because it is an essential trace element that plays fundamental roles in cell division and maturation and in the growth and function of many organ systems, including the neurologic system. Zinc deficiency may also influence child development by altering a child's ability to elicit or use nurturing interactions from caregivers. Low-birth-weight infants have been noted to have low zinc concentrations in cord blood, and zinc deficiency in childhood is associated with reduced immunocompetence and increased infectious disease morbidity (Sazawal et al., 2001). With a small liver and thus very limited hepatic stores of zinc and increased requirements for catch-up growth, they are at risk for zinc deficiency. Healthy infants are usually able to get an adequate amount of zinc from breast-feeding during the first 6 months of life, as long as the mother's milk supply is adequate and breast milk is not displaced by complementary foods. However, infants who are small for gestational age and premature infants may benefit from zinc supplementation in addition to the zinc they receive from breast-feeding. During the second 6 months of life, when complementary foods are introduced, the risk for zinc deficiency increases because most traditional complementary foods are low in bioavailable zinc (Black, 2003).

Zinc deficiency is regarded as a major public health problem with multiple health consequences. Zinc deficiency appears to be widespread in low-income countries because of low dietary intake of zinc-rich animal source foods and a high consumption of cereal grains and legumes, which contain inhibitors of zinc. The prevalence of zinc deficiency throughout childhood is estimated to be high, primarily related to the low consumption of foods high in bioavailable zinc. Children in poor countries are also frequently affected by diarrhea, which causes excess fecal losses of zinc (Penny et al., 2004). In such settings zinc supplementation trials among nutritionally deficient infants have demonstrated beneficial effects on mortality and on health indicators, including growth, diarrhea, and pneumonia morbidity (Brown, Peerson, Rivera, & Allen, 2002). Improved zinc status has been associated with improved appetites in young stunted children. Randomized trials are necessary to examine the specificity of zinc deficiency on children's behavior and development (Sanstead, Frederickson, & Penland, 2000; Bhatnagar & Taneja, 2001). Most of the research linking zinc to child development has not addressed the possibility of interactions with other micronutrient deficiencies.

The small, rapidly exchangeable pool of zinc is dependent on a steady source of zinc from the diet. The optimal source of zinc is from animal sources, such as beef, lamb, and oysters, which are also important sources of iron and vitamin B_{12}. This suggests that children who are zinc deficient are also likely to be deficient in iron and vitamin B_{12}. All three micronutrients have been associated with deficits in cognitive functioning. However, it is possible that simultaneous administration of multiple other micronutrients could interfere with zinc absorption or utilization. For example, adverse reactions between iron and zinc have been described (Penny et al., 2004).

Selenium

Selenium is a trace mineral involved in the regulation of thyroid hormone metabolism, healthy immune function, antioxidant activity, and prevention of coronary artery disease. Recognition of selenium's importance in the diet has long been impeded by fear of its toxicity and potential carcinogenic effects.

The quality of biomarkers of dietary intake of selenium and selenium status is quite favorable relative to that of most trace minerals. These biomarkers are in increasing demand principally because of the antioxidant role of this micromineral. Plasma selenium responds rapidly to selenium supplementation and is regarded as a biomarker of short-term selenium status, although in reasonably stable circumstances it also provides a biomarker of long-term intake. Whole blood selenium is of potential value as a biomarker of relatively long-term intake and status. Hair selenium has also been used to assess selenium status. Selenium homeostasis is regulated by excretion via the kidneys with increased intakes resulting in increased urinary metabolites (Hendler & Rorvik, 2001).

A limited number of studies identified children with severe neurodevelopmental delays and elevated liver function tests after developing intractable seizures during the first year of life. At the time of seizures, evidence of systemic selenium deficiency was documented. Findings support the hypothesis that the presence of selenium depletion in the brain among patients with epilepsy constitutes an important trigger of intractable seizures and neuronal damage (Ramaekers, Calomme, Berghe, & Makropoulos, 1994).

The amount of selenium found in foods is based on the concentration of selenium in the soil in which they were grown. Because of the uneven distribution of selenium in the soil throughout the world, disorders of deficiency and excesses have been reported. China, for example, is known to have the lowest and highest concentrations of soil selenium in the world. Reported adverse reactions to toxic levels of selenium are skin rash, brittle hair and nails, garlic-like breath, irritability, nausea, and vomiting (Kleinman et al., 2003).

Iodine

Iodine is required for the production of thyroid hormones, which are necessary for normal brain development and cognition. Iodine deficiency is the main cause of potentially preventable mental deficit in childhood and causes goiter and hypothyroidism in people of all ages. Environmental iodine deficiency causes a wide spectrum of devastating mental and physical disorders, collectively described as iodine deficiency disorders, which are a major public health problem all over the world (Chandra, Tripathy, Ghosh, Debnath, & Mukhopadhyay, 2005). Although endemic goiter is the most visible consequence of iodine deficiency, the most significant and profound consequences are on the developing brain. Congenital hypothyroidism and endemic iodine deficiency are a common cause of mental retardation (Simsek, Karabay, Safak, & Kocabay, 2003). Impaired intellectual development of people living in iodine-deficient regions is of particular concern, especially when all the adverse effects can be prevented by long-term sustainable iodine prophylaxis. Information processing, fine motor skills, and visual problem solving are improved by iodine repletion in moderately iodine-deficient school children (Zimmermann et al., 2006). Adverse effects of supplementation are generally minor and transient, including adolescent acne, rashes, arrhythmias, numbness, weakness in the hands, hypothyroidism, hyperthyroidism, parotitis (iodide mumps), and small bowel lesions. Children with cystic fibrosis appear to have an exaggerated susceptibility to the goitrogenic effect of high doses of iodide. High-quality controlled studies investigating long-term outcome measures are needed to address the best form of iodine supplementation in different population groups and settings (Angermayr & Clar, 2004).

The mean serum thyroid-stimulating hormone is increased in iodine deficiency, although absolute values may remain within the normal range. Thyroid function tests provide useful functional biomarkers of longer term iodine intake and iodide status. Urinary iodine is the standard biochemical indicator used worldwide that shows the current state of iodine nutrition. It is also a valuable indicator for the assessment of iodine deficiency disorders because 90% of the body's iodine is excreted through the urine (Hambridge, 2003; Chandra et al., 2005). Urine iodine excretion reflects intake within the past few days.

Percutaneous absorption of topically applied substances and the potential for systemic toxicity are important considerations in the child. Most cases of percutaneous drug toxicity have been reported in newborns, although cases in infants and young children have also been noted. Iodine-containing compounds such as povidone-iodine have long been used for topical antisepsis, and it has been suggested they may carry a significant risk to infants. Percutaneous toxicity is of greatest concern in the premature infant, in whom immaturity of the epidermal permeability barrier results in disproportionately increased absorption. Immature drug metabolism capabilities may further contribute to the increased risk in this population. Elevations in both plasma and urinary iodine have been documented in premature infants exposed to these agents. The potential for transient hypothyroxinemia and hypothyroidism has been a concern of many clinicians. This concern stems from the known risks of abnormal thyroid function in the infant, including growth and motor retardation, cognitive delay, and intraventricular hemorrhage. The surface area of the treated skin seems to correlate directly with the risk (Mancini, 2000). In addition to iodized salts, rich sources of iodine include fish and sea vegetables. Iodine is also available in animal products such as eggs, milk, meat, and poultry.

Chromium

Chromium is believed to be an essential trace mineral in human nutrition. Evidence suggests that it plays an important role in normal carbohydrate metabolism. The mechanism of chromium's possible glucose regulatory activity is not well understood. It has also been suggested that chromium may decrease hepatic extraction of insulin and improve glucose tolerance. It has been found that patients receiving long-term total parenteral nutrition without chromium develop glucose intolerance, weight loss, and peripheral neuropathy. These symptoms reverse when patients are given intravenous chromium chloride (Hendler & Rorvik, 2001). Suggestive but poorly substantiated evidence that chromium deficiency may be widespread, especially in individuals with some degree of glucose intolerance, points to a need for reliable biomarkers of dietary chromium and chromium status. It has been concluded that plasma chromium is unlikely to offer a useful indicator in part because normal values are so near the limit of detection. There are conflicting data on the relationship of urine chromium excretion to dietary intake. Only one study, in which controlled quantities of dietary chromium were given, provided some evidence for deterioration in glucose tolerance with a severely chromium-restricted diet (Hambridge, 2003).

The efficiency of absorption of chromium from inorganic or organic compounds is minimal at approximately 2%. Chromium is distributed to various tissues in the body but appears to have a preference for bone, spleen, liver, and kidney. Most ingested chromium is excreted in the feces. Chromium that has been absorbed is excreted mainly in the urine. There is much that remains unknown regarding the pharmacokinetics of chromium. Dietary intake is approximately 25 mg/day, with the recommended adequate daily dietary intake being 10 to 120 mg for children under the age of 7 (Hendler & Rorvik, 2001).

Good food sources of chromium include whole grains, cereals, mushrooms, brown sugar, and brewer's yeast. Fruits and vegetables are generally poor sources of chromium, as are most refined foods.

Summary

Generally, healthy infants and toddlers can achieve recommended levels of vitamins and minerals from food alone. Dietetic professionals should encourage caregivers to use foods rather than supplements as the primary source of nutrients in a child's diet. Vitamin and mineral supplements can help infants and toddlers with special nutrient needs or marginal intakes achieve adequate intakes, but care must be taken to ensure that supplements do not lead to excessive levels. This is especially important for nutrients that are widely used as food fortifiers, including vitamin A, zinc, and folate.

Despite the success of child survival programs, approximately 12 million children under 5 years old in developing countries still die of preventable causes, half of them of diarrheal diseases and respiratory infections. It is becoming clear that a large portion of the risk of infectious disease morbidity and mortality attributed to malnutrition may result primarily from deficiencies of a few critical micronutrients. Actions needed to control micronutrient deficiencies include prevention strategies, extensive nutrition, and health education through innovative materials to support program-specific problems and strengthening of various state government programs. Interventions to reduce infant and preschool morbidity are a public health priority globally.

Issues to Debate

1. Should the United States provide formula, food, and/or vitamins to poor counties? Why or why not?
2. What would be the cost of providing food/formula/vitamins and health care to the world's children?
3. What would be the cost of *not* providing food/formula/vitamins and health care to the world's children?

References

Adams, J. B., George, F., & Audhya, T. (2006). Abnormally high plasma levels of vitamin B_6 in children with autism not taking supplements compared to controls not taking supplements. *Journal of Alternative and Complementary Medicine, 12,* 59–63.

Ahmed, M., & Jenkins, H. R. (2004). Vitamin B-12 in Crohn's disease patients with small bowel surgery. *Archives of Disease in Childhood, 89,* 293.

American Academy of Pediatrics Committee on Fetus and Newborn. (2003). Controversies concerning vitamin K and the newborn. *Pediatrics, 112,* 191–192.

Angermayr, L., & Clar, C. (2004). Iodine supplementation for preventing iodine deficiency disorders in children. *Cochrane Database of Systematic Reviews*, (2), CD003819.

Atkinson, S. A. (2001). Special nutritional needs of infants for prevention of and recovery from bronchopulmonary dysplasia. *Journal of Nutrition, 131*, 942S–946S.

Barnes, C., Newall, F., Ignjatovic, V., Wong, P., Cameron, F., Jones, G., et al. (2005). Reduced bone density in children on long-term warfarin. *Pediatric Research, 57*, 578–581.

Berseth, C. L., Van Aerde, J. E., Gross, S., Stolz, S., Harris, C. L., & Hansen, J. W. (2004). Growth, efficacy and safety of feeding an iron-fortified human milk fortifier. *Pediatrics, 114*, 699–706.

Black, M. M. (2003). Evidence linking zinc deficiency with children's cognitive and motor functioning. *Journal of Nutrition, 133*, 1473S–1476S.

Black, M. M., Sazawal, S., Black, R. E., Khosla, S., Kumar, J., & Menon, V. (2004). Cognitive and motor development among small-for-gestational-age infants: Impact of zinc supplementation, birth weight, and caregiving practices. *Pediatrics, 113*, 1297–1305.

Briefel, R., Hanson, C., Fox, M. K., Novak, T., & Ziegler, P. (2006). Feeding Infants and Toddlers Study: Do vitamins and mineral supplements contribute to nutrient adequacy or excess among US infants and toddlers? *Journal of the American Dietetic Association, 106*(1 Suppl. 1), S52–S65.

Brown, K. H., Peerson, J. M., Rivera, J., & Allen, L. H. (2002). Effect of supplemental zinc on the growth and serum zinc concentrations of prepubertal children: A meta-analysis of randomized controlled trials. American *Journal of Clinical Nutrition, 75*, 1062–1071.

Cashman, K. D. (2005). Vitamin K status may be an important determinant of childhood bone health. *Nutrition Reviews, 63*, 284–289.

Chakravarty, I., & Sinha, R. K. (2002). Prevalence of micronutrient deficiency based on results obtained from the national pilot program on control of micronutrient malnutrition. *Nutrition Reviews, 60*(5 Pt. 2), S53–S58.

Chandra, A. K., Tripathy, S., Ghosh, D., Debnath, A., & Mukhopadhyay, S. (2005). Iodine nutritional status and prevalence of goiter in Sundarban delta of South 24-Parganas, West Bengal. *Indian Journal of Medical Research, 122*, 419–424.

Chaudhuri, A. (2005). Why we should offer routine vitamin D supplementation in pregnancy and childhood to prevent multiple sclerosis. *Medical Hypotheses, 64*, 608–618.

Chavasse, R. J., Francis, J., Balfour-Lynn, I., Rosenthal, M., & Bush, A. (2004). Serum vitamin D levels in children with cystic fibrosis. *Pediatric Pulmonology, 38*, 119–122.

Commission on the Nutrition Challenges of the 21st Century. (2000). Ending malnutrition by 2020: An agenda for change in the millennium. *Food and Nutrition Bulletin, 21*, 1–88.

Cunningham-Rundles, S., McNeeley, D. F., and Moon, A. (2005). Mechanisms of nutrient modulation of the immune response. *Journal of Allergy and Clinical Immunology, 115*, 1119–1128.

Dhonukshe-Rutten, R. A., van Dusseldorp, M., Schneede, J., de Groot, L. C., & van Staveren, W. A. (2005). Low bone mineral density and bone mineral content are associated with low cobalamin status in adolescents. *European Journal of Nutrition, 44*, 341–347.

Domellof, M., Lonnerdal, B., Abrams, S. A., & Hernell, O. (2002). Iron absorption in breast-fed infants: Effects of age, iron status, iron supplementation and complementary foods. *American Journal of Clinical Nutrition, 76*, 198–204.

Eitenschenck, L., Armari-Alla, C., Plantaz, D., Pagnier, A., & Ducros, V. (2005). Belated decompensation of an Imerslund-Grasbeck disease. *Archives of Pediatrics, 12*, 1729–1731.

Fawzi, W., Msamanga, G., Spiegelman, D., & Hunter, D. J. (2005). Studies of vitamins and minerals and HIV transmission and disease progression. *Journal of Nutrition, 135*, 938–944.

Fisher, J. O., Mitchell, D. C., Smiciklas-Wright, H., Mannino, M. L., & Birch, L. L. (2004). Meeting calcium recommendations during middle childhood reflects mother-daughter beverage choices and predicts bone mineral status. *American Journal of Clinical Nutrition, 79*, 698–706.

Forastiere, F., Pistelli, R., Sestini, P., Fortes, C., Renzoni, E., Rusconi, F., et al. (2000). Consumption of fresh fruit rich in vitamin C and wheezing symptoms in children. *Thorax, 55*, 283–288.

French, A. E., Grant, R., Weitzman, S., Ray, J. G., Vermeulen, M. J., Sung, L., et al. (2003). Folic acid food fortification is associated with a decline in neuroblastoma. *Clinical Pharmacology and Therapeutics, 74*, 288–294.

Gartner, L. M., Greer, F. R., & Section on Breastfeeding and Committee on Nutrition. (2003). Prevention of rickets and vitamin D deficiency: New guidelines for vitamin D intake. *Pediatrics, 111*, 908–910.

Greer, F. R. (2004). Issues in establishing vitamin D requirements for infants and children. *American Journal of Clinical Nutrition, 80*(6 Suppl.), 1759S–1762S.

Hambridge, M. (2000). Human zinc deficiency. *Journal of Nutrition, 130*(Suppl. 5), 1344S–1349S.

Hambridge, M. (2003). Biomarkers of trace mineral intake and status. *Journal of Nutrition, 133*, 948S–955S.

Hendler, S. S., & Rorvik, D. (2001). PDR for Nutritional Supplements. Montvale, NJ: Medical Economics Company.

Hollis, B. W., & Wagner, C. L. (2004). Assessment of dietary vitamin D requirements during pregnancy and lactation. *American Journal of Clinical Nutrition, 79*, 717–726.

Huiming, Y., Chaomin, W., & Meng, M. (2005). Vitamin A treating measles in children. Cochrane Database of Systematic Reviews, 19(4), CD001479.

James, S. J., Cutler, P., Melnyk, S., Jernigan, S., Janak, L., Gaylor, D. W., et al. (2004). Metabolic biomarkers of increased oxidative stress and impaired methylation capacity in children with autism. *American Journal of Clinical Nutrition, 80*, 1611–1617.

Juval, R., Osmamy, M., Black, R. E., Dhingra, U., Sarkar, A., Dhingra, P., et al. (2004). Efficacy of micronutrient fortification of milk on morbidity in pre-school children and growth—a double blind randomized controlled trial. *Asia Pacific Journal of Clinical Nutrition, 13*(Suppl.), S44.

Kapil, U., and Bhavna, A. (2002). Adverse effects of poor micronutrient status during childhood and adolescence. *Nutrition Reviews, 60*(5 Pt. 2), S84–S90.

Kim, S., Kim, J., & Keen, C. (2005). Comparison of dietary patterns and nutrient intakes of elementary school children living in remote rural and urban areas in Korea: Their potential impact on school performance. *Nutrition Research, 25*, 349–363.

Kleinman, R. E., & American Academy of Pediatrics (AAP) Committee on Nutrition (2004). *Pediatric Nutrition Handbook (5th ed.).* Elk Grove Village, IL: American Academy of Pediatrics.

Korenke, G. C., Hunneman, D. H., Eber, S., & Hanefeld, F. (2004). Severe encephalopathy with epilepsy in an infant caused by subclinical maternal pernicious anemia: Case report and review of literature. *European Journal of Pediatrics, 163,* 96–201.

Kronn, D. F., Sapru, A., & Satou, G. M. (2000). Management of hypercholesterolemia in childhood and adolescence. *Heart Disorders, 2,* 348–353.

Kwan, M. L., Block, G., Selcin, S., Month, S., & Buffler, P. A. (2004). Food consumption by children and the risk of childhood acute leukemia. *American Journal of Epidemiology, 160,* 1098–1107.

Li, M., Eastman, C. J., Waite, K. V., Ma, G., Zacharin, M. R., Topliss, D. J., et al. (2006). Are Australian children iodine deficient? Results of the Australian National Iodine Nutrition Study. *Medical Journal of Australia, 184,* 165–169.

Libermann, S., & Branning, N. (1997). *The Real Vitamins and Minerals Book* (2nd ed.). Garden City Park, NY: Avery.

Liu, S., West, R., Randell, E., Longerich, L., O'Connor, K. S., Scott, H., et al. (2004). A comprehensive evaluation of food fortification with folic acid for the primary prevention of neural tube defects. *BMC Pregnancy and Childbirth, 4,* 20.

Lumley, J., Watson, L., Watson, M., & Bower, C. (2000). Periconceptional supplementation with folate and/or multivitamins for preventing neural tube defects. *Cochrane Database of Systematic Reviews,* (2), CD001056.

Mahan, L. K., & Escott-Stump, S. (2000). *Krause's Food, Nutrition, and Diet Therapy* (10th ed.). Philadelphia: W. B. Saunders.

Mancini, A. J. (2000). Skin. *Pediatrics, 113,* 1114–1119.

Marcellini, M., Di Ciommo, V., Callea, F., Devito, R., Comparcola, D., Sartorelli, M. R., et al. (2005). Treatment of Wilson's disease with zinc from the time of diagnosis in pediatric patients: A single-hospital 10-year follow-up study. *Journal of Laboratory and Clinical Medicine, 145,* 139–143.

Merialdi, M., Caulfield, L. E., Zavaleta, N., Figueroa, A., Costigan, K. A., Dominici, F., et al. (2004). Randomized controlled trial of prenatal zinc supplementation and fetal bone growth. *American Journal of Clinical Nutrition, 79,* 826–830.

Miller, A. L. (2003). The methionine-homocysteine cycle and its effects on cognitive diseases. *Alternative Medicine Reviews, 8,* 7–19.

Milne, E., de Klerk, N. H., van Bockxmeer, F., Kees, U. R., Thompson, J. R., Baker, D., et al. (2006). Is there a folate-regulated gene-environment interaction in the etiology of childhood acute lymphoblastic leukemia? *International Journal of Cancer, 119,* 229–232.

Monsen, A. L., Refsum, H., Markestad, T., & Ueland, P. M. (2003). Cobalamin status and its biochemical markers MMA and homocysteine in different age groups from 4 days to 19 years. *Clinical Chemistry, 49,* 2067–2075.

Morgan, J. (2005). Nutrition for toddlers: The foundation for good health—toddler's nutritional needs: What are they and are they being met? *Journal of Family Health Care, 15,* 56–59.

Mughal, Z. (2002). Rickets in childhood. *Seminars in Musculoskeletal Radiology, 6,* 183–190.

Muntjewerff, J. W., Van der Put, N., Eskes, T., Ellenbroek, B., Steegers, E., Blom, H., et al. (2003). Homocysteine metabolism and B-vitamins in schizophrenic patients: Low plasma folate as a possible independent risk factor for schizophrenia. *Psychiatry Research, 121,* 1–9.

Murphy, S. P., Gewa, C., Liang, L., Grillenberger, M., Bwibo, N. O., and Neumann, C. G. (2003). School snacks containing animal source foods improve dietary quality for children in rural Kenya. *Journal of Nutrition, 133,* 3950S–3956S.

Neumann, C. G., Gewa, C., & Bwibo, N. O. (2004). Child nutrition in developing countries. *Pediatric Annals, 33,* 658–674.

Pawley, N., & Bishop, N. J. (2004). Prenatal and infant predictors of bone health: The influence of vitamin D. *American Journal of Clinical Nutrition, 80*(6 Suppl.), 1748S–1751S.

Penland, J. G. (2000). Behavioral data and methodology issues in studies of zinc nutrition in humans. *Journal of Nutrition, 130,* 147S–153S.

Penny, M. E., Marin, R. M., Duran, A., Peerson, J. M., Lanata, C. F., Lonnerdal, B., et al. (2004). Randomized controlled trial of the effect of daily supplementation with zinc or multiple micronutrients on the morbidity, growth and micronutrient status of young Peruvian children. *American Journal of Clinical Nutrition, 79,* 457–465.

Persad, V. L., Van den Hof, M. C., Dube, J. M., & Zimmer, P. (2002). Incidence of open neural tube defects in Nova Scotia after folic acid fortification. *CMAJ: Canadian Medical Association Journal, 167,* 241–245.

Pollitt, E. (2001). The developmental and probabilistic nature and functional consequences of iron-deficiency anemia in children. *Journal of Nutrition, 131,* 669S–675S.

Powers, H. J. (2003). Riboflavin (vitamin B-2) and health. *American Journal of Clinical Nutrition, 77,* 1352–1360.

Prabhu, S. S., & Dalvi, B. V. (2000). Treatable cardiomyopathies. *Indian Journal of Pediatrics, 67*(3 Suppl.), S7–S10.

Prousky, J. E. (2003). Pellegra may be a rare secondary complication of anorexia nervosa: A systematic review of the literature. *Alternative Medicine Reviews, 8,* 180–185.

Ramaekers, V. T., & Blau, N. (2004). Cerebral folate deficiency. *Developmental Medicine and Child Neurology, 46,* 843–851.

Ramaekers, V. T., Calomme, M., Berghe, V., & Makropoulos, W. (1994). Selenium deficiency triggering intractable seizures. *Neuropediatrics, 25,* 217–223.

Ray, P. E., Suga, S., Liu, X. H., Huang, X., & Johnson, R. J. (2001). Chronic potassium depletion induces renal injury, salt sensitivity, and hypertension in young rats. *Kidney International, 59,* 1850–1858.

Rodriguez, A., Hamer, D. H., Rivera, J., Acosta, M., Salgado, G., Gordillo, M., et al. (2005). Effects of moderate doses of vitamin A as an adjunct to the treatment of pneumonia in underweight and normal-weight children: A randomized, double-blind, placebo-controlled trial. *American Journal of Clinical Nutrition, 82,* 1090–1096.

Salamoun, M. M., Kizirian, A. S., Tannous, R. I., Nabulsi, M. M., Choucair, M. K., Deeb, M. E., et al. (2005). Low calcium and vitamin D intake in healthy children and adolescents and their correlates. *European Journal of Clinical Nutrition, 59,* 177–184.

Samour, P. Q., & King, K. (2005). *Handbook of Pediatric Nutrition* (3rd ed.). Sudbury, MA: Jones and Bartlett.

Sanstead, H. H., Frederickson, C. J., & Penland, J. G. (2000). Zinc nutriture as related to brain. *Journal of Nutrition, 130,* 140S–146S.

Sazawal, S., Black, R. E., Menon, V. P., Dinghra, P., Caulfield, L. E., Dhingra, U., et al. (2001). Zinc supplementation in infants born small for gestational age reduces mortality; a prospective, randomized, controlled trial. *Pediatrics, 108,* 1280–1286.

Scarfone, R. J. (1999). Use of magnesium sulfate in the treatment of children with acute asthma. *Clinical Pediatric Emergency Medicine, 1,* 6–12.

Simsek, E., Karabay, M., Safak, A., & Kocabay, K. (2003). Congenital hypothyroidism and iodine status in Turkey: A comparison between the data obtained from an epidemiological study in school-aged children and neonatal screening for congenital hypothyroidism in Turkey. *Pediatric Endocrinology Reviews: PER, 1*(Suppl. 2), 155–161.

Svahn, J., Schiaffino, M. C., Caruso, U., Calvillo, M., Minniti, G., & Dufour, C. (2003). Severe lactic acidosis due to thiamine deficiency in a patient with B-cell leukemia lymphoma on total parenteral nutrition during high-dose methotrexate therapy. *Journal of Pediatric Hematology/Oncology, 25,* 965–968.

Tanner, E. M., & Finn-Stevenson, M. (2002). Nutrition and brain development: Social policy implications. *American Journal of Orthopsychiatry, 72,* 182–193.

Uriu-Adams, J. Y., & Keen, C. L. (2005). Copper, oxidative stress, and human health. *Molecular Aspects of Medicine, 26,* 268–298.

Wang, J. Y., Wang, Y. L., Zhou, S. L., & Zhou, J. F. (2004). May chronic childhood constipation cause oxidative stress and potential free radical damage to children? *Biomedical and Environmental Sciences: BES, 17,* 266–272.

Wharton, B., & Bishop, N. (2003). Rickets. *Lancet, 362,* 1389–1400.

Yoshii, A., Takeoka, M., Kelly, P. J., & Krishnamoorthy, K. S. (2005). Focal status epilepticus as atypical presentation of pyridoxine-dependent epilepsy. *Journal of Child Neurology, 20,* 696–698.

Zacharin, M. (2004). Current advances in bone health of disabled children. *Current Opinion in Pediatrics, 16,* 545–551.

Zimmermann, M. B., Connolly, K., Bozo, M., Bridson, J., Rohner, F., & Grimci, L. (2006). Iodine supplementation improves cognition in iodine-deficient schoolchildren in Albania: A randomized, controlled, double-blind study. *American Journal of Clinical Nutrition, 83,* 108–114.

Zinc Investigators' Collaborative Group. (2000). Therapeutic effects of oral zinc in acute and persistent diarrhea in children in developing countries: Pooled analysis of randomized controlled trials. *American Journal of Clinical Nutrition, 72,* 1516–1522.

Special Topics in School-Aged Nutrition: Pediatric Vegetarianism and Childhood Overweight

Reed Mangels, PhD, RD, Inger Stallmann-Jorgensen, MS, RD, LD,

Edna Harris-Davis, MS, MPH, RD, LD

CHAPTER OUTLINE

Reader Objectives

After studying this chapter and reflecting on the contents, you should be able to

1. Describe the similarities and differences between lacto-ovo-vegetarian, lacto-vegetarian, vegan, macrobiotic, fruitarian, and raw foods diets.
2. List potential health and nutritional benefits of vegetarian diets for the pediatric population.
3. Describe possible motivations for following a vegetarian diet.
4. Contrast growth of lacto-ovo-vegetarian, vegan, and nonvegetarian children and adolescents.
5. Identify key nutrients for vegetarian infants, children, and adolescents and suggest acceptable food sources for each nutrient.
6. Identify major nutritional issues for pediatric vegetarians and describe appropriate approaches for working with these issues.
7. Describe specific considerations for counseling vegetarians of various ages and their families.
8. List the growing problems related to overweight in children.
9. Describe the paradigm shift that occurred over the years to cause increased rates of overweight children.
10. Articulate some steps that families may take to help prevent overweight in children.

Pediatric Vegetarianism

Reed Mangels, PhD, RD

Today, about a million school-aged children in the United States consistently follow a vegetarian diet (Vegetarian Resource Group, 2001) and say that they never eat meat, fish, or poultry. Many more children and adolescents eat a mostly vegetarian diet that may include limited amounts of animal products (Perry, McGuire, Neumark-Sztainer, & Story, 2002). Attitudes toward vegetarian diets for children have changed markedly. In the 1970s vegetarian diets were labeled a form of child abuse (Roberts, West, Ogilvie, & Dillon, 1979). Compare this with the 2003 statement by the American Dietetic Association and Dietitians of Canada that states, "appropriately planned vegan, lacto-vegetarian, and lacto-ovo-vegetarian diets satisfy nutrient needs of infants, children, and adolescents and promote normal growth" (Mangels, Messina, & Melina, 2003).

Types of Vegetarian Diets

When working with vegetarians it is important to understand what a vegetarian diet is and to realize there are several different kinds of vegetarians. In the broadest sense a **vegetarian** is a person who does not eat meat, fish, or poultry (Mangels et al., 2003). **Lacto-ovo-vegetarians** include dairy products and eggs in their diets. **Lacto-vegetarians** include dairy products but not eggs. **Vegans** avoid eating any animal products.

Other types of vegetarian (or near-vegetarian) diets that may be encountered include **macrobiotic,** raw foods, and **fruitarian** diets (Messina, Mangels, & Messina, 2004). Macrobiotic diets are based largely on grains along with vegetables, especially **sea vegetables;** beans; fruits; nuts; soy products; and possibly fish. A number of studies have reported serious nutrient deficiencies with long-term consequences in children following macrobiotic diets (Dagnelie, van Staveren, Vergote, Burema, et al., 1989; Dagnelie, Vergote, et al., 1990; Louwman et al., 2000; Dhonukshe-Rutten, van Dusseldorp, Schneede, de Groot, & van Staveren, 2005). Depending on food and supplement choices, with careful planning, macrobiotic diets can be used by children (Mangels & Messina, 2001; Messina, Mangels, & Messina, 2004). Practitioners of a raw

Vegetarian: A person who does not eat meat, fish, or fowl or products containing those foods.

Lacto-ovo-vegetarian: A vegetarian who eats dairy products and eggs.

Lacto-vegetarian: A vegetarian who eats dairy products but not eggs.

Vegan: A vegetarian who avoids all animal products, including dairy products and eggs.

Macrobiotic: A person following a vegetarian or near-vegetarian diet based largely on grains, legumes, and vegetables; may include limited amounts of fish.

Fruitarian: A person following a diet based on fruits, nuts, and seeds that often includes vegetables that are botanically fruits like avocado and tomatoes.

Sea vegetables: Wild ocean plants, including nori, kelp, hijiki, and dulse, that are often purchased in dried form.

foods diet consume foods only in their raw state. Foods used include fruits, vegetables, nuts, seeds, sprouted grains, and sprouted beans; raw dairy products may be used. Fruitarian diets are based on fruits, nuts, and seeds and often include vegetables that are botanically fruits like avocado and tomatoes. Use of extremely restrictive diets such as raw foods and fruitarian diets has not been studied in infants and children. These diets can be very low in protein, energy, some vitamins, and minerals and cannot be recommended for infants and children (Messina, Mangels, & Messina, 2004). Some self-described vegetarians eat fish, chicken, or even meat (Barr & Chapman, 2002; Perry et al., 2002). These practices can have a significant impact on food choices and nutrient intake, so individual assessment of the diets of vegetarian clients is essential.

How Many Vegetarians Are There?

Approximately 2% of children and adolescents in the United States consistently follow a vegetarian diet, whereas about 0.5% consistently follow a vegan diet, according to a Roper Poll conducted in 2000 (Vegetarian Resource Group, 2001). Similar results were obtained in a poll conducted in 1995 (Vegetarian Resource Group, 2001).

Vegetarianism and Cultural Diversity
Seventh-Day Adventists
Did you know?
- Seventh-day Adventists (SDAs) are a conservative religious group with more than 13 million members worldwide.
- SDAs are strongly encouraged to abstain from meat. About 27% are lacto-ovo-vegetarians, 3% are vegans, and 20% eat meat less than once a week.
- They tend to have healthy life-styles, eating more fruits and vegetables and exercising more frequently than their neighbors.
- Less than 2% use any form of tobacco; less than 10% use alcohol, and those who do generally drink only small amounts.
- SDAs have been studied extensively and have provided a wealth of information about the health advantages of a healthy life-style. Significant findings include
  - Lower rates of coronary disease than non-SDAs with even lower rates in vegetarian SDAs.
  - Lower incidence of lung, colon, stomach, bladder, and other cancers than non-SDAs.
  - SDAs live longer than non-SDAs; vegetarian SDAs live longer than nonvegetarian SDAs.
  - Vegetarian SDAs weigh less than nonvegetarian SDAs.
  - Vegetarian SDAs are less likely to develop diabetes, hypertension, and arthritis than nonvegetarian SDAs.

Compiled from Fraser, G. E. (2003). *Diet, Life Expectancy, and Chronic Disease: Studies of Seventh-Day Adventists and Other Vegetarians.* New York: Oxford University Press.

Reasons for Vegetarianism
Children and adolescents have a variety of motivations for following a vegetarian diet. Some are members of vegetarian families. Others cite an assortment of reasons, including health, animal welfare, and environmental concerns (Worsley & Skrzypiec, 1998; Larsson, Ronnlund, Johansson, & Dahlgren, 2003).

Health Benefits of Vegetarian Diets
There are numerous health benefits for adults following a vegetarian diet, including a lower body mass index (BMI), reduced risk of cardiovascular disease, lower blood pressure and lower rates of hypertension, reduced risk of type 2 diabetes, and a lower risk for prostate and colorectal cancer (Messina, Mangels, & Messina, 2004). Less is known about benefits for vegetarian children. Vegetarian children do tend to be leaner than nonvegetarian children (Hebbelinck & Clarys, 2001), and at least one study reported lower serum cholesterol concentrations in vegetarian children (Krajcovicova-Kudlackova, Simoncic, Bederova, Grancicova, & Megalova, 1997). Positive food patterns of vegetarian children and adolescents include greater consumption of fruits, vegetables, nuts, and legumes and lower consumption of sweets, fast food, and salty snack foods (Neumark-Sztainer, Story, Resnick, & Blum, 1997; Donovan & Gibson, 1996; Perry et al., 2002; Larsson & Johansson, 2005). In addition, diets of vegetarian children and adolescents tend to be lower in cholesterol, saturated fat, and total fat and higher in fiber than diets of nonvegetarians (Thane & Bates, 2000; Larsson & Johansson, 2002; Perry et al., 2002).

Growth and Energy Needs of Vegetarian Children

A limited number of studies have examined growth of vegetarian children in developed countries. Many of these studies were conducted more than 20 years ago when many foods frequently used by vegetarian families, such as fortified soy milk and veggie burgers, were much less available than today. Generally, studies of lacto-ovo-vegetarian school-aged children and adolescents show that their height is similar and their weight is similar to or slightly lower than nonvegetarians (Sabaté, Linsted, Harris, & Johnston, 1990; Sabaté, Linsted, Harris, & Sanchez, 1991; Nathan, Hackett, & Kirby, 1997; Hebbelinck & Clarys, 2001). Some studies have suggested that vegetarian girls enter puberty later than nonvegetarians and therefore are shorter than similarly aged nonvegetarian girls (Kissinger & Sanchez, 1987; Sabaté, Llorca, & Sanchez, 1992), whereas other studies have not found this (Hebbelinck & Clarys, 2001). Vegan children tend to be leaner than nonvegetarian children but are typically within normal ranges of standards for height and weight (Sanders, 1988; Sanders & Manning, 1992). Markedly lower heights and weights have been reported in children following macrobiotic diets (Dagnelie, van Staveren, van Klaveren, & Burema, 1988; Dagnelie, van Staveren, Vergote, Burema, et al., 1989), with lower heights persisting even after some relaxation of dietary practices (van Dusseldorp et al., 1996).

Lacto-ovo-vegetarian and vegan diets can support appropriate growth and development of children. If a child's growth rate is below what is expected, an increased energy intake may be necessary. This can be accomplished by providing concentrated energy sources, including soy products and other legumes, nuts and nut butters, and oils. In addition, some children may benefit from a somewhat lower fiber intake (Mangels, Messina, & Melina, 2003).

Nutritional Considerations

Key nutrients for vegetarian children and adolescents include protein, iron, zinc, calcium, vitamin D, vitamin B_{12}, and omega-3 fatty acids. In the nonvegetarian diet these nutrients are frequently largely obtained from animal products, so questions have been raised about their adequacy in vegetarian or vegan diets. Other nutrients, including folate, vitamin C, and vitamin A (as beta-carotene), are generally not considered problematic for vegetarians due to many vegetarians' higher consumption of fruits and vegetables.

Protein

Protein is rarely below recommendations in vegetarian children's diets that contain adequate energy and a variety of plant foods (Dagnelie, van Staveren, Verschuren, & Hautvast, 1989; Thane & Bates, 2000; Leung et al., 2001). The Institute of Medicine (IOM, Food and Nutrition Board, 2002) concluded that the protein requirement for vegetarians who consume a variety of plant proteins is not different from that of nonvegetarians. Plant proteins contain varying amounts of essential amino acids. For example, compared with the Amino Acid Scoring Pattern developed by the Food and Nutrition Board and IOM, wheat is low in lysine (IOM, 2002). Chickpeas and other legumes are relatively low in the sulfur amino acids (methionine and cysteine). By eating a variety of protein sources over the course of a day, differences in amino acid content are satisfied (Young & Pellett, 1994; Mangels, Messina, & Melina, 2003).

Iron and Zinc

Iron intakes of vegetarian children and adolescents vary. Some studies reported iron intakes by vegetarian children that are similar to or higher than those of nonvegetarian children (Houghton et al., 1997; Thane & Bates, 2000; Larsson & Johansson, 2002; Perry et al., 2002), whereas others identified lower iron intakes in vegetarians (Donovan & Gibson, 1995, 1996). Lower hemoglobin and ferritin levels have been reported in vegetarian children (Donovan & Gibson, 1995, 1996; Nathan, Hackett, & Kirby, 1996; Thane & Bates, 2000; Thane, Bates, & Prentice, 2003), suggesting that iron is not as well absorbed from a vegetarian diet.

Non-heme iron is the only form of iron found in vegetarian diets. Inhibitors and enhancers affect the absorption of non-heme iron. **Phytate,** found in whole grains, legumes, and to a lesser extent vegetables (Hallberg & Hulthen, 2000), is the main inhibitor of iron absorption in vegetarian diets. Although no information is available with regard to the phytate content of pediatric vegetarian diets, adult vegan diets may contain two to three times as much phytate as nonvegetarian diets; lacto-ovo-vegetarian diets have a phytate content intermediate between vegan and nonvegetarian diets (Ellis et al., 1987; Hunt, Matthys, & Johnson, 1998).

Because of the lower **bioavailability** of iron from vegetarian diets, a separate iron Recommended Dietary Allowance (RDA) has been established for vegetarians that assumes an iron bioavailability of 10% compared with 18% for nonvegetarian diets (IOM, Food and Nutrition Board, 2001). Adjustments do not need to be made to the RDA for infants from birth to 12 months (IOM, Food and Nutrition Board, 2001), because recommendations for infants from birth to 6 months are based on the iron content of breast milk. The RDA for infants ages 7 to 12 months is based on a bioavailability of 10% rather than

Non-heme iron: The form of iron found in plants and the portion of iron from animal foods that is not part of hemoglobin or myoglobin.

Phytate: A phosphorus-containing compound found in whole grains and dried beans that binds with minerals, particularly iron and zinc, and interferes with their absorption.

Bioavailability: A measure of how available to the body a nutrient is after it is ingested.

TABLE 7.1	Iron RDA for Vegetarian Children and Adolescents*	

Age, Gender	Iron RDA (mg/d)
1–3 yr, M/F	12.6
4–8 yr, M/F	18
9–13 yr, M/F	14.4
14–18 yr, M	19.8
14–18 yr, F	27

*Values calculated based on 1.8 times RDA for nonvegetarians.
From IOM (2001).

the higher bioavailability that is used for other age groups (IOM, Food and Nutrition Board, 2001). Iron recommendations for older vegetarian children can be found in **Table 7.1**.

Iron absorption from a vegetarian diet can be enhanced even in the presence of phytate by consuming a vitamin C source at the same time as the iron source (Hallberg & Hulthen, 2000; Sandstrom, 2001). Leavening of bread reduces its phytate content and enhances iron absorption (Hunt, 2002). Iron sources for vegetarian children include iron-fortified breakfast cereals, soy foods, dried beans, and whole grains. **Table 7.2** provides more information about vegetarian iron sources, and **Table 7.3** shows a sample menu that would meet a vegetarian adolescent girl's high iron requirements. Laboratory assessment of iron status is appropriate if a child's diet is low in iron and iron supplements are not regularly used.

TABLE 7.2	Food Sources of Iron* for Vegetarians	

Food, Standard Amount	Iron (mg)	Calories
Fortified ready-to-eat cereals (various), ~1 oz	1.8–21.1	54–127
Fortified instant cooked cereals (various), 1 packet	4.9–8.1	Varies
Soybeans, mature, cooked, 1/2 cup	4.4	149
Pumpkin and squash seed kernels, roasted, 1 oz	4.2	148
White beans, canned, 1/2 cup	3.9	153
Blackstrap molasses, 1 T	3.5	47
Lentils, cooked, 1/2 cup	3.3	115
Spinach, cooked from fresh, 1/2 cup	3.2	21
Kidney beans, cooked, 1/2 cup	2.6	112
Chickpeas, cooked, 1/2 cup	2.4	134
Prune juice, 3/4 cup	2.3	136
Cowpeas, cooked, 1/2 cup	2.2	100
Tomato puree, 1/2 cup	2.2	48
Lima beans, cooked, 1/2 cup	2.2	108
Soybeans, green, cooked, 1/2 cup	2.2	127
Navy beans, cooked, 1/2 cup	2.1	127
Refried beans, 1/2 cup	2.1	118
Tomato paste, 1/4 cup	2.0	54

*Food sources of iron ranked by milligrams of iron per standard amount; also calories in the standard amount. Adapted from DHHS and USDA. (2005, 2010). Dietary Guidelines for Americans. Washington, DC: DHHS and USDA. Nutrient values from Agricultural Research Service (ARS) Nutrient Database for Standard Reference, Release 17. Foods are from ARS single nutrient reports, sorted in descending order by nutrient content in terms of common household measures. Food items and weights in the single nutrient reports are adapted from those in 2002 revision of USDA Home and Garden Bulletin No. 72, Nutritive Value of Foods. Mixed dishes and multiple preparations of the same food item have been omitted from this table.

Limited information suggests that the zinc content of diets of vegetarian children is similar to that of nonvegetarian children (Sanders, 1995; Thane & Bates, 2000). However, because phytate inhibits zinc absorption, vegetarian children are likely to have higher requirements for zinc than nonvegetarian children. The IOM has not specified a zinc RDA for vegetarians but suggests that the dietary requirement for zinc may be as much as 50% greater for vegetarians, especially for those relying mainly on grains and legumes (IOM, Food and Nutrition Board, 2001). Techniques that can enhance zinc absorption include using yeast-leavened breads, using fermented soy products like tempeh and miso, and soaking dried beans and discarding the soaking water before cooking the beans (Gibson, Yeudall, Drost, Mtitmunit, & Cullinan, 1998). Zinc supplements should be considered for children on vegan diets, especially diets based on high-phytate cereals and legumes (Allen, 1998).

Calcium and Vitamin D

Children following lacto-ovo-vegetarian diets tend to have adequate intakes of calcium and vitamin D because of their use of dairy products (Thane & Bates, 2000; Perry et al., 2002). Limited data suggest that calcium intakes of vegan children are lower than recommendations (Messina, Mangels, & Messina, 2004). Rickets, due to a deficiency of vitamin D, has been seen in some children following macrobiotic diets (Dagnelie, Vergote, et al., 1990) and in infants and toddlers fed unfortified soy or rice milk (Carvalho, Kenney, Carrington, & Hall, 2001; Imataka, Mikami, Yamanouchi, Kano, & Eguchi, 2004). Adequate calcium and vitamin D are important for all children to promote bone growth and to reduce risk of fracture (Black, Williams, Jones, & Goulding, 2002; Kalkwarf, Khoury, & Lanphear, 2003). There is no evidence that vegan children need less calcium than nonvegetarians, and increased calcium intakes (342 vs. 1,056 mg/day) have been shown to improve bone mineral status of children on near-vegan diets (Dibba, Prentice, & Ceesay, 2000). The adequate intake for calcium is 500 mg/day for 1- to 3-year-olds, 800 mg/day for 4- to 8-year-olds, and 1,300 mg/day for 9- to 18-year-olds (IOM, Food and Nutrition Board, 1997).

There are a number of reliable sources of calcium for children and adolescents who limit or avoid dairy products. These include soy milks and juices that have been fortified with calcium (Heaney, Dowell, Rafferty, & Bierman, 2000;

TABLE 7.3	Example of an Iron-Rich Menu	
		Iron (mg)
1 cup oatmeal		1.6
1/4 cup raisins		1.4
8 oz fortified soy milk		0.7
6 oz orange juice		0.3
2 slices whole-wheat toast		1.7
Bean burrito:		
1 flour tortilla		1.0
1/2 cup kidney beans		2.6
2 T salsa		0.0
1 cup watermelon chunks		0.4
Stir-fry:		
3/4 cup tofu		10.0
1 cup cooked broccoli		1.0
1 cup brown rice		1.0
1/2 cup cooked carrots		0.3
3/4 cup strawberries		0.6
1 cup fortified soy milk		0.7
Trail mix:		
1/4 cup pumpkin seeds		8.5
2 T sunflower seeds		0.6
1/4 cup dried apricots		0.9
Total		33.3

From U.S. Department of Agriculture, Agricultural Research Service. (2005). USDA Nutrient Database for Standard Reference, Release 18, and manufacturers' information.

Heaney, Rafferty, & Bierman, 2005). Low-oxalate vegetables, like kale, broccoli, and collard greens, contain generous amounts of well-absorbed calcium (Weaver & Plawecki, 1994), and although these foods may not be the major source of calcium in children's diets, they can significantly increase calcium intake. Tofu processed with calcium sulfate, almonds, almond butter, and dried figs are other sources of calcium (Mangels et al., 2003). Vegan products that have been developed to resemble dairy products, such as soy yogurt and soy cheese, do not always contain the same amount of calcium as their dairy counterparts. Label reading is essential to determine the nutrient content of these products. **Table 7.4** provides more information about nondairy sources of calcium for vegetarians.

TABLE 7.4

TABLE 7.4 Nondairy Food Sources of Calcium* for Vegetarians

Food, Standard Amount	Calcium (mg)	Calories
Fortified ready-to-eat cereals (various), 1 oz	236–1,043	88–106
Soy beverage, calcium fortified, 1 cup	368	98
Tofu, firm, prepared with nigari,[†] 1/2 cup	253	88
Collards, cooked from frozen, 1/2 cup	178	31
Molasses, blackstrap, 1 T	172	47
Spinach, cooked from frozen, 1/2 cup	146	30
Soybeans, green, cooked, 1/2 cup	130	127
Turnip greens, cooked from frozen, 1/2 cup	124	24
Oatmeal, plain and flavored, instant, fortified, 1 packet prepared	99–110	97–157
Cowpeas, cooked, 1/2 cup	106	80
White beans, canned, 1/2 cup	96	153
Kale, cooked from frozen, 1/2 cup	90	20
Okra, cooked from frozen, 1/2 cup	88	26
Soybeans, mature, cooked, 1/2 cup	88	149
Beet greens, cooked from fresh, 1/2 cup	82	19
Pak-choi, Chinese cabbage, cooked from fresh, 1/2 cup	79	10
Dandelion greens, cooked from fresh, 1/2 cup	74	17

*Nondairy food sources of calcium ranked by milligrams of calcium per standard amount; also calories in the standard amount. The bioavailability may vary. Both calcium content and bioavailability should be considered when selecting dietary sources of calcium. Some plant foods have calcium that is well absorbed, but the large quantity of plant foods that would be needed to provide as much calcium as in a glass of milk may be unachievable for many. Spinach, Swiss chard, beet greens, and rhubarb are high oxalate vegetables, and the calcium in these foods is largely unavailable. Many other calcium fortified foods are available, but the percentage of calcium that can be absorbed is unavailable for many of them.

[†]Calcium sulfate and magnesium chloride.

Adapted from DHHS and USDA. (2005, 2010). Dietary Guidelines for Americans. Washington, DC: DHHS and USDA.

Nutrient values from Agricultural Research Service (ARS) Nutrient Database for Standard Reference, Release 17. Foods are from ARS single nutrient reports, sorted in descending order by nutrient content in terms of common household measures. Food items and weights in the single nutrient reports are adapted from those in 2002 revision of USDA Home and Garden Bulletin No. 72, Nutritive Value of Foods. Mixed dishes and multiple preparations of the same food item have been omitted from this table.

Fortified soy milks and juices also frequently contain vitamin D. Some breakfast cereals are fortified with vitamin D as well. Although cutaneous synthesis can be an important vitamin D source, factors like age, limited sunlight exposure, skin tone, season, and sunscreen use can lead to concerns about adequate vitamin D production (Holick, 2004). Vitamin D supplements can also be used to ensure adequate vitamin D intakes.

Vitamin B$_{12}$

Vitamin B$_{12}$ is found in significant amounts only in foods derived from animals or in fortified foods. Lacto-ovo-vegetarians who consume an adequate amount of cow's milk, yogurt, or eggs regularly can meet recommendations for vitamin B$_{12}$. Vegans must obtain their vitamin B$_{12}$ from fortified foods (some brands of soy milk, breakfast cereals, meat analogs, and nutritional yeast) or from vitamin B$_{12}$ supplements. **Table 7.5** provides information about recommendations, food sources, and serving sizes of vitamin B$_{12}$–rich foods. Foods such as sea vegetables, fermented soy products, and Spirulina are sometimes promoted as sources of vitamin B$_{12}$; these cannot be counted on as reliable sources because they have

TABLE 7.5	Recommendations, Food Sources, and Serving Sizes of Vitamin B_{12}–Rich Foods	
Age Group	Vitamin B_{12} RDA (AI/day)	Servings of Vitamin B_{12}–Rich Foods
0–6 mo	0.4 (AI)	Vitamin B_{12} should be obtained from breast milk, infant formula, or supplements
7–12 mo	0.5 (AI)	Vitamin B_{12} should be obtained from breast milk, infant formula, or supplements
1–3 yr	0.9	1
4–8 yr	1.2	1.5
9–13 yr	1.8	2
14–18 yr	2.4	3

AI, adequate intake. From IOM (2001).

been shown to contain analogs of vitamin B_{12} that can interfere with the absorption of active vitamin B_{12} (van den Berg, Dagnelie, & van Staveren, 1988; Dagnelie, van Staveren, & van den Berg, 1991; Watanabe et al., 1999).

Adequate vitamin B_{12} is especially important during pregnancy and lactation because the maternal diet during these times is the major influence on the infant's vitamin B_{12} status (IOM, Food and Nutrition Board, 1998). Breast-fed infants whose mothers do not consume dairy products, vitamin B_{12}–fortified foods, or vitamin B_{12} supplements regularly need vitamin B_{12} supplements at the adequate intake level from birth (IOM, Food and Nutrition Board, 1998).

Although the RDA for vitamin B_{12} is extremely low, failure to achieve an adequate intake can lead to serious consequences. Marginal vitamin B_{12} status in adolescents has been associated with impaired cognitive function (Louwman et al., 2000) and gait disturbances (Licht, Berry, Brooks, & Younkin, 2001), and vitamin B_{12} deficiency in infants and children has led to failure to thrive, developmental delay, and seizures (Centers for Disease Control and Prevention, 2003).

Vegetarians eating few or no animal foods and not using vitamin B_{12}–fortified foods or vitamin B_{12} supplements should have their **cobalamin** status assessed (CDC, 2003). Serum or urine methylmalonic acid is one test for cobalamin deficiency; holotranscobalamin II, total homocysteine, and serum B_{12} also can be used (Hermann & Geisel, 2002).

Omega-3 Fatty Acids

Vegetarian diets are generally low in **alpha-linolenic acid,** an omega-3 fatty acid, whose essential role appears to be as a precursor for the synthesis of the long chain omega-3 fatty acids, **eicosapentaenoic acid (EPA)** and **docosahexaenoic acid (DHA)**. DHA is found in high concentrations in the membrane lipids of the brain and the retina (IOM, 2002) and appears to play a role in visual and cognitive performance (Birch, Garfield, Hoffman, Uauy, & Birch, 2000; SanGiovanni, Parra-Cabrera, Colditz, Berkey, & Dwyer, 2000), although results of supplementation studies are mixed (McCann & Ames, 2005). Unless vegetarians eat eggs or generous amounts of sea vegetables, their diets will also lack direct sources of EPA and DHA. Requirements for alpha-linolenic acid may be higher for many vegetarians than for nonvegetarians because vegetarians must rely on conversion of alpha-linolenic acid to EPA and DHA rather than obtaining these **n-3 fatty acids** from their diet (Davis & Kris-Etherton, 2003). The conversion of alpha-linolenic acid to EPA and subsequently to DHA is very limited (Davis & Kris-Etherton, 2003; Francois, Connor, Bolewicz, & Connor, 2003).

Vegetarians' lower dietary intakes of EPA and DHA are reflected in blood and breast milk concentrations. Adult lacto-ovo-vegetarians and vegans have lower blood concentrations of EPA and DHA than non-vegetarians (Krajcovicova-Kudlackova, Simoncic, Babinska, &

Cobalamin: Vitamin B_{12}.

Alpha-linolenic acid: An essential 18-carbon omega-3 fatty acid.

Eicosapentaenoic acid (EPA): A 20-carbon omega-3 fatty acid found in fish oil.

Docosahexaenoic acid (DHA): A 22-carbon omega-3 fatty acid found in fish oil.

n-3 fatty acid: A polyunsaturated fatty acid in which the first double bond is three carbons from the methyl end of the carbon chain. Important sources in the U.S. diet include certain fish tissues, canola and soybean oils, and seeds and nuts such as flax seeds and walnuts.

Bederova, 1995; Geppert, Kraft, Demmelmair, & Koletzko, 2005; Rosell et al., 2005), and adolescent vegans have lower concentrations than lacto-ovo-vegetarians or nonvegetarians (Krajcovicova-Kudlackova, Simoncic, Bederova, & Klvanova, 1997). Breast milk concentrations of alpha-linolenic acid, EPA, and DHA reflect the amounts present in the mother's diet and are lower in breast milk of vegetarian and vegan women (Sanders & Reddy, 1992; Uauy et al., 1996). Breast-fed infants of vegetarian and vegan women have lower plasma and red blood cell DHA concentrations than breast-fed infants of nonvegetarian women (Sanders & Reddy, 1992).

DHA supplements derived from microalgae are one option for vegetarians (Conquer & Holub, 1996; Davis & Kris-Etherton, 2003; Geppert et al., 2005). Because some EPA can be synthesized from alpha-linolenic acid, good sources of alpha-linolenic acid such as flaxseed and flaxseed oil, canola oil, soybean oil, walnuts, and soy products should be promoted (Mangels, Messina, & Melina, 2003). The conversion of alpha-linolenic acid to EPA can be enhanced by limiting use of oils high in linoleic acid and transfats (Davis & Kris-Etherton, 2003).

Nutritional Counseling of Vegetarian Infants, Children, and Adolescents and Their Families

The Position of the American Dietetic Association and Dietitians of Canada: Vegetarian Diets states, "Dietetics professionals have an important role in supporting clients who express an interest in adopting vegetarian diets or who already eat a vegetarian diet" (Mangels, Messina, & Melina, 2003, p. 759). Families with vegetarian infants, children, and adolescents seek nutrition

> ### CRITICAL **Thinking**
>
> **Critical Thinking About a Vegetarian Diet for a Child**
>
> - What tools and techniques would you use to assess a 3-year-old vegan's nutritional status?
> - What are some "red flags" for an eating disorder in a vegetarian adolescent? What would you do if you suspected that a client had an eating disorder?
> - Why is it important to ask a vegetarian client to tell you specifically about foods eaten and avoided rather than relying on their characterization of their diet as "vegetarian"?
> - When would you recommend supplements for a vegetarian child? Which supplements and what amounts? Would your recommendations differ for a lacto-ovo-vegetarian and a vegan child?

counseling for a variety of reasons. Perhaps a child or adolescent has decided to become vegetarian but the rest of the family wants to continue eating meat. Perhaps a health care provider has referred the family because of concerns about dietary adequacy. Perhaps a family that is already following a vegetarian diet is seeking advice on dietary modifications to improve their diet or to cope with a condition such as renal disease or diabetes. In any case, dietetics professionals need to be able to provide information about food sources of key nutrients for infants, children, and adolescents; to adapt guidelines for individuals with allergies, chronic diseases, or other factors necessitating dietary modifications; to assist with meal planning, food purchases, and food preparation decisions; and to give current information about vegetarian nutrition for the pediatric age group (Mangels, Messina, & Melina, 2003).

Infants and Toddlers

In early infancy, vegetarian infants do not differ from nonvegetarian infants in terms of feeding practices. Exclusive breast-feeding for 6 months and breast-feeding with complementary foods until at least 12 months of age are the ideal feeding patterns for infants (Dobson & Murtaugh, 2001).

> **● Learning Point** If there is any question about adequate vitamin B_{12} in a lactating woman's diet, a vitamin B_{12} supplement is recommended for her infant.

Commercial infant formula is recommended for infants who are not breast-fed or who are weaned before 1 year of age. Lacto-ovo-vegetarian families who use infant formula can use a cow milk–based formula, whereas for vegan families who use infant formula, soy formulas are the only option. Commercial soy beverages do not provide adequate nutrition for infants and should not be used, except for small amounts in cooking, during the first year (Messina, Mangels, & Messina, 2004). Other formulas such as those based on rice, nut, or seed milks; nondairy creamer; cereal gruels; or mixtures of fruit or vegetables juices should not be used to replace breast milk or commercial infant formula (Mangels & Messina, 2001). After the first year, either fortified full-fat soy milk or whole cow's milk can be used as the primary beverage for a child who is growing normally and eating a variety of foods (Mangels & Messina, 2001).

Solid foods can be introduced to vegetarian infants in the same order that they would be introduced to nonvegetarian infants (Scott, 2003). At around 7 to 8 months when higher protein foods would typically be introduced, vegetarian infants can start to eat cooked and pureed legumes, well-mashed tofu, or soy yogurt. Infants in lacto-ovo-vegetarian families can also have pureed cottage cheese, yogurt mixed with mashed fruit, or egg yolks. Foods that will eventually play a significant role in the diets of vegetarian children (e.g., legumes, tofu, and leafy green vegetables) should be introduced in infancy so that the child becomes familiar with the flavor of these foods.

As toddlers are weaned from breast milk or infant formula, energy intake may decrease. Foods that are both nutrient and energy dense, like soy products, bean spreads, and avocado, are often recommended to maintain energy intake during weaning.

Meal Planning Guidelines

A variety of meal planning guidelines have been developed for vegetarian children and adolescents (Truesdell & Acosta, 1985; Messina & Mangels, 2001; Stepaniak & Melina, 2003; Messina, Melina, & Mangels, 2003; Messina, Mangels, & Melina, 2004). The ideal plan should achieve the following goals (Messina, Melina, & Mangels, 2003):

- Meet the needs of different types of vegetarian diets
- Help vegetarians meet the most recent nutrient recommendations
- Focus on specific nutrients identified as being of special importance to vegetarians
- Include a wide variety of foods
- Meet the needs of different age groups

Childhood Overweight

Inger Stallmann-Jorgensen, MS, RD, LD,
Edna Harris-Davis, MS, MPH, RD, LD

Obesity and obesity-related diseases are some of the biggest health challenges of the 21st century. The rapidly increasing rate of excessive weight in children is especially alarming. Thus, now is the time for health care professionals to accept the urgent challenge of addressing overweight and obesity through prevention-based approaches. To maximize effectiveness, overweight and obesity prevention efforts must target children and their families and focus on policy and environmental interventions.

The topic of overweight children is a large and complex issue; it is not possible to address every aspect of the problem and its prevention and treatment in this chapter. Rather, the aim of this chapter is to provide an overview of overweight children and to guide the entry-level practitioner in addressing this challenging health issue.

Assessment of Overweight Children

In the pediatric population the BMI is used as a screening tool and is not a diagnosis for overweight children. The CDC revised and published the growth charts for children ages 2 to 20 years: BMI-for-Age, Weight-for-Age, and Stature-for-Age. The BMI-for-Age nutrition status indicators for At Risk for Overweight and Overweight children are ≥85th percentile to <95th percentile and ≥95th percentile, respectively (CDC, n.d.) (see Appendix 1). There is evidence that many overweight children will become obese adults (Serdula et al., 1993; Freedman, Khan, Dietz, Srinivasan, & Berenson, 2001). However, the BMI-for-Age assessment should be applied carefully so as to not label children as obese in error. It is important to determine whether a child indeed has extra fat mass and not extra muscle mass, particularly across genders and ethnicity (Ellis, Abrams, & Wong, 1999; Taylor, Jones, Williams, & Goulding, 2002). In addition, labeling as "obese" carries a stigma for many people. Therefore, as CDC has defined them, the terms "overweight" and "at-risk for overweight" should be used when addressing the pediatric population and to establish some consistency when making comparisons between various groups of children, particularly in research literature.

Overweight Rates in the United States

For adults, there has been a rapid increase in our nation's prevalence rate of overweight status over the past two decades. The United States is not alone in facing this serious health problem. Obesity

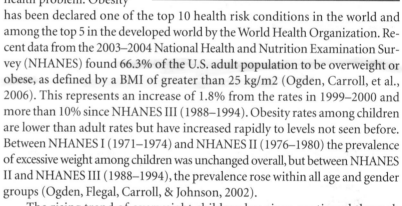

● **Learning Point** Even if the overweight status does not track into adulthood, there may be long-lasting medical and psychosocial effects in overweight children (Hill & Trowbridge, 1998).

has been declared one of the top 10 health risk conditions in the world and among the top 5 in the developed world by the World Health Organization. Recent data from the 2003–2004 National Health and Nutrition Examination Survey (NHANES) found 66.3% of the U.S. adult population to be overweight or obese, as defined by a BMI of greater than 25 kg/m2 (Ogden, Carroll, et al., 2006). This represents an increase of 1.8% from the rates in 1999–2000 and more than 10% since NHANES III (1988–1994). Obesity rates among children are lower than adult rates but have increased rapidly to levels not seen before. Between NHANES I (1971–1974) and NHANES II (1976–1980) the prevalence of excessive weight among children was unchanged overall, but between NHANES II and NHANES III (1988–1994), the prevalence rose within all age and gender groups (Ogden, Flegal, Carroll, & Johnson, 2002).

The rising trend of overweight children has since continued through NHANES 1999–2000, 2001–2002, and 2003–2004. Compared with 1988–1994 data, overweight rates in NHANES 2003–2004 increased by 6.9% for 12- to 19-year-olds, 7.5% for 6- to 11-year-olds, and 6.7% for 2- to 5-year-olds. Most recent rates now stand at 17.4% for 12- to 19-year-olds, 18.8% for 6- to 11-year-olds, and 13.9% for 2- to 5-year-olds for all racial/ethnic and gender groups combined. When children and adolescents (2 to 19 years of age) who are at risk

Health Disparities in Cultural Diversity

Ethnic, cultural, gender, genetic, socioeconomic, and regional differences exist that influence which children are at risk for being overweight. Especially boys of Hispanic-American origin, African-Americans, and those residing in the South experience higher rates of being overweight (Strauss & Pollack, 2001; Nelson, Chiasson, & Ford, 2004). The ethnic differences in the degree to which certain population groups are affected by overweight prevalence may exacerbate long-term health outcomes and economic disparities that already exist in the United States (Strauss & Pollack, 2001).

for excessive weight are included, the overall prevalence rate is 33.6%. However, the increases in over-weight rates have not occurred to the same extent among all age and race groups. Most affected by the rising trend in rates of at-risk for overweight and overweight combined are Mexican-American boys ages 6 to 11 (47.9%) and 2 to 5 (38.5%), followed by non-Hispanic African-American girls ages 6 to 11 (45.6%), 12 to 19 (42.1%), and 2 to 5 (27%). Thus, for some of these groups, almost half of the children and youth are either at risk for or are overweight (Ogden, Carroll, et al., 2006). The trend for increasing overweight prevalence among children is illustrated in **Figure 7.1**.

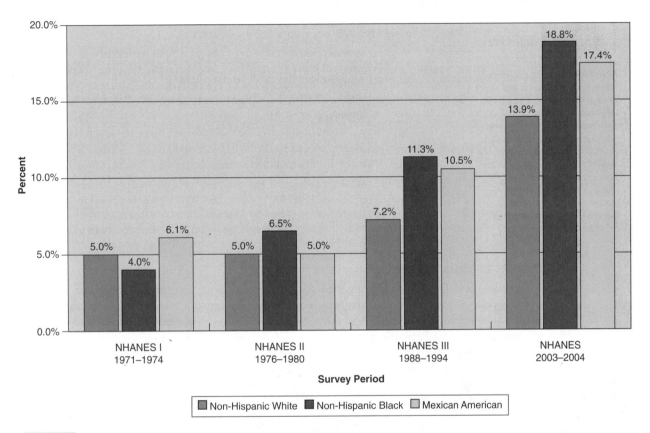

Figure 7.1   Prevalence of Overweight Among U.S. Children and Adolescents (Aged 2–19 Years), National Health and Nutrition Examination Surveys. *Source:* National Health and Nutrition Examinations Survey. Available at nutrition.gov.

Health Effects of the Overweight

The recent trends of overweight children are especially disturbing because of the predicted health consequences of being overweight. Freedman et al. (2001) studied the longitudinal relationship between children's BMI and their adult levels of lipids, insulin, and blood pressure. The mean time interval between first and follow-up measurements was 17 years. Over this time period 77% of overweight children remained so as adults. The persistence of excessive weight, once it occurs, is of great concern because being overweight is more strongly linked to chronic disease than is living in poverty, smoking, or drinking. The impact of obesity on overall health has been likened to aging by 20 years (Hill, Wyatt, Reed, & Peters, 2003). "Childhood obesity precedes insulin resistance/hyper-insulinemia and strongly predicts the risk of developing a constellation of metabolic, hemodynamic, thrombotic, and inflammatory disorders of syndrome X" (Berenson, 2002).

Although there is well-justified concern for overweight in children tracking into adulthood and increasing the risk of adult health problems, one must not ignore the acute, both physical and psychological, health issues that affect the overweight child. Many body functions are affected by being overweight, including the nervous, pulmonary, cardiovascular, skeletal, gastrointestinal, endocrine, and reproductive systems. In addition, overweight children suffer from mental health problems, such as depression, anxiety, lowered self-esteem, and sometimes eating disorders (Erickson, Robinson, Haydel, & Killen, 2000; Raman, 2002; Hassink, 2003). Pediatricians are diagnosing the most obese children and adolescents with hypertension, dyslipidemia, and non–insulin-dependent diabetes (NIDDM).

Environmental Influences on Overweight Children

Dietary Guidelines for Physical Exercise

The Dietary Guidelines Advisory Committee recommends that children engage in at least 60 minutes of physical activity on most (preferably all) days of the week. Physical activity may include short bouts (i.e., 10 minutes each) of moderately intense activity. In this way exercise can be accumulated through 3 to 6 bouts over the course of the day. The accumulated total of physical activity is what is important for health.

Societal Factors Influencing Overweight Children

Some overweight people have experienced discrimination because of the negative attitudes and judgmental behaviors of others who may see them as lazy and lacking will power. Such attitudes have contributed to a social stigma and caused psychological pain for those suffering from the condition. Viewing overweight children, within a construct of "personal responsibility," has allowed past treatment interventions to focus on the child and perhaps the family unit. Experience shows that this treatment model often fails because many overweight children have grown up to be overweight adults. Today, it is widely recognized that the micro-environment (home and family setting) and the macro-environment in which it is imbedded promote either healthy weight or overweight. Thus, altering both the micro- and macro-environments is vital to prevention and treatment of overweight in children. The dynamics between individuals and their near, intermediate, and distal environments influence their food choices and physical activity levels, both of which play important roles in the development of overweight (Booth et al., 2001).

Overweight Status and Energy Balance

The environmental factors underlying the recent increase in obesity rates in the United States are multiple; however, diet and physical activity play a crucial role. Basic to this concept is the fact that to maintain a stable weight, energy intake and output must be balanced. Thus, when physical activity level is low, weight status can be maintained with a diet appropriately lower in calories. However, if an adjustment is not made to keep energy intake and expenditure in balance, through either increased physical activity or decreased energy intake or a combined approach, excessive weight gain is the result. The alarming rise in overweight among U.S. children begs the question: What changes have occurred in our life-styles that could have contributed to this problem?

Dietary Trends Affecting Overweight Status in Children

Historical Perspective

Today's life-styles are very different from the life-styles of our hunter-gatherer ancestors. Genetically, humans evolved during the Paleolithic period 2.6 million to 10,000 years ago and were biologically adapted to survive under the prevailing conditions of that time. Today's Western-style diet is in sharp contrast to the diet of the hunter-gatherers, yet our human genome has changed little since that period to help us adapt to our present-day life-styles. Now, most of us "dwell in mechanized urban settings, leading sedentary lives and eating a highly processed, synthetic diet" (O'Keefe & Cordain, 2004). The differences in today's diets from that of the hunter-gatherers are that they consumed foods higher in fiber content and lower in energy density and with a different diet composition of the long chain fatty acids. The long chain fatty acids of the n-6 and n-3 families were consumed in a ratio of about 1:1. Today's Western-type diet can provide less of the omega-3 fatty acids with an n-6 to -n-3 ratio of 1:15–17 (Simopoulos, 2002). The diet of the hunter-gatherer was rich in plant foods, supplemented by fish and lean meats and nuts. Indications are that these early ancestors did not experience obesity. Changes in agricultural practices, as well as food processing and manufacturing, have resulted in a vastly different food supply that has evolved over a relatively short time. The development of agricultural societies led to diets based on grains. With this change from a plant-based to a grain-based diet, vitamin and mineral deficiencies began to appear as evidenced by studying bones and teeth. Our natural preference for foods that are calorie dense is rooted in the conditions of our ancestors in which obtaining food for survival through hunting, fishing, and gathering food required high levels of physical activity and a correspondingly high expenditure of energy.

In contrast, obtaining food today means a car ride to the grocery store and little connection between energy intake and expenditure (O'Keefe & Cordain, 2004). The typical American diet today is lower in fiber and plant foods, higher in meat, and high in highly refined carbohydrates (i.e., of high glycemic load) and possibly contains a much higher ratio of the n-6 relative to the n-3 long chain fatty acids. Sources of n-3 fatty acids that are diminished in our typical diet include fish, shellfish, wild game, and plant foods. Potassium intakes are much lower today, whereas sodium intakes are much higher than in the diets of our distant ancestors. In short, most people consume a diet they were not genetically designed to eat. Calcium is an important mineral for human health, yet calcium intakes are not adequate for adolescent girls, older women, and older men. Although calcium intake has increased a little for women aged 20 to 74 since NHANES III, recommendations for milk and dairy intake are not met by 70% of the population over 2 years of age, according to the NHANES 1999–2000 data (Briefel & Johnson, 2004). Researchers contend that these dietary changes, combined with sedentary life-styles, play a significant role in the etiology of chronic diseases affecting developed countries: heart disease, diabetes, cancer, and obesity (Simopoulos, 1999; Conner, 2000).

Changes in the Food Environment

One of the most noticeable changes affecting our food environment during the past two decades is the rapid growth in the number of restaurants and, especially, of fast food establishments, currently numbering about 250,000 outlets nationally. Fast food restaurants are found throughout our communities, even inside public schools and hospitals. The effective marketing and advertising of these restaurants to adults and children have fueled the growth of this industry. Unfortunately, fast food restaurant fare is usually high in calories, fat, salt, and sugars and low in fiber content (Bowman, Gortmaker, Ebbeling, Pereira, & Ludwig, 2004). This is especially true for menu items offered as special value promotions. Often, the more healthful selections on fast food menus are more expensive and are not subject to the low-price offers that might otherwise encourage customers to buy them.

Fast food items are convenient and relatively low cost. These factors appeal to working and single parents, and the percentage of children eating fast food meals will likely increase (Bowman et al., 2004). The amount of food dollars spent outside the home has increased significantly to now make up about 46% of total household food budgets. Fast food meals consume about 34% of the family food dollar. Meals eaten outside the home tend to be of large portion sizes and higher energy content and include fewer fruits and vegetables than meals eaten in the home. As a result, the increase in out-of-home meal consumption may have a negative impact on diet quality and on the obesity and health risk of children and their families (Nicklas, Baranowski, Cullen, & Berenson, 2001; American Dietetic Association, 2002).

Product innovations launched during the past two decades have included many products designed to lower the fat content of popular foods to address consumers' concerns about dietary fat and unwanted weight gain. In spite of an explosive growth in low-fat food products in many food categories, these food supply changes have seemingly not had the desired effect on our obesity rates. Many food manufacturers offset the lower fat content of the reformulated foods by increasing sugar and carbohydrate contents to maintain product acceptance by consumers. In the end, the caloric content of the lower-fat product is often similar to the original version. There is also concern that so-called low-fat foods may encourage the consumer to actually eat more calories overall because the low-fat food provides a "license to eat more" (Kurtzweil, 1996).

Energy intakes in children's diets have remained fairly stable since 1971–1974 (NHANES I), except for increases for children ages 1 to 2 years and for adolescent girls ages 12 to 19 years. The macronutrient composition of children's diets has changed, reflecting changes in the food supply. Fat intake as a percentage of energy intake fell from 38% to 33% since 1973, whereas carbohydrate and protein intakes increased. Still, about 75% of children did not meet the fat intake recommendations in 1994 (Munoz, Krebs-Smith, Ballard-Barbash, & Cleveland, 1997; Nicklas et al., 2001).

Children's diets have changed in respect to the types of carbohydrate they consume. In a 1998 round-table and national briefing on child nutrition, the director of the National Institute of Child Health and Human Development was quoted as saying that children's diets are characterized by "too much energy . . . too much sugar, and too little fiber" (fruits and vegetables) and could be described as an inverted MyPyramid (McBean & Miller, 1999). Easily digestible highly refined carbohydrates from foods and beverage sources have increased in consumption recently. Much scientific interest has been focused on the possible role of high **glycemic index** foods in the childhood and adult obesity epidemic. An effect of the glycemic index of breakfast foods on subsequent unrestricted food intake at lunch has been studied. Lunch intake after a breakfast of foods high in glycemic index (i.e., a meal of high **glycemic load**) was greater than after a breakfast of low glycemic load (Warren, Henry, & Simonite, 2003). In a review of the high glycemic index foods, hunger, and obesity connection, Roberts (2000) concluded that compared with similar low glycemic index carbohydrates, high glycemic index carbohydrates promote a more rapid return of the hunger sensation and increase subsequent caloric intake. Foods of high glycemic index may, therefore, contribute to maintenance of excess weight in the obese and to weight gain in susceptible individuals. Many children start their day with high sugar content breakfast cereals of high glycemic index. Over the longer term, a diet of high glycemic load could lead to higher energy intake and contribute to excess weight gain (Augustin, Franceschi, Jenkins, Kendall, & La Vecchia, 2002).

Glycemic index: The effect of carbohydrate in a food on blood glucose, as a percentage of the effect of an equal amount of glucose.

Glycemic load: Calculated by multiplying the glycemic index by the amount of carbohydrate provided by a food and dividing the total by 100. Dietary glycemic load is the sum of the glycemic loads for all foods consumed in the diet.

High sugar beverage intake is linked with fast food consumption because soft drinks are usually marketed and bundled with meal packages in fast food restaurants. Twice as many children and adolescents drank carbonated soft drinks if they had consumed fast foods on one of two survey days than if they did not (Paeratakul, Ferdinand, Champagne, Ryan, & Bray, 2003). So-called super-sized meal offers upgrade beverage serving size along with food portions. "Super-sizing" of meal packages may have contributed to increased intakes of sweetened beverages by children. Between 1977–1979 and 1994 the proportion of children who consumed soft drinks on a given day increased by 74% for boys and 65% for girls. High consumption of soft drinks among children and adolescents has been shown to be associated with higher energy intake (Harnack, Stang, & Story, 1999). An association between schoolchildren's sugar-sweetened drink consumption and their BMI has been demonstrated, although more research is ongoing. For example, a study conducted prospectively over 19 months showed that for each additional serving of sugar-sweetened beverage consumed, both BMI and propensity to become obese increased. This was after controlling for anthropometric, demographic, dietary, and life-style variables (Ludwig, Peterson, & Gortmaker, 2001).

The typical 12-fluid-ounce can of soda is rapidly being replaced by the 20-fluid-ounce bottle at convenience stores and in vending machines, encouraging increased consumption of these drinks. Many brands offer a 32-fluid-ounce version that is packaged in a bottle shape that is easy to tote around, thereby encouraging frequent and increased consumption. Average portion sizes of soft drinks have increased by 12% to 18% for persons ages 2 and older (Briefel & Johnson, 2004). Soft drink consumption (per capita) has increased about 500% over the past 50 years, with adolescents consuming between 36 and 58 g of sugar daily from this source (Ludwig et al., 2001).

Food portions have increased as well. Most consumers recognize portion inflation among baked goods, such as bagels and muffins. Also, hamburger sandwiches are both larger and offered with two and three servings of meat with cheese.

Regulation of Energy Intake

Although very young children possess innate abilities to regulate energy intake based on their needs, children tend to lose some of this ability as they age and become more responsive to environmental influences and increasingly take their behavioral cues from their surroundings. Children vary in their ability to self-regulate energy intakes (Johnson, 2000), but children who have experienced so-called restrictive feeding practices appear to be less able to respond appropriately to internal signs of hunger and satiety and may be more susceptible to overeating (Birch & Fischer, 1998). Also, as children learn from their environment, food portion sizes influence their intake. Thus, children may overeat when presented with excessive food and beverage portions, risking excessive weight gain over time.

Family Eating Environment

Genetic differences are estimated to account for about 30% to 50% of the variance of BMI within a population, but these estimates do not describe the complex interactions taking place between genetics and the environment (Allison & Faith, 2000). For example, parents contribute both genetics and environment to the equation. Their own eating behaviors help shape the child's eating environment and to an extent may be influenced by the parents' own genetic makeup. In turn, the child's or adolescent's eating environment helps to shape the development of the child's own eating behaviors. These learned (eating) behaviors in turn influence whether any genetic predispositions toward obesity are expressed in the child (Birch & Fischer, 1998).

Parents who are struggling with personal weight issues may hamper their children's ability to self-regulate energy intake. Because many adults suffer from overweight or obesity (National Center for Health Statistics, 1999), some parents are understandably concerned about their children's risk of also becoming overweight or obese. Aiming to avoid overweight in their children, parents may impose greater restrictions on their children's intake. If these same parents exhibit uninhibited eating styles themselves, they serve as poor role models. These behaviors in combination can cause the transfer of eating styles that pose an increased risk for the development of an overweight child. As a result, well-intentioned parents may actually produce the very outcome they sought to avoid (Johnson, 2000). A common strategy used to control children's intake is to restrict their access to high-calorie foods or to use favorite foods as a reward to shape behavior. At first, these behaviors may seem reasonable enough; however, restricting certain foods has been shown to increase the child's desire to consume these foods. When available, these desirable foods will likely be consumed in greater amounts. Again, such family dynamics around food may set up patterns of poor self-control of energy intake in the child (Fischer & Birch, 1999).

An optimal environment for children to develop self-control of energy intake is when parents provide nutritious food and allow children to determine if and how much to eat. These principles of division of responsibility are discussed extensively elsewhere (Satter, 1987, 1999, 2000; Johnson & Birch, 1994).

Household Food Insecurity

Although seemingly paradoxical, low-income compared with higher-income households appear to experience increased rates of overweight individuals. Proposed mechanisms for this effect include higher intakes of cheaper, more calorie-dense foods that may lead to excessive energy intakes (Alaimo, Olson, & Frongillo, 2001; Drewnowski & Specter, 2004). Persons from low-income, food-insecure households may overeat during periods of relative abundance and gain weight as a result. Food insecurity in low-income households appears to play a role in the increased overweight rates among older white girls (8 to 16 years of age) compared with children from low-income households that do not experience food insecurity (Alaimo et al., 2001). However, family participation in programs like the National School Breakfast and Lunch Programs and the Supplemental Nutrition Assistance Program (Food Stamps) may be protective for these girls. Girls who participated in all three programs had 68% reduced odds of becoming overweight when compared with nonparticipants from families experiencing food insecurity (Jones, Jahns, Laraia, & Haughton, 2003). In contrast, a more recent study found a 42.8% increase for young girls and a 28.8% decrease for young boys in the predicted probability of obesity with participation in the Supplemental Nutrition Assistance Program for the previous 5 years. This study did not control for food insecurity within households, which may help to explain the differing results (Gibson, 2004). Additional retrospective longitudinal studies that included assessment of food security and hunger status of each household member might help explain why some children are affected more than others. This is important because not all members of a household may experience food insecurity to the same extent. A better understanding of these dynamics can focus attention on those within a household who may be at a greater risk of being overweight.

Breast-Feeding

New mothers returning to work may decide against breast-feeding or may nurse their infants for only a very limited time because of the real and/or perceived obstacles to breast-feeding their infants while working outside the home. This is unfortunate, because breast milk is the ideal food for infants. Evidence is emerging that breast-feeding may offer some protection against obesity (Armstrong & Reilly, 2002). Proposed mechanisms for this effect include more normal growth patterns (lower early weight gain), possibly associated with lower basal insulin levels in the breast-fed versus the formula-fed infant, and the inherent control of food intake maintained by the breast-fed infant (Dietz, 2001).

Breast-feeding on demand is thought to teach infants to regulate their intakes appropriately, based on internal cues for hunger and satiety and in response to their individual growth needs. Formula-fed infants may have fewer opportunities to develop this important skill. Reasons for this may be that parents or caregivers may want to follow a set feeding schedule or may encourage the infant to consume a certain amount of formula. Both of these feeding behaviors override the infant's internal cues and may result in overfeeding and lessen the infant's ability to self-regulate energy intake (Birch & Fischer, 1998).

Physical Inactivity Affecting Overweight Status in Children

Physical inactivity among children is one of the major health concerns regarding overweight children. Children learn physical inactivity from their adult role models and environment through limited access to recreational activities in their community, lack of safe neighborhoods, and, perhaps, unlimited access to television viewing and other media outlets, including computers. In addition, many newly developed communities are poorly planned when "built-in" access to physical activity is left out of the design. Often, children are bused to school because walking to school is not an option due to safety issues and distance. Sidewalks were once common, but now some urban and suburban developments have shaped many residential areas into "unwalkable" communities. Although further research is needed for a better understanding of the influence of the human-built environment on physical activity, it appears clear that urban sprawl has affected land use, transportation, and health, particularly children's health (Frumkin, 2002).

School Physical Education

At school, children are challenged to find opportunities to be physically active on a daily basis. Often, school academic curriculums and programs take priority over physical education and recess time. Physical education curriculums and recess have slowly diminished over the past few years (Burgenson, Wechsler, Brener, Young, & Spain, 2001).

Data from the Youth Risk Behavior Surveillance System show that 55.7% of students nationwide were enrolled in physical education classes 1 or more days in an average week, whereas only 28.4% of students nationwide attended physical education classes 5 days in an average week. Of the 55.7% of students enrolled in physical education classes nationwide, 80.3% of students actually exercised or played sports more than 20 minutes. Improvements in physical education are also needed to decrease inappropriate teaching practices, such as prohibiting physical activity as a form of punishment or physical activity games that may cause embarrassment or aggressive behavior (i.e., dodge ball) (Burgenson et al., 2001). Although some physical education improvements are needed, a nationwide effort to establish laws or policies to increase student enrollment and participation in daily physical education is desirable, especially in the older student population. The goal is for children to establish healthy life-style habits that may carry over into adulthood.

Because most children spend much of their waking hours in school, it is a threat to children's health and fitness when the school schedule and curriculum do not include daily opportunities for physical activity. Advocacy for increasing student participation in daily recess and physical activity should be a top priority of schools and health and community leaders to help prevent overweight children.

Television Viewing

Television viewing and other media outlets to an extent have displaced a more natural environment of family interactions for growing children, such as learning and playing. Children who spend more time in sedentary activities tend to weigh more and to be at greater risk of being overweight. Several studies conclude that children who watch 4 or more hours of television each day are more likely to be overweight than those who watch less television (Gortmaker et al., 1996; Andersen, Crespo, Bartlett, Cheskin, & Pratt,

1998; Dowda, Ainsworth, Addy, Saunders, & Riner, 2001). In addition, African-American (30%) and Hispanic-American (22%) children are both more likely than white (12%) children to spend more than 5 hours a day watching television. Similarly, African-American (69%) and Hispanic-American (60%) children are more likely than white (48%) children to have a television in their bedroom (Kaiser Family Foundation, n.d.).

One cross-sectional study failed to find a relationship between television viewing and overweight status in adolescent girls (Robinson et al., 1993). Another study questioned the leisure activities in the United States, indicating that U.S. children overall are less active than children in other countries and cultures (Crawford et al., 2004). The trend toward increasingly sedentary life-styles is obvious to many older adults, as they compare the children's activity level in this current generation with that of children two or three generations earlier. Learning, playing, and physical activity were an integral part of family life, and television viewing was a special occasion. However, today, television viewing is a prominent part of family life, and it is a sedentary behavior.

Excessive television viewing not only leaves less time for positive family interactions and activities, but the actual programs and advertisements may be questionable for young viewers. Granted, there are many educational and worthwhile programs to watch on television. Unfortunately, not all programs and advertisements have children's health as a priority. One major challenge is the multimillion-dollar advertising industry that promotes products between and during television programming (Borzekowski & Robinson, 2001). Appealing and enticing advertising segments are targeted at children to increase their desire to choose unhealthy foods. Food products advertised directly to young children during children's television programming have contributed to an impressive growth in sales of high-sugar breakfast cereals and snack foods. The young consumers predictably request these products (or may even purchase these themselves) during trips to the grocery store, because they recognize their favorite cartoon characters on the colorful packages strategically placed at their eye level when riding in the grocery cart. Excessive television viewing by children creates a cycle of physical inactivity and high calorie consumption due to the influence of television food advertising; this combination of factors adds up to a perfect formula for fueling the rising trend of overweight status in children.

> **Obesigenic:** An environment that encourages obesity by features, including unlimited quantities of a variety of foods high in caloric density together with minimal need of energy expenditure.

An important part of treating overweight children is to decrease sedentary behavior and increase physical activity (Steinbeck, 2001). These are important factors in the intervention process; however, children are still challenged with real barriers to being physically active existing in their physical environment. Limited access to safe physical activity in the community, unlimited television viewing, fewer opportunities for physical activity in the schools, and adults who may not view physical activity as a priority are important barriers to physical activity. Thus, U.S. children live in an **obesigenic** society with various barriers that make healthy living choices, such as daily physical activity, difficult to achieve.

Opportunities to Intervene and Prevent Childhood Obesity

Health care practitioners are challenged to think of new and creative ways to address the problem of childhood obesity within existing venues and frameworks. To be most successful and cost effective, the emphasis must be on population-based approaches and prevention, as traditional and clinic-based services alone clearly have failed to adequately address the obesity epidemic. Thus, the health care practitioner should examine existing nutrition, social, and other programs and seize opportunities to intervene to prevent overweight in children. Some suggestions for opportunities are listed below.

Nutrition Programs

Supplemental Nutrition Assistance Program for Women, Infants, and Children

Developing policies and conducting outreach activities to recruit pregnant women into prenatal care during the first trimester promotes early intervention and nutrition care for the expectant woman. This may improve nutrition delivery to her unborn child and help to avoid under- or over-nutrition, thereby lowering the risk of future obesity in the child (Dietz, 2004). Some clinics conduct grocery store tours to teach shopping skills to participants in the Supplemental Nutrition Assistance Program (SNAP) for Women, Infants, and Children (WIC) to help them establish healthy eating patterns.

It is important to assess monitoring systems and develop policies or protocols to identify participant children older than 2 years of age who exhibit rapid weight gain and to target efforts to ensure they receive culturally appropriate interventions and guidance intervention to lower their risk of becoming overweight. Training clinic health care practitioners in anticipatory guidance and counseling will enable the team to provide infant and child feeding and physical activity advice consistent with evidence-based obesity prevention strategies and to serve as positive role models. The clinic environment should convey clear and consistent messages to encourage healthy eating and physical activity for both program participants and staff; this would include policies and environmental interventions that promote, support, and protect breast-feeding.

Social Programs

Preschool and Day Care

Policies to support healthy eating and physical activity should include strategies such as these: (1) serving healthy menu items within a positive eating environment for children, (2) opportunities for and encouragement of children (and adult caregivers) to be physically active daily, and (3) training of childcare providers and the food service team in obesity prevention strategies through nutritious food choices and daily physical activity appropriate for the children's age and development. Grants can provide resources to fund environmental intervention (i.e., playground, equipment for physical activity, and policy interventions for staff and parents to attend training in overweight prevention for children). Involving families and staff in fun events that encourage adoption of healthy living practices, such as less sedentary behavior and more physical activity, can help to reinforce the message.

School Systems

Advocating for daily recess and active physical education for all children through school boards, parent and teacher organizations, school administrators, and elected officials can help to bring needed changes to our children's daily environment. Such improvements should include policies that limit competitive foods and beverages and serve fruits and vegetables daily on the breakfast and lunch menus, nutrition standards for food and beverages sold from vending machines and school stores, and a unified message for healthy eating and physical activity throughout the school (no candy fundraisers, no food or candy rewards for good behavior in the classroom, healthy snacks at parties and school events, and a campus that is friendly to physical activity, providing walkways, bicycle racks, and safe outdoor play equipment). Promotion of school breakfast and lunch program participation can help to ensure appropriate nutrition for students within the school, whereas nutrition education curricula from pre-kindergarten through 12th grade (50 hours a year minimum has been suggested) can influence student eating behaviors outside the school as well (American Dietetic Association, Society for Nutrition Education, and the American School Food Service Association, 2003). Systems to assess children's health and behaviors (i.e., height and weight, BMI, blood pressure, fruit and vegetable consumption, television viewing, transportation modes to school, and actual physical activity during recess and physical education classes) are important to monitor progress and regress in these health promotion efforts and target areas for change.

After-School Care

The after-school setting offers opportunities for promotion of healthy eating and adequate physical activity that are very similar to those in childcare and school settings: staff training to support obesity prevention efforts, consistent messages regarding a healthy life-style, limited availability of competitive foods of low nutritional quality, and an environment friendly to physical activity for all children and youth. Again, grants can help provide funds to make environmental improvements as needed.

Other Possible Venues

Children of low-income households who participate in federal and state-supported summer food service programs may secure a nutritious alternative to the fast food and snacks of low nutritional quality that often compose a significant part of their diet between school years. Advocating for a healthy environment in various settings for children, such as Boys and Girls Clubs, YMCA/YWCA, and summer camps, can help children establish and maintain healthy life-styles year round. Directors and staff in these settings who are trained in overweight prevention strategies can strengthen their influence on the health behaviors of the children and youth in their care when they model healthy behaviors themselves.

Programs and Resources That Support Evidence-Based Practices in Preventing Childhood Obesity

The CDC Nutrition, Physical Activity and Obesity Prevention Program established three evidence-based goals to prevent and control obesity (CDC, 2003):

1. To increase physical activity
2. To reduce television viewing
3. To improve nutrition through increased breast-feeding and increased fruit and vegetable consumption

Although research is limited on successful practices in various settings, programs and resources that may be used by a health care practitioner when addressing overweight children follow.

Physical Activity

KidsWalk-to-School

KidsWalk-to-School is a community-based program developed by the CDC Nutrition and Physical Activity Program. It "encourages children to walk to and from school in groups accompanied by adults" (CDC, n.d.). This program mobilizes community members, such as school staff, the Parent Teacher Association, police departments, businesses, civic associations, and other groups to work together to increase safe routes to and from school for children to walk or ride their bicycles. The program raises community awareness of the importance of daily physical activity for children and the barriers to activity they encounter. In this way the program helps to change an "unwalkable" community into a "walkable" community, bringing about an environmental intervention. This program supports the Healthy People 2010 objectives related to children's trips to school by walking or bicycling (U.S. Department of Health and Human Services, 2000).

Television Viewing

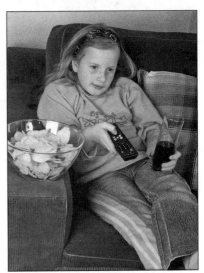

 The Center for Screen-Time Awareness (formerly the TV Turnoff Network) encourages children and adults to turn off the television and replace that time with enjoyable family activities that promote healthy living. It sponsors two programs: TV Turnoff Week and More Reading, Less TV. TV Turnoff Week is held during the last week of April of every year. TV Turnoff Week encourages physical activity, such as gardening, skating, dancing, walking, bicycling, or playing a sport, along with other nonphysical activities. More Reading, Less TV encourages reading as a replacement to television viewing among children and adults. Because of the link between excessive television viewing and increased BMI in children, decreasing television viewing may encourage children to be more physically active (Center for Screen-Time Awareness, n.d.). This program supports the Healthy People 2010 objectives related to increasing the number of adolescents watching 2 hours or less of television on school days (U.S. Department of Health and Human Services, 2000).

Nutrition

Breast-Feeding

Breast-feeding may serve as an early intervention to prevent childhood obesity, and breast-feeding promotion can occur in various settings. For instance, the health care practitioner may develop a breast-feeding coalition that focuses on developing breast-feeding policies in work sites, hospitals, and community sites. In addition, coalition members may monitor and evaluate the interventions implemented. Or, a health care practitioner may collaborate with partners or participate in coalitions to increase breast-feeding awareness and promotion through World Breastfeeding Week, health fairs, or other community events. In addition, a health care practitioner may train nutritionists, nurses, doctors, and other medical professionals on breast-feeding management and supportive ways to increase breast-feeding initiation and duration rates.

In a clinical setting a health care practitioner may provide one-on-one breast-feeding education, counseling, and support for pregnant and lactating women to increase the breast-feeding initiation and duration rates. This initiative supports the Healthy People 2010 objectives related to increasing the proportion of women who breast-feed their babies (U.S. Department of Health and Human Services, 2000).

Promoting Healthy Eating Practices

Beyond breast-feeding, healthy eating habits among toddlers and children are vitally important, because these lay the foundation for lifelong eating patterns. There are good sources of information on healthy eating practices among toddlers. An example is Children's Healthcare of Atlanta (Buechner, 2001), which has developed a Stress-Free Feeding© curriculum that advocates healthy eating habits and environments for both the parent and child. This initiative supports the Healthy People 2010 objective (developmental) related to increasing the proportion of children and adolescents who consume meals and snacks that are of good overall dietary quality (U.S. Department of Health and Human Services, 2000).

Fruits and Veggies–More Matters

The Produce for Better Health Foundation is a consumer education foundation that chairs the national Fruits and Veggies—More Matters program (formerly called the 5-A-Day for Better Health Program). The 5-A-Day for Better Health Program was the nation's largest public-private nutrition education initiative. Researchers have studied the relationship between fruit and vegetable intake and weight maintenance and loss, especially in the pediatric population. For example, one study found that families who increased fruit and vegetable intake tended to consume fewer calories and were better able to mange their

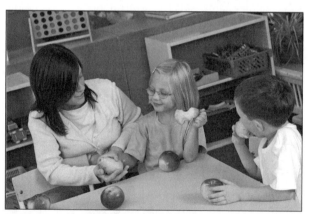

weight than those families who focused on decreasing fat and sugar intake in their diet. In addition, fruit and vegetable campaigns are timely and useful because they have adaptable toolkits and other promotional items that fit various settings. In particular, "There's a Rainbow on My Plate" is a good resource found at www.pbhfoundation.org/educators/teachers/rainbow. This toolkit is designed to educate children on the importance of healthy eating by consuming a variety of colorful fruits and vegetables. This initiative supports the Healthy People 2010 objective related to persons 2 years and older who consume 2 servings of fruit and 3 servings of vegetables daily (U.S. Department of Health and Human Services, 2000).

The programs and resources discussed above are only a few avenues to explore and recommend to partners and perhaps focus groups. To accomplish the ultimate goal of healthy children in healthy communities, the health care practitioner should be resourceful when suggesting programs, initiatives, and campaigns related to overweight children. The practitioner should have a "toolbox" ready when entering various settings: coalition, community, school, work site, health care facility, or other organizations. This toolbox of information and resources will vary depending on the target population. Nevertheless, health care practitioners must be creative and timely in sharing their vision and potential solutions to address childhood obesity. The authors encourage health care practitioners and students to research other resources and participate in Internet "listservs" for best practices and new findings in preventing and controlling overweight status among children.

Summary

Vegetarian diets can be healthful and nutritionally adequate for infants, children, and adolescents and can provide health and nutritional benefits. Key nutrients for vegetarian children and adolescents include protein, iron, zinc, calcium, vitamin D, vitamin B_{12}, and omega-3 fatty acids. A vegetarian diet can meet requirements for all these nutrients, although in some instances fortified foods or supplements can be especially useful in meeting recommendations. Dietetics professionals play key roles in counseling vegetarian children and adolescents and their families.

Health care practitioners may use existing nutrition and social programs as opportunities to promote evidence-based strategies to prevent obesity in children. Because many nutrition and social programs have a narrow focus, population-based services are essential to help communities, schools, work sites, other organizations, and families to adopt healthy behaviors. Healthy eating among children cannot be addressed without addressing the family as a whole and the environment. As discussed earlier, almost 65% of adults are overweight or obese, and this is a risk factor for their children to become overweight. Indeed, childhood obesity is a major public health concern; however, preventive efforts must target the parents and caregivers as well as the children. Improving family interaction through healthy eating practices and physical activity is essential to preventing childhood obesity. Healthy life-style behaviors can be taught in parenting classes, discussed during doctor's office visits, and presented at work sites, health fairs, parent-teacher organizations, and other sites. In addition, population-based services and partners can develop and implement policy and environmental interventions that make it convenient for families to include healthy eating practices and daily physical activity.

Issues to Debate

1. How would you advise a vegetarian family whose 12-year-old wants to begin eating meat?
2. Read the following two articles and discuss whether or not milk and dairy products are necessary for bone health in growing children and adolescents.
   - Lanou, A. J., Berkow, S. E., & Barnard, N. D. (2005). Calcium, dairy products, and bone health in children and young adults: A reevaluation of the evidence. *Pediatrics, 115,* 736–743.
   - Greer, F. R. (2005). Bone health: It's more than calcium intake. *Pediatrics, 115,* 792–794.
3. What suggestions could you make to the adolescent and the adolescent's nonvegetarian parents when the adolescent wants to be a vegetarian who will not eat dairy products, eggs, beans, tofu, or most vegetables?
4. Would it ever be appropriate to tell a vegetarian family that their children have to eat meat?
5. Physical activity and exercise are equally important as healthy eating in the pediatric population. How would you include physical activity as an intervention for children if you have limited training in this area?
6. What power (if any) does the government have to influence factors that impact childhood obesity?
7. Discuss how the media may promote childhood obesity and how it may be used to prevent this problem.
8. What should the health care practitioner consider when he or she plans or implements childhood obesity prevention interventions for families in clinic settings or special programs?

Case Studies

(Answers to all case studies are in the Instructor's Manual available at jbpub.com.)

Case Study: Overweight Vegetarian

Jacob is a 16-year-old lifelong lacto-ovo-vegetarian. His father has recently discovered he has elevated cholesterol. Jacob also has borderline high cholesterol and is about 20 pounds above ideal weight.

A typical intake for a day for Jacob includes the following:

Continued

- Breakfast: three scrambled eggs with melted cheese, three slices of toast with butter, and chocolate milk
- Lunch: three slices of cheese pizza, french fries, and a milkshake
- Dinner: A large serving of macaroni and cheese, two slices of bread and butter, whole milk, and a bowl of ice cream
- Snacks include potato chips, soft drinks, and candy bars

Case Study: An Underweight Vegetarian

Mollie is a 15-year-old dedicated cross-country runner. During the season (now), she runs 50 to 60 miles weekly. She has been a lacto-ovo-vegetarian for the past 2 years. She doesn't drink much milk, however, because she is lactose intolerant.

Mollie's parents are concerned because she has unintentionally lost 5 lb in the past month. Mollie is 5'5" and weighs 105 lb (BMI = 18). Mollie is concerned because she seems to get sick easily and doesn't have as much energy as she would like.

Mollie says she just doesn't have time to eat well. A typical day includes the following diet:
- Dry cereal with fruit for breakfast
- A veggie burger and fries for lunch
- A big salad with cheese cubes and beans and salad dressing along with a couple of rolls for dinner
- Snacks include air-popped popcorn and iced tea
- Her estimated calorie requirement is 2,200 kcal, whereas her estimated intake is 1,500 kcal.

Websites

American Dietetic Association: A New Food Guide for North American Vegetarians
    www.eatright.org/cps/rde/xchg/ada/hs.xsl/governance_5105_ENU_HTML.htm
American Dietetic Association and Dietitians of Canada Position Paper on Vegetarian Diets www.eatright.org/cps/rde/xchg/ada/hs.xsl/
    advocacy_933_ENU_HTML.htm
Vegetarian Baby www.vegetarianbaby.com/
Vegetarian Nutrition Dietetic Practice Group www.andrews.edu/NUFS/Vegan%20Children.html
Vegetarian Resource Group www.vrg.org/nutrition/pregnancy.htm; www.vrg.org/nutrition/teennutrition.htm; www.vrg.org/
    nutshell/kids.htm
Vegetarian Society of the UK www.vegsoc.org/info/childre1.html

Professional Organizations

American Academy of Pediatrics www.aap.org; www.pediatrics.org
American Dietetic Association www.eatright.org
American Medical Association http://ama-assn.org
American Nurse Association www.ana.org
American Psychological Association www.apa.org
American Public Health Association www.apha.org
Society of Nutrition Education www.sne.org

Statistical or Surveillance Systems

Behavioral Risk Factor Surveillance System www.cdc.gov/brfss
    • Combined Health Information Database www.cehn.org/cehn/resourceguide/chid.html
    • Kaiser Family Foundation, State Health Facts www.statehealthfacts.kff.org
Maternal and Child Health Data www.doh.wa.gov/cfh/mch/mch_assessment/mchdatareport/mch_data_report_home.htm
National Center for Health Statistics www.cdc.gov/nchs
Pediatric Nutrition Surveillance System www.cdc.gov/nccdphp/dnpa/PedNSS.htm
U.S. Census Bureau, Statistical Abstract of the United States: 2001 http://www.census.gov/compendia/statab/
Weight-Control Information Network, Statistics Related to Overweight and Obesity www.niddk.nih.gov/health/nutrit/pubs/
    statobes.htm
Youth Behavioral Risk Factor Surveillance System www.cdc.gov/HealthyYouth/yrbs/index.htm

Policy and Environmental Interventions

Center for Nutrition Policy and Promotion www.usda.gov/cnpp

Center for Science in the Public Interest (CSPI), School Nutrition Kit www.cspinet.org/nutritionpolicy

The Community Tool Box http://ctb.ku.edu

National Association of State Boards of Education—Fit, Healthy and Ready to Learn: A School Health Policy Guide nasbe.org/.../396-fit-healthy-and-ready-to-learn-a-school-health-policy-guide

National Recreation and Park Association www.nrpa.org

Nutrition

Children's Healthcare of Atlanta www.choa.org

CSPI Nutrition Policy Project www.cspinet.org/schoolfoods

CSPI School Foods Tool Kit www.cspinet.org/schoolfoodkit/

Dietary Guidelines for Americans http://www.health.gov/dietaryguidelines/

Food and Nutrition Information Center http://fnic.nal.usda.gov

Fruits and Veggies—More Matters http://www.fruitsandveggiesmatter.gov/

Junior Master Gardner http://jmgkids.us

National Dairy Council www.nationaldairycouncil.org

1% or less Campaign—School Kit www.cspinet.org/kids

3-A-Day www.3aday.org

Exercise

Heart N' Parks Program www.nhlbi.nih.gov/health/prof/heart/obesity/hrt_n_pk/index.htm

National Association for Sports and Physical Education www.aahperd.org/naspe

National Park and Recreation Association www.nrpa.org

P.E. 4 Life www.pe4Life.com

President's Council on Physical Fitness and Sports www.fitness.gov

Take 10! www.take10.net

Media

Center for Screen-Time Awareness www.tvturnoff.org

Youth Media Campaign www.cdc.gov/youthcampaign

School Resources

Action for Healthy Kids www.actionforhealthykids.org/about.php

CDC, Healthy Youth! http://apps.nccd.cdc.gov/shi

Center for Health and Healthcare in Schools www.healthinschools.org

National Association of State Boards of Education
www.nasbe.org/healthy_schools/hs/bytopics.php?topicid=3115&catexpand=acdnbtm_catc

Planet Health www.planethealth.com/

SPARK Program www.sparkpe.org

USDA Team Nutrition, www.fns.usda.gov/tn

Community Resources

ACES—Active Community Environments www.cdc.gov/nccdphp/dnpa/aces.htm

Association for Community Health Improvement www.communityhlth.org

Community Preventive Services, The Community Guide www.thecommunityguide.org

Community Service Block Grant www.csd.ca.gov/Programs/Community%20Services%20Block%20Grant%20(CSBG).aspx

North Carolina Prevention Partners www.ncpreventionpartners.org

Other Resources

APHA Food and Nutrition Section on Overweight in Childhood http://www.apha.org/membergroups/newsletters/ sectionnewsletters/food/winter09/default.htm#{AF1EB750-28BE-4FF9-B7A6-8352665D632A}

Bright Futures www.brightfutures.org

Centers for Disease Control and Prevention (CDC) www.cdc.gov

Centers for Disease Control and Prevention, Evaluation Working Group www.cdc.gov/eval/index.htm

Center for Science in the Public Interest (CSPI) www.cspinet.org

Cooperative State Research, Education, and Extension Service www.csrees.usda.gov

Healthy People 2010 www.healthypeople.gov

Maternal and Child Health Bureau www.mchb.hrsa.gov

National Institutes of Health health.nih.gov

U.S. Department of Health and Human Services www.hhs.gov

U.S. Department of Health and Human Services, GrantsNet www.hhs.gov/grantsnet/

YMCA of the USA www.ymca.org

References

Pediatric Vegetarianism

Allen, L. H. (1998). Zinc and micronutrient supplements for children. American *Journal of Clinical Nutrition, 68(Suppl.)*, 495S–498S.

Barr, S. I. (1999). Vegetarianism and menstrual cycle disturbances: Is there an association? *American Journal of Clinical Nutrition, 70(Suppl.)*, 549S–554S.

Barr, S. I., & Chapman, G. E. (2002). Perceptions and practices of self-defined current vegetarian, former vegetarian, and non-vegetarian women. *Journal of the American Dietetic Association, 102*, 354–360.

Birch, E. E., Garfield, S., Hoffman, D. R., Uauy, R., & Birch, C. G. (2000). A randomized controlled trial of early dietary supply of long-chain polyunsaturated fatty acids and mental development in term infants. *Developmental Medicine and Child Neurology, 42*, 174–181.

Black, R. E., Williams, S. M., Jones, I. E., & Goulding, A. (2002). Children who avoid drinking cow milk have low dietary calcium intakes and poor bone health. *American Journal of Clinical Nutrition, 76*, 675–680.

Carvalho, N. F., Kenney, R. D., Carrington, P. H., & Hall, D. E. (2001). Severe nutritional deficiencies in toddlers resulting from health food milk alternatives. *Pediatrics, 107*, E46.

Centers for Disease Control and Prevention (CDC). (2003). Neurologic impairment in children associated with maternal dietary deficiency of cobalamin—Georgia, 2001. *Morbidity and Mortality Weekly Report, 52*, 61–64.

Conquer, J. A., & Holub, B. J. (1996). Supplementation with an algae source of docosahexaenoic acid increases (n-3) fatty acid status and alters selected risk factors for heart disease in vegetarian subjects. *Journal of Nutrition, 126*, 3032–3039.

Dagnelie, P. C., van Staveren, W. A., & van den Berg, H. (1991). Vitamin B-12 from algae appears not to be bioavailable. *American Journal of Clinical Nutrition, 53*, 695–697.

Dagnelie, P. C., van Staveren, W. A., van Klaveren, J. D., & Burema, J. (1988). Do children on macrobiotic diets show catch-up growth? *European Journal of Clinical Nutrition, 42*, 1007–1016.

Dagnelie, P. C., van Staveren, W. A., Vergote, F. J. V. R. A., Burema, J., Van't Hof, M. A., van Klaveren, J. D., et al. (1989). Nutritional status of infants aged 4 to 18 months on macrobiotic diets and matched omnivorous control infants: A population-based mixed-longitudinal study. II. Growth and psychomotor development. *European Journal of Clinical Nutrition, 43*, 325–338.

Dagnelie, P. C., van Staveren, W. A., Vergote, F. J. R. V. A., Dingjan, P.G., van den Berg, H., & Hautvast, J. G. A. J. (1989). Increased risk of vitamin B-12 and iron deficiency in infants on macrobiotic diets. *American Journal of Clinical Nutrition, 50*, 818–824.

Dagnelie, P. C., van Staveren, W. A., Verschuren, S. A. J. M., & Hautvast, J. G. A. J. (1989). Nutritional status of infants aged 4 to 18 months on macrobiotic diets and matched omnivorous control infants: A population-based mixed longitudinal study. I. Weaning pattern, energy and nutrient intake. *European Journal of Clinical Nutrition, 43*, 311–323.

Dagnelie, P. C., Vergote, F. J. R. V. A., van Staveren, W. A., van den Berg, H., Dingjan, P. G., & Hautvast, J. G. A. J. (1990). High prevalence of rickets in infants on macrobiotic diets. *American Journal of Clinical Nutrition, 51*, 202–208.

Davis, B., & Kris-Etherton, P. (2003). Achieving optimal essential fatty acid status in vegetarians: Current knowledge and practical implications. *American Journal of Clinical Nutrition, 78(Suppl.)*, 640S–646S.

Dhonukshe-Rutten, R. A., van Dusseldorp, M., Schneede, J., de Groot, L. C., & van Staveren, W. A. (2005). Low bone mineral density and bone mineral content are associated with low cobalamin status in adolescents. *European Journal of Nutrition, 44*, 341–347.

Dibba, B., Prentice, A., & Ceesay, M. (2000). Effect of calcium supplementation on bone mineral accretion in Gambian children accustomed to a low-calcium diet. *American Journal of Clinical Nutrition, 71*, 544–549.

Dobson, B., & Murtaugh, M. A. (2001). Position of the American Dietetic Association: Breaking the barriers to breastfeeding. *Journal of the American Dietetic Association, 101*, 1213–1220.

Donovan, U. M., & Gibson, R. S. (1995). Iron and zinc status of young women aged 14 to 19 years consuming vegetarian and omnivorous diets. *Journal of the American College of Nutrition, 14*, 463–472.

Donovan, U. M., & Gibson, R. S. (1996). Dietary intakes of adolescent females consuming vegetarian, semi-vegetarian, and omnivorous diets. *Journal of Adolescent Health, 18*, 292–300.

Ellis, R., Kelsay, J. L., Reynolds, R. D., Morris, E. R., Moser, P. B., & Frazier, C. (1987). Phytate: zinc and phytate x calcium: zinc millimolar ratios in self-selected diets of Americans, Asian Indians, and Nepalese. *Journal of the American Dietetic Association, 87*, 1043–1047.

Francois, C. A., Connor, S. L., Bolewicz, L. C., & Connor, W. E. (2003). Supplementing lactating women with flaxseed oil does not increase docosahexaenoic acid in their milk. *American Journal of Clinical Nutrition, 77*, 226–233.

Geppert, J., Kraft, V., Demmelmair, H., & Koletzko, B. (2005). Docosahexaenoic acid supplementation in vegetarians effectively increases omega-3 index: A randomized trial. *Lipids, 40*, 807–814.

Gibson, R. S., Yeudall, F., Drost, N., Mtitmunit, B., & Cullinan, T. (1998). Dietary interventions to prevent zinc deficiency. *American Journal of Clinical Nutrition, 68(Suppl.)*, 484S–487S.

Hallberg, L., & Hulthen, L. (2000). Prediction of dietary iron absorption: An algorithm for calculating absorption and bioavailability of dietary iron. *American Journal of Clinical Nutrition, 71*, 1147–1160.

Heaney, R. P., Dowell, M. S., Rafferty, K., & Bierman, J. (2000). Bioavailability of the calcium in fortified soy imitation milk, with some observations on method. *American Journal of Clinical Nutrition, 71*, 1166–1169.

Heaney, R. P., Rafferty, K., & Bierman, J. (2005). Not all calcium-fortified beverages are equal. *Nutrition Today, 40*, 39–45.

Hebbelinck, M., & Clarys, P. (2001). Physical growth and development of vegetarian children and adolescents. In J. Sabate (Ed.), *Vegetarian Nutrition* (pp. 173–193). Boca Raton, FL: CRC Press.

Hermann, W., & Geisel, J. (2002). Vegetarian lifestyle and monitoring vitamin B_{12} status. *Clinica Chimica Acta; International Journal of Clinical Chemistry, 26*, 47–59.

Holick, M. F. (2004). Sunlight and vitamin D for bone health and prevention of autoimmune diseases, cancers, and cardiovascular disease. *American Journal of Clinical Nutrition, 80* (6 Suppl.), 1678S–1688S.

Houghton, L. A., Green, T. J., Donovan, U. M., Gibson, R. S., Stephen, A. M., & O'Connor, D. L. (1997). Association between dietary fiber intake and the folate status of a group of female adolescents. *American Journal of Clinical Nutrition, 66*, 1414–1421.

Hunt, J. R. (2002). Moving toward a plant-based diet: Are iron and zinc at risk? *Nutrition Review, 60*, 127–134.

Hunt, J. R., Matthys, L. A., & Johnson, L. K. (1998). Zinc absorption, mineral balance, and blood lipids in women consuming controlled lacto-ovo vegetarian and omnivorous diets for 8 wk. *American Journal of Clinical Nutrition, 67*, 421–430.

Imataka, G., Mikami, T., Yamanouchi, H., Kano, K., & Eguchi, M. (2004). Vitamin D deficiency rickets due to soybean milk. *Journal of Paediatrics and Child Health, 40*, 154–155.

Institute of Medicine (IOM), Food and Nutrition Board. (1997). *Dietary Reference Intakes for Calcium, Phosphorus, Magnesium, Vitamin D, and Fluoride.* Washington, DC: National Academy Press.

Institute of Medicine (IOM), Food and Nutrition Board. (1998). *Dietary Reference Intakes for Thiamin, Riboflavin, Niacin, Vitamin B6, Folate, Vitamin B12, Pantothenic Acid, Biotin, and Choline.* Washington, DC: National Academy Press.

Institute of Medicine (IOM), Food and Nutrition Board. (2001). *Dietary Reference Intakes for Vitamin A, Vitamin K, Arsenic, Boron, Chromium, Copper, Iodine, Iron, Manganese, Molybdenum, Nickel, Silicon, Vanadium, and Zinc.* Washington, DC: National Academy Press.

Institute of Medicine (IOM), Food and Nutrition Board. (2002). *Dietary Reference Intakes for Energy, Carbohydrate, Fiber, Fat, Fatty Acids, Cholesterol, Protein, and Amino Acids.* Washington, DC: National Academy Press.

Janelle, K. C., & Barr, S. I. (1995). Nutrient intakes and eating behavior scores of vegetarian and nonvegetarian women. *Journal of the American Dietetic Association, 95*, 180–186, 189.

Kalkwarf, H. J., Khoury, J. C., & Lanphear, B. P. (2003). Milk intake during childhood and adolescence, adult bone density, and osteoporotic fractures in US women. *American Journal of Clinical Nutrition, 77*, 257–265.

Kissinger, D. G., & Sanchez, A. (1987). The association of dietary factors with the age of menarche. *Nutrition Research, 7*, 471–479.

Krajcovicova-Kudlackova, M., Simoncic, R., Babinska, K., & Bederova, A. (1995). Levels of lipid peroxidation and antioxidants in vegetarians. *European Journal of Epidemiology, 111*, 207–211.

Krajcovicova-Kudlackova, M., Simoncic, R., Bederova, A., Grancicova, E., & Megalova, T. (1997). Influence of vegetarian and mixed nutrition on selected haematological and biochemical parameters in children. *Die Nahrung, 41*, 311–314.

Krajcovicova-Kudlackova, M., Simoncic, R., Bederova, A., & Klvanova, J. (1997). Plasma fatty acid profile and alternative nutrition. *Annals of Nutrition Metabolism, 41*, 365–370.

Larsson, C. L., & Johansson, G. K. (2002). Dietary intake and nutritional status of young vegans and omnivores in Sweden. *American Journal of Clinical Nutrition, 76*, 100–106.

Larsson, C. L., & Johansson, G. K. (2005). Young Swedish vegans have different sources of nutrients than young omnivores. *Journal of the American Dietetic Association, 105*, 1438–1441.

Larsson, C. L., Ronnlund, U., Johansson, G., & Dahlgren, L. (2003). Veganism as status passage: The process of becoming a vegan among youths in Sweden. *Appetite, 41*, 61–67.

Leung, S. S., Lee, R., Sung, S., Luo, H. Y., Kam, C. W., Yuen, M. P., et al. (2001). Growth and nutrition of Chinese vegetarian children in Hong Kong. *Journal of Paediatrics and Child Health, 37*, 247–253.

Licht, D. J., Berry, G. T., Brooks, D. G., & Younkin, D. P. (2001). Reversible subacute combined degeneration of the spinal cord in a 14-year-old due to a strict vegan diet. *Clinical Pediatrics, 40*, 413–415.

Louwman, M. W. J., van Dusseldorp, M., van de Vijver, F. J. R., Thomas, C. M., Schneede, J., Ueland, P. M., et al. (2000). Signs of impaired cognitive function in adolescents with marginal cobalamin status. *American Journal of Clinical Nutrition, 72*, 762–769.

Mangels, A. R., & Messina, V. (2001). Considerations in planning vegan diets. I. Infants. *Journal of the American Dietetic Association, 101*, 670–677.

Mangels, A. R., Messina, V., & Melina, V. (2003). Position of the American Dietetic Association and Dietitians of Canada: Vegetarian diets. *Journal of the American Dietetic Association, 103*, 748–765.

Martins, Y., Pliner, P., & O'Connor, R. (1999). Restrained eating among vegetarians: Does a vegetarian eating style mask concerns about weight? *Appetite, 32*, 145–154.

McCann, J. C., & Ames, B. N. (2005). Is docosahexaenoic acid, an n-3 long-chain polyunsaturated fatty acid, required for development of normal brain function? An overview of evidence from cognitive and behavioral tests in humans and animals. *American Journal of Clinical Nutrition, 82*, 281–295.

Messina, V., & Mangels, A. R. (2001). Considerations in planning vegan diets: Children. *Journal of the American Dietetic Association, 101*, 661–669.

Messina, V. K., Mangels, R., & Messina, M. (2004). *The Dietitian's Guide to Vegetarian Diets* (2nd ed.). Sudbury, MA: Jones and Bartlett.

Messina, V., Melina, V., & Mangels, A. R. (2003). A new food guide for North American vegetarians. *Journal of the American Dietetic Association, 103*, 771–775.

Nathan, I., Hackett, A. F., & Kirby, S. (1996). The dietary intake of a group of vegetarian children aged 7–11 years compared with matched omnivores. *British Journal of Nutrition, 75*, 533–544.

Nathan, I., Hackett, A. F., & Kirby, S. (1997). A longitudinal study of the growth of matched pairs of vegetarian and omnivorous children, aged 7–11 years, in the north-west of England. *European Journal of Clinical Nutrition, 51*, 20–25.

Neumark-Sztainer, D., Story, M., Resnick, M. D., & Blum, R. W. (1997). Adolescent vegetarians: A behavioral profile of a school-based population in Minnesota. *Archives of Pediatric and Adolescent Medicine, 151*, 833–838.

Perry, C. L., McGuire, M. T., Newmark-Sztainer, D., & Story, M. (2001). Characteristics of vegetarian adolescents in a multiethnic urban population. The *Journal of Adolescent Health, 29*, 406–416.

Perry, C. L., McGuire, M. T., Neumark-Sztainer, D., & Story, M. (2002). Adolescent vegetarians. How well do their dietary patterns meet the Healthy People 2010 objectives? *Archives of Pediatric and Adolescent Medicine, 156*, 431–437.

Roberts, I. F., West, R. J., Ogilvie, D., & Dillon, M. J. (1979). Malnutrition in infants receiving cult diets: A form of child abuse. *British Medical Journal, 1*, 296–298.

Rosell, M. S., Lloyd-Wright, Z., Appleby, P. N., Sanders, T. A., Allen, N. E., & Key, T. J. (2005). Long-chain n-3 polyunsaturated fatty acids in plasma in British meat-eating, vegetarian, and vegan men. *American Journal of Clinical Nutrition, 82,* 327–334.

Sabaté, J., Linsted, K. D., Harris, R. D., & Johnston, P. K. (1990). Anthropometric parameters of schoolchildren with different life-styles. *American Journal of Diseases of Children, 144,* 1159–1163.

Sabaté, J., Linsted, K. D., Harris, R. D., & Sanchez, A. (1991). Attained height of lacto-ovo vegetarian children and adolescents. *European Journal of Clinical Nutrition, 45,* 51–58.

Sabaté, J., Llorca, C., & Sanchez, A. (1992). Lower height of lacto-ovovegetarian girls at preadolescence: An indicator of physical maturation today? *Journal of the American Dietetic Association, 92,* 1263–1264.

Sanders, T. A. B. (1988). Growth and development of British vegan children. *American Journal of Clinical Nutrition, 48,* 822–825.

Sanders, T. A. B. (1995). Vegetarian diets and children. *Pediatric Clinics of North America, 42,* 955–965.

Sanders, T. A. B., & Manning, J. (1992). The growth and development of vegan children. *Journal of Human Nutrition and Dietetics, 5,* 11–21.

Sanders, T. A. B., & Reddy, S. (1992). The influence of a vegetarian diet on the fatty acid composition of human milk and the essential fatty acid status of the infant. *Journal of Pediatrics, 120,* S71–S77.

Sandstrom, B. (2001). Micronutrient interactions: Effects on absorption and bioavailability. *British Journal of Nutrition, 85*(Suppl. 2), S181–S185.

SanGiovanni, J. P., Parra-Cabrera, S., Colditz, G. A., Berkey, C. S., & Dwyer, J. T. (2000). Meta-analysis of dietary essential fatty acids and long-chain polyunsaturated fatty acids as they relate to visual resolution acuity in healthy preterm infants. *Pediatrics, 105,* 1292–1298.

Scott, M. (2003). Nutrition for the full-term infant. In N. Nevin-Folino (Ed.), *Pediatric Manual of Clinical Dietetics* (2nd ed., pp. 55–71). Chicago: American Dietetic Association.

Stepaniak, J., & Melina, V. (2003). *Raising Vegetarian Children.* Chicago: Contemporary Books.

Thane, C. W., & Bates, C. J. (2000). Dietary intakes and nutrient status of vegetarian preschool children from a British national survey. *Journal of Human Nutrition and Dietetics, 13,* 149–162.

Thane, C. W., Bates, C. J., & Prentice, A. (2003). Risk factors for low iron intake and poor iron status in a national sample of British young people aged 4–18 years. *Public Health Nutrition, 6,* 485–496.

Truesdell, D. D., & Acosta, P. B. (1985). Feeding the vegan infant and child. *Journal of the American Dietetic Association, 85,* 837–840.

Uauy, R., Peirano, P., Hoffman, D., Mena, P., Birch, D., & Birch, E. (1996). Role of essential fatty acids in the function of the developing nervous system. *Lipids, 31,* S167–S176.

van den Berg, H., Dagnelie, P. C., & van Staveren, W. A. (1988). Vitamin B12 and seaweed. *Lancet, 1,* 242–243.

van Dusseldorp, M., Arts, I. C. W., Bergsma, J. S., de Jong, N., Dagnelie, P. C., & van Staveren, W. A. (1996). Catch-up growth in children fed a macrobiotic diet in early childhood. *Journal of Nutrition, 126,* 2977–2983.

Vegetarian Resource Group. (2001 Jan/Feb). How many teens are vegetarian? How many kids don't eat meat? *Vegetarian Journal.*

Watanabe, F., Katsura, H., Takenaka, S., Fujita, T., Abe, K., Tamura, Y., et al. (1999). Pseudovitamin B (12) is the predominant cobalamide of an algal health food, Spirulina tablets. *Journal of Agricultural and Food Chemistry, 47,* 4736–4741.

Weaver, C. M., & Plawecki, K. L. (1994). Dietary calcium: Adequacy of a vegetarian diet. *American Journal of Clinical Nutrition, 59*(Suppl.), 1238S–1241S.

Worsley, A., & Skrzypiec, G. (1998). Teenage vegetarianism: Prevalence, social and cognitive contexts. *Appetite, 30,* 151–170.

Young, V. R., & Pellett, P. L. (1994). Plant proteins in relation to human protein and amino acid nutrition. *American Journal of Clinical Nutrition, 59,* 1203S–1212S.

Childhood Obesity

Alaimo, K., Olson, C. M., & Frongillo, Jr., E. A. (2001). Low family income and food insufficiency in relation to overweight in US children. Is there a paradox? *Archives of Pediatric and Adolescent Medicine, 155,* 1161–1167.

Allison, D. B., & Faith, M. S. (2000). Genetic and environmental influences on human body weight: Implications for the behavior therapist. *Nutrition Today, 35,* 18–21.

American Dietetic Association. (2002). Position paper. The role of dietetics professionals in health promotion and disease prevention. *Journal of the American Dietetic Association, 102,* 1680–1687.

American Dietetic Association, Society for Nutrition Education, and the American School Food Service Association. (2003). Position paper. Nutrition services: An essential component of comprehensive school health programs. *Journal of the American Dietetic Association, 103,* 505–514.

Andersen, R. E., Crespo, C. J., Bartlett, S. J., Cheskin, L. J., & Pratt, M. (1998). Relationship of physical activity and television watching with body weight and level of fatness among children: Results from the Third National Health and Nutrition Examination Survey. *Journal of the American Medical Association, 279,* 938–942.

Armstrong, J., & Reilly, J. J. (2002). Breastfeeding and lowering the risk of childhood obesity. Child Health Information Team. *Lancet, 359,* 2003–2004.

Augustin, L. S., Franceschi, S., Jenkins, D. J.A., Kendall, C. W. C., & La Vecchia, C. (2002). Glycemic index in chronic disease: A review. *European Journal of Clinical Nutrition, 56,* 1049–1071.

Berenson, G. S. (2002). Childhood risk factors predict adult risk associated with subclinical cardiovascular disease: The Bogalusa Heart Study. *American Journal of Cardiology, 90*(Suppl.), 3L–7L.

Birch, L. L., & Fischer, J. O. (1998). Development of eating behaviors among children and adolescents. *Pediatrics, 101,* 539–547.

Booth, S. L., Sallis, J. F., Ritenbaugh, C., Hill, J. O., Birch, L. L., Frank, L. D., et al. (Working Group II). (2001). Environmental and societal factors affect food choice and physical activity: Rationale, influences, and leverage points. *Nutrition Reviews, 59*(3, part 2), S21–S39.

Borzekowski, D. L. G., & Robinson, T. N. (2001). The 30-second effect: An experiment revealing the impact of television commercials on food preferences of preschoolers. *Journal of the American Dietetic Association, 101,* 42–46.

Bowman, S. A., Gortmaker, S. L., Ebbeling, C. B., Pereira, M. A., & Ludwig, D. S. (2004). Effects of fast-food consumption on energy intake and diet quality among children in a national household survey. *Pediatrics, 113,* 112–118.

Briefel, R. R., & Johnson, C. L. (2004). Secular trends in dietary intake in the United States. *Annual Review of Nutrition, 24,* 401–431.

Buechner, J. (2001). Stress-free Feeding Curriculum and Video. Atlanta, GA: Children's Healthcare of Atlanta.

Burgenson, C. R., Wechsler, H., Brener, N. D., Young, J. C., & Spain, C. G. (2001). Physical education and activity: Results from the School Health Policies and Programs Study 2000. *Journal of School Health, 71,* 279–293.

Carter, J., Wiecha, J., Peterson, K., Gortmaker, S. L. (2001). *Planet Health: An Interdisciplinary Curriculum for Teaching Middle School Nutrition and Physical Activity.* Champaign, IL: Human Kinetics.

Center for Screen-Time Awareness. (n.d.). Retrieved June 30, 2007, from www.tvturnoff.org

Centers for Disease Control and Prevention (CDC). (n.d.). KidsWalk-to-School. Nutrition and physical activity. Retrieved June 30, 2007, from http://www.cdc.gov/nccdphp/dnpa/kidswalk/

Centers for Disease Control and Prevention (CDC). (2003). Resource guide for nutrition and physical activity interventions to prevent obesity and other chronic disease. Retrieved June 30, 2007, from http://www.cdc.gov/nccdphp/dnpa/obesity/resource_guide.htm

Conner, W. E. (2000). Importance of n-3 fatty acids in health and disease. *American Journal of Clinical Nutrition, 71,* 171S–175S.

Crawford, P., Gosliner, W., Anderson, C., Strode, P., Becerra-Jones, Y., Samuels, S., et al. (2004). Counseling Latina mothers of preschool children about weight issues: Suggestions for a new framework. *Journal of American Dietetic Association, 104,* 87–394.

Dietz, W. H. (2001). Breastfeeding may help prevent overweight children. *Journal of the American Medical Association, 285,* 2506–2507.

Dietz, W. H. (2004). Overweight in childhood and adolescence. *New England Journal of Medicine, 350,* 855–857.

Dowda, M., Ainsworth, B. E., Addy, C. L., Saunders, R., & Riner, W. (2001). Environmental influences, physical activity, and weight status in 8- to 16-year-olds. *Archives of Pediatric Adolescent Medicine, 155,* 711–717.

Drewnowski, A., & Specter, S. E. (2004). Poverty and obesity: The role of energy density and energy costs. *American Journal of Clinical Nutrition, 79,* 6–16.

Ellis, K. J., Abrams, S. A., & Wong, W. W. (1999). Monitoring childhood obesity: Assessment of weight/height$_2$ index. *American Journal of Epidemiology, 150,* 939–946.

Erickson, S. J., Robinson, T. N., Haydel, K. F., & Killen, J. D. (2000). Are overweight children unhappy? *Archives of Pediatric and Adolescent Medicine, 154,* 931–935.

Fischer, J. O., & Birch, L. L. (1999). Restricting access to palatable foods affects children's behavioral response, food selection, and intake. *American Journal of Clinical Nutrition, 69,* 1264–1272.

Freedman, D. S., Khan, L. K., Dietz, W. H., Srinivasan, S. R., & Berenson, G. S. (2001). Relationship of childhood obesity to coronary heart disease risk factors in adulthood: The Bogalusa Heart Study. *Pediatrics, 108,* 712–718.

Frumkin, H. (2002). Urban sprawl and public health. *Public Health Reports, 117,* 201–217.

Gibson, D. (2004). Long-term Food Stamp Program participation is differently related to overweight in young girls and boys. *Journal of Nutrition, 134,* 372–379.

Gortmaker, S. L., Must, A., Sobol, A. M., Peterson, K., Colditz, G. A., & Dietz, W. H. (1996). Television viewing as a cause of increasing obesity among children in the United States, 1986–1990. *Archives of Pediatric and Adolescent Medicine, 150,* 356–362.

Harnack, L., Stang, J., & Story, M. (1999). Soft drink consumption among US children and adolescents: Nutritional consequences. *Journal of the American Dietetic Association, 99,* 436–441.

Hassink, S. (2003). Problems in childhood obesity. *Primary Care Office Practice, 30,* 357–374.

Hill, J. O., & Trowbridge, F. L. (1998). Childhood obesity: Future directions and research priorities. *Pediatrics, 101*(Suppl.), 570–574.

Hill, J. O., Wyatt, H. R., Reed, G. W., & Peters, J. C. (2003). Obesity and the environment: Where do we go from here? *Science, 299,* 853–855.

Johnson, S. L. (2000). Improving preschoolers' self-regulation of energy intake. *Pediatrics, 106,* 1429–1435.

Johnson, S. L., & Birch, L. L. (1994). Parents' adiposity and children's eating style. *Pediatrics, 94,* 653–661.

Jones, S. J., Jahns, L., Laraia, B. A., & Haughton, B. (2003). Lower risk of overweight in school-aged food insures girls who participate in food assistance. *Archives of Pediatric and Adolescent Medicine, 157,* 780–784.

Kaiser Family Foundation. (n.d.). Kids & media @ the new millenium: A Kaiser Family Foundation report. Retrieved June 30, 2007, from http://www.kff.org

Kurtzweil, P. (1996). Taking the fat out of food. *FDA Consumer Magazine,* online version, USDA. Retrieved June 30, 2007, from http://www.fda.gov/fdac/features/696_fat.html

Ludwig, D. S., Peterson, K. E., & Gortmaker, S. L. (2001). Relation between consumption of sugar-sweetened drinks and childhood obesity: A prospective, observational analysis. *Lancet, 357,* 505–508.

McBean, L. D., & Miller, G. D. (1999). Enhancing the nutrition of America's youth. *Journal of the American College of Nutrition, 18,* 563–571.

Munoz, K. A., Krebs-Smith, S. M., Ballard-Barbash, R., & Cleveland, L. E. (1997). Food intakes of US children and adolescents compared with recommendations. *Pediatrics, 100,* 323–329.

National Center for Health Statistics. (1999). Prevalence of overweight and obesity among adults. Retrieved June 4, 2007, from www.cdc.gov/nchs/products/pubs/pubd/hestats/obese/obse99.htm

Nelson, J. A., Chiasson, M. A., & Ford, V. (2004). Overweight children in a New York City WIC population. *American Journal of Public Health, 94,* 458–462.

Nicklas, T. A., Baranowski, T., Cullen, K. W., & Berenson, G. (2001). Eating patterns, dietary quality, and obesity. *Journal of the American College of Nutrition, 20,* 599–608.

Ogden, C. L., Carroll, M. D., Curtin, L. R., McDowell, M. A., Tabak, C. J., & Flegal, K. M. (2006). Prevalence of overweight and obesity in the United States, 1999–2004. *Journal of the American Medical Association, 295,* 1549–1555.

Ogden, C. L., Flegal, K. M., Carroll, M. D., & Johnson, C. L. (2002). Prevalence and trends in overweight among US children and adolescents, 1999–2000. *Journal of the American Medical Association, 288,* 1728–1732.

O'Keefe, J. H., & Cordain, L. (2004). Cardiovascular disease resulting from a diet and lifestyle at odds with our Paleolithic genome: How to become a 21st century hunter-gatherer. *Mayo Clinical Proceedings, 79,* 101–108.

Paeratakul, S., Ferdinand, D. P., Champagne, C. M., Ryan, D. H., & Bray, G. A. (2003). Fast-food consumption among US adults and children: Dietary and nutrient intake profile. *Journal of the American Dietetic Association, 103,* 1332–1338.

Raman, R. P. (2002). Obesity and health risks. *Journal of the American College of Nutrition, 21,* 134S–139S.

Roberts, S. B. (2000). High-glycemic index foods, hunger and obesity: Is there a connection? *Nutrition Reviews, 58,* 163–169.

Robinson, T. N., Hammer, L. D., Killen, J. D., Kraemer, H. C., Wilson, D. M., Hayward, C., et al. (1993). Does television viewing increase obesity and reduce physical activity? Cross-sectional and longitudinal analyses among adolescent girls. *Pediatrics, 91,* 273–280.

Satter, E. (1987). *How to Get Kids to Eat . . . But Not Too Much.* Palo Alto, CA: Bull Publishing.

Satter, E. (1999). *Secrets of Feeding a Healthy Family.* Madison, WI: Kelcy Press.

Satter, E. (2000). *Child of Mine: Feeding with Love and Good Sense.* Palo Alto, CA: Bull Publishing.

Serdula, M. K., Ivery, D., Coates, R. J., Freedman, D. S., Williamson, D. F., & Byers, T. (1993). Do obese children become obese adults? A review of literature. *Preventive Medicine, 65,* 167–177.

Simopoulos, A. P. (1999). Evolutionary aspects of omega-3 fatty acids in the food supply. *Prostaglandins, Leukotrienes, and Essential Fatty Acids, 60,* 421–429.

Simopoulos, A. P. (2002). The importance of the ratio of omega-6/omega-3 fatty acids. *Biomedical Pharmacotherapy, 56,* 365–379.

Steinbeck, K. S. (2001). The importance of physical activity in the prevention of overweight and obesity in childhood: A review and an option. *Obesity Reviews, 2,* 117–130.

Strauss, R. S., & Pollack, H. A. (2001). Epidemic increase in overweight children, 1986–1998. *Journal of the American Medical Association, 286,* 2845–2848.

Taylor, R. W., Jones, I. E., Williams, S. M., & Goulding, A. (2002). Body fat percentages measured by dual-energy x-ray absorptiometry corresponding to recently recommended body mass index cutoffs for overweight and obesity in children and adolescents aged 3–18 y. *American Journal of Clinical Nutrition, 76,* 1416–1421.

U.S. Department of Health and Human Services. (2000). *Healthy People 2010* (2nd ed.). With Understanding and Improving Health and Objectives for Improving Health (2 vols.). Washington, DC: U.S. Government Printing Office.

Warren, J. M., Henry, C. J., & Simonite, V. (2003). Low glycemic index breakfasts and reduced food intake in preadolescent children. *Pediatrics, 112,* e414.

Special Topics in Preadolescence and Adolescent Nutrition: Dietary Guidelines for Athletes, Pediatric Diabetes, and Disordered Eating

*Pamela S. Hinton, PhD, and
Karen Chapman-Novakofski, RD, LDN, PhD*

CHAPTER OUTLINE

Reader Objectives

After studying this chapter and reflecting on the contents, you should be able to

1. Determine fuel utilization during exercise.
2. Describe optimal nutrition before, during, and after an endurance competition.
3. Describe the consequences of chronic undernutrition and how they differ between males and females.
4. Recognize the prevalence and incidence of pediatric diabetes in the United States.
5. Understand the pathogenesis of types 1 and 2 diabetes in children.
6. Identify risk factors for types 1 and 2 diabetes in children.
7. Recognize conditions associated with pediatric diabetes.
8. Understand management principles to achieve optimal glycemic goals.
9. Describe the similarities and differences among the three eating disorders defined by the American Psychiatric Association.
10. Know the medical consequences of eating disorders.
11. Describe effective treatment for eating disorders, including recommendations for nutrition interventions.
12. Know the prevalence, etiology, and recommended treatment practices for eating disorders in special populations.
13. Identify childhood eating disorders and explain how they differ from anorexia nervosa and bulimia nervosa.

Dietary Guidelines for Athletes

Pamela S. Hinton, PhD

Energy

Total energy expenditure is the sum of resting energy expenditure, dietary-induced thermogenesis, and physical activity and varies with gender, age, and body size. Typically, physical activity accounts for 10% to 15% of total energy expenditure, but athletes in strenuous training programs or who participate in endurance sports may increase total energy expenditure by 2- to 3-fold due to physical activity. For example, cyclists competing in stage races such as the Tour de France may expend up to 8,000 kcal/day (Saris, van Erp-Baart, Brouns, Westerterp, & ten Hoor, 1989). The Institute of Medicine recently published formulas for estimated energy requirements based on gender, age, weight, height, and physical activity **(Table 8.1)**.

Accurately determining energy needs from prediction equations is difficult. Interindividual variation in resting energy expenditure is large, and energy expended during physical activity varies with exercise duration and intensity. Tables of **metabolic equivalent** values for various activities can be used to estimate energy expenditure in physical activity and activities of daily living (Ainsworth, Jacobs, Leon, Richardson, & Montoye, 1993).

Even if we have an estimate of how many calories are needed to be in energy balance, the error associated with evaluating dietary intake is largely due to over- or under-reporting, various methods of food preparation, and accuracy of food composition tables. Changes in body weight and/or composition may be the best way for athletes to self-monitor their energy balance over time.

Metabolic equivalent: The ratio of the work metabolic rate to the resting metabolic rate. One metabolic equivalent is defined as 1 kcal/kg/h or 3.5 mL O_2 consumed/kg/min.

TABLE 8.1	Institute of Medicine Equations for Estimating Energy Requirements in Healthy Adults

Males
EER = 662 − 9.53 × age (yr) + PA × [5.91 × weight (kg) + 539.6 × height (m)]
Females
EER = 354 − 6.91 × age (yr) + PA × [9.36 × weight (kg) + 726 × height (m)]
PA = 1.25 if you are "active" and 1.48 if you are "very active"
EER, estimate energy requirement; PA, physical activity.

From Food and Nutrition Board (2003).

Carbohydrate

Dietary carbohydrates (sugar and starch) have a **metabolizable energy** density of 4 kcal/g and are readily digested and absorbed. During exercise, glucose is the preferred substrate for ATP production. For this reason, and to replenish hepatic and muscle glycogen, athletes should consume 60% to 75% of their energy from carbohydrate. It is recommended that endurance athletes consume from 6 to 10 g carbohydrate/kg body weight (BW) (American Dietetic Association, Dietitians of Canada, and the American College of Sports Medicine, 2000). This recommendation assumes that an athlete is not over- or underweight. For example, an athlete weighing 70 kg needs between 420 and 720 g carbohydrate/day (which is 1,680 to 2,880 kcal carbohydrate). To equate grams of carbohydrate to foods, a serving from the grains, breads, and cereals group contains approximately 15 g of carbohydrate. A serving is one slice of bread, 1 ounce of cereal, or 1/2 cup of cooked rice or pasta (U.S. Department of Health and Human Services [DHHS]). This recommendation applies only to athletes who are regularly depleting their glycogen stores (i.e., through 2 to 3 hours of aerobic exercise a day 5 to 7 days a week).

> **Metabolizable energy:** Gross energy in a food minus the energy lost in feces, urine, and combustible gases. The metabolizable energies for protein and carbohydrate are 4 kcal/g, and the metabolizable energy for fat is 9 kcal/g.

> **● Learning Point** Foods that have rapidly digestible carbohydrate and contain glucose have the highest glycemic indices. For example, Gatorade® has a GI of 80.

There are several reasons for the emphasis on dietary carbohydrates, especially for athletes. First, the central nervous system and red blood cells have a high glucose requirement. Red blood cells do not have mitochondria, so they cannot oxidize fat; ATP must be produced from glycolysis and anaerobic metabolism of pyruvate to lactate. Second, dietary carbohydrates are needed to replenish liver and muscle glycogen stores. Inadequate carbohydrate intake necessitates gluconeogenesis from dietary or endogenous amino acids because fat cannot be used to make glucose.

Glucose is by far the most abundant dietary monosaccharide; the most prevalent dietary disaccharides are sucrose (glucose + fructose), more commonly referred to as table sugar; lactose (glucose + galactose), which is milk sugar; and maltose (glucose + glucose). The mono- and disaccharides fall into the category of "sugars" and are sometimes referred to as "simple carbohydrates." The term "complex carbohydrate" is used to describe carbohydrates that are glucose polymers. Short chains of glucose molecules linked together, such as maltodextrin or dextrose, are used by the food industry as sweeteners. These are also the "complex carbohydrates" added to sports drinks. The most complex carbohydrate molecules are the polysaccharides, which typically contain 10,000 to 1,000,000 glucose molecules. Polysaccharides make up the starches that are present in grains, legumes, and some vegetables.

Carbohydrates differ not only in their complexity, but also in their effect on blood sugar (Foster-Powell, Holt, & Brand-Miller, 2002). The effect of carbohydrates on blood sugar is important for overall health, fueling muscle during exercise, and replenishing glycogen stores after exercise. The effect of a food on blood glucose concentrations depends on the type and amount of carbohydrate in the food and on how quickly that carbohydrate can be digested and absorbed. Some foods cause a rapid increase in blood glucose concentrations, whereas others produce a slower and more prolonged rise. The glycemic index (GI) is used to quantify the effect of a food on blood glucose and to make comparisons among foods. The GI is defined as the increase in blood glucose concentration above baseline during the 2 hours after eating a test food relative to the response to glucose for an equivalent amount of carbohydrate. The glycemic response to glucose is set at 100, and the GI for all other foods is less than 100.

The actual GIs of foods may vary from the published values because they are affected by multiple factors. The physical form of the food alters the GI. Breaking down the food matrix increases the GI. For example, the GI of potatoes is increased by 25% if the potatoes are mashed. And, thin linguini has a GI of 87, but thick linguini is lower, at 68. The ripeness of fruit also has an effect on the GI because as a fruit ripens the starch is converted into sugar. Under-ripe bananas have a GI of 30 versus 50 for a ripe banana. Food processing and cooking methods also alter the GI. Heating, moisturizing, and pressing foods make the starch easier to digest, increasing the GI. For example, raw carrots have a GI of 20, and peeling and boiling them increases the GI to 40.

The GI of a food assumes that only that food has been eaten. However, most humans do not eat single foods but eat meals and snacks composed of several foods. Protein and fat do not cause an increase in blood glucose; only foods containing carbohydrate have this effect. However, the GI of a food eaten alone is different from the same food eaten as part of a mixed meal of carbohydrate, protein, and fat. For example, a plain French baguette has a GI of 95; bread with butter has a GI of 60. Meals that are high in soluble fiber or have a high acid content also lower the GI because the rate of gastric emptying is decreased, slowing the increase in blood glucose.

Glycemic load is the net effect of a food on blood glucose concentrations. Glycemic load depends not just on the GI of that food, but on how much of it is eaten. For example, jelly beans have a GI of 80, but eating only five jelly beans causes a much smaller increase in blood glucose than eating a handful of peanut M&Ms®, which have a GI of 30.

Despite these limitations, the concept of GI still has some practical value for athletes. Even if the GI of a food cannot be accurately determined when it is consumed as part of a meal, foods can be categorized as generally high or low GI. For example, a dinner of whole wheat fettuccine with chunky tomato sauce and sautéed vegetables has a lower GI than Spaghettios® because of the whole grain flour, the size of the pasta, the greater acidity of the tomato sauce, and the fiber in the vegetables.

For overall health, most dietary carbohydrate should come from unrefined whole grains, legumes, and fresh fruits and vegetables (Murphy & Johnson, 2003). Unrefined grains are superior to refined varieties because they provide more fiber and vitamins. Unrefined grains also have lower GIs, which may reduce the risk of non–insulin-dependent (type 2) diabetes. High GI foods may contribute to insulin resistance because the rapid increase in blood glucose levels after eating these foods stimulates a greater insulin response than lower GI foods. Although somewhat controversial, there is evidence that high GI foods contribute to elevated blood triglycerides (fats), which is a risk factor for heart disease.

Protein

Dietary protein has a metabolizable energy density of 4 kcal/g. Protein in meat, dairy products, eggs, and legumes is digested into amino acids, which are used to repair or build new tissues. If energy or carbohydrate intake is insufficient, amino acids from dietary protein or catabolism of endogenous protein are used for gluconeogenesis in the liver. Athletes have slightly higher protein requirements (1.2 to 1.7 g/kg BW) than nonathletes (0.8 g/kg BW) (American Dietetic Association et al., 2000; Wolfe, 2000). Endurance athletes should consume 1.2 to 1.4 g protein/kg BW to maintain lean body mass, and strength-trained athletes 1.6 to 1.7 g/kg to maximize muscle hypertrophy. Athletes who follow vegetarian diets have greater protein

● **Learning Point** To put grams of protein into food terms, a serving from the protein food group is equivalent to ~20 g. A serving from this group is 2 to 3 ounces of cooked meat, 1 cup of cooked beans, 1/4 cup of peanut butter, or ⅔ cup of nuts. Excess dietary protein is metabolized to glucose and fatty acids and stored as glycogen and triglycerides in adipose tissue.

requirements (1.3 to 1.8 g/kg BW) because of the lower quality of plant-derived proteins. A 70-kg athlete who participates in a team sport like basketball or soccer needs 84 to 98 g protein/day.

Fat

Dietary fat has a metabolizable energy density of 9 kcal/g, making it a more concentrated source of energy than carbohydrate or protein. For this reason, and because of the association between diets high in fat and cardiovascular disease, some female athletes restrict their fat intake. However, dietary fat plays an essential role in maintaining health. It is needed for absorption of the fat-soluble vitamins (vitamins A, D, E, and K), and vegetable oils are excellent sources of the antioxidant vitamin E. Fatty acids are incorporated into cell membranes and are required for normal immune function. It is recommended that athletes consume moderate amounts of fat (20% to 25% of energy) and no less than 15% of their total energy from dietary fat, preferably polyunsaturated fats (American Dietetic Association et al., 2000). As an example, if an athlete needs 3,000 calories per day, at least 450 of those calories should be from fat. This would be equivalent to 50 g of fat (i.e., 300 calories divided by 9 calories per gram of fat). The easiest way to change the amount of dietary fat is to increase or decrease the amount of fat added to foods, like butter or cream cheese on bagels, dressing on salads, mayonnaise on sandwiches, and oil in cooking. One tablespoon of butter, cream cheese, dressing, or oil contains about 10 g of fat and 100 calories.

> **● Learning Point** There is no direct evidence that omega-3 fatty acids improve athletic performance in humans. In one study of highly trained soccer players, 10 weeks of omega-3 supplementation in the form of fish oil had no effect on maximal aerobic power, anaerobic power, or running performance (Raastad et al., 1997).

Athletes should make an effort to consume fats from different sources to ensure they consume adequate amounts of the essential fatty acids. Omega-3 fatty acids are more likely to be missing from the typical U.S. diet, whereas omega-6 fatty acids are plentiful in the food supply. Dietary sources of omega-3 fatty acids include fatty fish, walnuts, flaxseed, and canola oil. Eicosapentaenoic acid and docosahexaenoic acid are the most common omega-3 fatty acids in the diet; purified eicosapentaenoic acid and docosahexaenoic acid also are sold as dietary supplements. Regular consumption of omega-3 fatty acids may reduce the risk of developing cardiovascular disease by lowering serum cholesterol and triglycerides and by reducing inflammation in the lining of the blood vessels (Connor, 2000; James, Gibson, & Cleland, 2000).

Omega-3 fatty acids alter cell metabolism by activating genes that are needed for cellular transport and use of fat. Omega-3 fatty acids promote the cellular uptake of fat by increasing the activity of lipoprotein lipase (Park & Harris, 2003) and by increasing the amount of fatty acid binding protein, which carries fatty acids across the cell membrane into the cells. Omega-3 fatty acids also facilitate production of energy from fat due to increased hepatic carnitine palmitoyltransferase-2 activity (Ukropec et al., 2003) and accelerated transport of fatty acids into the mitochondria (Raastad, Hostmark, & Stromme, 1997).

Regardless of whether or not omega-3 fatty acids improve performance, they are needed to optimize health and may reduce the risk of osteoporosis (Watkins, Li, Lippman, & Seifert, 2001), rheumatoid arthritis, asthma, cancer, and heart disease (Connor, 2000). According to the Food and Nutrition Board of the Institute of Medicine (2003), adult males should consume 1.6 g/day and adult females 1.1 g/day. Four ounces of cold-water fish, such as salmon, swordfish, or bluefish, contain about 1.5 g omega-3 fatty acids. One ounce of walnuts or flaxseeds (or 1 tablespoon of the oil) has about 2 g of omega-3 fatty acids.

Vitamins and Minerals

Athletes often believe their vitamin and mineral needs are significantly higher than those of the typical non athlete, so they consume micronutrients in excess of the Recommended Daily Allowances (RDAs). What athletes do not realize is that RDAs are set above the mean requirement for the general population, so there is a "safety factor" built into them. For example, the RDA for iron for women ages 19 to 50 years is 18 mg/day, whereas the mean requirement is 8 mg/day (Food and Nutrition Board, Institute of Medicine, 2001).

> **● Learning Point** Most athletes meet their nutrient needs if they consume the RDAs, which usually can be achieved by eating a varied and balanced diet. The exceptions are athletes who restrict their food intake and vegetarian and vegan athletes. Iron, zinc, and calcium are the most common inadequate nutrient intakes in these populations.

Athletes may require more of some nutrients than nonathletes because of increased nutrient excretion, metabolic waste production, and tissue synthesis and repair. However, the increment is small relative to the safety factor.

Iron

In the general population of adults in the United States, 3% to 5% of women are anemic and 11% to 13% are iron deficient; less than 1% of men are iron deficient (Looker, Dallman, Carroll, Gunter, & Johnson, 1997). The reasons for the relatively high prevalence of iron deficiency in women are increased iron losses through menstrual blood flow and from lower dietary iron intake. Endurance athletes, regardless of gender, are more likely to become iron deficient than non athletes. A recent study of recreationally competitive runners, cyclists, and triathletes found 36% of women and 6% of men to be iron deficient but not anemic (Sinclair & Hinton, 2005). The increased prevalence of iron deficiency in endurance athletes is because of greater iron losses, primarily via sweat and occult gastrointestinal bleeding.

Iron plays a critical role in oxidative metabolism. Hemoglobin and myoglobin bind dioxygen via the porphyrin ring of heme. Hemoglobin carries oxygen from the environment to the tissues; myoglobin transfers oxygen from erythrocytes to muscle cells. The electron transport chain depends on heme-containing cytochromes (a, a_3, b, b_5, c, c_1) and on non-heme iron–sulfur enzymes (NADH dehydrogenase, succinate dehydrogenase, and ubiquinone-cytochrome c reductase).

Iron deficiency is a degenerative condition that progresses through three stages (Food and Nutrition Board, Institute of Medicine, 2001): depleted iron stores but with functional iron is unchanged, early functional iron deficiency without anemia, and iron deficiency anemia. The clinical indicators used to assess each stage of iron deficiency are shown in **Table 8.2**. The clinical signs and symptoms of iron depletion are determined by the severity of the deficiency. Early functional iron deficiency reduces endurance capacity and energetic efficiency during submaximal work in young women (Hinton, Giordano, Brownlie, & Haas, 2000; Brutsaert et al., 2003; Brownlie, Utermohlen, Hinton, Giordano, & Haas, 2002; Brownlie, Utermohlen, Hinton, & Haas, 2004). Based on animal studies, this deficit is due to decreased activity of iron-containing oxidative enzymes and cytochromes (Finch et al., 1976; Davies et al., 1984; Willis, Brooks, Henderson, & Dallman, 1987). The hallmark symptoms of anemia are fatigue, lack of energy, and apathy. Anemia impairs maximal work performance (maximal oxygen consumption) by reducing oxygen delivery to the body (Celsing, Ekblom, Sylven, Everett, & Astrand, 1988).

TABLE 8.2	Laboratory Measurements Commonly Used in the Evaluation of Iron Status	
Stage of Iron Deficiency	**Indicator**	**Diagnostic Range**
Depleted stores	Stainable bone marrow iron	Absent
	Total iron binding capacity	>400 μg/dL
	Serum ferritin concentration	<12 μg/L
Early functional iron deficiency	Transferrin saturation	<16%
	Free erythrocyte protoporphyrin	>70 μg/dL erythrocyte
	Serum transferrin receptor	>8.5 mg/L
Iron deficiency anemia	Hemoglobin concentration	<130 g/L male
		<20 g/L female
	Mean cell volume	<80 fL

From Food and Nutrition Board (2003).

Daily basal iron losses are small compared with total body iron (0.9 to 1.2 mg iron/day): 0.6 mg/day are lost from the gastrointestinal tract, mostly in sloughed mucosal cells; 0.08 mg/day are lost in urine; and 0.2 to 0.3 mg/day are lost through the skin. Menstruating women require an additional 0.6 to 0.7 mg/day to account for menstrual blood loss. The estimated average requirement for iron was set to maintain the functional iron pool with minimal iron stores (i.e., serum ferritin > 15 μg/L) using factorial modeling of basal and menstrual iron losses and iron accretion (Food and Nutrition Board, Institute of Medicine, 2001).

Increased iron losses and low dietary intake are associated with increased risk of iron deficiency. Blood donation results in a loss of 200 to 250 mg iron/0.5 L of blood. Intense endurance exercise increases whole body iron turnover and iron losses. The increased loss via the gastrointestinal tract, hematuria, and hemoglobinuria may elevate the estimated average requirement for athletes by 30% to 70% (Food and Nutrition Board, Institute of Medicine, 2001). Because of lower bioavailability of non-heme iron compared with heme iron, vegetarians have an iron requirement that is 1.8 times that of individuals who consume a mixed diet.

To avoid becoming iron deficient, endurance athletes, especially women, should pay attention to how much iron they consume and to the source of iron in their diet. The current daily recommended intake for women ages 18 to 50 years is 18 mg iron/day. This is difficult to achieve through diet alone because the amount of iron in the United States' food supply is about 6 mg per 1,000 calories. Iron from plant sources is non-heme iron, which is poorly absorbed. For example, a 1-cup serving of raw spinach contains 6 mg of iron, but only 2% to 15%, or 0.1 to 0.6 mg, of that is absorbed in the small intestine. In contrast, animal sources of iron (i.e., meat) contain heme iron, which has a higher bioavailability. A 3-ounce serving of steak contains 4 mg of iron, up to 50% of which is absorbed in the intestine, for an actual intake of 2 mg iron. Thus, women who follow a vegetarian diet must be especially careful to consume enough iron.

Supplemental ferrous iron is available in complexes with sulfate, succinate, citrate, lactate, fumarate, and gluconate. Iron supplements should be taken with ascorbic acid to enhance absorption. Hematocrit and hemoglobin respond to supplemental iron after about 2 weeks; it may take up to 12 months to replete iron stores. Unlike most other minerals, iron cannot be actively excreted from the body, so the potential for toxicity is high. Iron supplements should be used only under medical supervision.

Calcium

Calcium is another mineral that is likely to be lacking in the diets of athletes, particularly vegans and women. Studies of the diets of athletes have repeatedly shown that many women do not meet the recommended intake of 1,000 mg calcium/day, primarily because they

● Learning Point There is no advantage to taking more than 1,200 mg calcium/day (DHHS, n.d.).

do not consume 3 to 4 servings of dairy products. Women who are concerned about their body weight or about cardiovascular disease may avoid dairy products because they believe they are high in fat (Leachman Slawson et al., 2001; Turner & Bass, 2001).

Inadequate calcium intake contributes to loss of bone mineral and/or failure to maximize bone mineral density during skeletal growth, which increases the risk of osteoporosis. Low dietary calcium and/or vitamin D consumption causes mobilization of calcium from bone to maintain the concentration of calcium in blood, allowing muscle contraction and nerve impulse transmission to continue uninterrupted.

Individuals who are lactose intolerant because they do not have adequate amounts of lactase cannot consume dairy products. Recently, food manufacturers have begun fortifying other foods with calcium, and women can now choose calcium-fortified orange juice, breakfast cereal, and soy milk as alternatives to dairy products.

Calcium is also available in dietary supplements. Calcium derived from oyster shells, coral, bone meal, or dolomite is poorly absorbed because of poor solubility in the intestine. The best types of supplemental calcium are calcium carbonate or calcium citrate; both are available in chewable tablets or soft chews. Some chewable antacid tablets contain calcium carbonate and are cheaper than most other calcium supplements.

Fluid and Electrolytes

Dehydration due to an imbalance between fluid loss and intake is the most common cause of heat-related illness in athletes (Convertino et al., 1996). Athletes may lose water at a rate of 0.5 to 1.5 L/h and up to 6% to 10% of their body weight. Water is lost from all fluid compartments, resulting in decreased sweating and impaired heat dissipation. The decline in blood volume decreases blood pressure and cardiac output. Heart rate increases 3 to 5 beats/min for every 1% of body weight lost to compensate for decreased stroke volume. Skin blood flow also is decreased, further reducing the ability to decrease body temperature. Symptoms of heat-related illness are headache, nausea, dizziness, apathy, confusion, exhaustion, and chills. Performance declines markedly because of decreased muscle perfusion. Paradoxically, gastric emptying is slowed, impairing fluid absorption and restoration of fluid balance. The risk of heat-related illness is increased by exercise in hot and humid environments, diuretics use, and older age.

> **● Learning Point** Magnesium supplements should be used with caution. Because magnesium and calcium are chemically similar, magnesium can interfere with intestinal absorption of calcium and with calcium's function in the body. For example, magnesium can block calcium binding to muscle cells and inhibit normal muscle contraction.

A disproportionate amount of fluid lost in sweat is from the extracellular fluid compartment, the fluid outside of the cells, including the blood plasma. The average concentration of sodium in sweat is 1,150 mg/L but can vary greatly (from 450 to 2,300 mg/L) (Convertino et al., 1996). Assuming a sweat rate of 1.5 L/h, an athlete with sweat of average saltiness would lose about 1,700 mg sodium/h. Excessive sweating, combined with consumption of plain water in copious amounts (e.g., 10 L in 4 hours), results in a sodium deficit, referred to as **dilutional hyponatremia.** The symptoms of hyponatremia are disorientation, confusion, seizure, and coma. This condition is quite rare and most often occurs in marathon- and ultramarathon-type events lasting longer than 3 hours and in individuals who ingest large volumes of fluid without electrolytes.

Dilutional hyponatremia: Low blood sodium concentrations; typically resulting in athletes from sodium losses in sweat and excessive consumption of plain water during exercise.

Because potassium is located in the intracellular fluid, much smaller amounts are lost in sweat compared with sodium. The average potassium concentration in sweat is about 350 mg/L, so the quantity lost in sweat is negligible compared with the total amount of potassium in the body (180,000 mg for a typical adult male). The Institute of Medicine recommends a daily potassium intake of 4,700 mg/day, which can easily be achieved by consuming fresh fruits and vegetables (Food and Nutrition Board, Institute of Medicine, 2005).

Like potassium, the amount of magnesium lost in sweat is minimal. This is because most of the magnesium in the body is part of the bone mineral matrix or in the intracellular fluid of muscle cells. It is not necessary to replace magnesium while exercising, but it is important to consume adequate amounts of magnesium in the diet. The recommended intake is about 300 mg daily for adult females and about 400 mg daily for adult males (Food and Nutrition Board, Institute of Medicine, 1997). Nuts, legumes, whole grains, green leafy vegetables, and chocolate are good food sources of magnesium.

Preexercise Hydration

The first step in preventing dehydration is adequate hydration before exercise or competition. Ensure euhydration by drinking fluid volumes that produce colorless urine in the 24 hours before competition. Glycerol ingestion induces hyperhydration (Anderson, Cotter, Garnham, Casley, & Febbraio, 2001); however, the performance benefit of overhydration while competing in hot and humid conditions can be attributed to the volume of fluid consumed and not to glycerol per se (Marino, Kay, & Cannon, 2003). The day of the event, consumption of 16 ounces of fluid 2 to 3 hours before the start allows time for excretion of excess water in urine before the competition begins.

Hydration During Exercise

Ideally, athletes should drink 8 to 12 ounces of fluid every 15 to 20 minutes during exercise. If a training session or competition exceeds 1 hour, a commercial fluid replacement beverage that contains carbohydrates and sodium is superior to plain water. Exogenous carbohydrate maintains blood glucose concentrations, so glycogenolysis is delayed. Sodium increases the palatability of the beverage and enhances fluid consumption; replacing some of the sodium lost in sweat reduces the risk of hyponatremia. The recommended concentration of sodium in a fluid replacement beverage is 500 to 700 mg/L (Convertino et al., 1996). Most sports drinks contain sodium, although the amount varies from 300 to 650 mg/L. An alternative to commercial fluid replacement beverages is easily prepared by adding 1/4 to 1/2 teaspoon of salt to 1 L (32 ounces) of water, which is equivalent to about 600 and 1,200 mg sodium/L. Salt (sodium chloride) tablets are available, but 8 ounces of fluid (250 mL) must be consumed with every 200 mg of sodium so that the concentration of sodium in blood does not rise too rapidly. Salt tablets are more effective and better tolerated (they may cause gastrointestinal problems in some people) if they are crushed and mixed with water.

The fluid that is consumed must be emptied from the stomach and absorbed from the intestine to be of any benefit. The rate of gastric emptying can reach 1 L/h and is maximized when gastric volume is high (> 600 mL), solutions are hypotonic, and the carbohydrate concentration is 4% to 8% (Convertino et al., 1996). The rate of fluid absorption is negatively affected by high-intensity exercise (> 80% maximal oxygen consumption), carbohydrate concentrations that exceed 8%, and dehydration (> 4% BW) (Convertino et al., 1996).

Postexercise Hydration

Rehydration after exercise is important because most athletes do not consume enough fluids during exercise to replenish the fluid lost in sweat and respiration. In general, an athlete should consume 24 ounces of fluid for every pound of weight lost during an exercise session (Convertino et al., 1996). Excess fluid consumption offsets "obligatory urine losses" that occur when a large volume of water is consumed within a short period of time. Obligatory urine losses can be minimized by drinking a beverage that contains sodium (Shirreffs & Maughan, 1998) and by eating foods that are high in sodium after exercise, such as pretzels, pickles, pizza, cheese, tomato sauce, soy sauce, and ketchup.

Nutrition During Exercise

During prolonged exercise, depletion of glycogen stores is associated with the onset of fatigue (Costill et al., 1988; Sherman, Doyle, Lamb, & Strauss, 1993). By consuming carbohydrate (glucose) during exercise, the onset of fatigue may be delayed by providing the body with an alternate glucose supply, which spares muscle glycogen (Couture, Massicotte, Lavoie, Hillaire-Marcel, & Peronnet, 2002). The recommended carbohydrate intake during exercise is 30 to 60 g carbohydrate/h. Drinking 16 to 32 ounces of a 4% to 8% carbohydrate commercial fluid replacement beverage every hour meets this guideline. The potential for erosion of dental enamel is partially negated by increasing the pH and calcium concentration of the sports drink (Venables et al., 2005). Solutions that have a carbohydrate concentration greater than 8% slow gastric emptying, and those that exceed 10% cause a net efflux of water from the intestine, contributing to dehydration. Energy gels contain about 25 g carbohydrate per packet and can be used if consumed with water to avoid gastrointestinal distress. Note that the recommendation for carbohydrate consumption during exercise maintains blood glucose concentrations but does not replenish energy used during exercise.

Sports Beverages

Sports beverages or gels contain either simple sugars or short-chain complex carbohydrates that are rapidly digested into monosaccharides. The significant difference among products is what simple sugars they contain or result from enzymatic hydrolysis in the small intestine. Glucose and galactose are absorbed quickly against a concentration gradient, using Na^+/glucose cotransporters on the mucosal side of the enterocytes. This is an energy-consuming process because the intracellular concentration of Na^+ must be maintained via a serosal Na^+/K^+ ATPase. Glucose and galactose are transported out of the enterocyte into the blood via GLUT (glucose-lactate-uptake-transporters) at the serosal surface. Galactose, however, must be converted into glucose in the liver before it can be used to generate ATP, so a sports beverage with galactose does not increase the energy available to the muscle as quickly as a glucose-only beverage.

Fructose is absorbed by GLUT5 transporters, and its rate of absorption is slower than that of glucose and galactose. Fructose is phosphorylated to fructose-1 phosphate in cells. Most fructose is metabolized in the liver to glyceraldehyde and dihydroxyacetone phosphate. These intermediates can proceed through glycolysis to pyruvate and can be used in fatty acid synthesis or in gluconeogenesis. Aldolase B is the rate–limiting enzyme in fructose metabolism and has a much lower affinity for fructose-1 phosphate than for fructose-1,6 bisphosphate. As a result the aldolase B reaction proceeds very slowly and fructose-1 phosphate tends to accumulate in the liver after ingestion of a large amount of fructose. Other tissues also can metabolize fructose but do so at a rate that is even slower than the rate of hepatic metabolism. In extrahepatic tissues fructose must be phosphorylated by hexokinase to fructose-6 phosphate. The affinity of hexokinase is much greater for glucose than it is for fructose, so the phosphorylation of fructose proceeds very slowly. Because of the way it is metabolized, fructose is not an optimal carbohydrate source during exercise.

Use of dietary carbohydrate for energy during exercise is limited by the rate of absorption (i.e., how fast the sugar molecule gets across the intestine into the bloodstream). One way to increase the speed at which glucose is absorbed is to add a small amount of fructose (or sucrose) to the sports beverage. This strategy works because glucose and fructose are absorbed by different pathways (Jentjens, Achten, & Jeukendrup, 2004; Jentjens, Moseley, Waring, Harding, & Jeukendrup, 2004; Jentjens, Venables, & Jeukendrup, 2004). However, the fructose content should not exceed 2% to 3% because ingesting large amounts of fructose could overwhelm the absorptive capability of the intestine. Fructose that is not absorbed and remains in the gut can cause diarrhea, bloating, and intestinal cramps.

Some athletes drink soda pop as a carbohydrate replacement beverage during endurance events. A 12-ounce can of cola provides about 150 calories as sugar. Soda pop is not the optimal choice during exercise. The concentration of carbohydrate in soda pop is about 11%. Once the sugar concentration of the beverage exceeds 8%, gastric emptying is slowed, meaning it takes longer for the sugar to reach the bloodstream. This also has negative implications for rehydration during exercise. Most sodas are sweetened with high fructose corn syrup that is 55% fructose and 45% glucose by weight. When combined with glucose, small amounts of fructose (2% to 3%, i.e., 2 to 3 g fructose/100 mL) enhance fluid absorption. However, the concentration of fructose in soda pop sweetened with high fructose corn syrup is about 6.5%. This amount of fructose decreases the rate of fluid and carbohydrate absorption. To make matters worse, the fructose stays in the intestine and may cause gastrointestinal distress. The optimal rehydration solution not only contains glucose to maintain blood sugar, but contains sodium as well. A beverage that has 50 to 70 mg sodium/100 mL enhances fluid retention, increases voluntary fluid intake due to enhanced taste, and prevents low blood sodium levels. The concentration of sodium in cola is much less than this recommendation—about 10 mg sodium/100 mL.

Performance benefits have been demonstrated for consumption of sports beverages containing 4% to 8% carbohydrate during endurance exercise. Two recent studies demonstrated an additional benefit when protein was added to the carbohydrate-containing fluid replacement drink (Ivy, Res, Sprague, & Widzer, 2003; Saunders, Kane, & Todd, 2004). Subjects had increased endurance (time to fatigue) and reduced muscle damage with consumption of carbohydrate and protein compared with carbohydrate alone. The drinks were not isoenergetic, so it cannot be determined if the benefit was due to additional energy consumption or due to protein per se.

Nutrition After Exercise

After exercise, elevating blood glucose levels quickly is beneficial to replenish glycogen stores, so high GI foods are recommended. Athletes should aim to consume 1.5 g carbohydrate/kg BW in the first 30 minutes after exercise and again every 2 hours for 4 to 6 hours after exercise (American Dietetic Association et al., 2000). Insulin secretion is needed for glycogen synthesis. Insulin increases glucose uptake into the muscle via GLUT4 and stimulates glycogen synthase. Therefore, after exercise the greater insulin secretion associated with high GI foods is advantageous. For maximal glycogen repletion, the GI of a carbohydrate is more important than whether it is simple or complex. There are some complex carbohydrates that are also high GI–synthetic sweeteners like maltodextrin, for example. In contrast, most complex carbohydrates in fruits, vegetables, grains, and legumes are lower on the GI scale.

● **Learning Point** The best practical recommendation is to consume carbohydrates immediately after exercise and then a mixed diet containing carbohydrate, protein, and fat thereafter.

High GI foods that are consumed in the proximal postexercise period are not converted into fatty acids and stored in adipose tissue. After exercise, skeletal muscle uses fatty acids, not glucose, for energy so that the glucose is available for glycogen storage (Wolfe, Klein, Carraro, & Weber, 1990). This diversion of glucose toward glycogen synthesis and away from lipogenesis occurs because acetyl-CoA carboxylase and glycerol-3-phosphate acyltransferase are inhibited by AMPK phosphorylase (Rasmussen, Hancock, & Winder, 1998; Hildebrandt, Pilegaard, & Neufer, 2003; Ruderman et al., 2003). At the same time, the rate of fatty acid release from adipose into the blood is increased to supply the muscles. There also is an increase in fatty acid transport into the mitochondria of skeletal muscle for beta-oxidation to produce ATP. The rate of glucose transport into muscle also increases after exercise. The net result is that there is more glucose getting into the muscle where it is used in glycogen synthesis.

The effect of protein on glycogen repletion is equivocal due to differences in study design. Studies that compare isoenergetic postexercise carbohydrate with carbohydrate plus protein usually conclude that there is no advantage to adding protein (Jentjens, van Loon, Mann, Wagenmakers, & Jeukendrup, 2001). Studies that compare treatments that are equivalent in carbohydrate but differ in protein and, therefore, energy content generally find that carbohydrate plus protein is superior to carbohydrate alone (Ivy, Goforth, et al., 2002; Williams, Raven, Fogt, & Ivy, 2003). Other factors affecting the conclusion are the dose and timing of the supplements after exercise. Studies providing large amounts of carbohydrate every 30 minutes during recovery from exercise maximized glycogen repletion compared with studies with less frequent feedings. If glycogen repletion is maximized with carbohydrate alone, then it is not possible for protein to enhance the response. Studies that found added protein increased glycogen synthesis after exercise could not attribute the difference to increased insulin levels, so the mechanism of the effect remains unknown (Ivy, Goforth, et al., 2002).

The best dietary strategy to optimize replacement of IMTG (intramuscular lipid storage) stores without compromising glycogen repletion is somewhat controversial. High-carbohydrate diets, regardless of fat intake, seem to interfere with the restoration of intramuscular fat stores to preexercise levels (Johnson et al., 2003; van Loon et al., 2003). One study of highly trained cyclists found that intramuscular fat stores were replenished after 48 hours of a diet providing 39% of energy as fat and 49% as carbohydrate, but an isoenergetic low-fat diet providing 24% of energy as fat and 62% as carbohydrate was ineffective. However, there is a tremendous downside to consuming inadequate carbohydrates after exercise. Glycogen stores are then not repleted, and it is well established that preexercise glycogen levels are strongly associated with time to fatigue during endurance exercise.

Exercise increases the rates of protein breakdown and synthesis in skeletal muscle, and with adequate nutrition it has an anabolic effect on skeletal muscle (i.e., it results in a net increase in protein synthesis). Carbohydrate consumed after exercise is beneficial because it reduces the rate of protein degradation (Borsheim, Aarsland, & Wolfe, 2004; Borsheim, Cree, et al., 2004). However, to increase protein synthesis and achieve a net increase in muscle mass, it is important to consume protein after exercise. Studies have shown that consuming about 0.2 g protein/kg BW per hour during the first 2 to 3 hours after exercise results in net protein synthesis (Tipton, Ferrando, Phillips, Doyle, & Wolfe, 1999; Borsheim, Tipton, Wolf, & Wolfe, 2002; Tipton, Borsheim, Wolf, Sanford, & Wolfe, 2003).

Alcohol, Coffee, Soda, and Other Vices

Alcohol

Ethanol is metabolized in the liver to acetate and acetaldehyde. ATP can be generated from beta-oxidation of acetate. Acetate (like fatty acids) cannot be used to make glucose, so alcohol cannot be used to replenish glycogen stores. Dietary carbohydrate consumed with ethanol can be used in glycogen synthesis. This was shown in a study of well-trained cyclists who exercised for 2 hours to deplete their glycogen stores and then consumed one of three test meals to look at the effects of alcohol ingestion on glycogen synthesis in muscle (Burke et al., 2003). The three test meals were carbohydrate, providing 7 g carbohydrate and 24 kcal per kg BW; alcohol, providing 1 g carbohydrate, 1.5 g alcohol, and 24 kcal per kg BW; and carbohydrate + alcohol, providing 7 g carbohydrate, 1.5 g alcohol, and 34 kcal per kg BW. The alcohol, equivalent to about 10 drinks, was consumed in the first 3 hours after exercise. Muscle biopsies of the quadriceps muscle were taken 8 and 24 hours after exercise. Although both groups that consumed alcohol had lower blood glucose levels, at 8 and 24 hours after exercise, than the CHO group, muscle glycogen was lower only in the alcohol group.

The acute effects of alcohol ingestion on performance are mostly negative and are dose dependent. Psychomotor function is impaired, and small to moderate doses of alcohol (2 to 4 oz of alcohol) slow reaction time; interfere with eye–hand coordination, accuracy, and balance; and make performing gross motor skills more difficult. Alcohol causes vasodilation of blood vessels and loss of body heat, increasing the risk of hypothermia when exercising in the cold. Alcohol lowers blood glucose and decreases glucose uptake by skeletal muscle, so an athlete experiences earlier onset of fatigue.

Caffeine

Caffeine is a mild stimulant; it interferes with the binding of adenosine, a neurotransmitter with calming effects, to its receptor. Hence, the stimulatory effects on many systems of the body are neural activity in parts of the brain, heart rate and blood pressure, water excretion by the kidneys, and secretion of the "stress hormones" adrenaline and cortisol by the adrenal gland.

There is considerable evidence from scientific studies that caffeine improves athletic performance in sprints and in endurance events. Enhanced alertness and reaction time contribute to improvements in sprinting. During endurance events, caffeine improves performance by stimulating the release of fatty acids into the blood due to increased activity of hormone-sensitive lipase. This allows increased utilization of fat rather than glucose, so muscle glycogen is not depleted as rapidly and the onset of fatigue is delayed. The effects of caffeine on lipolysis are mediated, at least in part, via the sympathetic nervous system, as evidenced by partial abrogation of the caffeine effect with pharmacologic beta-adrenergic blockade (Van Baak & Saris, 2000). Caffeine also may improve performance during submaximal exercise through other mechanisms. Time to fatigue during performance of submaximal isometric contractions was increased with caffeine (6 mg/kg BW) due to maintenance of force output and not because of altered firing rates (Acheson et al., 2004).

Caffeine is metabolized rapidly by the body; peak blood levels occur 30 minutes after oral ingestion, and the half-life of caffeine is 4 hours. For this reason caffeine should be consumed within 1 hour of an athletic event to have an effect on performance. An effective dose is 2 to 9 mg caffeine/kg BW, and no additional benefit is derived from higher doses. The caffeine content of coffee varies significantly; an 8-ounce cup may contain 100 to 300 mg. Drinking 1 to 2 cups of coffee should not produce the adverse effects of excess caffeine consumption, such as anxiety, jitteriness, heart arrhythmias, dehydration, and dry mouth.

Athletes may develop a tolerance to caffeine, but the variation in individual response to the drug is large—some people develop tolerance and others remain responsive (Lovallo et al., 2004). The rate at which tolerance to caffeine develops and the magnitude of the effect varies with the physiologic response (Watson, Deary, & Kerr, 2002). For example, 400 to 500 mg of caffeine (2 to 3 cups of regular coffee) a day for 7 days results in complete tolerance of its sleep-disrupting effects. Regular consumption of caffeine, however, does not eliminate the hypertensive response. Caffeine was removed from the World Anti-Doping Agency's "Prohibited List" in 2005 (World Anti-Doping Agency, 2005).

Soda Pop

Endurance athletes abstain from carbonated beverages because they believe the carbon dioxide interferes with oxygen use. In reality, the potential negative effect of drinking carbonated beverages has nothing to do with oxygen transport or blood pH but with hydration. Most of the CO_2 in blood arises as a waste product of cellular metabolism. This carbon dioxide is dissolved in blood and carried as carbonic acid and bicarbonate to the lungs, where it is expired. When blood concentrations of CO_2 are high, the body responds by breathing more deeply and frequently to expire the excess CO_2.

The CO_2 in carbonated beverages has no effect on the amount of CO_2 in blood or on the acid-base balance of the blood. This is because the CO_2 that is in soda never gets into the circulation. Most of the carbonation is lost before it is even swallowed. The increased temperature of the mouth versus the environment causes a large amount of the dissolved gas to come out of solution. The physical process of swallowing also reduces the amount of CO_2 in solution. Any CO_2 that does make it to the stomach is released from the body via the mouth (sometimes audibly) as a "belch." This is because the low pH (acid) in the stomach also makes the CO_2 less soluble. Because a carbonated beverage helps create a sensation of fullness in the stomach that is out of proportion to the amount consumed, voluntary fluid intake may be reduced (Lambert, Bleiler, Chang, Johnson, & Gisolfi, 1993).

The main source of dietary phosphoric acid is soda pop. Because of the association between soda consumption and increased risk of bone fractures, the constituents of soda (caffeine, phosphoric acid, citric acid, and fructose) have been scrutinized for their potential to cause calcium loss from bone. Anyone who has ever soaked a bone in vinegar would agree that phosphoric acid probably causes a loss of calcium and a weakening of the bones. However, what is observed in the test tube is not always what happens in the body, which has the ability to maintain constant internal conditions, including acidity of the blood.

Heaney and Rafferty (2001) compared the effects of caffeine, phosphoric acid, and citric acid (consumed in soda) on calcium excretion in the urine. Subjects consumed 20 ounces of either caffeinated cola (Coke, containing caffeine and phosphoric acid), noncaffeinated cola (Coke-Free, phosphoric acid only), caffeinated noncola (Mountain Dew, caffeine and citric acid), or noncaffeinated noncola (Sprite, citric acid only). Neither phosphoric acid nor citric acid increased calcium loss. Consumption of the caffeinated sodas caused an increase in calcium excretion, but the effect was small (6 to 14 mg) compared with the recommended daily calcium intake (1,000 mg).

When the kidney's ability to excrete acid is compromised, as in chronic renal failure, and the body is exposed to very high acid loads, then appreciable amounts of calcium may be lost from bone. However, in a healthy individual the acid load that results from the phosphoric acid in 20 ounces of soda is very small (4.5 to 5.0 mEq), which is much less than the acid load produced during normal metabolism of food (50 to 100 mEq). Consuming seven 12-ounce colas per day only produces an acid load of about 20 mEq, which is well within the excretory capacity of the kidney.

Body Composition

Body weight and composition influence an athlete's performance because body size and relative muscle mass affect strength, speed, and appearance. Body fat increases body weight without increasing strength, thereby reducing the power-to-body weight ratio. In sports that require moving the body over long distances or against the gravitational force, such as running and cycling, a high power-to-weight ratio is advantageous. In "appearance" sports such as gymnastics, figure skating, diving, and dance, a lean physique also is desirable. However, being too lean can negatively affect performance and overall physical and psychological health. The physical risks associated with excessive leanness are overtraining syndrome, frequent illness and injury, and loss of bone mass. Unrealistic body weight or composition goals can lead to increased body dissatisfaction, disordered eating, and negative affect.

In setting body weight goals, athletes must consider gender, body composition, genetics, and overall physical and mental health. Five percent to 10% body fat may be appropriate for an elite male athlete, but the healthy range for a female athlete is 12% to 28%. Athletes may be classified as overweight based on standard height and weight tables when in fact they are lean, simply because they have more muscle mass than the "reference" man or woman. Each person has a set-point weight, which is largely determined by genetics, that the body maintains over time. Muscle mass, like body weight, is highly regulated (Keesey & Corbett, 1984). Attempts to achieve a body weight or muscle mass above or below the set-point range result in metabolic adaptations to maintain the set point (Loucks, 2004).

Guidelines to Increase Muscle Mass

With adequate energy and protein intake, resistance training causes an increase in muscle mass. Protein turnover in skeletal muscle is increased for up to 48 hours after resistance exercise. Exercise reduces nitrogen losses during fasting by suppressing protein breakdown, although protein balance remains negative. Consuming a mixture of carbohydrates and amino acids before or immediately after resistance training results in net protein synthesis. Mammalian target of rapamycin (mTOR) is a kinase that stimulates protein synthesis via transcription and translation of messenger RNAs coding translation proteins, ribosome biosynthesis, and cell proliferation; mTOR also inhibits autophagy. Growth factors, insulin, and amino acids activate mTOR (Deldicque, Theisen, & Francaux, 2005). Resistance exercise activates mTOR, whereas endurance exercise inhibits mTOR activity due to activation of AMPK by AMP (Atherton et al., 2005). This finding has practical applications for athletes who engage in endurance and strength training. Protein synthesis in response to resistance training can be maximized by allowing adequate recovery after endurance exercise in conjunction with dietary carbohydrate and protein.

A reasonable rate of weight gain is 0.5 kg/wk. This requires an additional 500 kcal/day, in addition to the energy required to maintain current body weight. To increase skeletal muscle mass, additional amino acids are required. Athletes who are involved in strenuous resistance training should consume 1.6 to 1.7 g protein/kg BW. Protein in food can be scored based on how closely the proportion of amino acids it contains matches the amino acid composition of muscle protein, correcting for digestibility of the protein. Proteins that are high quality have the right mix of amino acids and receive a score of 1.00, whereas proteins that are missing in an essential amino acid or are poorly digested receive a lower score. Typically, protein from animal sources like meat (0.9) and egg whites (1.0) is high quality, and protein from plant sources like beans (0.6) and wheat (0.4) is lower quality. For this reason vegetarians need to combine plant sources of protein so they get all the essential amino acids. Examples of complementary foods are beans and rice, peanut butter and wheat bread, and tofu and rice. Because of the lower protein quality of plant-based foods, vegetarian athletes should consume 1.6 to 1.7 g protein/kg BW; this is higher than the recommendation for nonvegetarians of 1.2 to 1.4 g/kg BW.

Weight Cycling

The information of the effects of weight cycling in athletes is limited. There is a positive association between "yo-yo dieting" and heart disease in populations with other risk factors for cardiovascular disease, such as smoking, excessive weight and **obesity,** and lack of physical activity (Petersmarck et al., 1999). Weight cycling in conjunction with ad libitum consumption of a high-fat diet increases transcription of lipogenic genes in adipose tissue: fatty acid synthase, acetyl CoA carboxylase, malic enzyme, pyruvate kinase, and lipoprotein lipase (Sea et al., 2000). The body weight changes that occur in athletes who are relatively lean, nonsmoking, and active are very different from the weight fluctuations in people who start out overweight or obese. Athletes

Obesity: Category of body weight above overweight; for children, a body mass index for age and gender percentile is used.

Weight and Fat Loss: Misconceptions and Bad Ideas

Low-Intensity Exercise Is Better for Burning Fat

Energy balance is where the rubber hits the road when it comes to weight loss. Although it is true that a greater proportion of the energy comes from fat oxidation during low-intensity exercise, the total energy used is less (if the duration is constant) during low- versus high-intensity exercise. It follows, then, that the absolute amount of fat oxidized is less during low- versus high-intensity activities. For example, riding at 10 mph uses 6 kcal/kg/h, and 80% of those kilocalories come from fat. One hour of cycling at 10 mph uses a total of 600 kcal, and 480 of those kilocalories are from fat. Contrast that with riding at 18 mph, which uses 12 kcal/kg/h but only 50% of the energy from fat. At the faster speed the total energy cost is 1,200 kcal, and 600 kcal come from fat.

Low-Carbohydrate Diets Increase Weight Loss

Low-carbohydrate, high-protein weight loss diets have increased in popularity recently, even among athletes. These diets restrict carbohydrate intake to 30 to 120 g/day. The RDA for carbohydrate was determined based on the carbohydrate requirement of the brain. For healthy adults the RDA is 130 g of carbohydrate per day (Food and Nutrition Board, Institute of Medicine, 2003).

Skeletal muscle can use fat for energy at rest or during exercise of low intensity. As exercise intensity increases, skeletal muscle relies increasingly on carbohydrate for energy. The primary source of carbohydrate during exercise is what is stored in the muscle as glycogen. Athletes need more carbohydrate than the brain's minimum requirement to replete their muscle and liver glycogen stores. Training and performance will decline significantly on a low-carbohydrate diet.

These diets are popular because, by design, they promote rapid weight loss. During the first 24 to 48 hours of a low-carbohydrate diet, glycogen stores that remain are used to fuel the brain. When glycogen is broken down, the water that is part of the glycogen is released and excreted in the urine. This water loss can be 3 to 4 pounds. With continued inadequate carbohydrate intake, catabolism of skeletal muscle ensues and the amino acids that make up muscle proteins are used in gluconeogenesis. Muscle is about 73% water. So catabolism of skeletal muscle results in a significant change in body weight due to the loss of body water. The number on the scale may drop rapidly on this diet, but losing water and not body fat will do nothing to enhance performance.

may experience in- and out-of-season fluctuations in body weight, but even then most athletes stay within the normal range of weight for height. In the general population weight cycling is prevalent among people who are overweight and have repeatedly tried and failed to maintain a lower body weight. As a result, it is difficult to separate the effects of weight cycling from the effects of being overweight with regard to a person's overall risk of cardiovascular disease. Studies that found a relationship between weight cycling and risk factors for heart disease or type 2 diabetes saw that relationship disappear when they factored in the effects of being overweight or obese (Petersmarck et al., 1999). The metabolic benefits of endurance training on risk factors for cardiovascular disease (triglycerides, total cholesterol, low-density and high-density lipoproteins, insulin, LPL—lipoprotein lipase—activity) do not persist with detraining (Petibois, Cassaigne, Gin, & Deleris, 2004).

Most of the information that exists on the health effects of weight cycling in athletes comes from wrestlers. During their competitive season wrestlers restrict their food intake and exercise to "make weight," often losing 5% to 10% of their normal weight. Several studies examined how body composition and metabolic rate change as wrestlers lose and regain weight (Steen, Oppliger, & Brownell, 1988; Melby, Schmidt, & Corrigan, 1990; McCargar & Crawford, 1992). Although the results are equivocal, resting metabolic rate decreases during the weight loss phase. Thyroid hormone levels also decrease during weight loss, suggesting that the brain perceives an energy shortage and sends out signals for the body to conserve energy (Loucks, Laughlin, et al., 1992). Once the competitive season is over and wrestlers are no longer in a chronic energy deficit, metabolic rate returns to normal.

Eating Disorders and the Female Athlete Triad

In an effort to achieve or maintain an unrealistically low body weight or percentage of body fat, some athletes restrict their food intake so severely that endocrine function is disrupted. The hypothalamus senses the energy deficit, and the secretion of gonadotropin-releasing hormone, thyrotropin-releasing hormone, corticotropin-releasing hormone, and growth hormone–releasing hormone are altered at different thresholds of energy availability (Loucks, Laughlin, et al., 1992; Laughlin & Yen, 1996; Loucks & Verdun, 1998; Loucks, 2004). As a result, secretion of luteinizing hormone, follicle-stimulating hormone, thyroid-stimulating hormone, and growth hormone (GH) is abnormal and production of reproductive hormones, thyroid hormone, and insulin-like growth factor I (IGF-I) is reduced (Laughlin & Yen, 1996; Waters, Qualls, Dorin, Veldhuis, & Baumgartner, 2001; Rickenlund, Thoren, Carlstrom, von Schoultz, & Hirschberg, 2004).

The sex hormones are decreased in both men (testosterone) and women (estrogen and progesterone). Women experience irregular (**oligomenorrhea**) or absent menstrual cycles (**amenorrhea**); men may notice a decline in sex drive. Thyroid hormone (triiodothyronine) is decreased in both genders, resulting in the signs and symptoms of decreased metabolic rate,

Oligomenorrhea: Irregular or infrequent menstruation in menarchal females; cycles occur at an interval of 35 days or greater, resulting in 4 to 9 cycles per year.

Amenorrhea: Absence of three consecutive menstrual cycles in a menarchal female.

such as **bradycardia,** hypotension, slowed respiration rate, and delayed reflexes. GH secretion is increased, but because of the energy-deficient state, the liver and other tissues are resistant to GH. As a consequence, hepatic production of IGF-I is decreased. In addition, the secretion of adrenocorticotropic hormone is increased, and serum cortisol concentrations are elevated.

Each of these hormonal changes has a negative impact on bone mineral content and density. Bone turnover becomes uncoupled when energy availability is 10 to 20 kcal/kg lean body mass per day (Ihle & Loucks, 2004). Hypoestrogenemia and hypercortisolemia accelerate bone resorption. Bone formation is slowed with low testosterone, thyroid hormone, and IGF-I. Osteopenia, osteoporosis, and fractures are consequences of chronic low energy intake. Measurable loss of bone mineral density is evident after missing only six consecutive menstrual cycles. Loss of bone mass is insidious because it is irreversible and often proceeds undetected for long periods of time (Keen & Drinkwater, 1997). In women, the constellation of disordered eating, amenorrhea, and osteopenia/osteoporosis has been labeled "the female triad" by the American College of Sports Medicine (Yeager, Agostini, Nattiv, & Drinkwater, 1993; Otis, Drinkwater, Johnson, Loucks, & Wilmore, 1997).

There are other negative consequences of chronic low energy availability. Protein turnover is slowed, making athletes more susceptible to injury, illness, and overtraining syndrome. In response to inadequate energy intake from the diet, the body has to rely on other energy sources. The body uses energy that is stored body fat and breaks down muscle, converting the protein into glucose. Proteolysis of skeletal muscle results in a loss of strength and power, with negative effects on performance.

Childhood Through Adolescence

Children and adolescents have higher energy and protein needs per kilogram of body weight than adults to support growth. Growth is relatively constant at a rate of approximately 5 to 6 cm and 2.5 kg/yr from age 4 until puberty. At puberty, androgens, estrogens, GH, and IGF-I cause increases in bone mineral, muscle mass, and sex-specific deposition of body fat (Rogol, 2000). The RDA for protein is 0.95 g/kg BW for children ages 9 to 13 years and 0.85 g/kg BW for teenagers, compared with 0.8 g/kg BW for adults (Food and Nutrition Board, Institute of Medicine, 2003). Greater than 90% of peak bone mass is acquired by age 18 years, and bone mass doubles between the onset of puberty and young adulthood. Thus, children and adolescents require more calcium than adults; the adequate intake for calcium is 1,300 mg/day for ages 9 to 18 years (Food and Nutrition Board, Institute of Medicine, 1997). Iron and zinc needs also are increased during adolescence to support an increase in skeletal muscle mass and an expansion in red blood cell number (Food and Nutrition Board, Institute of Medicine, 2001).

Special Focus on Children and Adolescents

Weight-bearing physical activity has a greater effect on bone mass in children and adolescents compared with adults. The effects of exercise on growth and development are closely related to the energy drain created by the physical activity. Growth and sexual maturation can be delayed by intense physical training before puberty. Weight and height growth velocities can be decreased in elite female athletes and menarche delayed 1 to 2 years compared with a population reference menarchal age of 13.0 years. Delayed menarche and hypoestrogenism compromise acquisition of bone mass and bone mineral. Exercise duration and training intensity were negatively associated with bone mass density (BMD) in elite female adolescent gymnasts, and the younger the athlete started training, the greater the effect on bone (Markou et al., 2004). A cross-sectional study of 5,461 girls aged 11 to 17 years found that girls who participated in at least 16 hours of exercise per week were at greater risk for stress fractures than those who participated in less than 4 hours per week. Each hour per week spent running, performing gymnastics, or cheerleading also increased the risk of stress fracture (Loud, Gordon, Micheli, & Field, 2005). Some catch-up growth may be possible if an athlete's training load is reduced. Because there are few longitudinal growth studies that follow athletes before the onset of training, it is difficult to determine the effects of slowed growth and delayed maturation on adult body size.

Normal growth and development in males are less affected by training than in females. This may be, in large part, due to selection bias. Physical maturity is an asset in most male sports where strength and power confer a competitive advantage. Wrestlers are unique because of the ubiquitous practice of losing weight through dietary restriction and excessive exercise to compete in lower competitive weight classes. Growth velocity is slowed during the season, and catch-up growth occurs during the off season. It is not clear if the short stature of wrestlers is due to growth restriction, selection bias, or a combination (Rogol, Clark, & Roemmich, 2000).

Children and adolescents also are more susceptible to heat-related illnesses because of a greater impairment of thermal regulation with dehydration (Bar-Or, 2001). Until puberty, children and adolescents sweat less than adults. In addition, children have a greater surface area–to–body weight ratio than adults and therefore receive greater exposure to solar radiation. Similar to adult athletes, children and adolescents do not consume adequate fluids during exercise to remain euhydrated. Provision of a flavored carbohydrate–electrolyte drink increases fluid consumption and reduces voluntary dehydration in children (Rivera-Brown, Gutierrez, Gutierrez, Frontera, & Bar-Or, 1999).

Oral contraceptive agents (OCAs) have benefits for female athletes: timing of the menstrual cycle around important competitions, reduced risk of iron deficiency anemia due to decreased blood loss via menstrual bleeding, and reduced loss of bone mass in estrogen-deficient athletes with amenorrhea (Bennell, White, & Crossley, 1999). Despite these potential benefits, plus the obvious one of birth control, many athletes (and their coaches) worry that taking the pill will cause weight gain, decrease aerobic capacity, and negatively affect fuel metabolism. However, there is very little evidence to support these fears (Bonen, Haynes, & Graham, 1991; Bryner, Toffle, Ullrich, & Yeater, 1996; Casazza, Suh, Miller, Navazio, & Brooks, 2002; Jankowski, Ben-Ezra, Gozansky, & Scheaffer, 2004). Only a few studies have investigated the effects of oral contraceptives on athletic performance, and only a fraction of these used highly trained athletes as subjects. It is important to recognize that the effects of OCAs in trained women may differ from those observed in sedentary women.

A recent study of endurance-trained athletes and sedentary control subjects examined the effects of 10 months of OCA treatment (both estrogen and progesterone) on body weight and composition, aerobic capacity (maximal oxygen consumption), muscular strength, and bone mineral density. Half of the athletes were regularly menstruating and the other half were either oligomenorrheic (having cycles at intervals > 6 weeks) or amenorrheic (having absence of menstrual cycles for at least 3 consecutive months) (Rickenlund, Carlstrom, et al., 2004). The women with irregular menstrual cycles gained weight (body weight increase from 124 to 128 pounds, on average) and increased their percentage of body fat (from 17% to 20%, on average) after OCA treatment. Despite this increase in body weight, relative maximal oxygen consumption did not change with OCA treatment (56.7 vs. 55.6 mL/kg/min). The bone mineral density of the women with oligomenorrhea and amenorrhea significantly increased with OCAs, and the improvement in BMD was greatest in individuals with the lowest initial BMD. Ten months of OCAs did not alter body weight, body composition, aerobic capacity, strength, or bone mineral density in the regularly menstruating women or in the sedentary control subjects.

Dietary Supplements as Ergogenic Aids

Supplement Labeling and Performance Claims

The laws regarding supplements put the burden of investigating the benefits and harms of dietary supplements on the consumer. Because of the way dietary supplements are regulated, at least in the United States, manufacturers may put essentially any performance-related claim on the label, even if it is unsubstantiated. Unlike food and drugs, supplements are not monitored by the U.S. Food and Drug Administration for ingredient content or purity. In other words, the ingredients on the label may or may not be present, and additional compounds not listed on the label may be included. For example, small amounts of anabolic steroids have been found in supplements that claim to increase muscle mass. Many supplements that are evaluated by consumer protection groups are found to contain much less of the active ingredient than what is listed on the label. Both practices are illegal, but without quality control of the supplement industry they take place nonetheless. Therefore, safety of dietary supplements is a concern. Between 1995 and 1999 there were 2,500 adverse events reported to the U.S. Food and Drug Administration by consumers, health care professionals, and poison control centers. It is estimated that this figure represents only 1% of the actual adverse events. A good source of reliable information on dietary supplements is the National Center for

Complementary and Alternative Medicine of the National Institutes of Health (www.nccam.nih.gov/health). Information on whether a supplement contains what is on the ingredient list can be found at www.ConsumerLabs.com.

Placebo Effect

The power of the mind cannot be underestimated. If an athlete believes that a supplement is going to help his or her performance, it probably will. However, if the ergogenic effects of that supplement were studied in a double-blind placebo-controlled trial (meaning subjects randomly receive the supplement or an identical-looking placebo treatment and neither the subjects nor the investigators know who gets what), a significant difference between the supplement and placebo may not be detected.

Dietary supplements range from the conventional (multivitamins) to the everyday (caffeine), exotic (Chinese herbs), weird (caterpillar fungus), disgusting (pituitary extract), and dangerous (ephedra). In general, supplements taken to correct a nutrient deficiency will benefit the deficient individual. With a few exceptions, there is little evidence from double-blind placebo-controlled studies to support the use of dietary supplements to enhance athletic performance. A search of PubMed, a database of peer-reviewed journal articles, using the phrase "supplements and sports" returned over 500 entries, with most of these studies finding no effect of supplements on performance.

Even among the few supplements for which a performance-enhancing effect has been repeatedly demonstrated, the magnitude of the effect is relatively small compared with the sum of the improvements that could be obtained from increased training or better equipment (Jeukendrup & Martin, 2001).

Vitamin and Mineral Supplements

Consuming excessive amounts of any nutrient (even water) can have detrimental effects. Vitamin and mineral excesses produce negative health consequences. Potential toxicity is greater for fat-soluble vitamins than for water-soluble vitamins because excess fat-soluble vitamins are stored in the liver and body fat, accumulating to toxic levels over time. For example, consuming just three to four times the RDA for vitamin A results in toxicity symptoms of loss of appetite, hair loss, and bone and muscle pain. Excess vitamin D causes calcification of the organs, high blood pressure, and kidney dysfunction. Large doses of water-soluble vitamins also can be harmful. For example, vitamin C normally acts as an antioxidant, preventing damage to the cell membrane by reacting with harmful molecules. However, at high levels ($>$ 50 times the RDA), vitamin C can act as a pro-oxidant, reacting with iron or copper to generate compounds that can cause cell damage. Megadoses of vitamin B6 can cause degeneration of nerves, resulting in unsteady gait, numbness in the extremities, and impaired tendon reflexes. Consuming more than the RDA for iron can result in iron toxicity. Because iron is a pro-oxidant, it damages cell membranes and can ultimately result in loss of organ function.

Consuming too much of one nutrient often creates a deficiency of another. This can happen in several ways. If two or more nutrients are absorbed by the same pathway (i.e., transport proteins) in the intestine, then there is competition among those nutrients for absorption. For example, zinc, copper, and iron are absorbed by the same pathway. So if large amounts of one of these minerals are consumed, that mineral monopolizes the transport system and less of the other two minerals is absorbed. If two nutrients have similar chemical properties, they can interfere with each other's function in biochemical reactions. For example, calcium and magnesium are similar chemically but have opposing actions on blood clot formation. Calcium is needed for the clotting process. At high doses, magnesium substitutes for calcium, inhibiting blood clot formation. Similarly, at very high doses, vitamin E interferes with the actions of vitamin K.

Consuming supplemental vitamins and minerals in excess of needs is a waste of money. Absorption and excretion of vitamins and minerals are highly regulated. In general, the more the body needs, the more is absorbed from the intestine. By limiting nutrient absorption to what is needed, the chances of toxicity are reduced. Likewise, if the vitamin or mineral is already adequate, then the excess that is consumed is either stored or excreted. However, these built-in safety mechanisms of absorption and excretion can be overwhelmed if nutrients are consumed in large amounts.

Creatine

Creatine is a nitrogen-containing compound that is made in the liver and kidneys from the amino acids arginine and glycine. About 1 to 2 g of creatine is synthesized in the human body per day, and the typical diet provides another 1 to 2 g/day from meat and fish. Skeletal muscle contains most of the body's creatine, but there is an upper limit to the amount of creatine that the muscle will retain. Any excess creatine consumed in the diet or from supplements is excreted by the kidneys. For this reason, individuals who consume adequate amounts of creatine in their diet are less likely to derive any benefit from taking additional creatine than vegetarians whose diets are lacking creatine. The effects of creatine supplementation on oxygen consumption during exercise depends on the exercise intensity, fitness of the subjects, and the proportions of type I and type II muscle fibers (which are related to cardiovascular fitness but also influenced by genetics) (Wyss & Kaddurah-Daouk, 2000; Jones, Carter, Pringle, & Campbell, 2002).

In individuals who respond to supplementation, the amount of creatine in skeletal muscle typically increases 15% to 20% and body weight increases 1 to 3 kg during the first 5 to 7 days of supplementation. Creatine is not anabolic; it does not stimulate muscle protein synthesis or muscle growth. The rapid weight gain associated with creatine supplementation is due to water retention in the muscle cells. When the muscle cells take in more creatine, they also have to retain more water to maintain the correct intracellular fluid pressure. The extra water not only decreases the power-to-weight ratio (by increasing weight and not power), but it may impair muscle function and cause muscle stiffness and cramping. Because body water will shift from the blood to the muscle cells, sweating and thermoregulation may be impaired. Athletes who supplement with creatine must be especially careful not to become dehydrated—they should consume copious fluids and refrain from strenuous exercise, especially in the heat.

Creatine is used by skeletal muscle to make phosphocreatine. During maximal anaerobic efforts, phosphocreatine allows the muscle to generate large amounts of ATP very rapidly. However, there is only enough phosphocreatine to last 30 seconds.

The idea behind "creatine loading" is that by increasing the amount of creatine in the muscle, there will be more phosphocreatine on hand to generate ATP. If there is more ATP available for use during maximal anaerobic efforts, then the muscle will have more energy and performance will improve. Creatine supplementation has been shown to improve performance in repeated cycling sprints and maximal weightlifting efforts. In other words, creatine does not increase maximal power or strength but allows an individual to achieve his or her maximum potential during repetitive tests separated by short rest intervals. Creatine does not increase endurance performance, because ATP is derived from aerobic metabolism of glucose and fat and not from phosphocreatine. There is not enough evidence supporting an ergogenic effect of creatine on endurance performance to endorse its use for that purpose; this position is consistent with that published by the American College of Sports Medicine (Terjung et al., 2000).

Glutamine

Glutamine is a conditionally essential amino acid, meaning that under normal circumstances the body can make what it needs. Skeletal muscle is the most significant source of glutamine in the body. When muscle is broken down in response to the stress hormone cortisol, glutamine is released from the muscle into the blood. During times of extraordinary stress, such as severe trauma, burns, or sepsis, the body's demand for glutamine exceeds its ability to make the amino acid and it becomes essential (Castell, 2003). In clinical studies of critically ill patients, providing supplemental glutamine improved patient outcome and survival. This is in large part because cells of the immune system use glutamine for energy. During times of stress, the immune system is activated, requiring more energy. Although not nearly as stressful as a burn injury or sepsis, exhaustive exercise (e.g., running a marathon) causes a short-term (< 12 hours) decrease in blood glutamine concentrations. Overtraining syndrome also produces a decrease in blood glutamine concentrations (Halson, Lancaster, Jeukendrup, & Gleeson, 2003).

Because athletes competing in endurance events often experience a mild decrease in immune function and an increase in upper respiratory tract infections after the event, the effect of glutamine supplementation on immune response has been studied in endurance athletes (Krzywkowski, Petersen, Ostrowski, Kristensen, et al., 2001; Krzywkowski, Petersen, Ostrowski, Link-Amster, et al., 2001; Krieger, Crowe, & Blank, 2004). One study found that runners who consumed glutamine immediately and 2 hours after a marathon had fewer self-reported upper respiratory tract infections in the week after the race. Consuming glutamine for 3 to 4 weeks before competition also reduced self-reported infections in marathon runners and triathletes. However, numerous other studies investigating the mechanism behind the beneficial effect of glutamine found no effect of glutamine supplementation on immune cell function.

It should be noted that glutamine is not stable in solution, and exposure to ultraviolet light degrades it as well. The effective dose (0.1 g glutamine/kg BW) should not be exceeded. Amino acids compete with each other for absorption in the intestine, and consuming an excess of one amino acid can create a deficiency of another. Excessive protein consumption unnecessarily stresses the kidneys, and excess amino acids that are not used in protein synthesis will be stored as adipose tissue.

Other Supplements

Nitric oxide is made in the body from L-arginine and oxygen. This gaseous signal molecule plays an important role in many physiologic processes, including smooth muscle contraction, immune function, and nervous system activity. Because nitric oxide is a potent vasodilator, it plays an important role in oxygen use during exercise. Exercise stimulates nitric oxide production in blood vessels that perfuse skeletal muscle and causes increased blood flow to the working muscle (Krzywkowski, Petersen, Ostrowski, Kristensen, et al., 2001; Krzywkowski, Petersen, Ostrowski, Link-Amster, et al., 2001; Miyauchi et al., 2003). Interestingly, nitric oxide decreases mitochondrial oxygen consumption by inhibiting several key enzymes involved in synthesis of ATP (Stamler & Meissner, 2001). The net result is that nitric oxide release acts to increase the oxygen available to muscle by increasing delivery and decreasing the rate at which it is used. Because nitric oxide is a gas, it is not commercially available in supplement form. Dietary supplements that claim to increase nitric oxide levels contain arginine.

Cordyceps sinensis, also known as Chinese caterpillar fungus, was popularized by the sudden success of Chinese female distance runners in the early 1990s. When Wang Junxia shattered the world record in the 10,000 m, her coach attributed her performance to a diet of turtle blood and caterpillar fungus. Needless to say, the success and running careers of the Chinese women were short-lived. Cordyceps is a black fungus that is a parasite for several species of caterpillar. The fungus kills the caterpillar and uses it for nutrients as it grows. Because cordyceps in nature is rare, a strain (Cs-4) that contains the active components is now cultivated for commercial purposes (Zhu, Halpern, & Jones, 1998a,b). Other than the success of the Chinese runners, there is very little evidence to support the claim that cordyceps improves performance. In fact, two recent studies of trained male cyclists found no effect of cordyceps supplementation on maximal oxygen consumption, ventilatory threshold, or performance compared with placebo (Parcell, Smith, Schulthies, Myrer, & Fellingham, 2004).

Ventilatory threshold: The workload or exercise intensity that causes the first rise in the ventilatory equivalent of oxygen without a concurrent rise in the ventilatory equivalent of carbon dioxide; occurs near the lactate threshold.

Sports During Pregnancy, Lactation, and Menopause

Pregnancy and Sports

The American College of Obstetrics and Gynecology recommends that all women with uncomplicated pregnancies participate in moderate physical activity for at least 30 minutes on most, if not all, days of the week (American College of Obstetricians and Gynecologists, 2002). Regular exercise has been shown to reduce the occurrence of physical complaints during pregnancy, to improve mood, and to shorten delivery time (Clapp, 2000). Women who are accustomed to exercising at high intensity and female athletes may continue to train vigorously during pregnancy, but they should be aware that some of the physiologic changes associated with pregnancy may require them to back off the intensity or modify the type of activity. Resting metabolic rate is increased during pregnancy, meaning the body requires more oxygen at rest. As the uterus grows during the second and third trimesters, it puts pressure on the diaphragm, increasing the work required to breathe. Because the body requires more oxygen and has to work harder to obtain that oxygen, less oxygen is available for exercise. For this reason, maximal workload may be reduced and exercise may feel more difficult at a given intensity during pregnancy. Another consequence of the elevated metabolic rate is an increased susceptibility to overheating and dehydration. There is some evidence that maternal overheating (core temperature above 39.2°C) during the first trimester may increase the risk of birth defects. Therefore, pregnant women should avoid exercising in hot, humid weather and consume adequate fluids in the event of fever. The weight gain associated with pregnancy changes a woman's center of gravity, which may preclude activities that require balance to avoid abdominal trauma.

Pregnant women require an additional 300 kcal/day for growth of the fetus and maternal tissues (Food and Nutrition Board, Institute of Medicine, 2003). Inadequate energy consumption during pregnancy results in a low-birth-weight infant, which increases the chances of neonatal complications. Hormones produced by the placenta (human placental lactogen, estrogen, progesterone) cause changes in maternal metabolism such that the mother preferentially uses fat for energy, which allows glucose to be used by the fetus. These metabolic changes cause pregnant women to have lower fasting glucose levels and to use more glucose during exercise than nonpregnant women. Therefore, adequate carbohydrate consumption is especially important during exercise.

Lactation

The American Academy of Pediatrics (2005) recommends that infants be breast-fed for at least 12 months. Breast-feeding not only benefits the infant but is advantageous for the mother as well. Exercise during lactation enhances cardiovascular fitness, decreases postpartum weight retention, improves postprandial insulin response, and increases high-density lipoprotein (Larson-Meyer, 2002). Lactating women may exercise without any adverse effect on milk volume or composition, infant feeding, or growth. Maximal, but not submaximal, exercise increases the concentration of lactic acid in breast milk for 0.5 to 1.0 hours after exercise. Whether the increased lactic acid concentration reduces milk consumption is controversial. Wright and colleagues (2002) in a well-controlled study suggested that the increase in lactic acid has no effect on milk consumption.

Menopause

Menopause is defined as the absence of regular menstrual cycles for 12 consecutive months. Typically, women experience menstrual cycle irregularity before cycles stop completely; changes in cycle length and frequency are common. During this perimenopausal period, estrogen concentrations also may be highly variable, and after 3 months of missed periods, estrogen declines significantly. Menopause, like puberty, is a time of hormonally driven changes in body shape and composition. During middle age, women gain an average of 0.5 kg (~1 lb.) per year, and menopause does not seem to increase this rate of weight gain. Women lose muscle mass and increase fat mass during menopause, but these changes seem to be due to a decrease in physical activity as women get older rather than an inevitable consequence of menopause. Even if total body fat does not increase after menopause, there is a shift in body fat distribution from the hips and thighs to the abdomen. In other words, the "pears" start to look more and more like "apples."

It is the accumulation of fat around the internal organs located in the abdomen that probably causes changes in fat and glucose metabolism. Postmenopausal women have higher total cholesterol, low-density lipoprotein (bad) cholesterol, and triglycerides (fat) and lower high–density lipoprotein (good) concentrations in blood than premenopausal women. These changes explain why the risk of cardiovascular disease increases in women after menopause. Women, especially those who gain abdominal fat, after menopause may become insulin resistant. These changes in body composition and metabolism result not only from the direct effects of lower estrogen, but also from estrogen-mediated changes in other hormones. GH and IGF-I exert anabolic effects on bone and muscle, and GH increases fat use as an energy source by stimulating release of fatty acids from body fat stores. Hypoestrogenemia reduces pulsatile release of GH, consequently lowering IGF-I secretion.

Exercise counteracts many of the unfavorable metabolic changes that occur after menopause by reducing weight gain, increasing fat utilization, maintaining skeletal muscle mass, improving cholesterol and triglycerides, and increasing the body's response to insulin. Strength training helps to prevent the decline in muscle mass and offsets the decline in metabolic rate. Strength training with weights also benefits the skeleton by stimulating bone growth resulting from the mechanical stress placed on the skeleton.

Adequate calcium intake is especially important for postmenopausal women. In addition to dairy products, some vegetables, fish with bones, and fortified foods (e.g., orange juice, cereal) are good sources of calcium. During the first 5 to 7 years of menopause women lose up to 20% of their skeletal mass (DHHS, n.d.). Consuming 1,200 mg calcium/day may minimize that loss.

Pediatric Diabetes

Karen Chapman-Novakofski, RD, LDN, PhD

Incidence and Prevalence

More than 150,000 children have **type 1 diabetes** in the United States, with 10,000 to 15,000 new cases diagnosed each year (Centers for Disease Control and Prevention, 2005). The incidence of type 1 diabetes peaks in children both between 5 and 7 years of age and at puberty

Type 1 diabetes: Diabetes due to a lack of endogenous insulin.

(Haller, Atkinson, & Schatz, 2005). Incidence rates vary considerably among countries, with a low incidence in China, Venezuela, and India at 0.1 per 100,000 and a high incidence in Sardinia and Finland at 50 cases per 100,000 persons per year. The United States has an incidence rate of approximately 16 per 100,000/year (LaPorte & Chang, 1995; Karvonen et al., 2000).

Until recently, children and adolescents diagnosed with diabetes were assumed to have type 1 of an autoimmune etiology. Currently, children are also being diagnosed with **type 2 diabetes**, ranging from 8% to 45% of cases reported (American Diabetes Association, 2000). There is some discrepancy in diagnosis, with one report from Chicago suggesting that 24% of African-American and Hispanic-American adolescents diagnosed with type 1 diabetes may instead have type 2 diabetes (Keenan et al., 1999). The incidence is higher among older children, those who are obese, and minorities (Aye & Levitsky, 2003).

Type 2 diabetes: Diabetes due to ineffective or low levels of insulin.

A report concerning national reference values for hemoglobin AIc levels among individuals aged 5 to 24 years concluded that, in general, higher hemoglobin AIc values were found in those aged 10 to 14 years old, in those who were overweight, in those with parental history of diabetes, and in those with a blood glucose level greater than 126 mg/dL. These differences were small and usually represented hemoglobin AIc levels within a normal range, but these values may reflect differences in metabolism (Saaddine et al., 2002).

Diagnosis of Diabetes in Children

The diagnosis of diabetes in children does not differ from that of adults. Symptoms of diabetes plus a random (nonfasting) blood glucose level of 200 mg/dL or greater, fasting plasma glucose level of 126 mg/dL or greater, or a 2-hour plasma glucose level of 200 mg/dL or greater during an oral glucose tolerance test are all diagnostic of diabetes. However, these criteria should be repeated on a different day to confirm results (American Diabetes Association, 2005).

● **Learning Point** The classic symptoms of type 1 diabetes are polyuria, polydipsia, polyphagia, and weight loss, with children often brought to the hospital with diabetic ketoacidosis.

Pathogenesis of Type 1 Diabetes in Children

The classic model for type 1 diabetes is the genetically susceptible child exposed to an environmental trigger that results in pancreatic beta cell autoimmunity and eventual self-destruction (Eisenbarth, 1986). The autoimmunity is specific to the pancreatic beta cells, but the mechanisms have yet to be identified. Typically, it is believed that symptoms do not occur until 80% to 90% of the beta cells have been destroyed, although more recent evidence suggests that symptoms may present themselves when only 40% to 50% have been destroyed (Haller et al., 2005).

Type 1 diabetes is a complex disease despite responding to genetic influences. Although having a first-degree family member with type 1 diabetes increases the risk of developing the condition, 85% of those diagnosed with type 1 diabetes have no family history of the disease (Hamalainen & Knip, 2002). Clearly, environmental influences are also important. Among those environmental factors, both viral and nonviral agents have been suggested. Prenatal rubella, maternal enterovirus infection, and common childhood diseases such as mumps, chickenpox, measles, and rotavirus have possible associations with autoimmunity and type 1 diabetes (Haller et al., 2005). Although there seems to be a protective effect of breast-feeding, the early introduction of cow's milk as a potential environmental trigger remains controversial (Bell, Grochoski, & Clarke, 2006). A role of possible allergens such as soy and wheat has been suggested but requires additional research (Norris et al., 2003; Ziegler, Schmid, Huber, Hummel, & Bonifacio, 2003). Many other perinatal factors have been proposed, including maternal-child blood group incompatibility, maternal preeclampsia, and maternal age (Haller et al., 2005). Additional research is needed to define the role of these factors in the pathogenesis of type 1 diabetes.

Type 1 diabetes is at times further classified as type 1A, which is classic type 1 diabetes, and type 1B, which is diabetes with no known etiology. In type 1B there is no evidence of autoimmunity (Botero & Wolfsdorf, 2005).

Diabetes and Cultural Diversity

The incidence and prevalence of type 1 diabetes varies dramatically around the globe. Type 1 diabetes is uncommon in China, India, and Venezuela. The incidence of type 1 diabetes in children is highest in Canada and the Scandinavian countries of Norway, Sweden, and Finland, followed by Greenland and Australia. However, the prevalence of type 1 diabetes is strongest in Southeast Asia, followed by European countries. Although type 2 diabetes in children is increasing, data are very limited on a global scale. It is known that type 2 diabetes incidence is steeply increasing in the United States and Japan (Kitagawa, Owada, Urakami, & Yamauchi, 1998). The variations in incidence and prevalence rates worldwide may reflect differences in gene susceptibility, environmental risk factors, or differences in the quality of data collection.

In the United States, the rates of type 2 diabetes are approximately 1.7 times higher for girls than for boys and may be linked to obesity (Artz, Haqq, & Freemark, 2005). Ethnic youth compose a substantial number of cases of type 2 diabetes. Among teenage youth, Pima Indians have a very high prevalence of almost 5.1% (Fagot-Campagna et al., 2000). The prevalence of impaired fasting glucose levels has been reported to be significantly different among ethnic groups for adolescents: 13% Hispanic-American, 7% non–Hispanic-American white, and 4% non-Hispanic African-American youth (Williams et al., 2005).

Pathogenesis of Insulin Resistance in Children

Insulin resistance is characterized by **hyperinsulinemia**. The increased levels of insulin attempt to compensate for a declining peripheral sensitivity to insulin to maintain blood glucose levels within a normal range. The hyperinsulinemia is often accompanied by an increase in pancreatic islet cell size and beta cell mass (Artz & Freemark, 2004). Insulin resistance may be defined as the inability of circulating insulin levels to promote peripheral glucose disposal and to suppress hepatic glucose production. Fasting insulin levels greater than 15 mU/mL, post–oral glucose tolerance test peak insulin levels greater than 150 mU/mL, or post–oral glucose tolerance test insulin levels at 120 minutes of greater than 75 mU/mL indicate insulin resistance (Reaven et al., 1993).

Hyperinsulinemia: Blood levels of insulin above the normal range.

Insulin resistance often manifests during puberty, although diagnosis of type 2 diabetes may occur in later years. The peak reduction in insulin sensitivity occurs at Tanner stage III, with a recovery by Tanner stage V. Theories explaining this transient decline in insulin sensitivity include changes in body fat, sex hormone changes, or variation in GH (Goran, Ball, & Cruz, 2003).

Although not all cases of hyperinsulinemia progress to impaired fasting glucose, or "prediabetes," hyperinsulinemia is a significant risk factor for impaired fasting glucose. With impaired fasting glucose there is a dysregulation of basal insulin secretion, most notably with a loss of first-phase glucose-dependent insulin secretion and an increase in the circulating ratio of proinsulin to insulin (Bergman, Finegood, & Kahn, 2002). Insulin resistance may progress to type 2 diabetes in children and is usually associated with obesity.

Other Diabetes Classifications in Children

Maturity-onset diabetes of the young occurs in only a small subset of these children (Botero & Wolfsdorf, 2005). Cases of maturity-onset diabetes of the young reflect a genetic defect that affects insulin secretion but not insulin action. Many other types of diabetes classification exist but are rare in children (American Diabetes Association, 2006).

Risk Factors for Diabetes

Genetics plays a significant role in the development of diabetes, with a higher incidence of diabetes in those with a family history of the disease. Genetic predisposition seems to be an important factor in determining when hyperinsulinemia occurs and when it progresses to diabetes. However, many pathways lead to insulin resistance, most notably many molecular pathways involved in energy homeostasis, lipid metabolism, insulin receptor signaling pathways, cytokine regulation, hormone-binding protein regulation, and protease regulators (Ten & Maclaren, 2004). Genetic involvement in any of these pathways, or a combination of these pathways, could lead to a predisposition to diabetes.

In addition to genetics, the development of diabetes is influenced by a number of factors associated with the incidence of diabetes. Infants who are small for gestational age are at increased risk of developing diabetes (Barker, 2000). This is particularly true when small-for-gestational-age infants undergo rapid postnatal weight gain, leading to obesity (Wilkin et al., 2002). Large-for-gestational-age infants are also at higher risk for insulin resistance, as are infants from mothers with gestational diabetes or type 1 diabetes (Sobngwi et al., 2003).

The environmental factors associated with increased incidence of pediatric diabetes focus on obesity development. Obesity develops when caloric intake exceeds caloric output in the form of physical activity. Few studies in children have examined the role of macronutrients and their respective contribution to obesity and insulin resistance. In adults, the reports concerning the relative importance of dietary fat are conflicting (Steyn et al., 2004). Longitudinal studies in children have not shown a significant relationship between macronutrient distribution and body composition or weight gain (Maffeis, Talamini, & Tato, 1998; Magarey, Daniels, Boulton, & Cockington, 2001). In fact, most studies fail to show a relationship between energy intake and obesity, although this may be due to inaccurate reporting, the difficulty of discerning relatively small increases in caloric intake in short time frames, and the limitations of cross-sectional studies (Rodriguez & Moreno, 2006).

Additional dietary factors that have been explored in relation to obesity include meal patterns, meal frequency, family dining frequency, snacking frequency, beverage consumption, fast food consumption, and portion sizes. None of these factors has been found to have a significant influence on obesity development, although each may play a role for the individual child (Marr, 2004; Ello-Martin, Ledikwe, & Rolls 2005; Taveras et al., 2005; Rodriguez & Moreno, 2006; Jeffery, Baxter, McGuire, & Linde, 2006). Children tend to eat foods that are accessible and in the quantities served, so food that is highly accessible and available in large quantities may contribute to increasing body weight.

Studies in adults have shown that increased physical activity can reduce the risk of type 2 diabetes, reducing insulin resistance and improving glucose tolerance. Fewer studies have been conducted in children, but those that have been done also support the finding that greater physical activity is related to an improved metabolic profile (Ku, Gower, Hunter, & Goran, 2000; Nassis et al., 2005). It is likely that a combination of higher caloric intake and lower physical activity contributes to the development of obesity in children. Central adiposity seems to be more influential on fasting insulin, whereas increased total body fat decreases insulin sensitivity (Goran et al., 2003).

Leptin is a peptide hormone secreted from adipose tissue that has a role in regulating food intake and energy expenditure. Preliminary studies in children with diabetes have found lower leptin levels at the time of diagnosis and before insulin therapy that rise with subsequent insulin regulation (Soliman et al., 2002).

Associated Clinical Conditions

Youth with type 2 diabetes may present with **acanthosis nigricans,** a velvety skin texture often found in intertriginous areas such as skin folds of the groin, axilla, and breasts as well as the nape of the neck. Acanthosis nigricans that is not associated with cancer may occur neonatally, in childhood, or in adults. The skin condition is often associated with obesity and is more prevalent in the African-American population (Hermanns-Lê, Scheen, & Pierard, 2004). Obese patients with acanthosis nigricans have been found to have hyperinsulinemia. Acanthosis nigricans has been reported to be closely associated with insulin resistance in Native American children as well (Copeland et al., 2006).

The mechanism by which hyperinsulinemia may cause acanthosis nigricans is complex and not completely understood. The process probably involves excess insulin binding to IGF receptors that increase fibroblast and keratinocyte proliferation. This increase may lead to subsequent defects in the skin tissue (Hermanns-Lê et al., 2004).

Polycystic ovarian syndrome is also associated with type 2 diabetes in young women. The diagnosis is difficult because polycystic ovarian syndrome is a clinical syndrome, but generally the presence of two of the following three conditions is diagnostic: oligo- or anovulation,

Acanthosis nigricans: A velvety skin texture often found in skinfold areas that is often associated with obesity and type 2 diabetes.

Polycystic ovarian syndrome: A clinical syndrome in women consisting of two of the following three conditions: oligo- or anovulation, hyperandrogenism, and polycystic ovaries.

hyperandrogenism, and polycystic ovarian syndrome (PCOS Consensus Workshop Group, 2004; Meurer, Kroll, Jamieson, & Yousefi, 2006). Usually manifested during adolescence, polycystic ovarian syndrome may originate in intrauterine development and has a strong genetic component (Xita & Tsatsoulis, 2006). Weight loss through life-style modification is recommended for improvement in insulin sensitivity and decreasing androgens. Oral contraceptives for managing menses and cyproterone acetate, an antiandrogen medication, for decreasing androgen levels may be beneficial. Indications for these and other oral hypoglycemic agents depend on the age of the child and the clinical severity (Evangelia, Erasmia, & Dimitrios, 2006).

Management

There are not as yet evidence-based guidelines for pediatric diabetes. However, the overall management goal in pediatric diabetes is similar to that for adults: near normalization of blood glucose levels for the prevention of complications and improvement in health. Glycemic goals and ways to achieve these goals differ for children because of emotional and physical issues. As always, glycemic goals must be individualized to reflect physical, emotional, health, and cultural needs of the individual. The benefits of achieving lower **glycemic control** should be weighed against the possibility of hypoglycemia in the child. In general, the guidelines in **Table 8.3** provide a framework. Self-monitoring of blood glucose is advisable and is especially necessary if the child is taking insulin. In addition, urinary ketone measurement is recommended if the child has a fever or is vomiting, if the blood glucose continues to rise in an ill child, if the child becomes unusually drowsy or has stomach pains, or if overnight insulin insufficiency is suspected (International Society for Pediatric and Adolescent Diabetes, 2000).

Glycemic control: Maintaining blood glucose within the target range.

TABLE 8.3	Blood Glucose and Hemoglobin A_{Ic} Goals for Children With Type 1 Diabetes		
	Blood Glucose Goal Range (mg/dl)		
	Before Meals	Bedtime/Night Time	Hemoglobin A_{Ic} (%)
Toddlers less than 6 years	100–180	110–200	7.7–8.5
Ages 6–12 years	90–180	100–180	<8.0
Ages 13–19 years	90–130	90–150	<7.5

Source: National Institutes of Health. National Diabetes Program. Available at: http://ndep.nih.gov/media/diabetes/youth/youth_FS.htm#IdentifyingType1. Retrieved 5/4/09.

The Role of Exercise

Exercise is an important part of a healthy life-style. National guidelines suggest that adolescents engage in physical activity for a minimum of 60 minutes most days (U.S. Department of Agriculture, Department of Health and Human Services, 2005). Increasing the amount of moderate to vigorous physical activity is supported by evidence-based data for disease prevention in youth (Strong et al., 2005). However, few intervention studies have been conducted on the effects of physical activity on prevention or treatment of chronic disease in youth (Cruz et al., 2005).

For the child with type 2 diabetes, regular physical activity may help to achieve a healthier body weight. For the child with type 1 diabetes, care should be taken to prevent hypoglycemia (U.S. Department of Health and Human Services, National Diabetes Education Program, 2006). Hypoglycemia may occur after prolonged moderate-intensity-aerobic exercise, as might occur in an after-school program, and may require more carbohydrate than a traditional 15 g for treatment (Diabetes Research in Children Network Study Group, 2006). Children on continuous subcutaneous insulin infusion may need to use a variety of strategies depending on the physical activity. The pump can be removed for intense exercise such as in organized sports, but it must be recognized that blood glucose may drop due to the intense exercise or rise due to the excitement of the game. There may also be a risk of nocturnal hypoglycemia after an eventful day of physical activity such as a soccer or basketball tournament. For prolonged although evenly exerted activities such as biking or hiking, the pump may be set at half the usual rate of infusion, although this should also be individually calibrated (Tamborlane, Fredrickson, & Ahern, 2003).

To reach national guidelines of physical activity for youth in general, families, schools, after-school programs, and youth sports and recreation programs should all be involved at the individual and community levels. To promote physical activity in youth, media campaigns and the communities' structural environment should be engaged (Centers for Disease Control and

Medical nutrition therapy is an important factor in achieving both glycemic control and normal growth and development. Macronutrient distribution is based on adult recommendations but should be tailored to meet individual needs. Total calories should be balanced between needs for growth and prevention of obesity. The Dietary Reference Intakes listed in **Table 8.4** are guidelines for estimating caloric needs (Institute of Medicine, 2005).

Initial education for the child with type 1 diabetes and his or her family may be in the medical center. Topics discussed are generally "survival strategies," such as how to store and inject insulin. After hospitalization in the case of the child with type 1 diabetes and certainly for the child with type 2 diabetes, outpatient education should be multidisciplinary and similar to that for adults. For the child with type 1 diabetes, carbohydrate counting education is essential for both the child and caregiver(s) if continuous subcutaneous insulin infusion or basal-bolus insulin regimens are to be successful. Insulin therapies need to be accompanied by self-management of blood glucose training and home glucose monitoring. Usually, families are taught "correction factors" to treat elevated blood glucose levels. A common correction factor can be estimated by dividing 1,600 by the total daily dose of insulin. The result approximates the glucose-lowering effect of additional insulin. For example, a child normally taking 27 units of insulin each day would have a correction factor of 1,600/27 = 60, meaning that the child should take an additional 1 unit of a rapid-acting insulin for every 60 mg/dL glucose above the target range (Haller et al., 2005).

For the child with type 2 diabetes, body weight reduction must be a goal without compromising normal growth and development. Increased physical activity with healthy eating patterns and amounts are preferable to very restricted diets. The scientific literature supporting particular interventions for overweight and obese youth are lacking. Multicomponent interventions for families of children aged 5 to 12 years and school-based interventions for older children are recommended for treating obesity (American Dietetic Association, 2006). If life-style modifications are not successful, medication may be pre-

TABLE 8.4	Estimated Energy Requirements for Children and Adolescents
3–8 years	
Boys	88.5 − (61.9 × age [yr]) + PA × (26.7 × weight [kg] + 903 × height [m]) + 20 kcal
Girls	135.3 − (30.8 × age [yr]) + PA × (10.0 × weight [kg] + 934 × height [m]) + 20 kcal
9–18 years	
Boys	88.5 − (61.9 × age [yr]) + PA × (26.7 × weight [kg] + 903 × height [m]) + 25 kcal
Girls	135.3 − (30.8 × age [yr]) + PA × (10.0 × weight [kg] + 934 × height [m]) + 25 kcal

PA = physical activity coefficient:
1.0 if sedentary
1.13 if low active
1.26 if active
1.42 if very active

Source: From Institute of Medicine (2005).

scribed. Currently, only insulin and metformin are approved by the U.S. Food and Drug Administration for children with type 2 diabetes (Botero & Wolfsdorf, 2005). Metformin is an oral hypoglycemic agent whose main site of action is the liver, where it decreases hepatic gluconeogenesis and increases hepatic glucose uptake. Because metformin does not affect insulin levels, the risk of hypoglycemia is minimized. Preliminary studies suggest that met for min may be beneficial in hyperinsulinemic euglycemic adolescents in reducing body weight and insulin levels, thereby possibly reducing the risk of subsequent diabetes development (Artz & Freemark, 2004).

The child with diabetes should be routinely screened for complications. Developing nephropathy should be monitored once the child is 10 years old and has had diabetes for 5 years. A random spot urine analyzed for the microalbumin-to-creatinine ratio is recommended. Blood pressure should be monitored and treated if persistently elevated, as should blood lipid levels. Regular ophthalmologic care should begin once the child with diabetes is 10 years old and has had diabetes for at least 3 years (American Diabetes Association, 2005).

As with adults, diabetes self-management education is essential for optimal care. However, in pediatric diabetes care, additional supportive measures are usually required to manage social issues of adolescents and the subsequent effect on glycemic control and general health (Berry, Urban, & Grey, 2006).

Disordered Eating

Pamela Hinton, PhD

Eating disorders are psychiatric disorders with significant medical and psychosocial complications affecting about 5 million Americans, primarily adolescent girls and young women. Three eating disorders have been identified by the American Psychiatric Association: anorexia nervosa (AN), bulimia nervosa (BN), and eating disorder not otherwise specified (EDNOS); the diagnostic criteria are outlined in the *Diagnostic and Statistical Manual of Mental Disorders* (American Psychiatric Association, 2000). Although behaviorally distinct, with AN characterized by severe dietary restriction and BN by binge eating and compensatory purging behaviors, the eating disorders share an excessive importance of body weight and shape to self-concept and self-esteem. Eating disorder diagnoses are mutually exclusive; however, an individual may meet diagnostic criteria for more than one disorder during the course of his or her illness.

Anorexia Nervosa

AN is characterized by a relentless pursuit of thinness **(Table 8.5)**. Individuals with AN may achieve very low body weights via severe restriction of the amount and types of food eaten and compulsive and excessive exercise. Patients with the binge eating–purging subtype of AN occasionally use self-induced vomiting, laxatives, or diuretics to control their body weight. AN is a progressive condition, in that the standard for "thin" is lowered over time and patients are never satisfied with their body weight or shape. As weight loss progresses, impaired cognitive function, depression, anxiety, and social isolation worsen. Academic and work performance and personal relationships are often sacrificed to spend time exercising or to avoid social situations that require eating.

Bulimia Nervosa

Individuals with BN also desire thinness, but their chronic dieting is interspersed with recurrent episodes of binge eating, followed by compensatory purging behaviors (e.g., self-induced vomiting) to "undo" the effects of the binge **(Table 8.6)**. As a result most patients with BN are of normal body weight. Feelings of guilt, shame, depression, anxiety, and negative ego-syntonicity increase in parallel with the frequency of binge–purge cycles. Poor impulse regulation often manifests as

TABLE 8.5	Diagnostic Criteria for Anorexia Nervosa	
Criterion	**Description**	
A	Refusal to maintain body weight at or above a minimally normal weight for age and height.	
B	Intense fear of gaining weight or becoming fat, even though underweight.	
C	Disturbance in the way in which one's body weight or shape is experienced, undue influence of body weight or shape on self-evaluation, or denial of the seriousness of the current low body weight.	
D	In postmenarchal females, amenorrhea, i.e., the absence of at least three consecutive menstrual cycles. (A woman is considered to have amenorrhea if her periods occur only after hormone [e.g., estrogen] administration.)	
AN subtypes Restricting type	During the current episode of anorexia nervosa, the person has not regularly engaged in binge eating or purging behavior (i.e., self-induced vomiting or the misuse of laxative, diuretics, or enemas).	
Binge eating– purging type	During the current episode of anorexia nervosa, the person has regularly engaged in binge eating or purging behaviors (i.e., self-induced vomiting or the misuse of laxative, diuretics, or enemas).	

From U.S. Department of Health and Human Services, National Institute of Mental Health (2001).

TABLE 8.6	Diagnostic Criteria for Bulimia Nervosa	
Criterion	**Description**	
A	Recurrent episodes of binge eating. An episode of binge eating is characterized by both of the following: 1. Eating, in a discrete period of time (e.g., within any 2-hour period), an amount of food that is definitely larger than most people would eat during a similar period of time and under similar circumstances. 2. A sense of lack of control over eating during the episode (e.g., a feeling that one cannot stop eating or control what or how much one is eating).	
B	Recurrent inappropriate compensatory behavior to prevent weight gain, such as self-induced vomiting; misuse of laxatives, diuretics, enemas, or other medications; fasting; or excessive exercise.	
C	The binge eating and inappropriate compensatory behaviors both occur, on average, at least twice a week for 3 months.	
D	Self-evaluation is unduly influenced by body shape and weight.	
E	The disturbance does not occur exclusively during episodes of anorexia nervosa.	
BN subtypes Purging type	During the current episode of bulimia nervosa, the person has regularly engaged in self-induced vomiting or the misuse of laxatives, diuretics, or enemas.	
Nonpurging type	During the current episode of bulimia nervosa, the person has used other inappropriate compensatory behaviors, such as fasting or excessive exercise, but has not regularly engaged in self-induced vomiting or the misuse of laxatives, diuretics, or enemas.	

From U.S. Department of Health and Human Services, National Institute of Mental Health (2001).

substance misuse and abuse and self-harming behavior in patients with BN. For some individuals BN is also a progressive condition with the need to binge–purge interfering with academic or work performance and relationships and characterized by stealing.

Eating Disorder Not Otherwise Specified

EDNOS diagnoses should not imply a less serious condition or one that is not worthy of intervention. Typically, EDNOS is nearly identical to AN or BN but without meeting all the diagnostic criteria for either AN or BN (Henig, 2004). All the criteria for AN are met except

- The individual has regular menses.
- The individual's current weight is in the normal range.

All the criteria for BN are met except

- Binge eating and inappropriate compensatory mechanisms occur at a frequency of less than twice a week or for a duration of less than 3 months
- Regular use of inappropriate compensatory behavior by an individual of normal body weight after eating small amounts of food
- Chewing and spitting out, but not swallowing, large amounts of food
- Purging disorder
- Binge eating disorder

For example, an individual may meet all the diagnostic criteria for AN except amenorrhea. As in AN and BN, undue influence of body weight or shape on self-worth is the core psychopathology of most individuals who receive an EDNOS diagnosis. Binge eating disorder (BED) is a subtype of EDNOS, defined by criteria that are for research purposes only **(Table 8.7)**.

TABLE 8.7	Research Criteria for Binge Eating
Criterion	**Description**
A	Recurrent episodes of binge eating characterized by both of the following: a. Eating, in a discrete period of time, an amount of food that is definitely larger than most people would eat during a similar period of time under similar circumstances. Not continual snacking or grazing. Objective definition of quantity. b. A sense of lack of control over eating during the episode.
B	Binge eating episodes are associated with three or more of the following: a. Eating much more rapidly than usual b. Eating until uncomfortably full c. Eating large amounts when not feeling physically hungry d. Eating alone because embarrassed about quantity e. Feeling disgusted with oneself, depressed, or very guilty after overeating
C	Marked distress regarding binge eating is present due to loss of control, implication for weight and health
D	Binge eating occurs, on average, at least 2 days a week for 6 months
E	Binge eating is not associated with the regular use of inappropriate compensatory behaviors and does not occur exclusively during the course of anorexia nervosa

From U.S. Department of Health and Human Services, National Institute of Mental Health (2001).

Psychiatric Comorbidity

Psychiatric comorbidity is high among individuals with eating disorders (Becker, Grinspoon, Klibanski, & Herzog, 1999; American Psychiatric Association, 2000; Fairburn & Harrison, 2003), but as demonstrated in the Minnesota Starvation Study, starvation causes significant changes in mood, personality, and cognition and behavior (Keys, Brozek, Henschel, Mickelsen, & Taylor, 1950). Thus it is sometimes difficult to differentiate between primary and secondary psychological disturbances. Depression is common in both AN and BN, but affect improves significantly with refeeding and reduction in binge–purge symptomology. Obsessive-compulsive disorder and anxiety disorders are common among individuals with eating disorders, but the obsessions (thoughts), compulsions (behaviors), and fears are often related to the eating disorder. A significant number of individuals with eating disorders also suffer from personality disorders, and cotreatment of personality disorders may preclude recovery from eating disorders. Cluster B (Antisocial, Borderline, Histrionic, Narcissistic) personality disorders are more common in individuals with BN; patients with AN are more likely to have Cluster C personality disorders (Avoidant, Dependent, Obsessive-Compulsive). Self-harming behaviors, substance misuse and abuse, and suicide are present at higher rates in patients with eating disorders compared with the general population. If psychology comorbidity is present, it is important to treat all pathologies; otherwise, diminution of the eating disorder may exacerbate symptoms of the remaining disorders.

> **Psychiatric comorbidity:** Presence of additional mental disorders, e.g., substance abuse or personality disorder.

Etiology and Course of Eating Disorders

Eating disorders have multifactorial etiologies. Sociocultural, genetic, family, and personality factors predispose an individual to engage in behavioral risk factors, such as dieting and excessive exercise, which universally precede a clinical eating disorder. Negative life events, role transitions, developmental milestones, sexual and physical abuse, and criticism of physical appearance often precipitate the progression from dieting to eating disorder (American Psychiatric Association, 2000; Fairburn & Harrison, 2003).

Based on physical and behavioral criteria, about 50% of individuals diagnosed with AN and BN achieve full recovery, which is usually defined based on physical and behavioral criteria (i.e., normal body weight, regular menses, and normalization of eating patterns). An additional 30% of eating disorder patients partially recover; for the remaining 20% of affected individuals the eating disorder becomes chronic. Protection, control, and positive social reinforcement are benefits that eating disorder individuals derive from their disorder, thus contributing to the chronicity of the conditions. AN has the highest mortality rate of any psychiatric illness; the adjusted mortality rate ranges from 1.2% to 12.8% and the suicide rate is 56.9% (Agras et al., 2004).

The single most important positive prognostic factor is a short interval between onset of the eating disorder and intervention; thus, less severe weight loss and symptomology also are positive prognostic indicators (American Psychiatric Association, 2000; Fairburn & Harrison, 2003; Agras et al., 2004). Younger age at onset of the eating disorder is also associated with increased likelihood of recovery. Recovery is very difficult after the eating disorder has become **ego-syntonic** and the behaviors entrenched. Psychiatric comorbidity, high vomiting frequency, self-harming behaviors, and substance abuse disorders are negative prognostic indicators (Fairburn & Harrison, 2003).

> **Ego-syntonic:** Consistent with self-concept.

Epidemiology

Eating disorders are disorders of Western societies, although there are isolated reports of self-imposed starvation of adolescents from non-Western societies. Food refusal and thinness have little meaning where food is scarce and malnutrition is endemic. Eating disorders are more common in whites than in other ethnic and racial minorities, and 90% of individuals with AN and BN are female. The disparity between whites and African-Americans is less for BED than for AN and BN. The onset of AN typically occurs during adolescence, compared with young adulthood for BN and middle age for BED. Worldwide, the estimated prevalence of AN is 0.7% in teenage girls and that of BN is 1% to 2% in females aged 16 to 35 years. The estimated combined prevalence of AN and BN in the United States is 3% among young women, and an additional 3% have EDNOS, affecting about 5 million Americans (Becker et al., 1999). The incidence of AN is 19 females and 2 males per 100,000 per year, compared with 29 females and 1 male for BN (Fairburn & Harrison, 2003). Approximately 40% of patients with BED are male.

It is thought that the incidence of both AN and BN has increased in the recent past. However, it is very difficult to accurately determine the frequency of eating disorders in the general population (Agras et al., 2004). Because of the reluctance to seek treatment, many eating disorders go undiagnosed in the community. In addition, there is bias in access to treatment, which in turn biases the reported prevalence of eating disorders among different ethnic and racial groups and between the genders. There are very few epidemiologic data regarding EDNOS, although these atypical eating disorders seem primarily to affect adolescents and young adult women (Fairburn & Bohn, 2005).

Medical Consequences of Eating Disorders

Routine laboratory tests include measurements of serum electrolytes, glucose, blood urea nitrogen, creatinine, and a complete blood count (American Psychiatric Association, 2000; American Dietetic Association, 2001). However, normal laboratory findings are common in patients with eating disorders. Additional laboratory tests, such as serum calcium, magnesium, and phosphorus; liver function tests; electrocardiogram; bone density assessment; and estradiol or testosterone levels, are warranted if the patient exhibits signs and symptoms of malnutrition (American Psychiatric Association, 2000; Fairburn & Harrison, 2003).

Most of the medical complications of AN are due to inadequate energy intake and thus are reversed upon refeeding (American Psychiatric Association, 2000; Fairburn & Harrison, 2003). The exception is loss of bone mineral density, which may persist after restoration of body weight (Heer, Mika, Grzella, Heussen, & Herpertz-Dahlmann, 2004). Fifty percent of women with AN have BMD that is more than two standard deviations below the average value for young adult women (Becker et al., 1999). Physical signs and symptoms and clinical abnormalities associated with AN are presented in **Table 8.8**.

TABLE 8.8	Medical Consequences of Eating Disorders

Physical symptoms
  Cold intolerance
  Gastrointestinal complaints
  Dizziness
  Amenorrhea
  Poor sleep with early morning waking
  Apathy, poor concentration
  Muscle pain
  Weakness, lassitude
Physical signs
  Emaciation; stunted growth and failure/regression of secondary sex characteristics
  Dry skin
  Lanugo
  Orange discoloration of palms and soles with hypercarotenemia
  Swelling of parotid and submandibular glands (vomiting)
  Erosion of inner surface of front teeth (perimylolysis, due to vomiting)
  Scarring on dorsum of hand (Russell's sign, due to self-induced vomiting)
  Esophagitis, gastroesophageal reflux, erythema of pharynx

Continues

Cold hands and feet, hypothermia, acrocyanosis
Bradycardia, orthostatic hypotension, cardiac arrhythmias
Edema
Muscle weakness
Cognitive impairment, depressed irritable mood
Abnormalities on physical investigation
  Endocrine
    Low luteinizing hormone, follicle-stimulating hormone, estradiol
    Low triiodothyronine, thyroxine in normal range, normal thyroid-stimulating hormone
    Mild hypercortisolemia
    Elevated GH
    Hypoglycemia
    Low leptin
  Cardiovascular
    Electrocardiographic abnormalities (especially prolonged Q-T interval)
  Gastrointestinal
    Delayed gastric emptying
    Decreased colonic motility
    Acute gastric dilation
  Hematologic
    Moderate normocytic normochromic anemia
    Mild leucopenia with relative lymphocytosis
    Thrombocytopenia
  Other metabolic abnormalities
    Hypercholesterolemia
    Hypercarotenemia
    Hypophosphatemia
    Dehydration
    Electrolyte disturbance: metabolic alkalosis and hypokalemia (vomiting); metabolic acidosis,
      hypokalemia and hyponatremia (laxative abuse)
  Other abnormalities
    Osteopenia and osteoporosis
    Enlarged cerebral ventricles and external cerebrospinal fluid spaces

From U.S. Department of Health and Human Services, National Institute of Mental Health (2001).

Orthostatic hypotension: A sudden fall in blood pressure that occurs when a person assumes a standing position, causing dizziness, lightheadedness, blurred vision, and syncope.

Acrocyanosis: Blueness of the extremities (the hands and feet), caused by narrowing (constriction) of small arterioles (tiny arteries) toward the end of the arms and legs.

Leucopenia: A decrease in the number of white blood cells circulating within the blood.

Apparently, low energy availability is sensed in the brain; leptin and ghrelin (De Souza, Leidy, O'Donnell, Lasley, & Williams, 2004) may be signals from the periphery to the brain of energy status. Hypothalamic release of thyrotropin-releasing hormone and gonadotropin-releasing hormone are suppressed, resulting in decreased production of thyroid hormone (triiodothyronine, thyroxine), estrogen, and progesterone. In contrast, hypothalamic secretion of growth hormone–releasing hormone and corticotropin-releasing hormone are elevated and, subsequently, so are GH and cortisol. Although GH secretion is increased, the liver and extrahepatic tissues become GH resistant, and systemic and local production of IGF-I is decreased. These hormonal alterations produce many of the physical signs and symptoms associated with AN:

- Low triiodothyronine results in cold intolerance, bradycardia, **orthostatic hypotension, acrocyanosis,** and delayed reflexes
- Low estradiol causes anovulatory amenorrhea, loss of BMD, hypertriglyceridemia and hypercholesterolemia, elevated adhesion molecule expression, and impaired flow-mediated dilation
- GH resistance and low IGF-I results in muscle atrophy, loss of BMD, stunting in growing adolescents, and possibly **leucopenia**

- Hypercortisolemia may contribute to loss of muscle mass and BMD as well as to immune modulation

Growth of fine downy hair (**lanugo**), dry skin, brittle hair, and electrocardiographic abnormalities, usually prolongation of the Q-T interval (Swenne, 2000), are characteristic signs of malnutrition.

Lanugo: Downy, very fine, soft, and usually unpigmented hair.

The focus of eating disorder treatment should be correcting the self-imposed starvation rather than correcting hormone abnormalities via replacement therapy (Fairburn & Harrison, 2003). However, because of the irreversible nature of the loss of BMD, use of anabolic and antiresorptive pharmacologic interventions may be warranted to treat osteopenia and osteoporosis (Miller et al., 2004). There is limited evidence that the combination of rhIGF-I and estradiol may ameliorate loss of BMD during AN (Grinspoon, Friedman et al., 2003; Grinspoon, Miller, Herzog, Clemmons, & Klibanski, 2003; Grinspoon, Miller, Herzog, Grieco, & Klibanski, 2004).

The primary medical complications of BN result from electrolyte and fluid imbalances due to self-induced vomiting and laxative and diuretic misuse. Frequent vomiting results in metabolic alkalosis and hypokalemia; laxative misuse creates metabolic acidosis, hypokalemia, and hyponatremia. Electrolyte abnormalities cause cardiac arrhythmias, which are potentially life-threatening in severely underweight individuals. Peripheral edema and dehydration also result from electrolyte imbalances. Chronic laxative use creates colonic dependence; constipation results when laxative use is stopped because of decreased intestinal motility. Physical symptoms resulting from self-induced vomiting include callous on the dorsum of the hand (Russell's sign), swelling of the submandibular and parotid glands, and erosion of dental enamel on the occlusal and lingual surfaces of the teeth.

Individuals with EDNOS experience medical complications of AN and BN, depending on the nature of their disordered eating behaviors. A diagnosis of EDNOS does not mean that physical health is not jeopardized. Patients with BED are typically overweight and at risk for chronic diseases associated with excess adiposity.

Treatment

Unfortunately, treatment of eating disorders, especially AN, is often dictated by insurance reimbursement rather than need or long-term efficacy. Treatment of AN is costly: Approximately 50% of patients require hospitalization, 50% are prescribed pharmacotherapy, and all require outpatient therapy. In the United States, short-term hospitalization to achieve nutritional stabilization or avert a medical crisis is the norm. However, in other countries, long-term hospitalization with weight restoration and psychotherapy is the standard (Agras et al., 2004).

Treatment Goals

Ideally, treatment should achieve three objectives (American Dietetic Association, 2001; Fairburn & Harrison, 2003). First, effective management of eating disorders fosters motivation to change disordered eating behaviors. The second goal is normalization of body weight, which not only improves physical health but also facilitates improvements in mood and responsiveness to psychotherapy. Patients with AN cannot respond to serotonin reuptake inhibitors during semistarvation because serotonin production is impaired by malnutrition. The third treatment goal is to help patients accord body weight and shape an appropriate level of significance in their self-evaluation, to reduce disordered eating and exercise patterns, and to improve psychosocial functioning. In the case of chronic eating disorders that are resistant to treatment, the goal of therapy is to minimize the negative physical, social, and emotional consequences of the eating disorder.

Eating disorder treatment programs generally use a multidisciplinary treatment team to achieve these therapeutic goals (American Psychiatric Association, 2000; Stewart & Williamson, 2004). A physician oversees the treatment plan and monitors the physical health of the patient. Psychotherapy, by a psychologist, psychiatrist, psychiatric nurse, or social worker trained in eating disorders, helps the patient address unresolved emotional issues, dysfunctional cognitive styles, problematic relationships, and psychiatric comorbidity. A nutritionist or registered dietitian with eating disorder expertise counsels the patient regarding healthful diet and modification of eating habits (American Dietetic Association, 2001).

Inpatient Treatment

Outpatient therapy is preferable to inpatient whenever possible because of the high monetary cost of hospitalization and to the perception by the patient that inpatient treatment is punitive (Agras et al., 2004; Stewart & Williamson, 2004). It sometimes is helpful to the patient to refer to "food as medicine." However, there are circumstances that necessitate inpatient treatment: significant medical risk, very low body weight ($<$ 75% ideal body weight), dehydration, electrolyte disturbances, cardiac dysrhythmia, physiologic instability, arrested growth, acute medical complications of malnutrition (**syncope**, seizures, cardiac failure, pancreatitis), acute psychiatric emergencies (suicidal ideation, self-harming behaviors), uncontrollable binge eating and purging, substance abuse, and circumstances that interfere with treatment (dysfunctional family, abusive relationship). Some patients requiring inpatient treatment may need 24-hour care because of their extreme medical instability (Becker et al., 1999; American Psychiatric Association, 2000; Fairburn & Harrison, 2003; Stewart & Williamson, 2004). Although body weight is often the primary admission criterion, it should not be the single determinant of inpatient treatment. Individuals with eating disorders are adept at artificially elevating their body weight to avoid hospitalization via hyperhydration, which can result in acute hyponatremia. The rate of readmission is relatively high: Approximately 20% of individuals treated in hospital settings will be admitted a second time (Stewart & Williamson, 2004).

Syncope: Temporary loss of consciousness.

Outpatient Treatment

Outpatient therapy for eating disorders may be associated with an eating disorder treatment program or may be physician monitoring of body weight and physical health, psychotherapy, and nutritional counseling. Outpatient day-care facilities are an alternative to inpatient treatment and also serve as a transition from inpatient care (American Psychiatric Association, 2000).

Therapeutic Alliance

Therapeutic alliance: Cooperation between the patient and the therapist to engage in treatment; dependent on good rapport between patient and therapist.

Successful treatment of eating disorders depends on the relationship between the treatment team and the affected individual (Stewart & Williamson, 2004), referred to as the **therapeutic alliance**. Unconditional positive regard, genuineness, warmth, and empathy foster a positive relationship. Validation of the patient's feelings and thoughts by the treatment team increases the patient's self-trust. The treatment plan always should encourage the patient's sense of responsibility and autonomy.

Medical Nutrition Therapy

Weight Gain Goal

Although low body weight is only a symptom of underlying psychopathology, it is the focus of nutritional interventions. Because body weight often is used as the criterion for admission to or release from inpatient treatment programs and because low body weight is associated with increased morbidity and mortality, it frequently is monitored. The perceived focus on weight gain and measurement of body weight can cause significant distress for eating disordered individuals because of their intense fear of becoming fat. In addition, patients may believe the cause of their eating disorder is going to be ignored and go untreated if they perceive the primary treatment focus is restoration of body weight. Because the eating disorder often arises out of an unmet need to be "taken seriously," patients need reassurance that they will continue to receive the psychological treatment and therapeutic support they need even if they gain weight.

To minimize the distress associated with determination of body weight, patients are often weighed with their back to the scale. It also is helpful to focus on improving overall health during refeeding and weight restoration. Monitoring clinical signs and symptoms associated with malnutrition can provide the patient empirical evidence that they are becoming "healthy" rather than "fat."

Target body weight usually is determined as 92% of ideal body weight, 90% of previous highest weight, and weight at which menstruation resumes (Stewart & Williamson, 2004). Often, patients are initially not told their target body weight or the energy prescription required to achieve their goal weight.

Refeeding

The desired rate of weight gain is 1 to 2 pounds per week in outpatient therapy and 2 to 3 pounds for inpatient treatment (American Dietetic Association, 2001). Paradoxically, initial weight gain often is difficult for patients with AN. Although resting metabolic rate is suppressed even when expressed relative to lean body mass in AN, there is evidence that patients become hypermetabolic during refeeding (de Zwaan, Aslam, & Mitchell, 2002). Up to 70 to 100 kcal/kg BW a day may be needed for individuals with AN to gain weight (American Psychiatric Association, 2000). However, because of the risk of refeeding syndrome, energy intake should be increased gradually—that is, by about 200 kcal/day for 1 week (American Dietetic Association, 2001). Refeeding syndrome is characterized by hypophosphatemia (Fisher, Simpser, & Schneider, 2000), hypomagnesemia (Birmingham, Puddicombe, & Hlynsky, 2004), hypokalemia, glucose intolerance, pancreatitis (Morris, Stephenson, Herring, & Marti, 2004), gastrointestinal dysfunction, cardiac arrhythmias, and congestive heart failure. Fluid retention and edema are common and complicate accurate determination of changes in body cell mass. The risk of refeeding syndrome is greater with enteral and parenteral tube feeding.

The goal is to first achieve an energy intake of 2,500 kcal/day for 1 week, regardless of weight changes. This is followed by an incremental increase over an additional week to 3,500 kcal/day. At this point energy intake is adjusted to achieve a rate of weight gain of at least 2 pounds per week. If the patient does not gain a minimum of 2 pounds per week after 2 weeks of inpatient therapy, bed rest or nasogastric tube feeding may be implemented (Stewart & Williamson, 2004).

Micronutrient Deficiencies

Surprisingly, vitamin and mineral inadequacies are uncommon in patients with eating disorders, possibly due to decreased requirements (American Dietetic Association, 2001). Poor intakes of iron, zinc, and calcium are frequently reported in AN. There also is evidence of poor folate and vitamin B_{12} status, as evidenced by low red blood cell folate in patients with AN. Abnormalities in carotenoid metabolism result in elevated serum carotene concentrations. To minimize loss of bone mineral, it is important to ensure that patients with eating disorders consume adequate calcium and vitamin D (American Dietetic Association, 2001).

Normalization of Eating and Exercise Patterns

A goal of medical nutrition therapy is to enable the patient to eat regular meals that meet nutrient needs and include a variety of foods (American Dietetic Association, 2001). In addition, individuals recovering from eating disorders need to learn to be sensitive to hunger and satiety cues. This often involves learning to "trust" one's body—that is, that eating when hungry will not lead to excessive weight gain. Individuals with eating disorders often believe their bodies are somehow defective and different, that they will become obese if they eat like "normal people." Normalization of eating patterns often requires giving up "forbidden" foods and idiosyncratic rituals around food preparation and eating. It is unrealistic to expect an individual recovering from an eating disorder to give up all their disordered eating behaviors at once. Change seems possible if it is incremental.

Patients with BN often present wanting to lose weight. Key to recovery from BN is the recognition that weight loss cannot be achieved by "dieting" and that dieting initiates the binge eating–purging cycle. Individuals recovering from BN must learn that eating regular meals will not "make them fat" but will, in fact, facilitate weight control by minimizing binge eating. Nutritionists should assist patients with BN in structuring their eating patterns to three regular meals and one to three snacks per day. Initially, energy intake should be determined by hunger, because hunger is positively associated with binge eating and purging. Normalization of eating patterns and cessation of vomiting and laxative abuse may cause significant fluid retention and edema, which may be troubling to patients. Chronic laxative users benefit from a high-fiber diet and adequate fluid intake to minimize constipation (American Dietetic Association, 2001).

Individuals recovering from eating disorders should be educated on benefits of exercise in addition to weight control, and they should be encouraged to view exercise as pleasurable rather than compulsory. Trying new activities or sports may foster adoption of this positive view of physical activity. As with hunger and satiety, individuals with eating disorders often ignore feelings of fatigue and pain, exercising when sick or injured. They should be encouraged to "listen" to their bodies and to have an integrated view of their bodies, rather than viewing the body as something to be mastered or controlled.

Psychotherapy

A variety of psychological treatments have been used in the treatment of eating disorders: psychodynamic, interpersonal, cognitive behavioral (CBT), cognitive analytical, behavioral, and family psychotherapy (Fairburn & Harrison, 2003). There are very few controlled outpatient treatment studies comparing modes of psychotherapy for AN. The existing data are limited by small sample sizes, high rates of attrition, lack of standardized treatment protocols, and variation in outcome variables. In early onset AN, family therapy appears to be effective, and thus it is used in treatment of adolescents with eating disorders. There is some support for modest efficacy of psychodynamic therapy, cognitive analytical therapy, and CBT in AN (Becker et al., 1999; Agras et al., 2004).

The evidence in support of the efficacy of CBT for BN is strong. CBT is short-term (20 weekly sessions), structured, and manual-based therapy that focuses on changing dysfunctional cognitive styles that lead to disordered eating and exercise behaviors. About one-third to one-half of patients who participate in CBT experience significant and sustained improvements in bulimic behaviors. Interpersonal therapy, which focuses on problematic relationships, was shown to be as effective as CBT in two short-term trials (Becker et al., 1999; Agras et al., 2004).

Psychotropic Medications

Antidepressants are the most common pharmacologic intervention for eating disorders (Becker et al., 1999; Fairburn & Harrison, 2003). Patients with AN and BN often experience significant depressive symptoms, and there is increased prevalence of depression in families of eating-disordered individuals. Recently, genetic linkage studies examined the association between variants of the serotonin receptor gene and AN. There is limited evidence that one variation of a serotonin receptor gene (5-HTR2A) is associated with AN (Kaye, Frank, Bailer, & Henry, 2005; Kaye, Frank, Bailer, Henry, Meltzer, et al. 2005; Klump & Gobrogge, 2005). Serotonin reuptake inhibitors increase the availability of serotonin within the brain. These antidepressants significantly improve mood and bulimic symptoms acutely, but the positive effect is not sustained. Furthermore, antidepressants are neither as effective as CBT nor do they consistently augment the effects of CBT. There is no empirical evidence supporting the use of antidepressants in treatment of AN, especially during semistarvation. Serotonin synthesis is sensitive to nutritional status, rendering serotonin reuptake inhibitors ineffective in malnourished individuals. Fluoxetine may prevent relapse in weight-restored individuals with AN (Becker et al., 1999).

Special Populations

Males

Eating disorders are less common in men than in women. It is estimated that the ratio of male to female cases of AN is 1:6 and for BN, 1:20. However, the true gender ratio is unknown, because eating disorders are more likely to go undiagnosed in men than in women. Eating disorders are more common in homosexual compared with heterosexual males because of the increased social value of thinness in the homosexual community. Except in certain subcultures (e.g., homosexual community, wrestlers, and jockeys) there is no positive reinforcement of thinness for males. In males with eating disorders, the etiology of the eating disturbance is more likely to be related to improving athletic performance, avoiding medical disease, and escaping peer teasing. There are subtle differences in the body dissatisfaction experienced between the genders. Women with AN are preoccupied with body weight, and men generally are dissatisfied with their body shape or size, rather than weight per se. Males with AN experience the same medical complications as females, including a decline in testosterone and loss of bone mineral density. Limited evidence has shown that treatment outcome is improved if therapy is limited to all-male patients and the treatment team includes some male members. Strength training, in combination with nutrition counseling, improves body dissatisfaction in males who are concerned with their body shape or size (Andersen, 1999).

Pregnant Women

Although fertility is reduced in women with AN, ovulation may still occur in some individuals. Women with eating disorders have increased complications during pregnancy and are more likely to have a low-birth-weight infant and to deliver prematurely (Helgstrand & Andersen, 2005; Kouba, Hallstrom, Lindholm, & Hirschberg, 2005). BN is associated with increased risk of miscarriage. Prenatal death is more common in infants born to mothers with AN (Becker et al., 1999; Fairburn & Harrison, 2003; Kouba et al., 2005). Pregnancy is a time when women are receptive to making significant life-style changes to increase their chances of delivering a healthy baby. Women with eating disorders experience a decrease in the severity of their illness during pregnancy. Unfortunately, the symptoms often recur after delivery when the developing infant is no longer in jeopardy (Rocco et al., 2005).

Athletes

As discussed previously, athletes may be at an increased risk for eating disorders than nonathletes. Some studies have reported increased body dissatisfaction, drive for thinness, and disordered eating in athletes compared with nonathletes. Other investigations, however, found that athletes have a more positive body image than nonathletes and are not at greater risk for eating disorder than nonathletes. The prevalence of eating disorders may vary with the nature of the sport; endurance and aesthetic sports have higher rates of eating disorders than sports where body weight, composition, and appearance do not play a central role in performance (Goodman, 2005; Sanford et al., 2005).

When counseling athletes with eating disorders, it is important that the nutritionist be trained in sports nutrition. Athletes discredit diet and exercise recommendations that are not made by a professional who understands sports. Athletes often believe they are "special" and have unique nutrient requirements. This is especially important regarding exercise counseling. For example, an athlete who has been participating in rigorous training will be highly critical of any suggestion that 20 to 30 minutes of moderate exercise 5 days per week is "normal" or adequate. When the health of an athlete is compromised, the team physician may determine that participation in organized practice and competition is contingent on maintenance of a minimal weight or percentage of body fat or on behavioral criteria. Athletes may be reluctant to admit to an eating disorder and to seek help because they fear losing their scholarship and disappointing their coach and teammates. Some coaches facilitate intervention and treatment, whereas others resist, believing their authority has been overstepped. It is helpful if sports medicine professionals and coaches view eating disorders in athletes as they would any other injury or illness that requires treatment and physician release before return to practice and competition (Goodman, 2005).

Patients with Insulin-Dependent Diabetes Mellitus

There is limited evidence that insulin-dependent diabetes mellitus increases the risk for eating disorders. It has been hypothesized that dietary interventions and weight gain associated with insulin treatment are etiologic factors (Verrotti, Catino, De Luca, Morgese, & Chiarelli, 1999). Individuals with insulin-dependent diabetes mellitus may not comply with insulin therapy to prevent weight gain. Poor glycemic control is associated with rapid progression of complications from diabetes and should be considered a warning sign of eating disorder.

Childhood Eating Disorders

Disordered eating is problematic in pediatric and adolescent populations. Neither the American Psychiatric Association nor the World Health Organization provides diagnostic criteria for the classification of problematic eating in children. However, clinicians and researchers have defined several types of disordered eating in children based on psychological and behavioral characteristics (Watkins, 2002).

Pervasive refusal syndrome is characterized by refusal to eat, drink, talk, walk, and perform self-care (Lask, 2004). Social withdrawal and resistance to treatment are remarkable and further aggravate a serious and potentially life-threatening condition. The average age at onset is 8 to 16 years, and far more girls are affected than boys. Affected children are usually high achievers with high self-expectations, fear of failure, and difficulty dealing with failure to achieve personal standards. There is limited evidence that family violence and sexual abuse also are causal factors. The onset of pervasive refusal syndrome is usually acute. Illness and injury are the most common precipitating factors. Treatment is multidisciplinary, and hospitalization in a child psychiatric unit is usually required. The goal of medical nutrition therapy is to reverse dehydration and electrolyte imbalances and to improve energy intake and nutritional status. Nasogastric tube feedings are almost always needed; resistance to the nasogastric tube feeding is not uncommon. Because affected children are immobile, they must be moved frequently to prevent bedsores and infections. Passive stretching and hydrotherapy prevent muscle stiffness and contractions. Psychotherapy, which often involves nonverbal communication, helps patients identify and express emotions and deal with concerns about returning to normal life. Family therapy may help resolve dysfunctional family interactions. Recovery from pervasive refusal syndrome is slow, typically requiring 1 year after identification and entering treatment, but most children have a complete recovery.

Children with food avoidance emotional disorder present with symptoms similar to AN, depression, or anxiety disorders. Although the apparent lack of appetite and inadequate food intake result from negative affect, these children are not preoccupied with body weight or shape.

Children with functional dysphagia and food phobias are fearful of certain foods or textures, usually lumpy or solid foods. Their fears are rooted in beliefs that the food is poisonous or will make them gag, choke, or vomit. The origin of the phobia may be a traumatic event or a misplaced association between the food and expected negative consequence of eating the feared food.

Another type of disordered eating in children is selective eating or extreme faddism. It is normal for preschool children to go on "food jags" where they will consume only five or six acceptable foods. During this phase children resist trying new foods and may gag if forced to eat a novel food. It is thought that children with selective eating have not progressed beyond the preschool stage characterized by food faddism. Because affected children consume their preferred foods, they are usually of normal height and weight. This problem, which is most common in children ages 7 to 11 years, improves with increased social interaction.

Summary

Children and adolescents have higher energy and protein needs per kilogram of body weight than adults to support growth. Because of this fact, nutrition during athletic performance must be properly planned and supported by diet. At puberty, androgens, estrogens, GH, and IGF-I cause increases in bone mineral, muscle mass, and sex-specific deposition of body fat. The RDA for protein is 0.95 g/kg BW for children aged 9 to 13 and 0.85 g/kg BW for teenagers, compared with 0.8 g/kg BW for adults. Greater than 90% of peak bone mass is acquired by age 18 years, and bone mass doubles between the onset of puberty and young adulthood. Thus children and adolescents require more calcium than adults; the adequate intake for calcium is 1,300 mg/day for ages 9 to 18 years. Iron and zinc needs also are increased during adolescence to support an increase in skeletal muscle mass and an expansion in red blood cell number.

Both the prevalence and severity of subsequent complications place type 1 and type 2 diabetes as significant diseases among the pediatric population. Whereas type 1 diabetes pathogenesis is autoimmune dysfunction that is believed to be triggered by environmental factors, type 2 diabetes focuses on obesity development. Associated with type 2 diabetes in youth is acanthosis nigricans, and in young or adolescent females, polycystic ovarian syndrome.

Treatment for both type 1 and type 2 diabetes in youth involves appropriate calories for achieving and maintaining a healthy weight while preventing obesity and allowing for growth. Adolescence can be difficult emotionally for children without a chronic disease; for those with diabetes the transition to adulthood can be especially challenging. The health care team needs to work with the family and child not only to achieve glycemic control, but also to maintain a healthy social and psychological environment.

Eating disorders are psychiatric disorders with significant medical and psychosocial complications, affecting about 5 million Americans—primarily adolescent girls and young women. Three eating disorders have been identified by the American Psychiatric Association: AN, BN, and EDNOS. Although behaviorally distinct, with AN characterized by severe dietary restriction and BN by binge eating and compensatory purging behaviors, the eating disorders share an excessive importance of body weight and shape to self-concept and self-esteem. Eating disorder diagnoses are mutually exclusive; however, an individual may meet diagnostic criteria for more than one disorder during the course of the illness. Treatment is multidisciplinary, and hospitalization in a psychiatric unit is usually required. The goal of medical nutrition therapy is to reverse dehydration and electrolyte imbalances and to improve energy intake and nutritional status.

Issues to Debate

1. Should coaches and schools be responsible for the proper nutrition of their child athletes?
2. Although several lawsuits and media attention have focused on the role of the fast food industry on the increasing obesity prevalence in the United States, others have professed that individuals have a right to eat where and what they want. With a strong link between obesity and type 2 diabetes, should children of parents who are obese and have type 2 diabetes receive health warnings about places to eat or particular foods they should avoid? Is it the business world, the community, the parents, or the child him- or herself who should be responsible for eating patterns?
3. Adolescents with type 1 diabetes take insulin and monitor their blood glucose. However, it is not uncommon to experience some episodes of hypoglycemia. Should these young adults be allowed to take driver's education? Is having blood glucose levels checked before driving an invasion of privacy?
4. Knowing the medical consequences of eating disorders, should children be placed in a medical facility against their will for treatment?

Websites

American Diabetes Association www.diabetes.org
American Dietetic Association www.eatright.org
International Society for Pediatric and Adolescent Diabetes www.ispad.org
Juvenile Diabetes Research Foundation International www.jdrf.org
National Diabetes Education Program www.ndep.nih.gov/diabetes/youth/youth.htm

References

Dietary Guidelines for Athletes

Acheson, K. J., Gremaud, G., Meirim, I., Montigon, F., Krebs, Y., Fay, L. B., et al. (2004). Metabolic effects of caffeine in humans: Lipid oxidation or futile cycling? *American Journal of Clinical Nutrition, 79,* 40–46.

Ainsworth, B. E., Jacobs, D. R., Jr., Leon, A. S., Richardson, M. T., & Montoye, H. J. (1993). Assessment of the accuracy of physical activity questionnaire occupational data. *Journal of Occupational Medicine, 35,* 1017–1027.

American Academy of Pediatrics. (2005). Breastfeeding and the use of human milk. *Pediatrics, 115,* 496–450.

American College of Obstetricians and Gynecologists. (2002). ACOG committee opinion. Exercise during pregnancy and the postpartum period. *International Journal of Gynaecology and Obstetrics, 77,* 79–81.

American Dietetic Association, Dietitians of Canada, and the American College of Sports Medicine. (2000). Position paper: Nutrition and athletic performance. *Journal of the American Dietetic Association, 100,* 1543–1556.

Anderson, M. J., Cotter, J. D., Garnham, A. P., Casley, D. J., & Febraio, M. A. (2001). Effect of glycerol-induced hyperhydration on thermoregulation and metabolism during exercise in heat. *International Journal of Sport Nutrition and Exercise Metabolism, 11,* 315–333.

Atherton, P. J., Babraj, J., Smith, K., Singh, J., Rennie, M. J., & Wackerhage, H. (2005). Selective activation of AMPK-PGC-1alpha or PKB-TSC2-mTOR signaling can explain specific adaptive responses to endurance or resistance training-like electrical muscle stimulation. *FASEB Journal, 19,* 786–788.

Bar-Or, O. (2001). Nutritional considerations for the child athlete. *Canadian Journal of Applied Physiology, 26*(Suppl.), S186–S191.

Bennell, K., White, S., & Crossley, K. (1999). The oral contraceptive pill: A revolution for sportswomen? *British Journal of Sports Medicine, 33,* 231–238.

Bonen, A., Haynes, F. W., & Graham, T. E. (1991). Substrate and hormonal responses to exercise in women using oral contraceptives. *Journal of Applied Physiology, 70,* 1917–1927.

Borsheim, E., Aarsland, A., & Wolfe, R. R. (2004). Effect of an amino acid, protein, and carbohydrate mixture on net muscle protein balance after resistance exercise. *International Journal of Sport Nutrition and Exercise Metabolism, 14,* 255–271.

Borsheim, E., Cree, M. G., Tipton, K. D., Elliott, T. A., Aarsland, A., & Wolfe, R. R. (2004). Effect of carbohydrate intake on net muscle protein synthesis during recovery from resistance exercise. *Journal of Applied Physiology, 96,* 674–678.

Borsheim, E., Tipton, K. D., Wolf, S. E., & Wolfe, R. R. (2002). Essential amino acids and muscle protein recovery from resistance exercise. *American Journal of Physiology. Endocrinology and Metabolism, 283,* E648–E657.

Brownlie, T., Utermohlen, V., Hinton, P. S., Giordano, C., & Haas, J. D. (2002). Marginal iron deficiency without anemia impairs aerobic adaptation among previously untrained women. *American Journal of Clinical Nutrition, 75,* 734–742.

Brownlie, T., Utermohlen, V., Hinton, P. S., & Haas, J. D. (2004). Tissue iron deficiency without anemia impairs adaptation in endurance capacity after aerobic training in previously untrained women. *American Journal of Clinical Nutrition, 79,* 437–443.

Brutsaert, T. D., Hernandez-Cordero, S., Rivera, J., Viola, T., Hughes, G., & Haas, J. D. (2003). Iron supplementation improves progressive fatigue resistance during dynamic knee extensor exercise in iron-depleted, nonanemic women. *American Journal of Clinical Nutrition, 77,* 441–448.

Bryner, R. W., Toffle, R. C., Ullrich, I. H., & Yeater, R. A. (1996). Effect of low dose oral contraceptives on exercise performance. *British Journal of Sports Medicine, 30,* 36–40.

Burke, L. M., Collier, G. R., Broad, E. M., Davis, P. G., Martin, D. T., Sanigorski, A. J., et al. (2003). Effect of alcohol intake on muscle glycogen storage after prolonged exercise. *Journal of Applied Physiology, 95,* 983–990.

Casazza, G. A., Suh, S. H., Miller, B. F., Navazio, F. M., & Brooks, G. A. (2002). Effects of oral contraceptives on peak exercise capacity. *Journal of Applied Physiology, 93,* 1698–1702.

Castell, L. (2003). Glutamine supplementation in vitro and in vivo, in exercise and in immunodepression. *Sports Medicine, 33,* 323–345.

Celsing, F., Ekblom, B., Sylven, C., Everett, J., & Astrand, P. O. (1988). Effects of chronic iron deficiency anaemia on myoglobin content, enzyme activity, and capillary density in the human skeletal muscle. *Acta Medica Scandinavica, 223,* 451–457.

Clapp, J. F., 3rd. (2000). Exercise during pregnancy: A clinical update. *Clinical Sports Medicine, 19,* 273–286.

Connor, W. E. (2000). Importance of n-3 fatty acids in health and disease. *American Journal of Clinical Nutrition, 71*(1 Suppl.), 171S–175S.

Convertino, V. A., Armstrong, L. E., Coyle, E. F., Mack, G. W., Sawka, M. N., Senay, L. C., Jr., et al. (1996). American College of Sports Medicine position stand. Exercise and fluid replacement. *Medicine and Science in Sports and Exercise, 28,* i–vii.

Costill, D. L., Flynn, M. G., Kirwan, J. P., Houmard, J. A., Mitchell, J. B., Thomas, R., et al. (1988). Effects of repeated days of intensified training on muscle glycogen and swimming performance. *Medicine and Science in Sports and Exercise, 20,* 249–254.

Couture, S., Massicotte, D., Lavoie, C., Hillaire-Marcel, C., & Peronnet, F. (2002). Oral [(13)C] glucose and endogenous energy substrate oxidation during prolonged treadmill running. *Journal of Applied Physiology, 92,* 1255–1260.

Davies, K. J., Donovan, C. M., Refino, C. J., Brooks, G. A., Packer, L., & Dallman, P. R. (1984). Distinguishing effects of anemia and muscle iron deficiency on exercise bioenergetics in the rat. *American Journal of Physiology, 246*(6 Pt. 1), E535–E543.

Deldicque, L., Theisen, D., & Francaux, M. (2005). Regulation of mTOR by amino acids and resistance exercise in skeletal muscle. *European Journal of Applied Physiology, 94,* 1–10.

Finch, C. A., Miller, L. R., Inamdar, A. R., Person, R., Seiler, K., & Mackler, B. (1976). Iron deficiency in the rat: Physiological and biochemical studies of muscle dysfunction. *Journal of Clinical Investigations, 58,* 447–453.

Food and Nutrition Board, Institute of Medicine. (1997). Dietary reference intakes for calcium, phosphorous, magnesium, vitamin D, and fluoride. Washington, DC: National Academy Press.

Food and Nutrition Board, Institute of Medicine. (2001). Dietary reference intakes for vitamin A, vitamin K, arsenic, boron, chromium, copper, iodine, iron, manganese, nickel, silicon, vanadium, and zinc. Washington, DC: National Academy Press.

Food and Nutrition Board, Institute of Medicine. (2003). Dietary reference intakes for energy, carbohydrate, fiber, fat, protein, and amino acids. Washington, DC: National Academy Press.

Food and Nutrition Board, Institute of Medicine. (2005). Dietary reference intakes for water, potassium, sodium, chloride, and sulfate. Washington, DC: National Academy Press.

Foster-Powell, K., Holt, S. H., & Brand-Miller, J. C. (2002). International table of glycemic index and glycemic load values: 2002. *American Journal of Clinical Nutrition, 76,* 5–56.

Halson, S. L., Lancaster, G. I., Jeukendrup, A. E., & Gleeson, M. (2003). Immunological responses to overreaching in cyclists. *Medicine and Science in Sports and Exercise, 35,* 854–861.

Heaney, R. P., & Rafferty, K. (2001). Carbonated beverages and urinary calcium excretion. *American Journal of Clinical Nutrition, 74,* 343–347.

Hildebrandt, A. L., Pilegaard, H., & Neufer, P. D. (2003). Differential transcriptional activation of select metabolic genes in response to variations in exercise intensity and duration. *American Journal of Physiology. Endocrinology and Metabolism, 285,* E1021–E1027.

Hinton, P. S., Giordano, C., Brownlie, T., & Haas, J. D. (2000). Iron supplementation improves endurance after training in iron-depleted, nonanemic women. *Journal of Applied Physiology, 88,* 1103–1111.

Ihle, R., & Loucks, A. B. (2004). Dose-response relationships between energy availability and bone turnover in young exercising women. *Journal of Bone and Mineral Research, 19*, 1231–1240.

Ivy, J. L., Goforth, H. W., Jr., Damon, B. M., McCauley, T. R., Parsons, E. C., & Price, T. B. (2002). Early postexercise muscle glycogen recovery is enhanced with a carbohydrate-protein supplement. *Journal of Applied Physiology, 93*, 1337–1344.

Ivy, J. L., Res, P. T., Sprague, R. C., & Widzer, M. O. (2003). Effect of a carbohydrate-protein supplement on endurance performance during exercise of varying intensity. *International Journal of Sport Nutrition and Exercise Metabolism, 13*, 382–395.

James, M. J., Gibson, R. A., & Cleland, L. G. (2000). Dietary polyunsaturated fatty acids and inflammatory mediator production. *American Journal of Clinical Nutrition, 71*(1 Suppl.), 343S–348S.

Jankowski, C. M., Ben-Ezra, V., Gozansky, W. S., & Scheaffer, S. E. (2004). Effects of oral contraceptives on glucoregulatory responses to exercise. *Metabolism, 53*, 348–352.

Jentjens, R. L., Achten, J., & Jeukendrup, A. E. (2004). High oxidation rates from combined carbohydrates ingested during exercise. *Medicine and Science in Sports and Exercise, 36*, 1551–1558.

Jentjens, R. L., Moseley, L., Waring, R. H., Harding, L. K., & Jeukendrup, A. E. (2004). Oxidation of combined ingestion of glucose and fructose during exercise. *Journal of Applied Physiology, 96*, 1277–1284.

Jentjens, R. L., van Loon, L. J., Mann, C. H., Wagenmakers, A. J., & Jeukendrup, A. E. (2001). Addition of protein and amino acids to carbohydrates does not enhance postexercise muscle glycogen synthesis. *Journal of Applied Physiology, 91*, 839–846.

Jentjens, R. L., Venables, M. C., & Jeukendrup, A. E. (2004). Oxidation of exogenous glucose, sucrose, and maltose during prolonged cycling exercise. *Journal of Applied Physiology, 96*, 1285–1291.

Jeukendrup, A. E., & Martin, J. (2001). Improving cycling performance: How should we spend our time and money? *Sports Medicine, 31*, 559–569.

Johnson, N. A., Stannard, S. R., Mehalski, K., Trenell, M. I., Sachinwalla, T., Thompson, C. H., et al. (2003). Intramyocellular triacylglycerol in prolonged cycling with high- and low-carbohydrate availability. *Journal of Applied Physiology, 94*, 1365–1372.

Jones, A. M., Carter, H., Pringle, J. S., & Campbell, I. T. (2002). Effect of creatine supplementation on oxygen uptake kinetics during submaximal cycle exercise. *Journal of Applied Physiology, 92*, 2571–2577.

Keen, A. D., & Drinkwater, B. L. (1997). Irreversible bone loss in former amenorrheic athletes. *Osteoporosis International, 7*, 311–315.

Keesey, R. E., & Corbett, S. W. (1984). Metabolic defense of the body weight set-point. *Research Publications—Association for Research in Nervous and Mental Disease, 62*, 87–96.

Krieger, J. W., Crowe, M., & Blank, S. E. (2004). Chronic glutamine supplementation increases nasal but not salivary IgA during 9 days of interval training. *Journal of Applied Physiology, 97*, 585–591.

Krzywkowski, K., Petersen, E. W., Ostrowski, K., Kristensen, J. H., Boza, J., & Pedersen, B. K. (2001). Effect of glutamine supplementation on exercise-induced changes in lymphocyte function. *American Journal of Physiology. Cell Physiology, 281*, C1259–C1265.

Krzywkowski, K., Petersen, E. W., Ostrowski, K., Link-Amster, H., Boza, J., Halkjaer-Kristensen, J., et al. (2001). Effect of glutamine and protein supplementation on exercise-induced decreases in salivary IgA. *Journal of Applied Physiology, 91*, 832–838.

Lambert, G. P., Bleiler, T. L., Chang, R. T., Johnson, A. K., & Gisolfi, C. V. (1993). Effects of carbonated and noncarbonated beverages at specific intervals during treadmill running in the heat. *International Journal of Sport Nutrition, 3*, 177–193.

Larson-Meyer, D. E. (2002). Effect of postpartum exercise on mothers and their offspring: A review of the literature. *Obesity Research, 10*, 841–853.

Laughlin, G. A., & Yen, S. S. (1996). Nutritional and endocrine-metabolic aberrations in amenorrheic athletes. *Journal of Clinical Endocrinology and Metabolism, 81*, 4301–4309.

Leachman Slawson, D., McClanahan, B. S., Clemens, L. H., Ward, K. D., Klesges, R. C., Vukadinovich, C. M., et al. (2001). Food sources of calcium in a sample of African-American and Euro-American collegiate athletes. *International Journal of Sport Nutrition and Exercise Metabolism, 11*, 199–208.

Looker, A. C., Dallman, P. R., Carroll, M. D., Gunter, E. W., & Johnson, C. L. (1997). Prevalence of iron deficiency in the United States. *Journal of the American Medical Association, 277*, 973–976.

Loucks, A. B. (2004). Energy balance and body composition in sports and exercise. *Journal of Sports Science, 22*, 1–14.

Loucks, A. B., Laughlin, G. A., Mortola, J. F., Girton, L., Nelson, J. C., & Yen, S. S. (1992). Hypothalamic-pituitary-thyroidal function in eumenorrheic and amenorrheic athletes. *Journal of Clinical Endocrinology and Metabolism, 75*, 514–518.

Loucks, A. B., & Verdun, M. (1998). Slow restoration of LH pulsatility by refeeding in energetically disrupted women. *American Journal of Physiology, 275*(4 Pt. 2), R1218–R1226.

Loud, K. J., Gordon, C. M., Micheli, L. J., & Field, A. E. (2005). Correlates of stress fractures among preadolescent and adolescent girls. *Pediatrics, 115*, e399–e406.

Lovallo, W. R., Wilson, M. F., Vincent, A. S., Sung, B. H., McKey, B. S., & Whitsett, T. L. (2004). Blood pressure response to caffeine shows incomplete tolerance after short-term regular consumption. *Hypertension, 43*, 760–765.

Marino, F. E., Kay, D., & Cannon, J. (2003). Glycerol hyperhydration fails to improve endurance performance and thermoregulation in humans in a warm humid environment. *European Journal of Physiology, 446*, 455–462.

Markou, K. B., Mylonas, P., Theodoropoulou, A., Kontogiannis, A., Leglise, M., Vagenakis, A. G., et al. (2004). The influence of intensive physical exercise on bone acquisition in adolescent elite female and male artistic gymnasts. *Journal of Clinical Endocrinology and Metabolism, 89*, 4383–4387.

McCargar, L. J., & Crawford, S. M. (1992). Metabolic and anthropometric changes with weight cycling in wrestlers. *Medicine and Science in Sports and Exercise, 24*, 1270–1275.

Melby, C. L., Schmidt, W. D., & Corrigan, D. (1990). Resting metabolic rate in weight-cycling collegiate wrestlers compared with physically active, noncycling control subjects. *American Journal of Clinical Nutrition, 52*, 409–414.

Miyauchi, T., Maeda, S., Iemitsu, M., Kobayashi, T., Kumagai, Y., Yamaguchi, I., et al. (2003). Exercise causes a tissue-specific change of NO production in the kidney and lung. *Journal of Applied Physiology, 94*, 60–68.

Murphy, S. P., & Johnson, R. K. (2003). The scientific basis of recent US guidance on sugars intake. *American Journal of Clinical Nutrition, 78*, 827S–833S.

Otis, C. L., Drinkwater, B., Johnson, M., Loucks, A., & Wilmore, J. (1997). American College of Sports Medicine position stand. The female athlete triad. *Medicine and Science in Sports and Exercise, 29,* i–ix.

Parcell, A. C., Smith, J. M., Schulthies, S. S., Myrer, J. W., & Fellingham, G. (2004). Cordyceps sinensis (CordyMax Cs-4) supplementation does not improve endurance exercise performance. *International Journal of Sport Nutrition and Exercise Metabolism, 14,* 236–242.

Park, Y., & Harris, W. S. (2003). Omega-3 fatty acid supplementation accelerates chylomicron triglyceride clearance. *Journal of Lipid Research, 44,* 455–463.

Petersmarck, K. A., Teitelbaum, H. S., Bond, J. T., Bianchi, L., Hoerr, S. M., & Sowers, M. F. (1999). The effect of weight cycling on blood lipids and blood pressure in the Multiple Risk Factor Intervention Trial Special Intervention Group. *International Journal of Obesity and Related Metabolic Disorders, 23,* 1246–1255.

Petibois, C., Cassaigne, A., Gin, H., & Deleris, G. (2004). Lipid profile disorders induced by long-term cessation of physical activity in previously highly endurance-trained subjects. *Journal of Clinical Endocrinology and Metabolism, 89,* 3377–3384.

Raastad, T., Høstmark, A.T., & Strømme, S.B. (1997). Omega-3 fatty acid supplementation does not improve maximal aerobic power, anaerobic threshold and running performance in well-trained soccer players. *Scandinavian Journal of Medicine & Science in Sports, 7,* 25–31.

Rasmussen, B. B., Hancock, C. R., & Winder, W. W. (1998). Post exercise recovery of skeletal muscle malonyl-CoA, acetyl-CoA carboxylase, and AMP-activated protein kinase. *Journal of Applied Physiology, 85,* 1629–1634.

Rickenlund, A., Carlstrom, K., Ekblom, B., Brismar, T. B., Von Schoultz, B., & Hirschberg, A. L. (2004). Effects of oral contraceptives on body composition and physical performance in female athletes. *Journal of Clinical Endocrinology and Metabolism, 89,* 4364–4370.

Rickenlund, A., Thoren, M., Carlstrom, K., von Schoultz, B., & Hirschberg, A. L. (2004). Diurnal profiles of testosterone and pituitary hormones suggest different mechanisms for menstrual disturbances in endurance athletes. *Journal of Clinical Endocrinology and Metabolism, 89,* 702–707.

Rivera-Brown, A. M., Gutierrez, R., Gutierrez, J. C., Frontera, W. R., & Bar-Or, O. (1999). Drink composition, voluntary drinking, and fluid balance in exercising, trained, heat-acclimatized boys. *Journal of Applied Physiology, 86,* 78–84.

Rogol, A. D. (2000). Sex steroid and growth hormone supplementation to enhance performance in adolescent athletes. *Current Opinion on Pediatrics, 12,* 382–387.

Rogol, A. D., Clark, P. A., & Roemmich, J. N. (2000). Growth and pubertal development in children and adolescents: Effects of diet and physical activity. *American Journal of Clinical Nutrition, 72*(2 Suppl.), 521S–528S.

Ruderman, N. B., Park, H., Kaushik, V. K., Dean, D., Constant, S., Prentki, M., et al. (2003). AMPK as a metabolic switch in rat muscle, liver and adipose tissue after exercise. *Acta Physiologica Scandinavica, 178,* 435–442.

Saris, W. H., van Erp-Baart, M. A., Brouns, F., Westerterp, K. R., & ten Hoor, F. (1989). Study on food intake and energy expenditure during extreme sustained exercise: The Tour de France. *International Journal of Sports Medicine, 10*(Suppl. 1), S26–S31.

Saunders, M. J., Kane, M. D., & Todd, M. K. (2004). Effects of a carbohydrate-protein beverage on cycling endurance and muscle damage. *Medicine and Science in Sports and Exercise, 36,* 1233–1238.

Sea, M. M., Fong, W. P., Huang, Y., & Chen, Z. Y. (2000). Weight cycling-induced alteration in fatty acid metabolism. *American Journal of Physiology. Regulatory, Integrative and Comparative Physiology, 279,* R1145–R1155.

Sherman, W. M., Doyle, J. A., Lamb, D. R., & Strauss, R. H. (1993). Dietary carbohydrate, muscle glycogen, and exercise performance during 7 d of training. *American Journal of Clinical Nutrition, 57,* 27–31.

Shirreffs, S. M., & Maughan, R. J. (1998). Volume repletion after exercise-induced volume depletion in humans: Replacement of water and sodium losses. *American Journal of Physiology, 274*(5 Pt. 2), F868–F875.

Sinclair, L. M., & Hinton, P. S. (2005). Prevalence of iron deficiency with and without anemia in recreationally active men and women. *Journal of the American Dietetic Association, 105,* 975–978.

Stamler, J. S., & Meissner, G. (2001). Physiology of nitric oxide in skeletal muscle. *Physiology Review, 81,* 209–237.

Steen, S. N., Oppliger, R. A., & Brownell, K. D. (1988). Metabolic effects of repeated weight loss and regain in adolescent wrestlers. *Journal of the American Medical Association, 260,* 47–50.

Terjung, R. L., Clarkson, P., Eichner, E. R., Greenhaff, P. L., Hespel, P. J., Israel, R. G., et al. (2000). American College of Sports Medicine roundtable. The physiological and health effects of oral creatine supplementation. *Medicine and Science in Sports and Exercise, 32,* 706–717.

Tipton, K. D., Borsheim, E., Wolf, S. E., Sanford, A. P., & Wolfe, R. R. (2003). Acute response of net muscle protein balance reflects 24-h balance after exercise and amino acid ingestion. *American Journal of Physiology. Endocrinology and Metabolism, 284,* E76–E89.

Tipton, K. D., Ferrando, A. A., Phillips, S. M., Doyle, D., Jr., & Wolfe, R. R. (1999). Postexercise net protein synthesis in human muscle from orally administered amino acids. *American Journal of Physiology, 276*(4 Pt. 1), E628–E634.

Turner, L. W., & Bass, M. A. (2001). Osteoporosis knowledge, attitudes, and behaviors of female collegiate athletes. *International Journal of Sport Nutrition and Exercise Metabolism, 11,* 482–489.

Ukropec, J., Reseland, J. E., Gasperikova, D., Demcakova, E., Madsen, L., Berge, R. K., et al. (2003). The hypotriglyceridemic effect of dietary n-3 FA is associated with increased beta-oxidation and reduced leptin expression. *Lipids, 38,* 1023–1029.

U.S. Department of Health and Human Services (DHHS). (n.d). *Bone Health and Osteoporosis: A Report of the Surgeon General.* Washington, DC: Office of the Surgeon General. Retrieved October 19, 2009, from http://www.surgeongeneral.gov/library/bonehealth/content.html

Van Baak, M. A., & Saris, W. H. (2000). The effect of caffeine on endurance performance after nonselective beta-adrenergic blockade. *Medicine and Science in Sports and Exercise, 32,* 499–503.

van Loon, L. J., Schrauwen-Hinderling, V. B., Koopman, R., Wagenmakers, A. J., Hesselink, M. K., Schaart, G., et al. (2003). Influence of prolonged endurance cycling and recovery diet on intramuscular triglyceride content in trained males. *Amer-*

ican Journal of Physiology. *Endocrinology and Metabolism, 285,* E804–E811.

Venables, M. C., Shaw, L., Jeukendrup, A. E., Roedig-Penman, A., Finke, M., Newcombe, R. G., et al. (2005). Erosive effect of a new sports drink on dental enamel during exercise. *Medicine and Science in Sports and Exercise, 37,* 39–44.

Waters, D. L., Qualls, C. R., Dorin, R., Veldhuis, J. D., & Baumgartner, R. N. (2001). Increased pulsatility, process irregularity, and nocturnal trough concentrations of growth hormone in amenorrheic compared to eumenorrheic athletes. *Journal of Clinical Endocrinology and Metabolism, 86,* 1013–1019.

Watkins, B. A., Li, Y., Lippman, H. E., & Seifert, M. F. (2001). Omega-3 polyunsaturated fatty acids and skeletal health. *Experimental Biology and Medicine, 226,* 485–497.

Watson, J., Deary, I., & Kerr, D. (2002). Central and peripheral effects of sustained caffeine use: Tolerance is incomplete. *British Journal of Clinical Pharmacology, 54,* 400–406.

Williams, M. B., Raven, P. B., Fogt, D. L., & Ivy, J. L. (2003). Effects of recovery beverages on glycogen restoration and endurance exercise performance. *Journal of Strength and Conditioning Research/National Strength & Conditioning Association, 17,* 12–19.

Willis, W. T., Brooks, G. A., Henderson, S. A., & Dallman, P. R. (1987). Effects of iron deficiency and training on mitochondrial enzymes in skeletal muscle. *Journal of Applied Physiology, 62,* 2442–2446.

Wolfe, R. R. (2000). Protein supplements and exercise. *American Journal of Clinical Nutrition, 72*(2 Suppl.), 551S–557S.

Wolfe, R. R., Klein, S., Carraro, F., & Weber, J. M. (1990). Role of triglyceride-fatty acid cycle in controlling fat metabolism in humans during and after exercise. *American Journal of Physiology, 258*(2 Pt. 1), E382–E389.

World Anti-Doping Agency. (2005). *The Prohibited List. World Anti-Doping Code.* Montreal, Canada: Author.

Wright, K. S., Quinn, T. J., & Carey, G. B. (2002). Infant acceptance of breast milk after maternal exercise. *Pediatrics, 109,* 585–589.

Wyss, M., & Kaddurah-Daouk, R. (2000). Creatine and creatinine metabolism. *Physiology Review, 80,* 1107–1213.

Yeager, K. K., Agostini, R., Nattiv, A., & Drinkwater, B. (1993). The female athlete triad: Disordered eating, amenorrhea, osteoporosis. *Medicine and Science in Sports and Exercise, 25,* 775–777.

Zhu, J. S., Halpern, G. M., & Jones, K. (1998a). The scientific rediscovery of an ancient Chinese herbal medicine: Cordyceps sinensis. Part I. *Journal of Aternative and Complementary Medicine, 4,* 289–303.

Zhu, J. S., Halpern, G. M., & Jones, K. (1998b). The scientific rediscovery of a precious ancient Chinese herbal regimen: Cordyceps sinensis. Part II. *Journal of Aternative and Complementary Medicine, 4,* 429–457.

Pediatric Diabetes

American Diabetes Association. (1999). Diabetes mellitus and exercise. *Diabetes Care* (Suppl.), S49–S53.

American Diabetes Association. (2000). Type 2 diabetes in children and adolescents. *Pediatrics, 105,* 671–680.

American Diabetes Association. (2005). Standards of medical care. *Diabetes Care, 28*(Suppl. 1), S4–S36.

American Diabetes Association. (2006). Diagnosis and classification of diabetes mellitus. *Diabetes Care, 29*(Suppl. 1), S43–S48.

American Dietetic Association. (2006). Position of the American Dietetic Association: Individual-, family-, school-, and community-based interventions for pediatric overweight. *Journal of the American Dietetic Association, 106,* 925–945.

Artz, E., & Freemark, M. (2004). The pathogenesis of insulin resistance in children: Metabolic complications and the roles of diet, exercise and pharmacotherapy in the prevention of type 2 diabetes. *Pediatric Endocrinology Reviews, 1,* 296–309.

Artz, E., Haqq, A., & Freemark, M. (2005). Hormonal and metabolic consequences of childhood obesity. *Endocrinology and Metabolism Clinics of North America, 34,* 643–658.

Aye, T., & Levitsky, L. L. (2003). Type 2 diabetes: An epidemic disease in childhood. *Current Opinion in Pediatrics, 15,* 411–415.

Barker, D. J. (2000). In utero programming of cardiovascular disease. *Theriogenology, 53,* 555–574.

Bell, S. J., Grochoski, G. T., & Clarke, A. J. (2006). Health implications of milk containing ß-casein with the A2 genetic variant. *Critical Reviews in Food Science and Nutrition, 46,* 93–100.

Bergman, R. N., Finegood, D. T., & Kahn, S. E. (2002). The evolution of beta cell dysfunction and insulin resistance in type 2 diabetes. *European Journal of Clinical Investigations, 32,* 35–45.

Berry, D., Urban, A., & Grey, M. (2006). Management of type 2 diabetes in youth (part 2). *Journal of Pediatric Health Care, 20,* 88–97.

Botero, D., & Wolfsdorf, J. I. (2005). Diabetes mellitus in children and adolescents. *Archives of Medical Research, 36,* 281–290.

Centers for Disease Control and Prevention. (2005). Diabetes projects. Retrieved June 28, 2006, from www.cdc.gov/diabetes/projects/cda2.htm

Centers for Disease Control and Prevention. (n.d.). National Center for Chronic Disease Prevention and Health Promotion. Healthy youth! Physical activity, promoting better health. Retrieved July 3, 2006, from http://www.cdc.gov/healthyyouth/physicalactivity/promoting_health/

Copeland, K., Pankratz, K., Cathey, V., Immohotichey, P., Maddox, J., Felton, B., et al. (2006). Acanthosis nigricans, insulin resistance (HOMA) and dyslipidemia among Native American children. *Journal of the Oklahoma State Medical Association, 99,* 19–24.

Cruz, M. L., Shaibi, G. Q., Weigensberg, M. J., Spruijt-Metz, D., Ball, G. D., & Goran, M. I. (2005). Pediatric obesity and insulin resistance: Chronic disease risk and implications for treatment and prevention beyond body weight modification. *Annual Reviews of Nutrition, 25,* 435–468.

Diabetes Research in Children Network Study Group. (2006). The effects of aerobic exercise on glucose and counterregulatory hormone concentrations in children with type 1 diabetes. *Diabetes Care, 29,* 20–25.

Ello-Martin, J. A., Ledikwe, J. H., & Rolls, B. J. (2005). The influence of food portion size and energy density on energy intake: Implications for weight management. *American Journal of Clinical Nutrition, 82*(1 Suppl.), 236S–241S.

Eisenbarth, G. S. (1986). Type 1 diabetes mellitus: A chronic autoimmune disease. *New England Journal of Medicine, 314,* 1360–1368.

Evangelia, Z., Erasmia, K., & Dimitrios, L. (2006). Treatment options of polycystic ovary syndrome in adolescence. *Pediatric Endocrinology Reviews: PER, 3*(Suppl. 1), 208–213.

Fagot-Campagna, A., Pettitt, D. J., Engelgau, M. M., Burrows, N. R., Geiss, L. S., Valdez, R., et al. (2000). Type 2 diabetes among North American children and adolescents: An epidemiologic review and a public health perspective. *Journal of Pediatrics, 136,* 664–672.

Goran, M. I., Ball, G. D., & Cruz, M. L. (2003). Obesity and risk of type 2 diabetes and cardiovascular disease in children and adolescents. *Journal of Clinical Endocrinology and Metabolism, 88,* 1417–1427.

Haller, M. J., Atkinson, M. A., & Schatz, D. (2005). Type 1 diabetes mellitus: Etiology, presentation, and management. *Pediatric Clinics of North America, 52,* 1553–1578.

Hamalainen, A. M., & Knip, M. (2002). Autoimmunity and familial risk of type 1 diabetes. *Current Diabetes Reports, 2,* 347–353.

Hermanns-Lê, T., Scheen, A., & Pierard, G. E. (2004). Acanthosis nigricans associated with insulin resistance: Pathophysiology and management. *American Journal of Clinical Dermatology, 5,* 199–203.

Institute of Medicine. (2005). Panel on Micronutrients, Subcommittees on Upper Reference Levels of Nutrients and of Interpretation and Use of Dietary Reference Intakes, and the Standing Committee on the Scientific Evaluation of Dietary Reference Intakes. Dietary reference intakes for energy, carbohydrates, fiber, fat, protein, and amino acids (macronutrients). Washington, DC: National Academy Press.

International Society for Pediatric and Adolescent Diabetes. (2000). Consensus guidelines for the management of type 1 diabetes mellitus in children and adolescents. Retrieved July 6, 2006, from http://www.diabetesguidelines.com/health/dwk/pro/guidelines/ispad/ispad.asp

Jeffery, R. W., Baxter, J., McGuire, M., & Linde, J. (2006). Are fast food restaurants an environmental risk factor for obesity? Retrieved July 10, 2006, from http://www.ijbnpa.org/content/3/1/2

Karvonen, M., Viik-Kajander, M., Moltchanova, E., Libman, I., LaPorte, R., & Tuomilehto, J. (2000). Incidence of childhood type 1 diabetes worldwide: Diabetes Mondiale (DiaMond) Project Group. *Diabetes Care, 23,* 1516–1526.

Keenan, H., Lipton, R., Zierold, K., Patel, A., Stolte, K., & Chambers, E. (1999). What proportion of diabetes in minority young people is actually type 2? *American Journal of Epidemiology, 149*(Suppl. 2), 11.

Kitagawa, T., Owada, M., Urakami, T., & Yamauchi, K. (1998). Increased incidence of non-insulin dependent diabetes mellitus among Japanese schoolchildren correlates with an increased intake of animal protein and fat. *Clinical Pediatrics, 37,* 111–115.

Ku, C. Y., Gower, B. A., Hunter, G. R., & Goran, M. I. (2000). Racial differences in insulin secretion and sensitivity in prepubertal children: Role of physical fitness and physical activity. *Obesity Research, 8,* 506–515.

LaPorte, R. E. M. M., & Chang, Y.-F. (1995). *Prevalence and Incidence of Insulin-Dependent Diabetes.* Bethesda, MD: National Institutes of Health.

Maffeis, C., Talamini, G., & Tato, L. (1998). Influence of diet, physical activity and parents' obesity on children's adiposity: A four-year longitudinal study. *International Journal of Obesity and Related Metabolic Disorders, 22,* 758–764.

Magarey, A. M., Daniels, L. A., Boulton, T. J., & Cockington, R. A. (2001). Does fat intake predict adiposity in healthy children and adolescents aged 2–15 y? A longitudinal analysis. *European Journal of Clinical Nutrition, 55,* 471–481.

Marr, L. (2004). Soft drinks, childhood overweight, and the role of nutrition educators: Let's base our solutions on reality and sound science. *Journal of Nutrition Education and Behavior, 36,* 258–265.

Meurer, L. N., Kroll, A. P., Jamieson, B., & Yousefi, P. (2006). Clinical inquiries. What is the best way to diagnose polycystic ovarian syndrome? *Journal of Family Practice, 55,* 351–352, 354.

Nassis, G. P., Papantakou, K., Skenderi, K., Triandafillopoulou, M., Kavouras, S. A., Yannakoulia, M., et al. (2005). Aerobic exercise training improves insulin sensitivity without changes in body weight, body fat, adiponectin, and inflammatory markers in overweight and obese girls. *Metabolism, 54,* 1472–1479.

Norris, J. M., Barriga, K., Klingensmith, G., Hoffman, M., Eisenbarth, G. S., Erlich, H. A., et al. (2003). Timing of initial cereal exposure in infancy and risk of islet autoimmunity. *Journal of the American Medical Association, 290,* 1713–1720.

PCOS Consensus Workshop Group. (2004). Revised 2003 consensus on diagnostic criteria and long-term health risks related to polycystic ovary syndrome (PCOS). *Human Reproduction, 19,* 41–47.

Pollock, M. L., Franklin, B. A., Balady, G. J., Chaitman, B. L., Fleg, J. L., Fletcher, B., et al. (2000). Resistance exercise in individuals with and without cardiovascular disease: Benefits, rationale, safety, and prescription. An advisory from the Committee on Exercise, Rehabilitation, and Prevention, Council on Clinical Cardiology, and American Heart Association. Position paper endorsed by the American College of Sports Medicine. *Circulation, 101,* 828–833.

Reaven, G. M., Chen, Y. D., Hollenbeck, C. B., Sheu, W. H., Ostrega, D., & Polonsky, K. S. (1993). Plasma insulin, C-peptide, and proinsulin concentrations in obese and nonobese individuals with varying degrees of glucose intolerance. *Journal of Clinical Endocrinology and Metabolism, 76,* 44–48.

Rodriguez, G., & Moreno, L. A. (2006). Is dietary intake able to explain differences in body fatness in children and adolescents? *Nutrition, Metabolism, and Cardiovascular Diseases, 16,* 294–301.

Saaddine, J. B., Fagot-Campagna, A., Rolka, D., Narayan, K. M., Geiss, L., Eberhardt, M., et al. (2002). Distribution of HbA(1c) levels for children and young adults in the U.S.: Third National Health and Nutrition Examination Survey. *Diabetes Care, 25,* 1326–1330.

Sobngwi, E., Boudou, P., Mauvais-Jarvis, F., Leblanc, H., Velho, G., Vexiau, P., et al. (2003). Effect of a diabetic environment in utero on predisposition to type 2 diabetes. *Lancet, 361,* 1861–1865.

Soliman, A. T., Omar, M., Assem, H. M., Nasr, I. S., Rizk, M. M., El Matary, W., et al. (2002). Serum leptin concentrations in children with type 1 diabetes mellitus: Relationship to body mass index, insulin dose, and glycemic control. *Metabolism, 51,* 292–296.

Steyn, N. P., Mann, J., Bennett, P. H., Temple, N., Zimmet, P., Tuomilehto, J., et al. (2004). Diet, nutrition and the prevention of type 2 diabetes. *Public Health Nutrition, 7,* 147–165.

Strong, W. B., Malina, R. M., Blimkie, C. J., Daniels, S. R., Dishman, R. K., Gutin, B., et al. (2005). Evidence based physical activity for school-age youth. *Journal of Pediatrics, 146,* 732–737.

Tamborlane, W., Fredrickson, L. P., & Ahern, J. H. (2003). Insulin pump therapy in childhood diabetes mellitus. *Treatments in Endocrinology, 2,* 11–21.

Taveras, E. M., Rifas-Shiman, S. L., Berkey, C. S., Rockett, H. R., Field, A. E., Frazier, A. L., et al. (2005). Family dinner and adolescent overweight. *Obesity Research, 13,* 900–906.

Ten, S., & Maclaren, N. (2004). Insulin resistance syndrome in children. *Journal of Clinical Endocrinology and Metabolism, 89,* 2526–2539.

U.S. Department of Agriculture, Department of Health and Human Services. (2005, 2010). Dietary guidelines for Americans. Retrieved July 3, 2009, from http://www.healthierus.gov/dietaryguidelines/

U.S. Department of Health and Human Services, National Diabetes Education Program. (2006). Overview of diabetes in children and adolescents. Retrieved July 3, 2009, from http://ndep.nih.gov/diabetes/pubs/Youth_FactSheet.pdf

Wilkin, T. J., Metcalf, B. S., Murphy, M. J., Kirkby, J., Jeffery, A. N., & Voss, L. D. (2002). The relative contributions of birth weight, weight change, and current weight to insulin resistance in contemporary 5-year-olds: The Early Bird Study. *Diabetes, 51,* 3468–3472.

Williams, D. E., Cadwell, B. L., Cheng, Y. J., Cowie, C. C., Gregg, E. W., Geiss, L. S., et al. (2005). Prevalence of impaired fasting glucose and its relationship with cardiovascular disease risk factors in US adolescents, 1999–2000. *Pediatrics, 116,* 1122–1126.

Xita, N., & Tsatsoulis, A. (2006). Review: Fetal programming of polycystic ovary syndrome by androgen excess: Evidence from experimental, clinical, and genetic association studies. *Journal of Clinical Endocrinology and Metabolism, 91,* 1660–1666.

Ziegler, A. G., Schmid, S., Huber, D., Hummel, M., & Bonifacio, E. (2003). Early infant feeding and risk of developing type 1 diabetes-associated autoantibodies. *Journal of the American Medical Association, 290,* 1721–1728.

Disordered Eating

Agras, W. S., Brandt, H. A., Bulik, C. M., Dolan-Sewell, R., Fairburn, C. G., Halmi, K. A., et al. (2004). Report of the National Institutes of Health workshop on overcoming barriers to treatment research in anorexia nervosa. *International Journal of Eating Disorders, 35,* 509–521.

American Dietetic Association. (2001). Position paper: Nutrition intervention in the treatment of anorexia nervosa, bulimia nervosa, and eating disorders not otherwise specified (EDNOS). *Journal of the American Dietetic Association, 101,* 810–819.

American Psychiatric Association. (2000). *Diagnostic and Statistical Manual of Mental Disorders* (4th ed.). Washington, DC: American Psychiatric Association.

Andersen, A. E. (1999). Gender-related aspects of eating disorders: A guide to practice. *Journal of Gender Specific Medicine, 2,* 47–54.

Becker, A. E., Grinspoon, S. K., Klibanski, A., & Herzog, D. B. (1999). Eating disorders. *New England Journal of Medicine, 340,* 1092–1098.

Birmingham, C. L., Puddicombe, D., & Hlynsky, J. (2004). Hypomagnesemia during refeeding in anorexia nervosa. *Eating and Weight Disorders, 9,* 236–237.

De Souza, M. J., Leidy, H. J., O'Donnell, E., Lasley, B., & Williams, N. I. (2004). Fasting ghrelin levels in physically active women: Relationship with menstrual disturbances and metabolic hormones. *Journal of Clinical Endocrinology and Metabolism, 89,* 3536–3542.

de Zwaan, M., Aslam, Z., & Mitchell, J. E. (2002). Research on energy expenditure in individuals with eating disorders: A review. *International Journal of Eating Disorders, 32,* 127–134.

Fairburn, C. G., & Bohn, K. (2005). Eating disorder NOS (EDNOS): An example of the troublesome "not otherwise specified" (NOS) category in DSM-IV. *Behaviour Research and Therapy, 43,* 691–701.

Fairburn, C. G., & Harrison, P. J. (2003). Eating disorders. *Lancet, 361,* 407–416.

Fisher, M., Simpser, E., & Schneider, M. (2000). Hypophosphatemia secondary to oral refeeding in anorexia nervosa. *International Journal of Eating Disorders, 28,* 181–187.

Goodman, L. R. (2005). The female athlete and menstrual function. *Current Opinion in Obstetrics and Gynecology, 17,* 466–470.

Grinspoon, S. K., Friedman, A. J., Miller, K. K., Lippman, J., Olson, W. H., & Warren, M. P. (2003). Effects of a triphasic combination oral contraceptive containing norgestimate/ethinyl estradiol on biochemical markers of bone metabolism in young women with osteopenia secondary to hypothalamic amenorrhea. *Journal of Clinical Endocrinology and Metabolism, 88,* 3651–3656.

Grinspoon, S., Miller, K., Herzog, D., Clemmons, D., & Klibanski, A. (2003). Effects of recombinant human insulin-like growth factor (IGF)-I and estrogen administration on IGF-I, IGF binding protein (IGFBP)-2, and IGFBP-3 in anorexia nervosa: A randomized-controlled study. *Journal of Clinical Endocrinology and Metabolism, 88,* 1142–1149.

Grinspoon, S., Miller, K. K., Herzog, D. B., Grieco, K. A., & Klibanski, A. (2004). Effects of estrogen and recombinant human insulin-like growth factor-I on ghrelin secretion in severe undernutrition. *Journal of Clinical Endocrinology and Metabolism, 89,* 3988–3993.

Heer, M., Mika, C., Grzella, I., Heussen, N., & Herpertz-Dahlmann, B. (2004). Bone turnover during inpatient nutritional therapy and outpatient follow-up in patients with anorexia nervosa compared with that in healthy control subjects. *American Journal of Clinical Nutrition, 80,* 774–781.

Helgstrand, S., & Andersen, A. M. (2005). Maternal underweight and the risk of spontaneous abortion. *Acta Obstetricia et Gynecologica Scandinavica, 84,* 1197–1201.

Henig, R. M. (2004, November 30). Sorry. Your Eating Disorder Doesn't Meet Our Criteria. *New York Times.*

Kaye, W. H., Frank, G. K., Bailer, U. F., & Henry, S. E. (2005). Neurobiology of anorexia nervosa: Clinical implications of alterations of the function of serotonin and other neuronal systems. *International Journal of Eating Disorders, 37*(Suppl.), S15–S19; discussion S20–S11.

Kaye, W. H., Frank, G. K., Bailer, U. F., Henry, S. E., Meltzer, C. C., Price, J. C., et al. (2005). Serotonin alterations in anorexia and bulimia nervosa: New insights from imaging studies. *Physiology & Behavior, 85,* 73–81.

Keys, A., Brozek, J., Henschel, A., Mickelsen, O., & Taylor, H. L. (1950). *The Biology of Human Starvation I–II.* Minneapolis: University of Minnesota Press.

Klump, K. L., & Gobrogge, K. L. (2005). A review and primer of molecular genetic studies of anorexia nervosa. *International Journal of Eating Disorders, 37*(Suppl.), S43–S48; discussion S87–S49.

Kouba, S., Hallstrom, T., Lindholm, C., & Hirschberg, A. L. (2005). Pregnancy and neonatal outcomes in women with eating disorders. *Obstetrics and Gynecology, 105,* 255–260.

Lask, B. (2004). Pervasive refusal syndrome. *Advances in Psychiatric Treatment, 10*, 153–159.

Miller, K. K., Grieco, K. A., Mulder, J., Grinspoon, S., Mickley, D., Yehezkel, R., et al. (2004). Effects of risedronate on bone density in anorexia nervosa. *Journal of Clinical Endocrinology and Metabolism, 89*, 3903–3906.

Morris, L. G., Stephenson, K. E., Herring, S., & Marti, J. L. (2004). Recurrent acute pancreatitis in anorexia and bulimia. *Journal of the Pancreas, 5*, 231–234.

Rocco, P. L., Orbitello, B., Perini, L., Pera, V., Ciano, R. P., & Balestrieri, M. (2005). Effects of pregnancy on eating attitudes and disorders: A prospective study. *Journal of Psychosomatic Research, 59*, 175–179.

Sanford, T. C., Davidson, M. M., Yakushoko, O. F, Martens, M. P., Hinton, P. S., & Beck, N. C. (2005). Clinical and subclinical eating disorders: An examination of collegiate athletes. *Journal of Applied Sport Psychology, 17*, 79–86.

Stewart, T. M., & Williamson, D. A. (2004). Multidisciplinary treatment of eating disorders. Part 1. Structure and costs of treatment. *Behavior Modification, 28*, 812–830.

Swenne, I. (2000). Heart risk associated with weight loss in anorexia nervosa and eating disorders: Electrocardiographic changes during the early phase of refeeding. *Acta Paediatrica, 89*, 447–452.

Verrotti, A., Catino, M., De Luca, F. A., Morgese, G., & Chiarelli, F. (1999). Eating disorders in adolescents with type 1 diabetes mellitus. *Acta Diabetologica, 36*, 21–25.

Watkins, B. L. B. (2002). Eating disorders in school-aged children. *Child and Adolescent Psychiatric Clinics of North America, 11*, 185–199.

Special Topics in Adult Nutrition: Chronic Disease Nutritional Assessment

Jennifer L. Bueche, PhD, RD, CDN

CHAPTER OUTLINE

Reader Objectives

After studying this chapter and reflecting on the contents, you should be able to

1. Outline the metabolic changes associated with the aging process and their impact on the nutritional requirements of adults throughout adulthood.
2. Refer to the Dietary Reference Intake to determine nutritional requirements for an individual or life stage group (specifically ages 19 to 30, 31 to 50, and 51 to 70).
3. Describe how to perform a nutritional assessment of an adult based on the American Dietetic Association Nutrition Care Process and Model.
4. Identify the chronic diseases in adulthood that are most related to diet, the resulting nutritional implications, and subsequent appropriate medical nutritional therapy.
5. Apply the American Dietetic Association Nutrition Care Process and Model to the case study provided.
6. Discuss the nutritional issues of epidemic proportion in the adult population and the recommended nutrition intervention.

This chapter begins by defining adulthood and outlining the metabolic changes associated with the aging process. These are important issues to understand because the maturation process greatly impacts the dietary recommendation and the nutritional requirements of adults throughout their life as they age. In 1997 the Recommended Daily Allowance (RDA) went through a major overhaul to incorporate not only prevention of disease but promotion of health. The Dietary Reference Intake (DRI) replaced the RDA and has been issued in stages since then (Appendix 2). This information is presented and discussed with regard to the life stage groups (i.e., ages 19 to 30, 31 to 50, and 51 to 70) that span most of the adult years. Next, this chapter reviews the components of the nutritional assessment process and introduces the new American Dietetic Association (ADA) Nutrition Care Process and Model. Given that this textbook takes an evidence-based approach, for each of the chronic diseases presented, the research literature was reviewed to provide evidence-based practice guidelines as they exist related to the four steps in the nutrition care process (nutrition assessment, nutrition diagnosis, nutrition intervention, and/or nutrition monitoring) and evaluation for each particular chronic disease state. In addition, overweight/obesity and osteoporosis have been highlighted given their rise to epidemic proportions in the adult population.

Definition of Adulthood

Adulthood can span 60 years depending on a person's genetic predisposition and the choices a person makes throughout his or her life, including how healthy he or she chooses to eat. Life expectancy in the United States is 77.6 years based on the latest data released in February 2005 by the National Center for Health Statistics, with women still living longer than men (80.1 years versus 74.8 years, respectively) (Kochanek, Murphy, Anderson, & Scott, 2004). Not surprising, given the obesity epidemic in this country and the ensuing health consequences, a potential decline in life expectancy has been predicted in the first half of this century (Olshansky et al., 2005). That is, for the first time in 1,000 years, children today will not live as long as their parents.

In this chapter the adult years are initially broken down into three phases, the young adult years, the middle adult years, and the older adult years, because they coincide with the life stage groups outlined by the DRI (i.e., ages 19 to 30, 31 to 50, and 51 to 70). This makes presenting nutritional requirements across such a large span of years much easier to manage.

Young Adult Years (Ages 19 to 30)

- Typically, growth and maturation are completed by early adulthood, although some males can grow slightly after age 20 (Brown et al., 2005).

- At this point the focus shifts to maintaining health and physical fitness and avoiding weight gain. This may be particularly challenging for college students, especially freshman, given the requirement to purchase an "all you care to eat" dining plan, a lack of involvement in sports because of time constraints, and competing with the net average weight gain of 15 pounds (Kelly, 2003; Levitsky & Youn, 2004).
- Bone density continues to develop until ages 30 to 35.
- Muscle mass continues to grow as long as muscles are used.
- Young adults tend to be very involved in their careers. If they are married with children both parents are juggling the demands of work, family, and day care.
- There are many different definitions of "family." Reproduction may or may not be seen as a priority. According to the latest reports from the Centers for Disease Control and Prevention, in 1970 the average age for a first-time mother was about 21; today that age is 25 to 29 years (Martin et al., 2005).
- Women of reproductive age have special nutrition needs that must be addressed at each stage: before conception, prenatal, and postnatal/lactation.
- Alcohol intake accounts for 5% of calorie intake between ages 20 and 34 (Kant, 2000).
- The **prevalence** of selected chronic conditions for 18- to 24-year-olds based on the top five conditions were asthma (13.7%), chronic joint symptoms (11.1%), sinusitis (8.3%), hay fever (5.7%), and doctor's diagnosis of arthritis (3.5%) (National Center for Health Statistics, 1984–1995).

> **Prevalence:** The percentage of a population that is affected with a particular disease at a given time.

Middle Adult Years (Ages 31 to 50)

- Beginning at about age 30, physiologic functions that impact mobility begin to decline at the rate of about 1% or more per year (Worthington-Roberts, 1996).
- Body composition begins to shift; weight may seem like it is harder to lose. Weight gain usually seen after age 40 in women and men goes hand in hand with hormonal changes and less exercise.
- Hormonal changes in men and women differ:
  - In men, testosterone levels begin to decline around ages 40 to 50, although sperm can fertilize eggs until much later. Decreased sperm production is linked to underweight status; malnutrition is linked to declining libido. National Health and Nutrition Examination Survey data show that as men age their calorie consumption decreases. Weight gain after 40 is more than likely due to less exercise.
  - In women, the reproductive cycle lasts approximately 40 years, with 13 menstrual cycles per year (minus those missed during pregnancy or for other reasons). Birth rates for women aged 35 to 39 are higher than they have ever been. The birth rate for women aged 40 to 44 has gone up more than 51% since 1990 (Martin et al., 2005).
- In 2002–2003 the prevalence of selected chronic conditions for 25- to 44-year-olds were as follows: chronic joint symptoms (17.9%), sinusitis (13.5%), asthma (9.9%), hay fever (9.5%), and doctor's diagnosis of arthritis (9.3%) (National Center for Health Statistics, 1984–1995). Comparing middle-aged adults to young adults, chronic joint symptoms replaced asthma as the top chronic health condition.

Older Adult Years (Ages 51 to 70)

- Typically, adults in this age group have more time to enjoy life with less responsibility in terms of raising children.
- Typically, there is more disposable income as careers are peaking.
- Many older adults enjoy the benefits of eating healthy and exercising. If they are not, it is more than likely because they are dealing with one or more chronic disease(s) (i.e., heart disease or diabetes).
- Muscle mass and strength decrease with age, but exercise can offset this decline (Chin et al., 2001). Lack of exercise results in loss of muscle mass, which in turn decreases overall lean muscle mass, increases body fat, and decreases metabolic rates leading to weight gain.

- The immune system weakens with age, and the ability to fight off infection becomes more and more difficult. This can be further compromised by an inadequate intake of nutrients or underlying chronic disease.
- Posture begins to deteriorate, which could be as a result of lack of exercise and poor muscle tone, bad habits, or bone loss.
- Major changes occur in the ability to taste and smell food. The senses are dulled; thus foods should have stronger smells and flavors to them so they will be more appealing.

- Saliva decreases, gastric secretions decline, and constipation, gas, and bloating can become more of a problem. Often the causes of these problems are incorrectly attributed to certain foods and the diet can become more and more restrictive as perceived intolerances increase.
- According to the latest National Health and Nutrition Examination Survey data, alcohol intake accounts for 3% of calorie intake between ages 51 and 64 (Kant, 2000).
- The prevalence of selected chronic conditions for 45- to 64-year-olds based on the top five conditions were chronic joint symptoms (33.7%), doctor's diagnosis of arthritis (29.5%), hypertension (29.5%), sinusitis (17.5%), and all types of heart disease (12.7%) (National Center for Health Statistics, 1984–1995).

Delaying the onset of disabilities caused by chronic disease in adulthood is referred to as compression of morbidity (Harvard Health Letter, 2002). Perhaps the overall goal should not necessarily be the number of years lived but the number of healthy good-quality years lived.

Nutritional Requirements for the Adult

Combining the tools of nutrition assessment and nutrition research currently available, nutritional requirements for the adult can be determined with confidence. The current Food and Nutrition Board was formed in 1993 and has been working on the DRI, which has been released in stages throughout the past few years. The DRI has become the overarching framework that encompasses four sets of standards: estimated average requirements, RDA, adequate intakes, and tolerable intake levels (upper levels).

Energy

The standard used to express energy needs, called estimated energy requirements, refers to the average needs based on height, age, gender, and activity level to promote weight maintenance. Excess energy consumed is not excreted like most vitamins and minerals; thus it is not desirable to consume excess calories in any form (i.e., protein, carbohydrate, fat, and/or alcohol).

● Learning Point The DRI: Estimated Energy Requirements for Men and Women 30 Years of Age were released in 2002 by the Food and Nutrition Board and allow for adjustment in kilocalories based on age. For each year below age 30, add 7 kcal/day for women and 10 kcal/day for men. For each year above 30, subtract 7 kcal/day for women and 10 kcal/day for men.

It is estimated that energy needs decrease by 6% between the ages of 51 and 74 years, and they decline a further 6% after the age of 74 years (Gary & Fleury, 2002). The doubly labeled water method revolutionized the understanding of energy requirement and energy balance in humans because for the first time this method could be applied to humans, allowing energy requirements and energy balance to be measured. The doubly labeled water method contains two stable isotopes, deuterium oxide and oxygen–18. After administering an oral dose of water labeled with both isotopes (thus the term "doubly labeled water") the deuterium is eliminated from the body as water and the oxygen–18 is eliminated as water and carbon dioxide. Periodic sampling of body water (urine, saliva, and plasma) is taken. The two isotopes are measured for 10 to 14 days, and the difference between the two elimination rates is the measure of carbon dioxide production. Carbon dioxide can then be equated to total energy expenditure (Schoeller, 1999).

It is interesting to note that National Health and Nutrition Examination Survey data on energy consumption indicates that older adults are often below the current RDA recommendation, with men ages 65 to 74 years consuming on average 1,800 kcal/day and women ages 65 to 74 years consuming on average between 1,300 and 1,600 kcal/day (Committee on Nutrition Services for Medicare Beneficiaries and Institute of Medicine, 2000).

Macronutrients

Protein recommendations are based on the RDA for protein (0.8 g protein/kg body weight) listed on the DRI based on a reference weight for each life stage group. The amount of protein recommended for women is the same for all three life stages (i.e., ages 19 to 30, 31 to 50, and 51 to 70) and is 46 g/day. For men the recommended amount of protein for all three life stages is 56 g/day.

The DRI for carbohydrate is based on the RDA, which is 130 g for both men and women for all three life stages. This amount is based on the lowest amount of glucose needed daily for normal brain function. An eating plan that simply meets the RDA for carbohydrates may be inadequate for other nutrients and fiber. In people over age 65, fasting blood glucose rises to a mean of 140 mg/dL, resulting in an increased **incidence** of non–insulin-dependent diabetes, which can be attributed to age, obesity, and decreased physical activity level. Thus, recommendations regarding amount and distribution of carbohydrate must be individualized at this point

Incidence: Rate of occurrence.

The grams of fat per day are not determinable but rather are recommended in terms of acceptable macronutrient distribution ranges. The acceptable macronutrient distribution ranges for fat are 20% to 35% kcal energy/day, for carbohydrate are 45% to 65% kcal energy/day, and for protein are 10% to 35% kcal energy/day. These recommendations meet the needs of nearly 98% of all healthy individuals of similar age and gender based on each life stage group.

Micronutrients

Most vitamin and mineral requirements for healthy people remain the same as they move throughout each life stage group. Micronutrient status changes with age for vitamin D, vitamin B_{12}, and calcium related to the decline in absorption, use, or activation of these nutrients. As people age they can become deficient in vitamin D for a number of reasons, such as their skin is less able to take up vitamin D from the blood, their skin is unable to make vitamin D when exposed to sunlight, they spend less time outdoors, and when outdoors they are more likely to protect themselves from the sun (Hanley & Davison, 2005). The adequate intake for vitamin D for adults aged 51 to 70 is 10 mg, as compared with 5 mg for adults ages 19 to 30 and 31 to 50.

Calcium needs increase with age for men and women to compensate for bone loss. Calcium recommendations increase by 200 mg/day for 51- to 70-year-olds. This increase compensates for the loss of ability to absorb calcium from the diet because of the loss of vitamin D receptors in the gut. Increased fiber reduces calcium absorption, as does gastrointestinal distress or inflammation. Vitamin B_{12} needs increase after the age of 50 because about 10% to 30% of older people may poorly absorb food-bound vitamin B_{12} because of reduced acid production by the stomach.

Almost one-third of all older individuals have been observed to have deficiencies of vitamins and trace elements (Russell, 1997). The need for iron is increased to 18 mg/day for women aged 19 to 50 years to make up for iron lost during menstrual blood loss. After menopause, iron requirements decrease to 8 mg/day because of the cessation of the menstrual cycle.

Water

Often overlooked as a nutrient, water should be considered one of the most important nutrients because you can survive only days without it compared with weeks or months without food (Mahan, 2004). The DRI recommendations are based on adequate intakes for generally healthy individuals who are adequately hydrated. It is well known that water requirements vary from individual to individual. Water recommendations take into consideration water from all sources, including all beverages and food. The water content of many foods is quite high (i.e., an apple is 84% water). Moisture in foods can contribute 20%

of the total water intake. For healthy men the recommendation of 3.7 L/day of water is the same for all three life stage groups. For healthy women the recommendation of 2.7 L/day of water is the same for all three life stage groups. No upper level has been set for water because of a lack of suitable data; however, caution is warranted in consuming levels above the recommended intakes. The RDA for an adult is approximately 1 mL water/kcal expended as long as kilocalorie needs are met (Food and Nutrition Board, National Research Council, & National Academy of Sciences, 1989).

Two other methods exist for determining water requirements in the clinical setting. The first method estimates fluid requirements starting with 100 mL/kg for the first 10 kg of body weight. For the second 10 kg of body weight another 50 mL/kg of water is added. For the remaining body weight 20 mL/kg is used if the person is less than 50 years old, and 15 mL/kg is used if the person is older than 50 years. The second method is expressed in mL/kg based on age: 40 mL/kg, 15 to 30 years old; 35 mL/kg, 25 to 55 years old; 30 mL/kg, 44 to 65 years old; and 25 mL/kg, more than 65 years old.

Fiber

Fiber recommendations, based on the average daily dietary fiber recommendations for 2002 (adequate intake), are 25 g for women (ages 19 to 50) and 38 g for men (ages 19 to 50) or 14 g of dietary fiber per 1,000 kcal. For women and men ages 51 to 70, average daily dietary fiber recommendations for 2002 (adequate intake) are 21 g and 28 g of fiber, respectively, per day. Daily median intakes are 12.1 to 13.8 g for women and 16.5 to 19.5 for men (Brown et al., 2005).

Nutritional Assessment in Chronic Disease

A relation between nutrition and overall health and the prevention of chronic disease has been well documented (Public Health Service, 1988; Food and Nutrition Board, Committee on Diet and Health, & National Research Council, 1989). In the adult years nutrition plays an important role in maintaining wellness and reducing risk of chronic disease. According to the Healthy People 2010 report issued by the U.S. Department of Health and Human Services, nutrition is one of the many factors affecting health and longevity of older people. This is especially true for older people who are minorities and of low income (U.S. Department of Health and Human Services, 2000). It is estimated that up to 60% of older people admitted to the hospital have protein energy malnutrition on admission or their nutritional status becomes compromised while hospitalized (Gallagher-Allred, Voss, Finn, & McCamish, 1996; Berry & Braunschwig, 1998; Gary & Fleury, 2002).

The physiologic changes in the adult and the assessment of energy expenditure in adults with chronic disease, two important knowledge and skill areas, are reviewed first before the discussion of nutrition assessment in chronic disease; that section follows below.

Physiologic Changes in the Adult: Nutritional Implications

Eighty-five percent of older adults have one or more nutrition-related problems (ADA, 2000). The most common are obesity, diabetes, cardiovascular disease, hypertension, arthritis, osteoporosis, and malnutrition. Many of these disorders put people at nutritional risk. Two major metabolic changes occur as people age. There is a decrease in lean body mass, with a 10% decrease in lean body mass from ages 25 to 60 years, another 10% decrease from ages 60 to 75 years, and another 20% to 25% decrease after age 75 (Chin et al., 2001). Basal metabolic rate also decreases with age and in response to the decrease in lean muscle mass and increase in adipose tissues. The challenge then becomes to make sure that nutrient needs are met with declining kilocalorie needs while maintaining weight. **Table 9.1** summarizes the numerous physiologic changes experienced by adults as they age. These physiologic changes individually or cumulatively over time could negatively impact overall nutritional health.

RDAs and related standards apply only to healthy people, but many older people may not be healthy, especially those with a chronic disease. In addition, many older people take medications that may negatively impact specific nutrients. The use of a supplement to help meet vitamin D, vitamin B_{12}, and calcium needs may be beneficial for older people who require such a low energy intake that they are not able to consume enough nutrient-dense foods to meet their requirements. Certain conditions that are more prevalent with age increase the need for specific vitamins and minerals. Some examples include decrease in immune function (increased need for vitamin B_6, vitamin E, and zinc), increased gastric pH (increases need for vitamin B_{12}, folic acid, calcium, iron, and zinc), and increase in oxidative stress (increases need for beta-carotene, vitamin C, and vitamin E) (Wardlaw, Hampl, & DiSilvestro, 2004). In fact, because of these conditions a balanced multivitamin and mineral supplement is recommended for all older adults by many nutrition experts.

Assessment of Energy Needs in Adults with Chronic Disease

The assessment of energy needs can be measured in a number of ways. Indirect calorimetry is a method for estimating energy production by measuring O_2 consumption and CO_2 production at a specific point in time, accurately determining resting metabolic rate (Mahan, 2004). Devices such as the Douglas bag or metabolic cart are the most useful in measuring resting metabolic rate. Indirect calorimetry data, such as the respiratory quotient, tell clinicians the net substrate oxidation of fat, carbohydrate, and protein, allowing for precise changes in nutrition support when necessary (Brandi & Calafa, 1997). New technology allows the production of smaller, handheld versions of the larger, costly, less accessible models. Indirect calorimetry, although still used, is not used as a routine assessment of energy expenditure in clinical dietetic practice. Assessment of energy needs is most often determined by using energy prediction equations, because they are practical and their accuracy rate is enough to provide a starting point in which adjustments (increases or decreases) can be made based on the patient's metabolic response to total kilocalories and diet composition provided. The following equations are currently used in clinical practice to determine energy needs:

TABLE 9.1	Physiologic Changes Experienced with Aging

Decline in dental health
Reduced thirst sensation
Fall in gastrointestinal function
Changes in liver, gallbladder, and pancreatic function
Decline in kidney function
Reduced immune function
Reduced lung function
Reduced hearing and vision
Reduced cardiovascular health

TABLE 9.2	Harris-Benedict Equation

Men: BEE = 66.47 + 13.75 (wt in kg) + 5 (ht in cm) − 6.76 (age in yr)
Women: BEE = 655.1 + 9.56 (wt in kg) + 1.85 (ht in cm) − 4.68 (age in yr)

- Harris-Benedict equation (refer to **Table 9.2**): Harris and Benedict conducted a study in which 239 subjects (aged 15 to 74 years) had their basal metabolic rates measured. By today's standards these measurements would be referred to as resting metabolic rates. The Harris-Benedict equation was derived from this study and is still used today. It is well known, however, that the Harris-Benedict equation can overestimate energy needs by as much as 20% to 30%, with an accuracy rate of 69% (Frankenfield, Roth-Yousey, & Compher, 2005).
- Mifflin–St. Jeor equation: Body composition has changed a great deal since 1919 when the Harris-Benedict equation first was derived. The Mifflin–St. Jeor equation was developed in 1990 and has been shown to report resting metabolic rate 82% of the time in nonobese adults. The Mifflin–St. Jeor equation has an overestimation error of 15% and an underestimation error of 18%. Once resting metabolic rate is calculated, it is then multiplied by activity or injury and stress factors to determine the total energy required.
- Ireton-Jones equation: The Ireton-Jones equation provides estimated energy expenditure for hospitalized and critically ill patients who either are breathing spontaneously or are ventilator dependent. This equation takes into account age, weight (kg), and gender. The equation adjusts for trauma, burns, and/or obesity. The obesity adjustment should be used when the patient weighs more than 130% of his or her ideal body weight or has a **body mass index (BMI)** above 27 (Ireton-Jones, 1997).

Body mass index (BMI): Calculated by dividing weight in kilograms by height in meters squared (BMI 5 kg/m^2); shown in the research literature to be correlated with adiposity and increased risk of chronic disease.

Depending on the illness, calorie needs can rise substantially in the hospitalized patient. For this reason, it is critically important to assess the energy needs of each patient individually (Klipstein-Grobusch, Reilly, Potter, Edwards, & Roberts, 1995).

Nutritional Care Process and Model

Before the adoption of the ADA's final version of the Nutrition Care Process and Model, no standardized nutrition care process existed. Dietetic professionals strongly supported a standardized nutrition care process for use by registered dietitians and dietetic technicians because this standardized process would in effect promote the dietetic professional as the unique provider of nutrition care and enhance the practice of dietetics by improving outcomes and showing the value of dietetic services (Lacey, 2003).

Two very important systems that are not considered part of the Nutrition Care and Process Model but are critically important are the screening and referral system and the outcomes management system. Nutritional screening is not required to be done by a dietetic professional (a registered dietitian or dietetic technician); however, the process depends on accurate and timely nutritional screening. It is critical that the nutritional screening process be monitored and evaluated as part of the outcomes management system to ensure that those who are at nutritional risk are identified. The outcomes management system allows data to be collected and analyzed to determine where changes need to be made to improve overall quality of nutritional care provided.

It is important to distinguish between standardized process and standardized care. The Nutritional Care Process and Model does not attempt to standardize care (i.e., giving all patients the same care). Nutritional care still must be individualized. What the Nutritional Care Process and Model does do is provide a framework or guide based on a series of connected steps or actions in which nutrition care is provided. In a nutshell, the Nutritional Care Process and Model can be defined as "a systematic problem-solving method that dietetics professionals use to critically think and make decisions to address nutrition related problems and provide safe and effective quality nutrition care" (Lacey, 2003).

There are four steps in the nutrition care process: (1) nutrition assessment, (2) nutrition diagnosis, (3) nutrition intervention, and (4) nutrition monitoring and evaluation. There is a difference between medical nutrition therapy and the nutrition care process. Medical nutrition therapy (MNT) was redefined as part of the 2001 Medicare benefit legislation as "nutritional diagnostic, therapy, and counseling services for the purpose of disease management, which are furnished by a registered dietitian or nutrition professional" (Smith, 2003). Medical nutrition therapy is only one type of nutrition care. The Nutritional Care Process and Model is broader in scope and guides nutrition education and other preventative nutrition services.

Evidence-based practice is needed to determine which practices support outcomes (Myers, Pritchett, & Johnson, 2002). The government is looking to evidence-based practice as a way to improve the quality of medical care provided to patients while managing the rising costs of an overburdened nearly dysfunctional health care system (Smith, 2003). By applying evidence-based practice as a part of the Nutrition Care Process and Model, practitioners and educators can apply the best research knowledge to dietetics practice. Demonstrating the science behind dietary recommendation and validating nutritional assessment tools utilizing evidence-based analysis to further dietetics practice would strengthen the profession. The ADA has begun this process and has created evidence-based nutrition practice guidelines for numerous topic areas that can be accessed free by all ADA members through the Evidence Analysis Library on the ADA website (www.eatright.org).

Nutritional Assessment in Chronic Diseases

In this section we review the following chronic diseases: cardiovascular disease (coronary heart disease and cerebrovascular disease), cancer, chronic obstructive pulmonary disease (COPD), diabetes, chronic kidney disease, and HIV/AIDS. For each chronic disease reviewed, disease-specific considerations are addressed when conducting a nutritional assessment. Evidence analysis for evidence-based practice is presented for each chronic disease based on a thorough review of the current literature.

Cardiovascular Disease

Cardiovascular disease affects more than 13 million Americans and is still the number-one leading cause of death in the United States (Kochanek et al., 2004). Cardiovascular disease is a broad term that encompasses a number of conditions, such as coronary heart disease (often called heart disease), stroke, and any other conditions that affect the structure or function of the heart. If the heart does not receive adequate blood, the heart becomes starved of oxygen and the vital nutrients it needs to work properly. This could result in unstable angina (chest pain), damage to the heart muscle, and/or myocardial infarction; the severity and progression depends on the degree of blockage.

Symptoms are highly variable from person to person, more so when comparing symptoms for men versus women. Treatment for coronary artery disease involves an assessment of risk factors for determination of appropriate intervention as outlined by the latest report issued by the National Cholesterol Education Program (NCEP) Adult Treatment Panel III report recommendations (NCEP, 2001; National Heart, Lung, and Blood Institute & National Institutes of Health, 2002).

Nutritional Assessment in Coronary Heart Disease

Nutritional assessment should include evaluation of the following:

- Excess weight for height: BMI > 25 (overweight), BMI > 30 (obese)
- Excess abdominal fat: waist circumference of 35 inches for females, 40 inches or more for males, or waist-to-hip ratio of less than 0.8 for women and less than 1.0 for men
- Evidence of **hypertension** (blood pressure >140/90 mm Hg)
- Complete lipid profile, fasting preferred (total cholesterol, low-density lipoprotein and **high-density lipoprotein** cholesterol)
- Nonfasting total cholesterol, high-density lipoprotein if complete fasting lipid profile unavailable (proceed to lipoprotein profile if total cholesterol ≥ 200 mg/dL or high-density lipoprotein < 40 mg/dL)
- Plasma apolipoprotein B (an atherogenic lipoprotein)
- **Homocysteine** levels
- Evidence of diabetes, fasting blood sugar levels
- Evidence of atherogenic diet: evaluate dietary intake (saturated fat and trans-fatty acid intake, omega-3 fatty acid intake; overall diet quality particularly with regard to intake of fruits, vegetables, and whole grains)
- Physical activity level
- Smoking, tobacco use
- Family history of premature coronary heart disease
- Gender
- Age (men 45 years, women ≥ 55 years)

Hypertension: Systolic blood pressure above 140 mm Hg or diastolic blood pressure above 90 mm Hg.

High-density lipoproteins: Often referred to as "good cholesterol," these lipoproteins contain mostly protein with less cholesterol and triglyceride. High levels of high-density lipoproteins in the blood are associated with a decreased risk of coronary heart disease risk.

Homocysteine: An amino acid that can be measured in the blood and has been shown to be an independent risk factor for cardiovascular disease.

Evidence Analysis for Evidence-Based Practice in Coronary Heart Disease

The original NCEP guidelines followed the recommendations of the American Heart Association's Step I and Step II diets (NCEP, 1988). The new NCEP guidelines released in 2002 are evidence-based guidelines that result in reduction of low-density lipoprotein cholesterol levels and reduced risk of coronary heart disease (National Heart, Lung, and Blood Institute, & National Institutes of Health, 2002). The Therapeutic Lifestyle Changes diet lowers saturated fat and cholesterol intakes to levels of the previous Step II American Heart Association diet **(Table 9.3)**. If lipid levels are not achieved initially, plant stanols/sterols (2 g/day) and viscous (soluble) fiber (10 to 25 g/day), known to have low-density lipoprotein lipid-lowering effects, may be added to the diet.

The new NCEP Adult Treatment Panel III guidelines increase the emphasis on weight management and physical activity:

- Consume less than 200 mg of dietary cholesterol per day.
- Limit sodium intake to less than 2,400 mg a day.

TABLE 9.3 Therapeutic Lifestyle Changes Diet Guidelines

Food Group	Number of Servings	Serving Size
Lean meat, fish, poultry, and dry beans	No more than 6 oz/day	6 ounces maximum per day lean meat, poultry, and fish ½ cup cooked dry peas or beans ½ cup tofu
Eggs	No more than four yolks a week	Two egg whites = 1 whole egg in recipes
Egg substitute/egg whites	Unlimited	
Low-fat milk, yogurt, and cheese	2–3	1 cup fat-free or 1% milk 1 cup nonfat or low-fat yogurt 1 ounce of low-fat or fat-free cheese (≤3 g of fat in 1 ounce)
Fats and oils	No more than 6–8	1 teaspoon soft margarine or vegetable oil 1 tablespoon salad dressing 1 ounce nuts
Fruits	2–4	1 piece of fruit ½ cup diced fruit ¾ cup juice
Vegetables	3–5	1 cup leafy or raw ½ cup cooked ¾ cup juice
Breads, cereals, pasta, rice, and other grains	6–11	1 slice of bread ½ bun, bagel, or muffin 1 ounce dry cereal ½ cup cooked cereal, potatoes, pasta, rice, or other grains
Sweets and snacks	Now and then	

Adapted from the National Cholesterol Education Program (Adult Treatment Panel III). Serving sizes are based on the USDA's MyPyramid.

- Eat 25% to 35% or less of the day's total calories from fat.
- Consume less than 7% of the day's total calories from saturated fat.
- Eat just enough calories to achieve or maintain a healthy weight and reduce your blood cholesterol levels.
- The recommendations for cholesterol and sodium are the same for everyone on the Therapeutic Lifestyle Changes diet, regardless of caloric intake.
- The recommendations for saturated fat and total fat are based on the percentage of calories consumed and vary with intake.

Cholesterol-lowering medications may be necessary if diet alone does not adequately lower levels.

Cerebrovascular disease, or stroke, strikes about 700,000 Americans each year, although most survive, bringing the number of stroke survivors to close to 5 million who are managing their health today (http://www.webmd.com/diseases_and _conditions/stroke.htm). There are two types of stroke: ischemic and hemorrhagic. An ischemic stroke is caused by a blood clot that blocks the supply of blood to the brain. Most often this is due to atherosclerosis, which is caused by high blood pressure, diabetes, high cholesterol, or a combination of the three. Blood flow can also be interrupted by low blood pressure (hypotension), which may be a result of a heart attack, blood loss, or a severe infection. Clots can also break free as a result of procedure or surgery and cause a stroke. A hemorrhagic stroke is the result of bleeding in or around the brain as a result most often of a ruptured blood vessel or uncontrolled blood pressure.

Nutritional Assessment in Cerebrovascular Disease

Generally, the nutritional assessment for cerebrovascular disease is the same as that for coronary heart disease except that a patient's functional status needs to be determined, especially as it relates to his or her ability to meet nutritional needs orally. **Table 9.4** shows the recommended intakes of total fat and saturated fat.

TABLE 9.4	Maximum Daily Intake of Fat and Saturated Fatty Acid							
	Calorie Level							
	1,600	1,800	2,000	2,200	2,400	2,600	2,800	3,000
Total fat, g	44–62	50–70	56–78	61–86	67–93	72–101	78–109	83–117
Saturated fat, g	12	14	16	17	19	20	22	23

Recommended intake of total fat 25% to 35% and saturated fat < 7%.
(From the National Cholesterol Education Program (Adult Treatment Panel III).

Evidence Analysis for Evidence-Based Practice in Cerebrovascular Disease

Given the fact that evidence has already been presented above for the treatment of coronary heart disease (with the underlying cause of atherosclerosis), the focus here is on the evidence available to support prevention and control of hypertension, the other major underlying cause of strokes. The Trials of Hypertension Prevention and the Dietary Approaches to Stop Hypertension studies clearly demonstrated that dietary intervention prevented hypertension or lowered blood pressure in persons with high to normal blood pressure (Appel et al., 1997; Trials of Hypertension Prevention Collaborative Research Group, 1997). The Dietary Approaches to Stop Hypertension diet is used to prevent and control blood pressure and is based on a "heart healthy" diet with twice the average daily consumption of fruits and vegetables (available at http://www.nhlbi.nih.gov/health/public/heart/hbp/dash/new_dash.pdf).

Cancer

Cancer is a group of related diseases in which damage to the DNA of the cells causes uncontrolled growth and spread of abnormal cells. This abnormal cellular growth can have an effect on any one part of the body (breast, skin, lungs) or the whole body (**metastases**). Cancer is the second leading cause of death in the United States, with 1.2 million new cases diagnosed annually and nearly 9 million Americans with a history of cancer (Nutrition Screening Initiative, 2002; Kochanek et al., 2004). Given the fact that 35% of all cancers are diet related, cancer prevention depends to a large degree on the overall quality of diet and the ability to maintain a healthy weight.

Metastasis: Growth of malignant tissue that spreads to surrounding tissues or organs.

Nutritional Assessment

One of the most important markers of nutritional status is assessment of body weight, which can be represented by an unplanned weight loss or a BMI less than 22, a serum albumin less than 3.5, or a cholesterol level less than 150 mg/dL. The diet history is evaluated to determine adequacy of caloric intake and overall diet quality, especially with regard to protein and vitamin and mineral intake. Particular attention is paid to the use of vitamins and minerals and complementary and alternative therapies.

Evidence Analysis for Evidence-Based Practice

The main nutrition goal is to prevent or reverse nutrient deficiencies, to preserve lean body mass, to minimize nutrition-related side effects, and to maximize the quality of life. The role of nutrition is vitally important in the treatment of cancer patients. Much time is spent dealing with the common nutrition problems that occur as a result of the disease, treatment, or both. Common nutrition problems include anorexia/cachexia, nausea, vomiting, mucositis, esophagitis, xerostomia, dysgeusia, hypogeusia, diarrhea, and constipation. Recommendations for dealing with common nutrition problems are outlined in **Table 9.5**.

TABLE 9.5	Strategies to Improve Intake in Cancer Patients

Strategies to address anorexia/cachexia:
- Identify factors contributing to poor appetite.
- Keep high calorie/high protein foods/liquids on hand for when appetite is good:
  - Milkshakes, Carnation Instant Breakfast, peanut butter, fruited yogurt
- Discourage intake of high-fiber foods that can cause early satiety.
- Appetite stimulant if anorexia is longstanding or other strategies fail to improve condition

Strategies to address nausea
- Sip liquids at frequent intervals separately from solid foods to maintain hydration.
- Discourage fasting because it may cause hypoglycemia and increase nausea.
- Cold or room temperature foods may be better tolerated.
- Avoid high-fat, high-fiber, spicy, or gas-producing foods that may be poorly tolerated.

Strategies to address vomiting:
- Encourage adequate fluids to prevent dehydration.
- Start with low-fat fluids and advance as tolerated.
- Introduce dry starchy foods first when advancing.
- Introduce high-fiber and high-fat foods last.
- Avoid eating 1½ to 2 hours pre- and posttreatment.

Strategies to Address Mucositis:
- Encourage good oral hygiene practices.
- Use oral baking soda rinse:
  - 1 mL of baking soda to 250 mL of water
- Soft, moist, semisolid, or blended foods may be tolerated better than rough/crisp foods.
- Discourage intake of known irritants:
  - Tart or acidic foods, spicy or salty foods, very hot or cold foods, tobacco, alcohol, and alcohol-based items
- Recommend dunking or moistening dry foods:
  - Order extra gravy on trays.
- Alter temperature and consistency to individual tolerances.
- Reinforce use of analgesics as prescribed before meals to reduce pain associated with eating.

Strategies to address esophagitis:
- Same as strategies for mucositis plus the following:
  - Suggest the use of local anesthetic and analgesic before meals.
  - In cases of peptic esophagitis, antireflux and antacid therapy may be helpful.
  - Recommend regular antacids before and 1 hour after meals and before bed.

Strategies to address thick saliva/mucus:

- Beverages or foods that are slightly tart or carbonated may help to thin secretions.
- If milk products are found to affect mucus try soy-based items (such as soy milk) for tolerance.
- Mucous production may be minimized if clear fluids are consumed after milk products.
- Limit caffeine, alcohol, and spicy foods.
- Encourage a mouth rinse throughout the day.

Strategies to address xerostomia:
- Increased liquid consumption may provide symptomatic relief; however, liquids have no lubricating properties.
- Encourage consumption of foods such as gravies, sauces, and salad dressings (Italian).
- Mint or tart sugar-free gum/candy may stimulate saliva production.
- Discourage commercial mouthwashes and alcohol because they contribute to dryness.
- Citric-acid-containing beverages such as lemonade, orange-flavored soft drinks, frozen juice bars, and sherbets may help increase secretions.
- Recommend sugar-free or diet products to reduce the risk of dental decay and mouth infection.

Strategies to address dysgeusia:
- Determine specific taste or smell changes.
- Encourage fluids with meals to decrease unpleasant tastes.
- Reinforce proper oral care before and between meals.
- Tart foods can stimulate taste buds.
- Suggest mild-tasting foods such as biscuits, milk, pudding, and custards.
- If meat tastes bitter or metallic:
  - Serve meat cold or at room temperature.
  - Include meat in mixed dishes like casseroles.
  - Choose alternative protein sources from dairy group: cottage cheese, yogurt, custard.
  - Try tofu or eggs.
  - Marinate foods in pineapple or lime juice, vinegar, wine, or sweet and sour sauce.
  - Eat with plastic utensils in place of metal ones.
  - Cinnamon or sugar-free gum or mints may help mask the metallic taste.

Strategies to address hypogeusia:
- Reinforce proper oral care.
- Encourage experimenting with strong flavors and seasonings.
- Encourage liberal intake of "treats" or comfort foods.
- Emphasize a variety in colors and textures in a meal to encourage eating.

Strategies to address diarrhea:
- When appropriate use antidiarrheal agents as prescribed by physician first to avoid dietary limitations.
- Encourage energy-dense fluids to match output.
- Encourage potassium-rich foods.
- Try the following modifications one at a time to determine effectiveness:
  - Limit bowel stimulants (e.g., caffeine, alcohol, prunes).
  - Adjust fat intake as tolerated.
  - Restrict lactose.
  - Restrict fiber intake.
  - Limit gas-producing foods.
  - Limit foods or fluids that exacerbate symptoms (e.g., spices).

Strategies to address constipation:
- Encourage intake of naturally laxative foods such as prunes, rhubarb, papaya, and mango.
- Encourage physical activity as able.
- Advise the use of a bulk-forming laxative and reinforce the importance of adequate fluid intake.
- Daily use of stool softeners as necessary

Information adapted from the American Institute for Cancer Research (www.aicr.org)

Cancer cachexia: Irreversible weight loss (body fat and muscle stores) that accompanies advanced cancer despite adequate nutritional intake.

Nutritional recommendations for energy are highly variable and must be individualized. Protein requirements range from 1.2 to 2.0, with average protein requirements at 1.5 g/kg. Energy requirements are typically 25 to 30 kcal/kg or, if using an energy prediction equation, use an injury factor of 1.3 to 1.5 (Mahan, 2004). Patients with **cancer cachexia** exhibit a syndrome of irreversible weight loss, anorexia, asthenia, anemia, and abnormalities in protein, fat, and carbohydrate metabolism. This "wasting" is similar to what is experienced by patients with sepsis and inflammation (Mahan, 2004).

Alterations occur in glucose, protein, and lipid metabolism because of the metabolic demands of the cancerous tumor(s). Tumors exert a constant demand for glucose and amino acids. To keep up with this constant need for glucose, gluconeogenesis and lipolysis occur at a high rate at the expense of skeletal muscle and adipose tissue as the fuel source. Catabolism can be so great that visceral organ and other body proteins (albumin) are affected.

Antitumor therapy, such as chemotherapy, radiation, surgery, or immunotherapy, can contribute to nutritional alterations in patients by interfering with their ability to ingest, digest, and absorb adequately. Ideally, early intervention is the key to minimize weight loss and to prevent or correct nutritional deficiencies as soon as possible and if at all possible.

Chronic Obstructive Pulmonary Disease

COPD is a slow progressive obstruction of the airways of the lung. COPD affects more than 16 million Americans and is the fourth leading cause of death in the United States (Nutrition Screening Initiative, 2002; Kochanek et al., 2004). There are two categories of patients with COPD. Type 1, or emphysema, is seen in older patients who are thin and cachectic, with cor pulmonale that develops late in course. **Cor pulmonale** is a medical term used to describe enlargement and failure of the right side of the heart due to pulmonary hypertension from prolonged high blood pressure in the arteries or veins of the lungs. Type 2, or chronic bronchitis, is seen in patients with normal weight or excessive weight and prominent hypoxemia in which cor pulmonale develops early in the course of the disease.

Cor pulmonale: A heart condition characterized by enlargement of the right side of the heart (right ventricle) and failure due to pulmonary hypertension.

Nutritional Assessment

It is well known that the maintenance of a well-nourished nutritional state plays a key role in maintaining ventilatory muscle strength, improved immune response, and reduced risk of respiratory mortality (Whittaker, Ryan, Buckle, & Road, 1990; Rogers, Donahoe, & Constantino, 1992; Gray-Donald, Gibbson, Shapiro, Macklern, & Martin, 1996). Malnutrition, however, is common among patients with COPD (Schols, Mostert, Soester, Greve, & Wouters, 1989; Laaban et al., 1993). Given the degree of malnutrition in the COPD population, Thorsdottir, Gunnarsdottir, and Eriksen (2001) conducted a study to evaluate and develop a screening method for detecting malnutrition in patients with COPD based on previously published work by Elmore et al. (1994) and refinement of their previously published general screening tool (Thorsdottir, Eriksen, & Eysteinsdottir, 1999). Serum albumin, total lymphocyte count, BMI, and triceps skinfold thickness were sensitive measures in the identification of malnutrition. Triceps skinfold thickness and BMI were shown to be the best single parameters for detecting malnutrition, but neither one individually or together equaled the quality of the screening tool using the four-point criteria. Results of the study confirmed that patients with COPD are frequently malnourished and that the screening tool developed could identify 69% of malnourished patients.

In a study conducted by Soler-Cataluna et al. (2005), muscle mass depletion was estimated indirectly by determining the midarm muscle area (of the nondominant arm) and was determined to be a better predictor of mortality than BMI in COPD patients. This has important implications for nutritional screening given the obesity epidemic in this country because normal and overweight patients show muscle mass depletion (Schols, Soeters, et al., 1993). Adequacy of dietary intake and vitamins and minerals also needs to be addressed.

Evidence Analysis for Evidence-Based Practice

Identifying and correcting malnutrition is the main goal when working with patients with COPD. Energy needs are increased; however, changes must be made in balance. A balanced protein-to-fat-to-carbohydrate ratio (15% to 20%:30% to 45%:40% to 55% of calories) is needed to preserve the respiratory quotient. Patients' nutritional needs should be assessed on an individual basis; however, a study conducted by Thorsdottir and Gunnarsdottir (2002) recommended energy intakes to be above 140% of basal energy expenditure and protein consumption to be at least 1.2 g/kg body weight to avoid protein losses, prevent weight loss, and prevent worsening nutritional status.

Deficiency in lung elasticity and respiratory muscle results in hypoproteinemia and in calcium, magnesium, phosphorus, vitamin K, and vitamin C deficiencies. Intakes based on DRI should be provided, with magnesium and phosphorus levels monitored for patients receiving aggressive nutritional support. Increased vitamin D and vitamin K may be warranted based on results of **bone mineral density** tests, glucocorticoid medications, and adequacy of intake (Mahan, 2004). Lung function has been shown to be better when higher antioxidant levels are given (Hu & Cassano, 2000).

> **Bone mineral density:** A measurement of bone mass after development is complete; reported in grams per centimeter squared.

Diabetes

Diabetes is a serious chronic disease characterized by abnormalities in the metabolism of cholesterol, protein, and fat. The incidence of type 2 diabetes is tracking right along with the obesity epidemic and is fueling the diabetes epidemic (Cowie et al., 2003). Glucose intolerance or hyperglycemia is the common denominator, and the body does not produce or respond to insulin. Insulin is a hormone produced by the B cells of the pancreas, and it is the key that "unlocks" the cells so that the cell can then utilize glucose as a fuel source. Diabetes affects 16 million people, with more than 5 million undiagnosed; it is the sixth leading cause of death (Nutrition Screening Initiative, 2002; Kochanek et al., 2004). The three major forms of diabetes are type 1, type 2, and gestational diabetes, of which type 2 accounts for 90% to 95% of all cases.

> **Insulin resistance:** An impaired biological response to either exogenous or endogenous insulin; plays a role in the etiology of type 2 diabetes.

Nutritional Assessment

A body weight assessment should be conducted (i.e., assessment of height, weight, BMI, and waist circumference). Waist circumference more than 40 inches for men and more than 35 inches for women has been shown to increase **insulin resistance** (Centers for Disease Control and Prevention, 2002). Blood pressure should be checked to determine whether a patient is hypertensive as well (at least 140/90 mm Hg). Laboratory work should be reviewed and evaluated based on the following: hemoglobin A_{Ic} or **glycosylated hemoglobin (HbA$_{Ic}$)**, fasting glucose, urinary glucose or ketones, blood urea nitrogen, creatine, potassium, sodium, alanine and aspartate aminotransferases, lactic acid dehydrogenase, and lipid profile. Clinical signs of malnutrition and poor control need to be recognized and addressed. Adequacy of intake and compliance needs to be assessed based on established goals individualized for each patient.

> **Glycosylated hemoglobin (HbA$_{Ic}$):** A blood test that can reflect blood glucose control over a 3-month period. An A_{Ic} of 6% reflects an average plasma glucose level of about 120 mg/dL. In general, each 1% increase in A_{Ic} is a reflection of an increase in average glucose levels of about 30 mg/dL.

Evidence Analysis for Evidence-Based Practice

Although specific evidence-based nutrition principles and recommendations for the treatment and prevention of diabetes and related complications exist, they should be individualized based on each patient's usual intake and eating habits, metabolic profile, treatment goals, and desired outcomes (American Diabetes Association, 2002). The nutritional principles and recommendations are based on the following goals of medical nutrition therapy for diabetes as outlined in the 2002 American Diabetes Association Position Statement:

- Attain and maintain optimal metabolic outcomes, including
  - Blood glucose levels in the normal range or as close to normal as is safely possible to prevent or reduce the risk of complications for diabetes.
  - A lipid and lipoprotein profile that reduces the risk for macrovascular disease.
  - Blood pressure levels that reduce the risk for vascular disease.
- Prevent and treat the chronic complications of diabetes. Modify nutrient intake and life-style as appropriate for the prevention and treatment of obesity, dyslipidemia, cardiovascular disease, hypertension, and nephropathy.

- Improve health through healthy food choices and physical activity.
- Address individual nutritional needs, taking into consideration personal, ethnic, and cultural preferences, as well as life-styles, while respecting the individual's wishes and willingness to change.

In terms of specific dietary recommendations, evidence exists regarding the following:

- *Carbohydrates:* The total amount of carbohydrate in the meal or snack is more important than the source or type. Whole grains, fruits, vegetables, and low-fat milk are healthy choices. Sugar (sucrose) does not increase blood sugar levels any more than the same kilocalorie level of starch-containing food and as such does not need to be restricted in people with diabetes. If sucrose is consumed, it must be substituted for other carbohydrate sources. Nonnutritive sweeteners have been shown to be safe when consumed within the acceptable daily intake levels established by the U.S. Food and Drug Administration.
- *Protein:* There is no evidence to suggest that usual protein intakes (15% to 20%) need to be modified if renal function is not impaired.
- *Dietary fat:* Given the comorbidity of cardiovascular disease, a heart-healthy diet is warranted. Recommendations include less than 10% of total kilocalories from saturated fat, and for individuals with low-density lipoprotein cholesterol more than 100 mg/dL it is recommended that saturated fat consumption be lowered to less than 7% of total kilocalories. The recommendation for total cholesterol intake is less than 300 mg/day. For individuals with low-density lipoprotein cholesterol, more than 100 mg/dL cholesterol intake should be reduced to less than 200 mg/day.
- *Energy balance:* Weight loss, even modest weight loss, has been shown to improve insulin resistance and overall blood sugar control.
- *Micronutrients:* There is no clear evidence to support vitamin and mineral supplementation in people with diabetes unless they have known underlying vitamin and mineral deficiencies.
- *Alcohol:* The same guidelines apply to people with diabetes regarding alcohol intake based on the 2005 U.S. Dietary Guidelines. In addition to the fact that alcohol intake is limited to one drink for women and two drinks for men, to reduce the risk of hypoglycemia it is suggested that alcohol be consumed with food. (One drink is considered a 12-oz. beer, a 5-oz. glass of wine, or 1.5 oz. of 80-proof spirits.)
- Older adults with diabetes: Older adults require less kilocalories to meet their nutritional needs, and they are more likely to be undernourished. Caution should be used when prescribing weight-loss diets in this population.

Chronic Kidney Disease

Chronic kidney disease is the inability of the kidney to function normally. The primary function of the kidney is to maintain homeostatic balance with respect to fluids, electrolytes, and organic solutes and to remove waste from the body through the production of urine. The kidney filters approximately 1,600 L of blood per day and produces 1 to 2 L of urine per day. Symptoms of chronic kidney disease include severe headache, **dyspnea,** failing vision, poor appetite, nausea and vomiting, abdominal pain, and mouth ulcers. Dialysis is postponed for as long as possible.

Dyspnea: Shortness of breath.

Nutritional Assessment

Nutritional assessment of the patient with chronic kidney disease is very similar to a standard nutritional assessment, with some additional features based on the Kidney Dialysis Outcome Quality Initiative (K/DOQI) guidelines. In addition to evaluating the standard laboratory values available on admission, which would include albumin, the following laboratory values should be evaluated: serum prealbumin, predialysis serum creatinine, urea reduction ratio, serum bicarbonate, and lipid profile. The K/DOQI also recommends the use of the Subjective Global Assessment, a four-item, seven-point scale, to monitor nutrition status changes and patients' anthropometric measurements using each patient as his or her own control.

Evidence Analysis for Evidence-Based Practice

Current clinical practice guidelines for nutritional care in chronic kidney disease are based on recommendations by the 2002 National Kidney Foundation K/QODI guidelines that can be accessed online (www.kidney.org/professionals/kdoqi). The guidelines are evidence based, with the rationale for each guideline explained and referenced based on extensive literature review evaluated for quality and strength (Beto & Bansal, 2004).

More recently, under the 2003 K/DOQI guidelines, chronic kidney disease has been classified into five stages based on a **glomerular filtration rate** upon which to diagnose and base care in a uniform manner (Beto & Bansal, 2004). Stages 1 to 4 are predialysis, and stage 5 requires replacement therapy (dialysis) to sustain life. Dialysis therapies mimic the function of the kidneys to the extent possible, exchanging high levels of circulating products such as urea, phosphorus, and potassium that the kidney would normally remove using osmotic pressure to cross a barrier membrane to be removed from the body. There are two types of dialysis treatment: hemodialysis and peritoneal dialysis. Hemodialysis is artificial filtering of blood by a machine that requires permanent vein access through a fistula and the dialysis fluid similar to plasma. Peritoneal dialysis is artificial filtering of the blood by a hyperosmolar solution through the peritoneum.

> **Glomerular filtration rate:** The quantity of glomerular filtrate formed per unit in all nephrons of both kidneys.

In clinical nutrition practice, intervention needs to be matched to the function of the kidney based on biochemical data and corresponding K/DOQI nutritional guidelines. This can be challenging because the function of the kidneys changes day to day and compliance with the diet can be difficult because of all the restrictions that must be managed. The goals of nutritional intervention for stages 1 to 4 are to minimize tissue catabolism; maintain nutritional status, weight, appetite, electrolyte balance, and lean body mass; and postpone dialysis as long as possible.

HIV/AIDS

AIDS is a disease characterized by the transmission of a retrovirus called the human immunodeficiency virus by the exchange of bodily fluids through sexual contact, infected blood, contaminated needles, or mother-to-child transmission. AIDS was first described by the Centers for Disease Control and Prevention in 1981 and included severe depression of cellular immunity accompanied by unusual **opportunistic infections** such as *Pneumocystis carinii* pneumonia, cytomegalovirus, or Kaposi sarcoma (Gottlieb, Schanker, Saxon, Weisman, & Pozalski, 1981). HIV disease is currently the sixth leading cause of death for all races combined for the age group 25 to 44 years and ninth for the age group 45 to 64 years (Kochanek et al., 2004). AIDS is defined as an HIV infection with a CD4 cell count of 200 or less and the presence of at least one opportunistic infection, dementia, wasting syndrome, or malignant disease.

> **Opportunistic infections:** Infection by an organism that would not ordinarily cause disease but because of an impaired immune response the organism becomes pathogenic.

Nutritional Assessment

No nationally accepted standard of care for HIV/AIDS exists, but evidence does exist that medical nutrition therapy plays a critical role in increasing energy, protein, and micronutrient intake among HIV-positive and AIDS patients. In a joint position statement, the ADA and the Dietitians of Canada urged that nutrition referrals be made as soon as possible after the HIV-positive diagnosis to obtain the most benefit from medical nutrition therapy (ADA & the Canadian Dietetic Association, 1994). In 1996 the ADA developed an HIV/AIDS medical nutrition therapy protocol that recommended a baseline nutritional assessment and nutrition self-management training to include follow-up assessment and training for the patients one to two times a year when asymptomatic and consultations two to six times a year when patients became symptomatic or converted to AIDS (Journal of the American Dietetic Association, 2004). The ADA nutritional assessment should be comprehensive and include an evaluation of

HIV wasting syndrome:
Catabolic condition; loss of
body weight (body fat and
muscle stores); very similar
to cancer cachexia.

weight in terms of percentage of usual weight. Anthropometric measurements are useful because many patients have multiple clinic visits and/or hospitalizations, making it possible to have numerous measurements over a period of time. Visceral protein (i.e., albumin, prealbumin) should be monitored to observe changes in visceral protein stores. Patients should be evaluated for **HIV wasting syndrome,** which is characterized by an unintentional loss of 10% body weight over 6 months, loss of 5% lean body mass within 6 months, body cell mass less than 35% and BMI less than 27 (men), body cell mass less than 23% and BMI less than 27 (women), and BMI less than 20 (Polsky, Kotler, & Steinhart, 2001).

Evidence Analysis for Evidence-Based Practice

Studies indicate that weight determines outcome and mortality (Kotler, Tierney, Wang, & Pierson, 1989; Grunfeld & Feingold, 1992). Nutrient requirements need to be individualized for each patient and vary depending on health status. Keusch and Thea (1993) recommended using BEE $\times$ 1.3 for maintenance and BEE $\times$ 1.5 for weight gain in order to determine energy requirement. Additional kilocalories and protein need to be provided if fever is present, with energy requirements increasing by 13% and protein requirements increasing by 10% for every degree Celsius of temperature elevation above normal (Grunfeld & Feingold, 1992).

Nutritional Issues of Epidemic Proportion

Excessive Weight and Obesity

Excessive weight and obesity have reached epidemic proportions in the United States. The prevalence of obesity in the United States has increased at alarming rates in the past three decades (Kuczmarski, Flegal, & Campbell, 1994). Excessive weight is defined as a BMI greater than 25 but less than 30. People who have a BMI of 30 or higher are considered obese. Consider the following obesity data; although not in line with the data on young, middle, and older adults discussed earlier in the chapter, the data do differentiate between the first and second half of adulthood:

- Obesity data for 25- to 44-year-olds for 1999–2002 indicated that 34.2% of adults in this age group were overweight and 28.5% were obese. Even more concerning was the 7.8% increase in the percentage of adults who were classified as obese when compared with the previous 10-year span (1988–1994). This increase in the number of obese adults contributed in part to the increase in the overall percentage of adults who were overweight or obese; 62.8% for overweight/obese up from 51.7% in 1988–1994 (Flegal, Carroll, Ogden, & Johnson, 2002; Hedley, Ogden, Carroll, Curtin, & Flegal, 2004).
- Obesity data for 45- to 64-year-olds for 1999–2002 indicated that 35.7% of adults in this age group were overweight and 35.8% were obese. The increase in the percentage of adults in this age group who were overweight/obese was due to a 6.7% increase in the percentage of adults who were classified as obese. The overall percentage of adults who were overweight or obese was 71.5%, up from 65.5% in 1988–1994 (Flegal et al., 2002; Hedley et al., 2004).

Research in obesity has been extensive in the past two decades and has helped build our understanding of the genetic, psychological, metabolic, and environmental influences on body weight, which has served to increase our awareness of the complexities of weight management (ADA, 2002). The most-often-asked question is, what is the cause? We live in an environment that is conducive to obesity because of our sedentary life-style and the abundance of energy-dense foods (Wolf & Colditz, 1998; Allison, Fontaine, Manson, Steven, & Vanitallie, 1999). Data on weight-loss interventions indicate that they do not produce long-term results and have a success rate of about 5% (National Institutes of Health & National Heart, Lung, and Blood Institute, 1998). What then is the role of the dietitian? The dietitian can play a critical role as a facilitator of change through the counseling process to help the patient formulate reasonable goals that can be met and sustained with a healthy eating approach. In terms of the nation as a whole, public policy must be changed and a battle must be waged on all fronts (i.e., through the media, the food industry, etc.) if we are to win the war on obesity.

Osteoporosis

Osteoporosis, often called the "silent epidemic," is a disease that takes a lifetime to develop and consequently a lifetime to prevent. It is characterized by a decrease in bone mass and deterioration of bone tissue with no outward signs or symptoms until late in the disease, when bones become much more fragile and are apt to break. Osteoporosis affects 10 million Americans annually, 80% of whom are women; women are four times more likely than men to develop osteoporosis (Kaunitz, 2000). However, men can develop osteoporosis; in fact, one-third of men by the age of 75 develop osteoporosis (Nutrition Screening Initiative, 2002). Osteoporosis leads to 1.5 million fractures every year in the United States, most commonly of the vertebrae. Visible signs of osteoporosis are altered posture caused by deformity of the spine, such as increased thoracis kyphosis (humpback) described as a "widow's hump," or postural slumping due to acute pain and loss of height as a result of vertebral collapse fractures.

Controllable measures an individual can take to avoid osteoporosis are to ensure adequate consumption of calories and to take in enough calcium to promote optimum bone development in the first three decades of life. As was mentioned earlier in the chapter, older adults need additional vitamin D and calcium as they age. Many young adults, especially women, do not consume an adequate amount of calcium and may benefit from calcium and vitamin D supplementation. Calcium and vitamin D supplementation may be beneficial for people who have a family history of osteoporosis or who are exhibiting early signs of osteoporosis. Weight-bearing exercise has been shown to be especially beneficial in helping to reduce the loss of bone mass that happens as a natural part of the aging process. More and more evidence supports the role of antiresorptive therapy, which includes hormonal therapy (estrogen replacement therapy during menopause), bisphosphate therapy (Fosamax or Actonel), selective estrogen receptor modulators (Evista), and calcitonin (Miacalcin), in reducing the incidence of osteoporosis (National Institutes of Health Consensus Development Panel on Osteoporosis Prevention, 2001; Nutrition Action Healthletter, 2002).

Summary

Although genetic predisposition determines longevity to a degree, each person can choose to live a longer, healthier life by eating healthier and exercising. Nutrigenomics is a new and upcoming field that encompasses the study of nutrition and genetics. Thanks to the Human Genome Project, nutritional science is on the edge of a new frontier (Collins & McKusick, 2001). It may be possible someday to receive a nutrition prescription based on your genetic profile with nutrition recommendations that reflect the latest scientific evidence utilizing evidence-based analysis and practice guidelines. Nutrition experts have much work ahead of us if we are going to contribute to the impact of the obesity and osteoporosis epidemics in this country. At the same time we must pay close attention to what is fast becoming the next epidemic—type 2 diabetes. Although each person must take personal responsibility for the choices he or she makes, including food choices and how much to exercise, it is up to us as professionals to interpret the latest nutrition research and translate this information to the public and advocate for public policy that promotes an environment conducive to a healthier life.

Issues to Debate

1. What can the dietetics profession do to help people make better life-style choices?
2. How can some of these ideas be made a practical reality?
3. What is the responsibility of corporate America in keeping people healthy?

References

Allison, D. B., Fontaine, K. R., Manson, J. E., Steven, J., & Vanitallie, T. B. (1999). Annual deaths attributable to obesity in the United States. *Journal of the American Medical Association, 282,* 1530–1538.

American Diabetes Association. (2002). Position statement: Evidence-based nutrition principles and recommendations for the treatment and prevention of diabetes and related complications. *Journal of the American Dietetic Association, 102,* 109–120.

American Dietetic Association (ADA). (2000). ADA Reports: Position of the American Dietetic Association: Nutrition, aging and the continuum of care. *Journal of the American Dietetic Association, 100,* 580.

American Dietetic Association (ADA). (2002). Position of the American Dietetic Association: Weight management. *Journal of the American Dietetic Association, 102,* 1145–1155.

American Dietetic Association (ADA) & the Canadian Dietetic Association. (1994). Nutrition intervention in the care of persons with human immunodeficiency virus infection. *Journal of the American Dietetic Association, 94,* 129–132.

Appel, L. J., Moore, T. J., Obarzanek, E., Vollmer, W. M., Svetkey, L. P., Sacks, F. M., et al. (1997). A clinical trial of the effects of dietary pattern on blood pressure. *New England Journal of Medicine, 336,* 1117–1124.

Berry, J. K., & Braunschwig, C. A. (1998). Nutritional assessment of the critically ill patient. *Critical Care Nursing Quarterly, 21,* 33.

Beto, J. A., & Bansal, U. K. (2004). Medical nutrition therapy in chronic kidney failure. Integrating clinical practice guidelines. *Journal of the American Dietetic Association, 104,* 404–409.

Brandi, L. S., & Calafa, M. (1997). Indirect calorimetry in critically ill patients: Clinical applications and practical advice. *Nutrition, 13,* 349–358.

Brown, J. E., Isaacs, J. S., Krinke, U. B., Murtaugh, M. A., Sharbaugh, C., Stang, J., et al. (2005). *Nutrition Through the Life Cycle* (2nd ed.). Belmont, CA: Thomson Wadsworth.

Centers for Disease Control and Prevention (CDC). (2002). Basics about overweight and obesity. Retrieved from www.cdc.gov/nccdphp/dnpa/obesity/basics.htm

Chin, A., Paw, M. J., DeJong, N., Schouten, E. G., Hiddink, G. J., & Kok, F. J. (2001). Physical exercise and/or enriched foods for functional improvement in frail, independent living elderly: A randomized controlled trial. *Archives of Physical and Medical Rehabilitation, 82,* 811–817.

Collins, F. S., & McKusick, V. A. (2001). Implications of the Human Genome Project for medical science. *Journal of the American Medical Association, 285,* 540.

Committee on Nutrition Services for Medicare Beneficiaries and Institute of Medicine. (2000). *The Role of Nutrition in Maintaining Health in the Nation's Elderly.* Washington, DC: Author.

Cowie C. C., Rust K. F., Byrd-Holt D. D., Eberhardt M. S., Flegal K. M., Engelgau M. M., et al. (2006). Prevalence of diabetes and impaired fasting glucose in adults in the U.S. population: NHANES 1999–2002. *Diabetes Care, 29,* 1263–1268.

Elmore, M. F., Wagner, D. R., Knoll, D. M., Eizember, L., Oswall, M. A., Glowinski, E. A., et al. (1994). Developing an effective adult nutrition screening tool for a community hospital. *Journal of the American Dietetic Association, 94,* 1113–1118, 1121.

Flegal, K. M., Carroll, M. D., Ogden, C. L., & Johnson, C. L. (2002). Prevalence and trends in obesity among US adults, 1999–2000. *Journal of the American Medical Association, 288,* 1723–1727.

Fonesa, V., & Wall, J. (1995). Diet and diabetes in the elderly. *Clinical Geriatric Medicine, 11,* 613–624.

Food and Nutrition Board, Committee on Diet and Health, & National Research Council. (1989). *Diet and Health: Implications for Reducing Chronic Disease Risk.* Washington, DC: National Academy Press.

Food and Nutrition Board, National Research Council, & National Academy of Sciences. (1989). *Recommended Dietary Allowances.* Washington, DC: National Academy Press.

Frankenfield, D., Roth-Yousey, L., & Compher, C. (2005). Comparison of predictive equations for resting metabolic rate in healthy nonobese and obese adults: A systematic review. *Journal of the American Dietetic Association, 105,* 775–790.

Gallagher-Allred, C. R., Voss, A. C., Finn, S. C., & McCamish, M. A. (1996). Malnutrition and clinical outcomes: The case for medical nutrition therapy. *Journal of the American Dietetic Association, 96,* 361–367.

Gary, R., & Fleury, J. (2002). Nutritional status: Key to preventing decline in hospitalized older adults. *Topics in Geriatric Rehabilitation, 17,* 40–71.

Gottlieb, M. S., Schanker, H. M., Saxon, A., Weisman, J. D., & Pozalski, I. (1981). Pneumocystis pneumonia—Los Angeles. *Morbidity and Mortality Weekly Review, 30,* 250–252.

Gray-Donald, K., Gibbson, L., Shapiro, S. H., Macklern, P. T., & Martin, J. G. (1996). Nutritional status and mortality in chronic obstructive pulmonary disease. *American Journal of Respiratory and Critical Care Medicine, 153,* 961–966.

Grunfeld, C., & Feingold, K. R. (1992). Metabolic disturbances and wasting in the acquired immunodeficiency syndrome. *New England Journal of Medicine, 327,* 329–337.

Hanley, D. A., & Davison, K. S. (2005). Vitamin D insufficiency in North America. *Journal of Nutrition, 135,* 332–338.

Harvard Health Letter. (2002). Aging: Living to 100. What's the secret? *Harvard Health Letter, 27,* 1.

Hedley, A. A., Ogden, C. L., Carroll, M. D., Curtin, L. R., & Flegal, K. M. (2004). Overweight and obesity among US children, adolescents, and adults, 1999–2002. *Journal of the American Medical Association, 291,* 2847–2850.

Hu, G., & Cassano, P. (2000). Antioxidant nutrients and pulmonary function: The Third National Health and Nutrition Examination Survey. *American Journal of Epidemiology, 151,* 975.

Ireton-Jones, C. J. (1997). Why use predictive equations for energy expenditure assessment? *Journal of the American Dietetic Association, 9,* A44.

Journal of the American Dietetic Association. (2004). Position of the American Dietetic Association and Dietitians of Canada: Position paper. Nutrition Intervention in care of persons with HIV infection. *Journal of the American Dietetic Association, 104,* 1425–1441.

Kant, A. K. (2000). Consumption of energy-dense nutrient-poor foods by adult Americans: Nutritional and health implications. The third National Health and Nutrition Examination Survey, 1984–1994. *American Journal of Clinical Nutrition, 72,* 929.

Kaunitz, A. M. (2000). Osteoporosis: The silent epidemic. *Jacksonville Medicine, 51*(5).

Kelly, K. (2003). The "freshman 15." *U.S. News and World Report, 135,* 54.

Keusch, G. T., & Thea, D. M. (1993). Malnutrition in AIDS. *Medical Clinics of North America, 77,* 795.

Klipstein-Grobusch, K., Reilly, J., Potter, J., Edwards, C., & Roberts, M. (1995). Energy intake and expenditure in elderly patients admitted to hospital with acute illness. *British Journal of Nutrition, 73,* 323–324.

Kochanek, K. D., Murphy, S. L., Anderson, R. N., & Scott, C. (2004). *Deaths: Final Data for 2002.* Hyattsville, MD: National Center for Health Statistics.

Kotler, D. P., Tierney, A. R., Wang, J., & Pierson, R. N. (1989). Magnitude of body cell mass depletion and the timing of death from wasting in AIDS. *American Journal of Clinical Nutrition, 50,* 444–447.

Kuczmarski, R. J., Flegal, K. M., & Campbell, S. M. (1994). Overweight prevalence and trends for children and adolescents: The National Health and Nutrition Examination Surveys, 1963 to

1991. *Journal of the American Medical Association, 149,* 1085–1092.

Laaban, J. P., Kouchakji, B., Dore, M. F., Orvoen-Frija, E., David, P., & Rochemaure, J. (1993). Nutritional status of patients with chronic obstructive pulmonary disease and acute respiratory failure. *Chest, 103,* 1362–1368.

Lacey, K. P. E. (2003). Nutrition Care Process and Model: ADA adopts road map to quality care and outcome management. *Journal of the American Dietetic Association, 103,* 1061–1072.

Levitsky, D. A., & Youn, T. (2004). The more food young adults are served, the more they overeat. *Journal of Nutrition, 134,* 2436–2550.

Mahan, L. E. (2004). *Krause's Food, Nutrition, and Diet Therapy* (11th ed.). Philadelphia: W. B. Saunders.

Martin, J. A., Hamilton, B. E., Sutton, P. D., Ventura, S. J., Menacker, F., & Munson, M. L. (2005). *Births: Final Data for 2003.* Hyattsville, MD: National Center for Health Statistics.

Myers, E. F., Pritchett, E., & Johnson, E. Q. (2002). Evidence-based practice guides vs protocols: What's the difference? *Journal of the American Dietetic Association, 101,* 1085–1090.

National Center for Health Statistics. (1984–1995). Prevalence of Selected Conditions by Age and Sex: United States. Retrieved January 12, 2006, from http://www.cdc.gov/nchc/agingact.htm

National Cholesterol Education Program (NCEP). (1988). Report of the National Cholesterol Education Program Expert Panel on Detection, Education, and Treatment of High Blood Cholesterol in Adults. *Archives of Internal Medicine, 148,* 36–69.

National Cholesterol Education Program (NCEP). (2001). Executive summary of the third report of the National Cholesterol Education Program Expert Panel on Detection, Evaluation, and Treatment of High Blood Cholesterol in Adults (Adult Treatment Panel III). *Journal of the American Medical Association, 285,* 2486.

National Heart, Lung, and Blood Institute, & National Institutes of Health. (2002). *Third Report of the National Cholesterol Education Program Expert Panel on Detection, Evaluation, and Treatment of High Cholesterol in Adults (Adult Treatment Panel III).* Washington, DC: National Institutes of Health.

National Institutes of Health, & National Heart, Lung, and Blood Institute. (1998). Clinical guidelines on the identification, evaluation and treatment of overweight and obesity in adults—The evidence report. *Obesity Research, 6,* 121.

National Institutes of Health Consensus Development Panel on Osteoporosis Prevention, Diagnosis, and Treatment. (2001). Osteoporosis prevention, diagnosis, and treatment. *Journal of the American Medical Association, 285,* 785.

Nutrition Action Healthletter. (2002). Bare bones: How to keep yours strong. *Nutrition Action Healthletter, 29.*

Nutrition Screening Initiative. (2002). A Physician's Guide to Nutrition in Chronic Disease Management for Older Adults. Retrieved February 25, 2006, from http://www.aafp.org/x16105.xml

Olshansky, S. J., Ludwig, D. S., Passaro, D. J., Allison, D. B., Hershow, R. C., Butler, R., et al. (2005). A potential decline in life expectancy in the United States in the 21st century. *New England Journal of Medicine, 352,* 1138–1146.

Polsky, B., Kotler, D., & Steinhart, C. (2001). HIV-associated wasting in the HAART era: Guidelines for assessment, diagnosis and treatment. *AIDS Patient Care and STDs, 15,* 411.

Public Health Service. (1988). *The Surgeon General's Report on Nutrition and Health: Summary and Recommendations.* Publ. No. 88-50211. Washington, DC: Department of Health and Human Service, Public Health Service.

Rogers, R. M., Donahoe, M., & Constantino, J. (1992). Physiologic effects of oral supplemental feeding in malnourished patients with chronic obstructive pulmonary disease. *American Review of Respiratory Disease, 146,* 1511–1517.

Russell, R. (1997). New views on the RDAs for older adults. *Journal of the American Dietetic Association, 97,* 515–518.

Schoeller, D. A. (1999). Recent advances from application of doubly labeled water to measurement of human energy expenditure. *Journal of Nutrition, 129,* 1765–1768.

Schols, A. M. W. J., Mostert, R., Soester, P., Greve, L. H., & Wouters, E. M. F. (1989). Inventory of nutritional status in patients with COPD. *Chest, 96,* 247–249.

Schols, A. M. W. J., Soeters, P. B., Dingemans, A. M. C., Mostert, R., Frantzen, P. J., & Wouters, E. F. (1993). Prevalence and characteristics of nutritional depletion in patients with COPD eligible for pulmonary rehabilitation. *American Review of Respiratory Disease, 147,* 1151–1156.

Smith, R. (2003). Expanding medical nutrition therapy: An argument for evidence-based practices. *Journal of the American Dietetic Association, 103,* 313–314.

Soler-Cataluna, J. J., Sanchez-Sanchez, L., Martinez-Garcia, M. A., Sanchez, P. R., Salcedo, E., & Navarro, M. (2005). Mid-arm muscle area is a better predictor of mortality than body mass index in COPD. *Chest, 128,* 2108–2115.

Thorsdottir, I., Eriksen, B., & Eysteinsdottir, S. (1999). Nutritional status at submission for dietetic services and screening for malnutrition at admission to hospital. *Clinical Nutrition, 18,* 15–21.

Thorsdottir, I., & Gunnarsdottir, I. (2002). Energy intake must be increased among recently hospitalized patients with chronic obstructive pulmonary disease to improve nutritional status. (Research and Professional Briefs). *Journal of the American Dietetic Association, 102,* 247.

Thorsdottir, I., Gunnarsdottir, I, & Eriksen, B. (2001). Screening method evaluated by nutritional status measurements can be used to detect malnourishment in chronic obstructive pulmonary disease. *Journal of the American Dietetic Association, 101,* 648.

Trials of Hypertension Prevention Collaborative Research Group. (1997). Effects of weight loss and sodium reduction intervention on blood pressure and hypertension incidence in overweight people with high-normal blood pressure. *Archives of Internal Medicine, 157,* 657.

U.S. Department of Health and Human Services. (2000). *Healthy People 2010* (2nd ed.). With Understanding and Improving Health and Objectives for Improving Health. Washington, DC: U.S. Government Printing Office.

Wardlaw, G. M., Hampl, J. S., & DiSilvestro, R. A. (2004). *Perspectives in Nutrition* (6th ed.). New York: McGraw Hill.

Whittaker, J. S., Ryan, C. F., Buckley, P. A., & Road, J. D. (1990). The effects of refeeding on peripheral and respiratory muscle function in malnourished chronic obstructive pulmonary disease patients. *American Review of Respiratory Disease, 142,* 283–288.

Wolf, A. M., & Colditz, G. A. (1998). Current estimates of the economic cost of obesity in the United States. *Obesity Research, 6,* 97–106.

Worthington-Roberts, B. S. (1996). *Nutrition Throughout the Life Cycle* (3rd ed.). St. Louis: Mosby.

Special Topics in Adults and Chronic Diseases: Nutrition and Public Health

Judith Sharlin, PhD, RD

CHAPTER OUTLINE

Preventing Disease and Promoting Health

Chronic Diseases: The Leading Causes of Death and Disability

Risk Factors and Chronic Disease

Prevention Strategies

Primary Prevention: Health Promotion • Secondary Prevention: Risk Appraisal and Risk Reduction • Tertiary Prevention: Treatment and Rehabilitation • Implications of the Prevention Levels

Dietary Guidelines for Disease Prevention

Diet and Health: Nutrition Strategies and Risk Factors

Obesity • Cardiovascular Disease • Cancer • Diabetes • Osteoporosis • HIV/AIDS

Reader Objectives

After studying this chapter and reflecting on the contents, you should be able to

1. Identify the primary causes of death and disability in adults in the United States.
2. Describe primary, secondary, and tertiary levels of health prevention and health promotion and their relationship to nutrition program planning.
3. Identify risk factors for chronic diseases and their implications for nutrition.
4. Describe the dietary risk factors associated with the leading chronic diseases.
5. Discuss the common features of the dietary guidelines issued by the major U.S. health organizations.
6. Compare different dietary interventions a public health nutritionist or dietitian offers to the community, family, or an individual at risk.
7. Recognize the mission and role of public health nutrition in preventing disease and promoting adult health.
8. Name some of the public health nutrition programs that exist today for maintaining adult health.

Preventing Disease and Promoting Health

Growing scientific evidence reveals that nutrition or dietary intake in adults contributes significantly to preventing illnesses and premature deaths in the United States (Frazao, 1999). Life expectancy has increased dramatically over the past 100 years, and today the average life expectancy is nearly 78 years (U.S. Department of Health and Human Services [USDHHS], 2000b). Health and nutrition programs for adults aim at prevention and improving quality of life. However, chronic diseases account for 7 of every 10 deaths in the United States (McRobbie & Kolbe, 2009; USDHHS, 2004). The increasing cost of crisis medical care and the growing economic burden provide a cost-effective incentive for individuals and our nation to prevent chronic disease. Chronic diseases cost the United States 75% of the $1 trillion spent on health care annually (USDHHS, 2004). In spite of this, only 3% of the total annual health care expenditures in our nation were spent on prevention (Centers for Disease Control and Prevention [CDC], 1992). Nutrition interventions and policies target the factors related to adult health and aim to prevent chronic diseases that are the leading causes of death and disability.

Chronic Diseases: The Leading Causes of Death and Disability

To successfully create programs to promote health, longevity, and quality of life, we must examine the leading causes of death and disability. Data from the National Center for Health Statistics (NCHS) show that chronic diseases are the leading causes of death and disability **(Table 10.1)** (Xu et al., 2007). Cardiovascular diseases and cancer account for about half of all deaths in the United States (USDHHS, 2004).

A report on the health status of U.S. adults emphasized that increasing numbers of people still smoke, are physically inactive, and are overweight (NCHS, 2003). Mokdad, Marks, Stroup, and Gerberding (2004) noted that about half of the deaths among U.S. adults in 2000 could have been prevented. These findings revealed that 400,000 deaths occur each year because of poor diet and physical inactivity. (This number was found to be 20% less in a subsequent study [Mokdad, Marks, Stroup, & Gerberding, 2005].) It appears that the increasing trend of excessive weight and obesity will likely overtake tobacco as the leading preventable cause of mortality in the United States (Mokdad, Marks, Stroup, & Gerberding, 2004; USDHHS, 2002). Although mortality rates from heart disease, stroke, and cancer have declined, behavioral changes have led to an increased prevalence of obesity and diabetes (Koplan & Dietz, 1999; USDHHS, 2002). Dietary factors are now associated with 4 of the 10 leading causes of death: coronary heart

> **Learning Point** More than 60% of chronic disease mortality can be attributed to life-style factors such as diet, which can be modified (Krauss et al., 2000).

TABLE 10.1 Deaths and Percentage of Total Deaths for the 10 Leading Causes of Death: United States, 2003–2004

Cause of death (based on the *International Classification of Diseases, Tenth Revision,* 1992)	Rank	2004 Deaths	2004 Percent of Total Deaths	2003 Deaths	2003 Percent of Total Deaths
All causes		2,397,615	100.0	2,448,288	100.0
Diseases of heart (100–109,111,113,120–151)	1	652,486	27.2	685,089	28.0
Malignant neoplasms (C00–C97)	2	553,888	23.1	556,902	22.7
Cerebrovascular diseases (160–169)	3	150,074	6.3	157,689	6.4
Chronic lower respiratory diseases (J40–J47)	4	121,987	5.1	126,382	5.2
Accidents (unintentional injuries) (V01–X59,Y85–Y86)	5	112,012	4.7	109,277	4.5
Diabetes mellitus (E10–E14)	6	73,138	3.1	74,219	3.0
Alzheimer's disease (G30)	7	65,965	2.8	63,457	2.6
Influenza and pneumonia (J10–J18)	8	59,664	2.5	65,163	2.7
Nephritis, nephrotic syndrome and nephrosis (N00–N07,N17–N19, N25–N27)	9	42,480	1.8	42,453	1.7
Septicemia (A40–A41)	10	33,373	1.4	34,069	1.4

Source: National Vital Statistics Report. (Nov. 20, 2007). Deaths and Leading Causes for 2004. Vol. 56, No. 5.

disease (CHD), some types of cancer, stroke, and type 2 diabetes (NCHS, 1997). The Surgeon General's report in 1988 confirmed these findings: "For two out of three adult Americans who do not smoke and do not drink excessively, one personal choice seems to influence long-term health prospects more than any other, what we eat" (USDHHS, 1998).

Risk Factors and Chronic Disease

Chronic diseases, although prevalent and costly, are among the most preventable. Research has identified a Health Promotion and Preventive Action model for risk factors (Elo & Caltrop, 2002). In this model, risk factor identification, reduction, modification, and education are related to human health and developmental stages (Elo & Caltrop, 2002). **Risk factors** can be defined as those specific characteristics associated with an increased chance of developing a chronic disease. Risk factors that can be changed or modified, such as diet or physical activity, are those most commonly associated with life-style choices (Wimbush & Peters, 2000). There are four types of risk factors (USDHHS, 2000b):

Risk factors: Specific characteristics associated with an increased chance of developing a chronic disease.

1. Biological factors such as an individual's genetic makeup, family history, age, or gender
2. Environmental conditions, such as social and physical environment
3. Access to quality health care
4. Individual behavior and life-style factors such as smoking, exercise, and good eating habits

Healthy People 2010 (HP 2010) provides the most recent guidelines and recommendations for specific health objectives and goals for the nation (USDHHS, 2000b). HP 2010 reveals that individual biological behaviors and environmental factors are responsible for approximately 70% of all premature deaths (USDHHS, 2000b). Biological factors such as age or gender are not modifiable. However, the leading causes of death are associated with dietary factors, which are modifiable. The determinants of health illustrate how individual biology and behaviors influence health through the individual's social and physical environments (USDHHS, 2000b). Finally, health can be improved through policies and interventions with access to quality health care. Because the leading causes of illness and death in the United States, such as CHD, some types of cancer, stroke, type 2 diabetes, and atherosclerosis, are associated with dietary factors, we must address the concern that chronic diseases have resulted from dietary excesses and imbalance (USDHHS, 2000b). Furthermore, there is evidence that more intensive dietary counseling can lead to reduced intakes of dietary fat and cholesterol and increased fiber, fruit, and vegetable consumption (USDHHS & NHLBI, 2003).

> **● Learning Point** HP 2010 outlines 28 focus areas that include risk factors for chronic diseases and addresses nutrition and excessive weight, physical activity, tobacco use, cancer, diabetes, cardiovascular disease, and access to quality health care.

Prevention Strategies

Health promotion and disease prevention provide complementary interventions to change health risk factors. Prevention efforts in public health, community, and worksite settings are divided into three levels: primary prevention (health promotion), secondary prevention (risk appraisal and reduction), and tertiary prevention (treatment and rehabilitation) (Shamansky & Clausen, 1980; Kaufman, 1990; American Dietetic Association [ADA], 1998).

Primary Prevention: Health Promotion

Primary prevention strategies, or health promotion, encourage health-enhancing behaviors by giving individuals, families, and communities ways to reduce risk factors associated with disease and injury (ADA, 1998). Risk factors include environmental, economic, social, and biological aspects. Good examples of primary prevention strategies include nutrition and weight management classes in a community center for adults, environmental changes to provide nutritious choices in a school cafeteria vending machine, and local Fruits and Veggies: More Matters campaigns to increase the availability of fresh fruits and vegetables from farmers' markets (ADA, 1998). Primary prevention strategies seek to expand the positive potential of health (Brunner et al., 1997).

> **Primary prevention strategies:** Encourage health-enhancing behaviors by giving individuals, families, and communities ways to reduce risk factors associated with disease and injury.
>
> **Holistic approach:** Individual life-style factors, social and political issues, and access to quality health care.

A **holistic approach,** embracing individual life-style factors, the environment, and economic, social, and political factors, can help communities and private sector partners achieve health promotion and disease prevention goals. Providing information, available on food labels and through health messages to the public, is one effective method. These messages encourage consumers to apply the U.S. Dietary Guidelines, the Food Guide Pyramid, Dietary Reference Intakes, and the Dietary Guidelines Alliance's It's All About You campaign (U.S. Department of Agriculture [USDA] & USDHHS, 1992; Dietary Guidelines Alliance, 1996;). Voluntary community and health organizations, the federal government, worksite programs, and schools can reach consumers daily to promote nutrition interventions.

The media remain an effective means of communicating nutrition issues to the public (ADA, 1996). Programs to promote physical activity and fitness, good nutrition, and smoking cessation must be broadly accessible. Worksite nutrition-centered health promotion and disease prevention programs provide opportunities to harness social support and influence (ADA, Office of Disease Prevention and Health Promotion, Public Health Service, & USDHHS, 1993).

Motivations should be provided for food processors and vendors, restaurant chefs, and school and worksite cafeteria managers to prepare and serve foods lower in fat, calories, and sodium. Finally, legislation and regulations can be ratified to endorse more complete food and nutrition labeling. Food labels that provide short, unequivocal, positive messages aimed at a single behavior prove beneficial to consumers (Goldberg, 1992).

Secondary Prevention: Risk Appraisal and Risk Reduction

Secondary prevention includes risk appraisal and screening to emphasize early detection and diagnosis of disease (Shamansky & Clausen, 1980; ADA, 1998; Elo & Caltrop, 2002). Secondary prevention begins at the point where the pathology of a disease may occur. It encompasses diagnostic services that include screening, surveillance, and clinical examinations (Elo & Caltrop, 2002). Screening strategies include follow-up education, counseling, and health referral. One model for secondary prevention involving screening is a cholesterol screening program for early detection of cardiovascular problems, such as elevated blood pressure, elevated blood cholesterol, and high glucose levels (Sharlin, Posner, Gershoff, Zeitlin, & Berger, 1992). For people with an elevated blood cholesterol level, this means introducing "therapeutic life-style changes," such as reducing total and saturated fat in the diet, increasing physical activity, and reducing or maintaining a healthy weight. If this is not effective, or if low-density lipoprotein levels are abnormally high, drug therapy can be recommended by the physician.

Secondary prevention: Risk appraisal and screening to emphasize early detection and diagnosis of disease.

Strategies in secondary prevention are aimed at self-care for people with chronic diseases. An example of a secondary prevention program involving self-care is an educational and awareness program to teach a woman with a history of gestational diabetes how to control her weight through diet and exercise (Shamansky & Clausen, 1980; ADA, 1998).

Tertiary Prevention: Treatment and Rehabilitation

Tertiary prevention involves treatment and rehabilitation and is defined as the reduction in the amount of disability caused by a disease to achieve the highest level of function (Pender, 1996). Examples of tertiary diseases include diabetes, kidney disease, and angina. The goal of treatment and rehabilitation is the prevention of further disability and any secondary conditions that might result from the initial health problem.

Tertiary prevention: Treatment and rehabilitation; reduction in the amount of disability caused by a disease to achieve the highest level of function.

Examples of tertiary prevention programs include medical nutrition therapy (MNT) for people suffering from kidney disease, nutrition education about vitamin and mineral supplementation and feeding strategies to prevent further complications of wasting from HIV/AIDS, and cardiac rehabilitation through diet, exercise, and stress management. The ultimate goal of tertiary prevention is, through rehabilitation, to restore the individual to an "optimal" level of functioning, given the constraints of the disease (ADA, 1998).

Implications of the Prevention Levels

The prevention levels are useful concepts to help set objectives for public health programs concerned with adult health in communities, worksites, and other settings. Recent findings underscore the need to emphasize population-based prevention programs (Resnicow, Orlandi, Vaccaro, & Wynder, 1989; Wimbush & Peters, 2000). As discussed earlier, research points to a holistic approach that aims at health and prevention when using the level concept for public health programs. This approach is embraced in HP 2010 in terms of the nutrition and health objectives (USDHHS, 2000b). For each goal, the holistic approach involving individual life-style factors, environmental factors, social and political issues, and access to quality health care is addressed.

Public health endeavors focus on primary or secondary prevention. It is important to choose the appropriate prevention level when planning a public health program. This is illustrated with two different approaches for handling CHD risk factors: one intended to reduce the prevalence of high blood pressure and one to reduce obesity levels.

Almost all adults in the United States have had their blood pressure measured sometime in their lives. One study found that 90% of Americans had had their blood pressure measured in the past two years and could state whether it was normal or abnormally high (USDHHS, CDC, & NCHS, 2003). Over 90% of Americans are aware of the relationship between hypertension and stroke and hypertension and heart disease (USDHHS & National Heart, Lung, and Blood Institute, 2004). Almost 70% of people with hypertension know about high blood pressure, yet the same percentage (70%) do not have their blood pressure under control (less than 140/90 mm Hg) (CDC, 2006). Kannel et al. (1980) showed that systolic (higher number) blood pressure is a more important predictor of heart disease than diastolic blood pressure, especially in the elderly. In addition, ethnic disparities exist for prevalence rates of high blood pressure, and African-Americans in the United States have a greater prevalence of high blood pressure than do whites (CDC, 2006). These data suggest that to reduce mortality from hypertension, secondary prevention strategies should be directed toward persons with hypertension (especially those with elevated systolic pressures), African-Americans, and the elderly. This approach would be more effective than primary prevention strategies aimed at increasing public awareness.

In contrast, many U.S. adults are just beginning to be aware of the growing obesity epidemic and the significance of elevated body mass index (BMI) (30 and above) for the risk of death and illness (USDHHS, 2004). Americans understand the viability of lowering this risk factor associated with many chronic diseases. Extensive data exist to substantiate that making life-style changes such as engaging in regular physical activity and healthy eating could, at the very least, halt the continued growth of the obesity epidemic (USDHHS, 2004). Given the dramatic increases in overweight and obese U.S. adults between 1976–1980 and 1999–2000 (USDHHS, 2004), population-based efforts could be more efficient at reducing the obesity epidemic than efforts to identify those individuals at risk.

One primary prevention effort, called America on the Move (see americaonthemove.org), is a national initiative dedicated to helping individuals and communities become more physically active and to eat more healthfully. The program creates and supports an "integrated grassroots network" at the state level to build communities that support individual behavior changes. In addition, America on the Move involves public and private partnerships at the national, state, and local levels. It publicizes small behavioral changes such as cutting 100 calories a day and taking 2,000 steps daily.

Health promotion and chronic disease prevention programs should focus on coalition building between community-based nutrition and health professionals, government, local businesses, health agencies, and insurers (ADA, 1998). In this rapidly changing health care environment, continued training and research in public health program development is crucial to provide evidence of the efficacy of health prevention and promotion.

All levels of prevention should be addressed when devising strategies for dietary behavior changes for chronic disease prevention. However, for some diseases, the nutrition strategy may prove similar at each prevention level. Weight reduction, for example, may prevent the onset of hypertension or may be part of the treatment for type 2 diabetes. In the case of other diseases, such as cancer, nutrition strategies might vary with the prevention level.

Dietary Guidelines for Disease Prevention

Various health organizations and government agencies have issued dietary guidelines and recommendations based on current scientific evidence. In 1989 the National Research Council published its report *Diet and Health: Implications for Reducing Chronic Disease Risk,* providing evidence for the relationship between all major chronic conditions and diet (USDHHS, 2004). More recently, HP 2010 set forth a comprehensive health promotion and disease prevention program for the nation. HP 2010's comprehensive health agenda has two overarching goals: (1) to increase the quality and years of a healthy life and (2) to eliminate health disparities (USDHHS, 2000b). These goals embrace the dietary recommendations set forth by several government and health organizations.

> **Visit www.health.gov for more information about the National Research Council's report *Diet and Health: Implications for Reducing Chronic Disease Risk.***

In 2001 the U.S. Dietary Guidelines were assessed in terms of surveillance and research needs, especially related to risk for chronic diseases, such as cancer (American Institute of Cancer Research [AICR], 2001). In the same year, the revised Dietary Guidelines of the American Heart Association (AHA) gave greater emphasis to the diet as a whole and, specifically, to certain protective foods for chronic disease risk prevention (Kris-Etherton et al., 2001). Scientifically based dietary guidelines from the American Cancer Society (ACS) and the AICR reinforce these guidelines and further emphasize eating foods from plant sources (AICR, 2004). Dietary recommendations for women reiterated these health-promoting dietary guidelines (ADA & the Dietitians of Canada, 2004). In addition, the Alternate Healthy Eating Index was developed to target food choices and nutrient intake associated with chronic disease risk (McCullough et al., 2002).

The dietary guidelines from these major health organizations agree in their basic message. The AICR stated, "Our research has shown that a diet that prevents cancer can also prevent other chronic diseases . . . the United States Department of Agriculture (USDA) and other major health organizations are now largely in agreement about specific dietary guidelines that protect overall health" (AHA, 2004).

The AHA, the ACS, the American Diabetes Association, the AICR, and the North American Association for the Study of Obesity concur with the new dietary recommendations (AHA, 2004). In July 2004 the ACS, the American Diabetes Association, and the AHA collaborated to work on health promotion and disease prevention (Eyre, Kahn, & Robertson, 2004). In their collaborative efforts these organizations are making unified health statements concerning the prevention of heart disease, cancer, diabetes, and related risk factors. Furthermore, these organizations agree on the following dietary patterns, which may help reduce the risk of chronic diseases (AHA, 2004; Eyre et al., 2004):

- Consume a diet that emphasizes whole grains and legumes, vegetables, and fruits.
- Decrease saturated fat and dietary cholesterol; limit red meat and full-fat dairy products.
- Limit intake of foods and beverages high in added sugars.
- Limit overall intake of calories and engage in regular physical activity to maintain a healthy body weight.

In revising the Dietary Guidelines and the Food Guide Pyramid for 2006, the following revisions have been proposed (USDA, 2004):

- **Balance calories from foods and beverages according to the amount of calories expended and using the food guide to determine appropriate caloric requirements based on age and physical activity levels.**

- **Select nutritional goals for food intake patterns.**

- **Propose food intake patterns for educating the American public about healthful eating patterns.**

- **Use "cups" and "ounces" instead of "servings" in educational materials.**

- **Select appropriate illustrations of food patterns for consumer materials.**

Despite the evidence of the importance of diet to health, vegetable and fruit consumption among adults continues to be below recommended amounts: Fewer than 25% of U.S. adults consume five servings a day (ACS, 2009). According to the USDA's 1994–1996 Continuing Survey of Food Intakes by Individuals and the Food Guide Pyramid, only 3% of individuals meet four of the five recommendations for the intake of grains, fruits, vegetables, dairy products, and meats (USDA, 1998).

The current Dietary Guidelines for Americans were released in January 2005 by the USDHHS and the USDA. In the past a diet low in fat was recommended, but in 2000 this recommendation was changed to a diet "moderate" in total fat, and specifically low in saturated fat and cholesterol. The dietary guidelines have consistently encouraged the consumption of complex carbohydrates and fiber by eating more fruits, vegetables, and whole grains. In 2000 the guidelines separated the recommendations for eating fruits and vegetables and eating whole grains. The issue of safe foods was added. Two separate guidelines—"aiming for a healthy weight" and "increasing physical activity"—also were added in 2000.

In summary, diverse health organizations stress the similarities in the dietary recommendations for reducing disease risk. These recommendations are to eat less saturated fat and cholesterol (limit red meat and full-fat dairy products); increase consumption of fruits, vegetables, whole grains, and legumes; limit added sugar and sodium; drink alcohol in moderation; and increase physical activity. By using clear terms, public health nutrition and dietetic professionals can make the nutrition message easier for the public to understand, value, and implement. The Dietary Guidelines for Americans will be revised again for 2010; see http://www.cnpp.usda.gov/DietaryGuidelines.htm for updates.

Diet and Health: Nutrition Strategies and Risk Factors

Nutrition strategies are essential in the prevention and management of several chronic diseases and their risk factors.

Because many risk factors can be modified by healthy life-style changes, early recognition of the risk factors for chronic disease prevention is critical.

Obesity

Obesity has reached epidemic proportions in the United States. More than one-third of U.S. adults (over 66%), or over 72 million people, were obese in 2005–2006 (http://www.cdc.gov/obesity/data/trends/html). Rates of excessive weight and obesity are steadily growing in our country. More than 66% of the U.S. adult population was overweight or obese in 2003–2004, compared with 55% in 1988–1994 and 46% in 1976–1980 (USDHHS, 2000e; USDHHS, 2007). The National Institutes of Health (NIH) Expert Panel uses BMI for defining excessive weight and obesity (National Heart, Lung, and Blood Institute [NHLBI], 1998). The cut-off point for overweight status is a BMI of 25 kg/m^2. Obesity, defined as having a BMI of 30 kg/m^2 or greater, has doubled among adults since 1980. Extreme obesity (BMI of 40 kg/m^2 or higher) increased from 4.7% in 1999–2000 to 5.9% in 2003–2004 (Ogden, Carroll, & Flegal, 2008). The age-adjusted prevalence of overweight and obesity (BMI 25 kg/m^2 and higher) increased from 64.5% in 1999–2000 to 66.3% in 2003–2004. During the same time, obesity (BMI of 30 kg/m^2 or higher) increased from 30.5% to 34.3% (Ogden, Carroll, McDowell, & Flegal, 2007). Many diseases are associated with excessive weight and obesity, including CHD, stroke, high blood pressure, diabetes, arthritis-related disabilities, sleep apnea, gallbladder disease, and some cancers (USDHHS, 2000e).

The public health burden of excessive weight and obesity is overwhelming in terms of premature deaths and disability, lost productivity, and social stigmatization. Medical expenses for obesity accounted for 9.1% of total U.S. medical expenditures in 1998 and may have reached as high as $92.6 billion in 2002 (Finkelstein, Flebelkorn, & Wang, 2003). Another estimate places the total cost of obesity at $117 billion (USDHHS, 2004). Obesity rates are higher among certain population groups, such as Hispanic-Americans, African-Americans, Native Americans, and Pacific Islander-American women (USDHHS, 2000e). Research has reported, however, that overweight status has increased in all parts of the U.S. population (Mokdad, Bowman, et al., 2001; Flegal, Carroll, Ogden, & Johnson, 2002). The recent trend of overweight in the United States has become so severe that if it is not reversed in the next few years, poor diet and lack of physical exercise will likely become the leading preventable cause of mortality among adults (Mokdad, Marks, Stroup, & Gerberding, 2004).

Many factors contribute to excessive weight and obesity. For each individual, metabolic and genetic factors, as well as behaviors affecting dietary intake and physical activity, contribute to being overweight. Cultural, environmental, and socioeconomic influences also play a role. Most overweight and obese individuals eat more calories from food than they expend through physical activity. As body weight increases, so does the prevalence of health risks in an individual. For this reason, encouraging obese individuals to adopt new eating and physical activity habits is of vital importance.

Weight Management

The goals and outcomes of weight management programs should be guided by an assessment of an individual's weight (BMI) and health. The NHLBI guidelines recommend intervention for people who are overweight and have two or more risk factors associated with their weight (Kuczmarski & Flegal, 2000). Furthermore, according to the position paper of the ADA (2002) for weight management, assessment should incorporate the following areas: anthropometrics, medical causes, psychological causes, and nutritional causes.

For an individual, the goal of a weight management program should focus on the prevention of weight gain as well as weight loss. This recommendation encourages individuals to adopt healthier lifestyles, such as increasing physical activity and choosing less calorically dense foods. With this approach, weight loss will lead to reductions of health risks (Kassiger & Angell, 1998). A weight loss of as little as 10% can improve health risks associated with being overweight and obesity (NIH & NHLBI, 1998).

> ● **Learning Point** When developing a public health program, risk factor assessment needs to be addressed. The following criteria can be assessed:
> - The risk factor must have a strong association with the development of a chronic disease (e.g., obesity and heart disease).
> - The risk factor must affect a significant number of people.
> - The risk factor must be modifiable, so it can be reduced or changed.
> - The risk factor must have a modification that, when changed or reduced, results in decreased mortality.

> Visit www.nhlbi.gov for more information about the NHLBI's recommendations.

- *Anthropometrics:* The assessment of height, weight, BMI, and waist circumference (as waist measurement increases, so do health risks)

- *Medical causes:* Identifying potential causes, age at onset, obesity-associated complications, and severity of obesity

- *Psychological causes:* Eating disorders, possible psychological causes, and barriers to treatment

- *Nutritional causes:* Weight history, diet history, current eating patterns, nutritional intake, environmental factors, meals eaten away from home, exercise history, and motivation to change

For effective weight management programs, a multidisciplinary team should be involved, including a physician, a dietitian, an exercise physiologist, and a behavioral therapist. Health care professionals should be especially dedicated and sensitive to the needs of overweight and obese individuals. It is appropriate to discuss realistic goals of weight loss and maintenance so that shared responsibility for weight management can develop between the provider and individual. Goals might include the following (ADA, 2002):

- Prevention or cessation of weight gain in an individual who is continuing to see an increase in his or her weight
- Progress in physical and emotional health
- Small, realistic weight losses achieved through sensible eating and exercise
- Improvements in eating, exercise, and any behaviors apart from weight loss

Establishing both short- and long-term treatment goals and documenting measures before implementing the weight management plan and after the individual has started on the plan are important goals of care. Positive behavior changes, other than absolute weight, should be rewarded, because these can be very motivating.

Physical activity is highly recommended as an essential part of a weight management program. It is well established that to maintain weight loss, healthful dietary habits must be coupled with increased physical activity (USDHHS, 2000e). Physical activity contributes to weight loss not only by changing energy balance, but also by positively changing body composition by increasing lean body mass. Exercise decreases the risk of chronic disease and improves mood and quality of life. Many experts believe that physical inactivity is responsible for the increasing prevalence of excessive weight and obesity in the United States (USDHHS & NHLBI, 2001). Combining weight loss with regular physical activity reduces one's risk for chronic diseases such as heart disease and diabetes by reducing both blood cholesterol and blood glucose levels.

The biggest challenge in weight management is to maintain a healthy weight once it is achieved. It is essential to include physical activity in weight loss programs because regular physical activity is one of the best predictors of weight maintenance (Pavlou, Krey, & Stefee, 1989). Unfortunately, studies show that within five years, most people regain the weight they have lost (NIH Technology Assessment Conference Panel, 1993). The NIH recommends that both dietary and physical activity changes need to be continued indefinitely for weight loss to be maintained (NIH & NHLBI, 1998). A comprehensive life-style program that focuses on nutrition, exercise, cognitive behavioral changes, and medical monitoring has been shown to be most effective for long-term success (Jeffrey et al., 2000).

Because of the increased prevalence of overweight and obesity in the United States, weight management becomes crucial for primary prevention of many chronic diseases. It is the foundation of secondary and tertiary prevention of hypertension, high blood cholesterol, diabetes, arthritis, and some cancers. It is important for health care providers to lobby for public health policies that endorse the treatment and management of weight. Also, clients must be informed of the known healthy and positive outcomes achieved through weight management programs.

Cardiovascular Disease

Cardiovascular disease remains the nation's leading cause of death, accounting for more than 36% of all deaths in the United States. Despite a decline in heart-disease mortality, in 2005 one in three U.S. adults, or more than 864,000 Americans, died of cardiovascular disease (AHA, 2009). Three modifiable health behaviors—poor nutrition, lack of physical activity, and smoking—contribute greatly to the burden of heart disease.

Cardiovascular diseases include diseases of the heart and blood vessels: CHD, stroke, and peripheral vascular diseases. CHD is the most common form of cardiovascular disease and usually involves atherosclerosis and hypertension. Atherosclerosis is characterized by the buildup of plaques along the inner walls of the arteries, causing inadequate blood flow and leading to serious cardiovascular problems.

The consequences of cardiovascular disease are usually heart disease and stroke; these two diseases combined cause one death every 33 seconds (USDHHS, 2004). About 80 million U.S. adults live with the effects of heart disease and stroke. The annual cost of cardiovascular disease and stroke is estimated at $475 billion (CDC, National Center for Chronic Disease Prevention and Health Promotion, & U.S. Department of Health and Human Services, 2009). The death rate from cardiovascular disease fell by 17% in the last part of the 20th century; however, the number of deaths increased by 2.5% each year due to the growth and size of the population aged 65 years and older (CDC, 2006). The decrease in the mortality rates due to cardiovascular disease is attributed to primary prevention (i.e., a decrease in dietary intake of saturated fat), secondary prevention (i.e., early detection and treatment of hypertension), and improved medical and surgical treatments (AHA, 2004). In general, mortality and prevalence rates of cardiovascular disease could be improved by reducing the major risk factors: high blood pressure, high blood cholesterol, tobacco use, physical inactivity, and poor nutrition. Controlling one or more of these risk factors could have a major public health impact in our country.

Hypertension

High blood pressure, or hypertension, remains a "silent killer" in the United States, affecting about 73.6 million, or one in three, Americans (CDC, 2009). High blood pressure is a major independent risk factor for cardiovascular disease. Hypertension increases the risk of heart attack, heart failure, stroke, and kidney disease (USDHHS, NIH, NHLBI, & NHBPEP, 2003). This is significant because heart disease and stroke are, respectively, the first and third leading causes of death in the United States (USDHHS, 2007).

> **● Learning Point** A usual food intake in the United States, complete with convenience and fast foods, may provide 10,000 to 20,000 mg of sodium per day. Visit www.nhlbi.nih.gov/guidelines/hypertension/ for more information about the Seventh Report of the Joint National Committee on Prevention, Detection, Evaluation, and Treatment of High Blood Pressure.

In the latest classification of blood pressure for adults, normal blood pressure is considered to be less than 120/80 mm Hg, and prehypertension is designated as 120 to 139 systolic or 80 to 89 mm Hg diastolic pressure (USDHHS, NIH, & NHLBI, 2003). High blood pressure for adults is defined as a systolic pressure of 140 mm Hg or higher or a diastolic pressure of 90 mm Hg or higher.

A recent finding has determined that systolic blood pressure is a more important predictor of CHD in older adults than diastolic blood pressure (Systolic Hypertension in the Elderly Program, 1991).

The number of people who were able to control their high blood pressure through life-style changes and the use of antihypertensive drugs rose from about 16% in 1971–1972 to about 65% in 1988–1994 (NHLBI, 1998). The age-adjusted death rate attributed to hypertension rose by about 36.4% from 1991 to 2001, with the actual number of deaths increasing by 53% (Eyre et al., 2004). From 1995 to 2005 the death rate from high blood pressure increased 25% and the actual number of deaths rose 56.4% (AHA, 2009). Among people with high blood pressure, 69% are being treated, 45% have it under control, and 54.6% do not have their high blood pressure under control (AHA, 2009). Significant disparities exist among persons diagnosed with hypertension; for example, African-Americans have high blood pressure at an earlier age and in general have higher blood pressures (USDHHS, 2000c). Twenty-two percent of U.S. adults are unaware they have hypertension (AHA, 2009).

The latest guidelines for the treatment of hypertension are found in the Seventh Report of the Joint National Committee on Prevention, Detection, Evaluation, and Treatment of High Blood Pressure (USDHHS, NIH, & NHLBI, 2003). This report advocates major life-style modifications shown to lower blood pressure, enhance antihypertensive drug efficacy, and decrease cardiovascular risk. General lifestyle modifications include weight reduction for overweight or obese individuals (the goal is for a BMI of 18.5 to 24.9) (Trials of Hypertension Prevention Collaborative Research Group, 1997; He, Whelton, Appel, Charleston, & Klag, 2000), the adoption of the Dietary Approaches to Stop Hypertension (DASH) eating plan (Sacks et al., 2001), reducing sodium intake (Chobanian & Hill, 2000), increasing physical activity (Whelton, Chin, Xin, & He, 2002), and moderating alcohol consumption (Xin et al., 2001).

The DASH eating plan is a diet rich in calcium and potassium, consisting of fresh fruits, vegetables, and low-fat dairy products (Sacks et al., 2001; Vollmer et al., 2001). The DASH eating plan advocates a low sodium intake; intakes of 1,600 mg have been found to be as effective as single drug therapy in lowering blood pressure (Sacks et al., 2001). Other specific life-style modifications include reducing sodium to 2,400 mg a day, engaging in regular aerobic physical activity at least 30 minutes a day (most days of the week), and limiting alcohol consumption (two drinks a day for men and one drink a day for women) (USDHHS, NIH, & NHLBI, 2003). The report's guidelines recommend these life-style modifications for all individuals. For those people who have not achieved the goal blood pressure (< 140/90 mm Hg), antihypertensive drugs, such as thiazide-type diuretics, may also be recommended (Psatsy et al., 1997).

Cholesterol

High blood cholesterol is one of the major independent risk factors for heart disease and stroke (USDHHS, 2004). Modifying this risk factor is effective in reducing cardiovascular disease mortality. Animal, epidemiologic, and metabolic research show that having elevated blood cholesterol levels is associated with cardiovascular disease. In spite of recommended dietary guidelines and medications available, about 45% of U.S. adults have total blood cholesterol levels of 200 mg/dL or greater and almost 33% have a low density lipoprotein (LDL) cholesterol of 130 mg/dL or higher (NCHS, 2007). Between 1999–2000 and 2005–2006, mean serum total cholesterol levels in adults aged 20 and older declined from 204 mg/dL to 199 mg/dL (NCHS, 2007).

● **Learning Point** Statin drugs lower blood cholesterol by inhibiting 5-hydroxy-3-methylglutaryl coenzyme A reductase, a liver enzyme that is responsible for producing cholesterol.

● **Learning Point** The decision to go on drug therapy for high LDL levels depends on a multitude of risk factors and is decided between the physician and the patient.

● **Learning Point** Nutritionists also need to consider prevailing eating and ethnic habits when counseling people to lower blood cholesterol levels. In terms of adhering to the ATP III protocol guidelines (and the update), patients and health care providers are key players in realizing the benefits of cholesterol-lowering and in attaining the highest possible levels of CHD risk reduction.

Research in the 1980s showed that lowering high blood cholesterol significantly reduces the risk for heart attacks and reduces overall mortality rates. As a result, the National Cholesterol Education Program was launched in 1985 (Cleeman & Lenfant, 1998). Since its inception, the percentage of people who have had their cholesterol checked more than doubled, from 35% in 1983 to 75% in 1995 (NHLBI, 1995). Current guidelines recommend that all adults, aged 20 or older, have their blood cholesterol levels checked every five years as a preventive measure (USDHHS, 2000c). Nevertheless, over 80% of adults who have high blood cholesterol do not have it under control.

In terms of dietary trends and blood cholesterol levels, as dietary consumption of total fat, saturated fat, and cholesterol declined in the 1980s and 1990s, average blood cholesterol levels in adults declined from 213 mg/dL in 1978 to 203 mg/dL in 1991 (Cleeman & Lenfant, 1998). Research shows that as little as a 10% decrease in total cholesterol levels can reduce the incidence of CHD by almost 30% (USDHHS, 2004).

In 2001 the National Cholesterol Education Program released updated clinical guidelines in its report of the Expert Panel on the Detection, Evaluation and Treatment of High Blood Cholesterol in Adults, referred to as the Adult Treatment Panel (ATP) III (USDHHS & NHLBI, 2001). This report updates the recommendations made in ATP II and I for people with high blood cholesterol levels and reinforces findings from studies that confirm elevated LDL cholesterol to be a major cause of CHD. The guidelines in ATP III focus on strategies to lower LDL cholesterol and on primary prevention in persons with multiple risk factors (USDHHS, NIH, & NHLBI, 2003). In 2004 an update was added to the National Cholesterol Education Program guidelines on cholesterol management that advised physicians to consider new, more intensive medical treatments, such as statin drugs for people at high and moderately high risk for a heart attack (Grundy et al., 2004).

The ATP III report recommends a complete lipoprotein profile that includes total cholesterol, LDL cholesterol, high-density lipoprotein (HDL) cholesterol, and triglycerides as the preferred test rather than screening for total cholesterol and HDLs alone. For LDL-lowering therapy, a person's risk status needs to be assessed based on multiple risk factors, including cigarette smoking, hypertension, low HDL, family history of premature CHD, and age. Diabetes is considered as a CHD equivalent in assessing a person's risk. In addition, the current guidelines use the Framingham scoring projections of 10-year absolute CHD risk to identify people who need more intensive therapy and those with multiple metabolic risk factors. The National Cholesterol Education Program defines high-risk patients as those who have CHD, diabetes, or multiple (two or more) risk factors, such as hypertension or smoking, which gives them a greater than 20% chance of having a heart attack within 10 years (USDHHS & NHLBI, 2001). Very high-risk patients are those who have cardiovascular disease together with either multiple risk factors (especially diabetes) or badly controlled risk factors (e.g., smoking), or metabolic syndrome (a constellation of risk factors associated with obesity). For moderately high-risk and high-risk persons, the ATP III report and update recommend drug therapy in addition to therapeutic life-style changes, which include intensive use of nutrition, weight control, and physical activity (USDHHS & NHLBI, 2001; Grundy et al., 2004).

The specific parts of therapeutic life-style changes include the following: reducing intakes of saturated fat to less than 7% of total calories and decreasing cholesterol to less than 200 mg/day. Total fat from calories can be in the 25% to 35% range, as long as saturated and trans-fatty acids are kept low. Individuals are encouraged to use plant stanols and sterols in their diet (2 g/day). Small amounts of plant sterols, or phytosterols, occur naturally in pine trees and foods like soybeans, nuts, grains, and oils. Increasing soluble fiber to 10 to 25 g/day is also recommended with weight reduction and increased physical activity. Because excessive weight and obesity are considered major underlying risk factors for CHD, weight reduction enhances LDL-lowering interventions.

In comparing the recommendations set forth in the ATP III report to the more recent updates, more intensive treatment options are delineated for very high-risk individuals. For high-risk patients, the goal in both reports remains an LDL level of less than 100 mg/dL; for very high-risk patients, a therapeutic option is to treat with statins to lower levels to less than 70 mg/dL. The update lowers the threshold for drug therapy to an LDL of 100 mg/dL or higher and recommends drug therapy for those high-risk people whose LDL is 100 to 129 mg/dL.

In ATP III, for moderately high-risk persons the LDL treatment goal is less than 130 mg/dL and drug therapy is recommended if LDL levels are 130 mg/dL or higher. In the update, there is a therapeutic option to set the treatment goal at LDL less than 100 mg/dL and to use statin drug therapy if LDL is 100 to 129 mg/dL to reach the goal. In the update, when LDL drug therapy is used it is advised that enough medication be used to achieve at least a 30% to 40% reduction in LDL levels. In both reports, anyone with LDL above the goal is a candidate for therapeutic life-style changes. In the update, any person at high or moderately high risk who has life-style-related risk factors should follow therapeutic life-style changes, regardless of LDL level (USDHHS & NHLBI, 2001; Grundy et al., 2004).

As individuals learn about their risk factors and begin therapeutic life-style changes, more registered dietitians and nutritionists will be asked to help people make necessary dietary changes. ATP III guidelines recommend that physicians refer individuals to dietitians for MNT (USDHHS & NHLBI, 2001). Referral to a dietitian is recommended at all stages in the model of therapeutic life-style changes. The guidelines challenge public health providers to provide diet and exercise recommendations that will make a difference to those with elevated blood cholesterol levels.

Both screening for risk factors and compliance in adopting the lipid-lowering guidelines are essential. In reality, fewer than 50% of those persons eligible for meeting the criteria actually receive treatment (USDHHS & NHLBI, 2001).

Physical Activity

Research demonstrates that virtually all individuals benefit from regular physical activity. Yet, more than 60% of U.S. adults are not regularly physically active (USDHHS, 1996). According to recent research, the prevalence of regular leisure-time physical activity among adults is 30.8% (CDC, 2007). Twenty-five percent of all adults are not active at all. Inactivity increases with age and is more common among women than men. Also, those with lower incomes and less education exercise less than those with higher incomes or education (USDHHS, 1996). Thus, physical inactivity is a prevalent risk in the United States. People who are sedentary are almost twice as likely to develop CHD as people who engage in regular physical activity (USDHHS, 2000f). The risk imposed by physical inactivity is almost as high as other well-known CHD risk factors, such as high blood cholesterol, high blood pressure, or smoking (USDHHS, 1996, 2000f). Even moderate physical activity produces significant health benefits, such as a decreased risk of CHD (NIH Consensus Development Panel on Physical Activity and Cardiovascular Health, 1996).

Research shows that moderate physical activity, such as walking 30 minutes a day five times a week, is more likely to be adopted and maintained than vigorous activity (Pate et al., 1995).

There are many health benefits to be gained from regular physical activity. It enhances cardiovascular function, reduces very low-density lipoprotein levels, raises HDL cholesterol, and can lower LDL cholesterol levels (USDHHS & NHLBI, 2001). Physical activity lowers blood pressure and reduces insulin resistance. Overall, physical activity improves muscle function, cardiovascular function, and physical performance and aids in weight management (USDHHS, 1996). Nutritionists should become aware of the different types of physical activity, especially moderate levels of activity, that can lower an individual's risk for cardiovascular disease.

Smoking

Cigarette smoking is responsible for more than 440,000 deaths each year and is the single largest preventable cause of death and disease among U.S. adults (USDHHS, 2004). Public health professionals, concerned about the risk factors for cardiovascular disease, need to discuss smoking with clients because it is a leading risk factor. Of the estimated 12 million deaths from smoking, almost half (5.5 million) are deaths from cardiovascular diseases (USDHHS, 2004). In 2003 an estimated 1.1 million Americans had a new or recurrent heart attack. Cigarette smoking results in a 2- to 3-fold risk of dying from coronary heart disease. Smoking-related CHD may also contribute to congestive heart failure, causing 4.6 million to suffer from this disease (USDHHS, 2004). Smoking approximately doubles a person's risk of stroke, which is the third leading cause of death in the United States. However, the risk of stroke decreases when an individual stops smoking. Nonsmokers exposed to secondary smoke increase their risk of heart disease by 25% to 30% (USHHS, 2006).

Smoking cessation is also effective in preventing heart disease. In fact, after just 1 year of smoking abstinence, people who quit smoking have a 50% lower risk of death from CHD than those who continue to smoke (USDHHS, 1990). Studies have shown that secondhand smoke exposure causes heart disease among adults, with an estimated 35,000 deaths each year (Glanz & Parmely, 1995; USDHHS, 2004).

Smoking is a modifiable risk factor, and its modification is effective in preventing cardiovascular disease mortality. Smoking cessation is particularly important in people with other cardiovascular risk factors, such as high blood pressure and elevated blood cholesterol, because these risk factors work synergistically. Cigarette smoking is also a risk factor for other leading causes of death and disability, including several kinds of cancer and chronic lung diseases (USDHHS, OSG, 2004).

Trends

Progress has been made in decreasing mortality and risk factors for cardiovascular diseases. Between 1987 and 1996 the age-adjusted death rate for CHD declined by 22.2%, whereas deaths caused by stroke declined by 13.2% (CDC, 1999). However, the HP 2010 objectives on CHD and stroke were not reached. Hypertension rates climbed from 11% to 29%. The prevalence of high blood cholesterol, however, declined from 26% to 19% between 1988 and 1994. There was a slight decline in smoking between 1995 and 1999–2000, yet deaths from smoking, poor diet, and physical inactivity still accounted for almost one-third of all deaths in the United States (Mokdad, Marks, Stroup, & Gerberding, 2004).

Results from epidemiologic studies suggest that diets rich in fruits, vegetables, whole grains, and low-fat dairy foods are associated with a lower risk of mortality from many chronic diseases, including heart disease (McCullough et al., 2002). This nutritional pattern is supported by all the major health organizations. Nevertheless, a large gap remains between recommended dietary patterns and what U.S. adults actually eat. Only about one-fourth of U.S. adults eat the recommended five or more servings of fruits and vegetables each day (USDHHS, 2004). Recent research on frequency of fruit and vegetable consumption shows little change from 1994 to 2000 (Serdula et al., 2004). Caloric intake from total fat declined from 36% to 34% from 1976 to 1994 but fell short of the target goal of 30% set by HP 2010 (USDHHS,

2000c). According to data from the National Health and Nutrition Examination Surveys, decreases in calories from dietary fat and dietary cholesterol coincided with decreases in blood cholesterol levels (Ernst, Sempos, Briefel, & Clark, 1997).

From 1950 to 1996 age-adjusted death rates from cardiovascular diseases declined 60% (CDC, 1999). Although this is a positive trend, other health indicators have not improved significantly. Increasing prevalence rates in obesity and the continued high levels of blood pressure and stroke pose a continued public health challenge (CDC, 1999).

Cancer

Cancer is an umbrella term used to describe a large group of diseases characterized by uncontrolled growth and spread of abnormal cells (ACS, 2009). Cancer is the second leading cause of death in the United States, causing 1 in every 4 deaths. In 2006 an estimated 560,000 Americans died from this disease (ACS, 2009). According to the ACS (2009) about one-third of cancer deaths are preventable and are attributed to dietary factors, physical inactivity, being overweight, or obesity. For U.S. adults who do not smoke, dietary choices and physical activity are the most modifiable determinants of cancer risk. All cancers caused by cigarettes and the heavy use of alcohol could be prevented. The National Cancer Institute estimates that about 9.6 million Americans who had been diagnosed with cancer at some point in their lives were alive in 2000 (ACS, 2009). This estimate includes people living with cancer and those who were cancer free (Ries et al., 2003). The five-year relative survival rate for all cancers is 63%, or about 4 in 10 persons, which represents people who are living five years after diagnosis of cancer (ACS, 2009).

Age-standardized death rates from all cancers decreased by 7.2% between 1991 and 2000 (Ries et al., 2003). Compared with the peak rate of 215.1 deaths per 100,000 in 1991, the cancer death rate decreased 16% to 180.7 in 2006. Despite this decrease in the death rate from cancer, the total number of people who develop or die from cancer each year continues to increase because of our aging population (Stewart, King, Thompson, Friedman, & Wingo, 2004). The overall decrease in death rates from cancer is due to a decline in smoking and more effective detection and screening. The recent decrease in deaths from breast cancer in white women, for example, is due to a greater use of breast screening in regular medical care. Cancer death rates vary by gender, race, and ethnicity. For example, African-Americans are more likely to die from cancer than are whites (Key, Allen, Spencer, & Travis, 2002).

Although inherited genes play a significant role in cancer risk, they explain only part of all cancer incidences (ACS, 2009). Most of the variation in cancer incidence cannot be explained by inherited factors. The predominant causes of cancer are external factors such as cigarette smoking, diet or nutrition, weight, and physical inactivity (Key et al., 2002; ACS, 2009). These factors act to modify the risk of cancer at all stages. It is estimated that more than 50% of all cancers could be prevented through dietary improvements, such as reducing total fat and increasing fruit and vegetable consumption, and smoking cessation (Willett, 1996; USDHHS, 2004). Doll and Peto (1981) estimated that about 10% to 70% of deaths from cancer were attributable to diet. However, recent evidence showing actual causes of death in the United States found that 14% of cancer deaths occurring in 1990 could be attributed to diet (McGinnis & Foege, 1993). The science of nutrition and cancer is evolving but still is not as developed as that of diet and cardiovascular disease. Many large-scale studies are currently under way to further elucidate the relationship between various nutrients and cancer (McGinnis & Foege, 1993). Future research points to the areas of diet and gene interactions and biomarkers for cancer that will further our understanding in this area (Mandelson et al., 2000).

Current dietary recommendations are based on evidence from the ACS, the AICR/World Cancer Research Fund, and the Harvard Cancer Prevention Study (Food and Nutrition Science Alliance [FANSA], 2004; (ACS, 2009). In 2001 the ACS updated its guidelines on nutrition and physical activity after reviewing current scientific evidence (Byers et al., 2002). In general, the current dietary guidelines support the existing 2005 Dietary Guidelines for Americans and also encourage the consumption of plant-based diets, without relying on processed foods. The guidelines endorse eating a diet that promotes healthy weight control along with physical activity (FANSA, 2004; ACS, 2009). See the 2010 Dietary Guidelines for Americans at www.dietaryguidelines.gov for updates. For cancer prevention the ACS recommends that individuals eat five or more servings of fruits and vegetables a day. Fruit and vegetable consumption may protect against cancers of the mouth and pharynx, esophagus, lung, stomach, colon, and rectum (ACS, 2009). In 2007 about 1 in 4 adults was eating the recommended amount. There has been little improvement in U.S. fruit and vegetable consumption since the mid-1990s, however. Nutrition and food scientists agree on the following recommendations to lower cancer risk (ACS, 2009):

- Eat a plant-based diet that includes a wide variety of fruits, vegetables, whole grains, beans, and legumes. The recommendation is to choose whole grains over refined sources and eat 3 to 5 servings of vegetables and 2 to 4 servings of fruits per day.
- Eat less fat from all food sources.
- Limit excess calories and maintain a healthful weight throughout life. Eat a sound diet and incorporate moderate or vigorous physical activity 5 days a week or more to further reduce risks of cancer.
- Drink alcohol in moderation.

Nutrition supplements are not universally recommended for cancer prevention. Instead, the cancer prevention benefits of diet are considered among the best due to the interactions of many vitamins, minerals, and other plant-derived substances found naturally occurring in foods (ACS, 2009). However, the possible benefits of supplemental folate, calcium, and selenium are noted (Byers et al., 2002; ACS, 2009). By eating whole foods and following the cancer prevention dietary recommendations along with physical activity, the protection of the body's cells may take place during the initiation, promotion, and progression stages of cancer. These food substances may repair damage that has already occurred in cells. Some literature sources state that individuals do not need to be concerned about the pesticide residues on fruits and vegetables, because the benefits of eating fruits and vegetables far outweigh any potential risk (AICR, 2004). More long-term studies may help to state this definitively.

The study of diet and cancer prevention is relatively new. Dietitians and other public health care professionals need to stay abreast of these discoveries to give appropriate guidance to individuals at risk. The basis of MNT should include those recommendations set forth by the ACS and the World Cancer Research Fund/AICR (AICR, 2004; ACS, 2009).

Diabetes

Diabetes is a serious, costly, and increasingly common chronic disease that poses a significant public health challenge. In 2003–2004 diabetes was the sixth leading cause of death in the United States (Xu et al., 2007). About 18 million Americans have diabetes, and over 5 million of these people are unaware they have the disease (Xu et al., 2007). Type 2 diabetes, once referred to as adult onset diabetes, may account for about 90% to 95% of all diagnosed cases of diabetes (NIDDK, 2004). The total prevalence of diabetes in the United States is expected to more than double from 2005 to 2050—from 5.6% to 12%. (Narayan et al., 2006). By 2050 an estimated 29 million Americans are expected to have a diagnosis of diabetes. The increase in the number of cases has been particularly high within certain ethnic and racial groups in the United States (CDC, 2004b).

● Learning Point The Diabetes Prevention Program, a major large-scale study of over 3,000 people at high risk for developing diabetes, confirmed that positive lifestyle changes such as diet, weight loss of 5% to 7%, and moderate-intensity physical activity (such as walking 30 min/day) can delay onset of diabetes and found a 58% reduction in the development of diabetes over a three-year period. The findings from this study, sponsored by the NIH, showed that exercise, a healthy diet, and weight loss can reduce the risk of developing diabetes by as much as 71% in high-risk individuals (Diabetes Prevention Program Research Group, 2003).

Medical complications of type 2 diabetes include heart disease, kidney failure, leg and foot amputations, and blindness. Each year about 12,000 to 24,000 people become blind because of diabetic eye disease (USDHHS, 2004). Most deaths caused by diabetes are due to diabetes-associated cardiovascular disease. The presence of diabetes in adults is associated with a 2- to 4-fold increase in CHD compared with nondiabetic adults. Almost three-fourths of adults with diabetes have hypertension (USDHHS, 2004). Diabetes is the cause of 44% of end-stage renal disease cases. Severe forms of nervous system damage occur in 60% to 70% of diabetic adults. Approximately 60% of all nontraumatic amputations in the United States occur in people with diabetes (USDHHS, 2000f). Periodontal or gum disease is also more common among diabetics. As a result diabetes is a costly disease, with the total attributable costs (direct and indirect) estimated at $174 billion annually (NIDDK, 2007).

Type 2 diabetes is associated with the following factors:

- *Age:* Diabetes is most common in people over 60 years of age (USDHHS, 2000f).
- *Ethnicity:* Deaths from diabetes are twice as high for African-Americans than for whites, Native Americans, and Hispanic-Americans; certain Pacific Islander-American and Asian-American populations also have higher rates.
- *Genetics and family history:* Genetic markers that indicate a greater risk for type 2 diabetes have been identified.
- *Obesity:* The increased prevalence of obesity among adults is positively associated with the increased rates of diabetes (Mokdad, Ford, et al., 2000). Data from clinical trials strongly support the potential of moderate weight loss to reduce the risk of type 2 diabetes (Diabetes Prevention Program Research Group, 2003).
- *History of gestational diabetes in women:* Gestational diabetes is a form of glucose intolerance that develops in some women during pregnancy. Obesity is associated with gestational diabetes. Women with a family history of gestational diabetes and Hispanic-American and African-American women are at an increased risk (Franz et al., 2004).
- *Impaired glucose metabolism:* People with prediabetes, or who are at increased risk of developing diabetes, have impaired fasting blood glucose. Research studies suggest that weight loss and increased physical activity among people with prediabetes may return glucose levels to normal and prevent the onset of diabetes (CDC, 2004b).
- *Physical inactivity:* If you are at higher risk and fairly inactive or exercise fewer than 3 times a week, you are more likely to develop type 2 diabetes.

In the United States recent life-style changes such as decreased physical activity and increased energy consumption, which contribute to the increased prevalence rates of obesity, are also strong risk factors for diabetes (Diabetes Prevention Program Research Group, 2003). Positive life-style changes such as healthful diet, weight loss of 5% to 7%, and moderate-intensity physical activity (e.g., walking 30 minutes a day) can delay the onset of diabetes.

MNT is an essential part of diabetes management for adults. Objectives for MNT include the following (Franz et al., 2004):

- Attaining and maintaining optimal metabolic outcomes, including normalizing blood glucose levels, maintaining a lipid profile that reduces vascular disease risk, and normalizing blood pressure levels
- Preventing, delaying, and treating the onset of complications by modifying nutrient intake and life-style to prevent and treat obesity, cardiovascular disease, hypertension, and nephropathy
- Optimizing health through sensible food choices and physical activity
- Addressing personal and cultural preferences as well as life-style factors, including a person's willingness to change, when determining individual nutritional needs

In terms of specific nutrients and dietary recommendations for type 2 diabetes, studies in healthy subjects and those at risk for type 2 diabetes support the importance of including foods containing complex carbohydrates in the diet, particularly those from whole grains, fruits, vegetables, and low-fat milk (Franz et al., 2004). Reduced intake of total fat, especially saturated fat, may reduce the risk of diabetes.

In summary, life-style changes such as reduced energy intake, increased physical activity, and nutrition education (with the goal of promoting weight loss) represent essential aspects of type 2 diabetes management for adults. HP 2010 (USDHHS, 2000a) discusses the challenges of diabetes and the preventive interventions aimed at them: primary prevention, screening and early diagnosis, access, and quality of care. This includes secondary and tertiary prevention, such as glucose control and decreasing complications from diabetes (USDHHS, 2000a). For dietitians, public health professionals, and educators, many opportunities exist to contribute to the effective management of diabetes.

Osteoporosis

As one grows, bones develop and become larger, heavier, and denser. At approximately age 30 years, peak bone mass is achieved in both men and women. After this time period adults begin to lose bone mass, and this continues as they get older. Osteoporosis, or porous bone disease, develops when bone loss reaches the point of causing fractures under common everyday stresses. Because of increased bone fragility, there is a greater susceptibility to fractures of the hip, spine, and wrist. Both men and women suffer from osteoporosis.

Osteoporosis currently affects 44 million Americans, or 55% of people aged 50 and older, 68% of whom are women (NIH, 2003; National Osteoporosis Foundation, 2008). These rates correspond to one in two women and one in four men, aged 50 and older, who will experience an osteoporosis-related fracture in their lifetime (NIH, 2003). Osteoporosis causes significant disability with important economic consequences, costing about $19 billion each year in direct expenditures (hospitals and nursing homes) (NIH, 2001). Experts predict that by 2025 these costs will rise to about $25.3 billion (National Osteoporosis Foundation, 2008). Of the 2 million fractures occurring each year due to osteoporosis, over 300,000 are hip fractures, 547,000 are vertebral fractures, and 450,000 are wrist fractures. Of the 300,000 annual hip fractures, 24% result in death following complications from the fracture (National Osteoporosis Foundation, 2008).

> For those living in colder climates without much sunshine, vitamin D supplementation is suggested to accompany calcium intake.

Osteoporosis is often called the "silent disease" because it can occur without any overt symptoms. The technical standard for measuring bone mineral density is dual-energy x-ray absorptiometry. A low bone mass density is a strong predictor of fracture risk (National Osteoporosis Foundation, 2008). Bone density tests can detect osteoporosis before a fracture occurs and can serve as a predictor for future fracture risks.

The chances of developing osteoporosis are greatest in white women beyond menopause. Women have less bone tissue and lose bone more easily than men because of the hormonal changes involved in menopause. Those individuals who have a low dietary intake of calcium and vitamin D over a lifetime, who are physically inactive, who are cigarette smokers, who are excessive alcohol drinkers, who are thin and small-framed, and who have a family history of osteoporosis are at increased risk (NIH, 2003; National Osteoporosis Foundation, 2008). In addition, white and Asian-American women are at highest risk, whereas African-American and Hispanic-American women have lower risks (National Osteoporosis Foundation, 2008). Excessive intake of protein, sodium, and caffeine also contribute to being at risk for osteoporosis. Anorexia nervosa, the use of certain medications, and low testosterone levels in men are also risk factors for osteoporosis.

The five factors that can be modified to prevent osteoporosis are (1) a diet rich in calcium and vitamin D, (2) weight-bearing exercise, (3) a healthy life-style that excludes smoking and excessive alcohol intake, (4) routine bone density measurements, and (5) the use of medication, when appropriate (National Osteoporosis Foundation, 2008).

Nutrition is an important modifiable risk factor in terms of both bone health and the prevention and treatment of osteoporosis. An adequate amount of calcium and vitamin D contributes significantly to bone health. Low calcium and vitamin D intakes are associated with low bone mass, rapid bone loss, and high fracture rates (Heany, 2002). Bone is a living, growing tissue, and 99% of the body's calcium is found in bone. Throughout one's lifetime, bone formation and resorption occurs. This process, known as bone turnover, is responsive to dietary calcium regardless of age. Dietary calcium works to strengthen bone by suppressing bone resorption and parathyroid hormone (Heany, 2002).

According to the NIH (2001), calcium is the most important nutrient for the prevention of osteoporosis. In spite of this, actual calcium intakes for most of the U.S. population are considerably lower than the current Dietary Reference Intake (Standing Committee on the Scientific Evaluation of Dietary Reference Intakes, Food and Nutrition Board, Institute of Medicine, 1997). Many studies have shown that adult skeletal health is improved by increasing dairy foods or calcium intake in the diet (Dairy Council, 2004). The DASH diet, used to treat hypertension, is a low-fat diet, rich in calcium, and has been shown to reduce bone turnover and reduce the risk of osteoporosis (Sacks et al., 2001). Calcium requirements can be met with low-fat dairy products; however, low consumption of milk and other dairy products in the U.S. diet is mainly responsible for low calcium intakes among U.S. adults (Dairy Council, 2004). Other foods contain calcium, such as dark leafy greens, but these foods usually provide less calcium per serving than milk, and most Americans do not eat these vegetables often. For individuals who do not consume enough calcium in their diets, calcium supplements are recommended.

Vitamin D also plays an important role in calcium absorption and bone health. Vitamin D is a major determinant of intestinal calcium absorption. When skin is exposed to sunlight, the body synthesizes vitamin D. However, studies show decreased production of vitamin D in the elderly and individuals who are housebound, especially in the winter months (NIH, 2003). Because of inadequate intake of vitamin D in a high proportion of older adults, the most recent Dietary Reference Intake increased the vitamin D requirements for people 50 years and older (Standing Committee on the Scientific Evaluation of Dietary Reference Intakes, Food and Nutrition Board, Institute of Medicine, 1997). Low-fat and non-fat milk, excellent sources of calcium, are fortified with 100 IU of vitamin D per serving.

In conclusion, osteoporosis is a serious public health disease and is largely preventable. Starting early in life both females and males should be advised on how to incorporate sources of calcium into their diets. The use of low-fat and non-fat dairy foods should be recommended, and if persons cannot consume dairy products, other food sources and calcium supplements are necessary. Adequate vitamin D intake needs to be addressed, as well. Public health nutritionists should encourage individuals to participate regularly in physical activity. Modifiable life-style factors should be discussed to promote bone health throughout life.

HIV/AIDS

In 1981 a new infectious disease, AIDS, was first identified in the United States. A few years later HIV was discovered, and this was identified as the viral agent that causes AIDS. HIV/AIDS has affected almost every ethnic, socioeconomic, and age group in the United States (CDC, 2001).

AIDS, a deadly disease, is the end stage of HIV infection. The infection progresses to overwhelm the immune system and leaves individuals defenseless against numerous other infections and diseases. HIV is spread through direct contact with contaminated body fluids, through sexual intercourse, through direct blood contact, or from mother to infant. In 1996, death rates from AIDS in the United States declined for the first time (CDC, 2001). Nevertheless, HIV/AIDS remains a significant cause of illness, disability, and death in the United States. According to the CDC, in 2006 the estimated number of diagnosed AIDS cases was about 1,106,400 (CDC, 2008). Death rates from AIDS have dropped dramatically in the United States due to the introduction of antiretroviral therapies (CDC, 2001).

Health complications for people with HIV/AIDS are immune dysfunction and its associated complications, which include malnutrition and wasting. HIV targets the immune system, rendering an individual susceptible to infections and disease. The CDC defines AIDS-related wasting syndrome as a 10% weight loss in a 6-month period accompanied by diarrhea or fever for more than 30 days (USDHHS, 2000d). Malnutrition and its complications can reduce one's tolerance to medications and other therapies. Malnutrition occurs in the form of tissue wasting, fat accumulation, increased lipid levels, and risk of other chronic disease. The ADA and the Dietitians of Canada (2000) strongly support nutrition evaluation and MNT as parts of the ongoing health care of HIV-infected individuals. In terms of MNT, this includes early assessment and treatment of nutrient deficiencies, the maintenance and restoration of lean body mass, and continued support for performing daily activities and maintaining quality of life.

According to the ADA and the Dietitians of Canada (2000), nutrition education and guidance should incorporate the following aspects:

- Healthful eating principles
- Water and food safety issues
- Perinatal and breast-feeding issues
- Nutrition management for symptoms such as anorexia, swallowing problems, diarrhea, and so on
- Food–medicine interactions
- Psychosocial and economic issues

- Alternative feeding methods (supplementation, tube feeding, or parenteral nutrition)
- Additional therapies, including physical activity and disease management
- Guidelines for evaluating nutrition information, diet claims, and individual mineral and vitamin supplementation
- Strategies for treatment of altered fat metabolism

In addition, it is important for an HIV-infected individual to have adequate access to food, health care, and other support systems. The maintenance and restoration of nutrition stores are interrelated with recommended medical therapies; therefore, it is essential that a public health nutritionist be an active participant in the health care team to provide optimal MNT.

Issues to Debate

1. What would you propose should be incorporated into public health programs that focus on nutrition as an important preventive factor in illness, disability, and death?
2. What advice would you give to the individual in the community with regard to preventing chronic disease risk factors such as obesity, physical inactivity, and smoking to reduce society's financial burden?
3. What proportion of public funds designated for nutrition services should be given for primary, secondary, and tertiary prevention versus acute medical care?
4. Programs such as for-profit weight loss centers are proliferating in the United States. What are positive and negative aspects of this trend compared with public health weight-management programs?

Websites

Alternate Healthy Eating Index www.hsph.harvard.edu/nutritionsource/pyramids.html
American Cancer Society www.cancer.org
American Diabetes Association www.diabetes.org
American Dietetic Association www.eatright.org
American Heart Association www.americanheart.org
American Institute for Cancer Research www.aicr.org
America on the Move www.americaonthemove.org
North American Association for the Study of Obesity www.naaso.org
U.S. Dietary Guidelines www.health.gov/dietary guidelines/

References

American Cancer Society (ACS). (2009). *Cancer Statistics 2009.* Atlanta, GA: ACS.

American Dietetic Association (ADA). (1996). Position paper: Nutrition education for the public. *Journal of the American Dietetic Association, 96,* 1183–1187.

American Dietetic Association (ADA). (1998). Position paper: The role of nutrition in health promotion and disease prevention programs. *Journal of the American Dietetic Association, 98,* 205–208.

American Dietetic Association (ADA). (2002). Position paper: Weight management. *Journal of the American Dietetic Association, 102,* 1145–1155.

American Dietetic Association (ADA) & the Dietitians of Canada. (2000). Position paper: Nutrition intervention in the care of persons with human immunodeficiency virus infection. *Journal of the American Dietetic Association, 100,* 708–717.

American Dietetic Association (ADA) & the Dietitians of Canada. (2004). Position paper: Nutrition and women's health. *Journal of the American Dietetic Association, 104,* 984–1001.

American Dietetic Association (ADA), the Office of Disease Prevention and Health Promotion, Public Health Service, & the

U.S. Department of Health and Human Services. (1993). *Worksite Nutrition: A Guide to Planning, Implementation, and Evaluation* (2nd ed.). Chicago: ADA.

American Heart Association (AHA). (2004). AHA comment, May 31, 2004. Health agencies applaud HHS/USDA new dietary guidelines. Retrieved June 29, 2004, from www.american heart.org

American Heart Association (AHA). (2009). *Heart Disease and Stroke Statistics: 2009 Update.* Dallas, TX: AHA.

American Institute of Cancer Research (AICR). (2001). The dietary guidelines: Surveillance issues and research needs. *Journal of Nutrition, 131*(Suppl.), 3154S–3155S.

American Institute of Cancer Research (AICR). (2004). Retrieved May 26, 2004, from www.aicr.org

Brunner, E., White, I., Thorogood, M., Bristow, A., Curle, D., & Marmot, M. (1997). Can dietary interventions change diet and cardiovascular risk factors? A meta-analysis of randomized controlled trials. *American Journal of Public Health, 87,* 1415–1422.

Byers, T., Nestle, M., McTiernan, A., Doyle, C., Currie-Williams, A., Gansler, T., et al. (2002). American Cancer Society guidelines on nutrition and physical activity for cancer prevention: Reducing the risk of cancer with healthy food choices and physical activity. *Cancer Journal for Clinicians, 52,* 92–111.

Centers for Disease Control and Prevention (CDC). (1999). Decline in deaths from heart disease and stroke—United States, 1990–1999. *Morbidity and Mortality Weekly Report, 48,* 649–656.

Centers for Disease Control and Prevention (CDC). (2001). Cases of HIV infection and AIDS in the United States, 2002. HIV/AIDS surveillance report. Addendum, 2002. *14*(2). Retrieved October 26, 2009 from http://www.cdc.gov/Hiv/topics/surveillance/resources/reports/2002report/default.htm

Centers for Disease Control and Prevention. (2009a). *The Burden of Chronic Diseases and Their Risk Factors: National and State Perspectives 2004.* Atlanta: U.S. Department of Health and Human Services. Retrieved October 20, 2009, from http://www.cdc.gov/nccdphp/burdenbook2004

Centers for Disease Control and Prevention (CDC). (2009b). *National Diabetes Fact Sheet: General Information and National Estimates on Diabetes in the United States.* Atlanta: U.S. Department of Health and Human Services, Centers for Disease Control and Prevention.

Centers for Disease Control and Prevention (CDC). (2006). *Fact Sheet: High Blood Pressure.* Retrieved October 20, 2009, from http://www.cdc.gov/DHDSP/library/fs_bloodpressure.htm

Centers for Disease Control and Prevention (CDC). (2006). Tobacco-related mortality. Retrieved June 15, 2009, from http://www.cdc.gov/tobacco/data_statistics/fact_sheets/health_effects/tobacco_related_mortality/

Centers for Disease Control and Prevention (CDC). (2007). Behavioral risk factor surveillance system (BRFSS) [information on prevalence and trends data, physical activity, year 2007]. Retrieved from http://apps.nccd.cdc.gov/brfss/page.asp?yr=2007&state=All&cat=PA#PA

Centers for Disease Control and Prevention (CDC). (2008). HIV prevalence estimate—United States, 2006. *Morbidity and Mortality Weekly Report 57*(39), 1073–1076.

Centers for Disease Control and Prevention (CDC), National Center for Chronic Disease Prevention and Health Promotion, & U.S. Department of Health and Human Services. (2009). Preventing heart disease and stroke: Addressing the nation's leading killers. Retrieved October 11, 2009, from http://www.cdc.gov/nccdphp/publications/AAG/dhdsp.htm

Centers for Disease Control and Prevention (CDC) & National Center for Health Statistics. (1992). Effectiveness in disease and injury prevention; estimated national spending on prevention. United States, 1988. *Morbidity and Mortality Weekly Report, 41,* 529–531.

Chobanian, A. V., & Hill, M. (2000). National Heart, Lung, and Blood Institute Workshop on Sodium and Blood Pressure: A critical review of current scientific evidence. *Hypertension, 35,* 858–863.

Cleeman, J. L., & Lenfant, C. (1998). The National Cholesterol Education Program: Progress and prospects. *Journal of the American Medical Association, 280,* 2099–2104.

Dairy Council. (2004). The benefits of dairy foods in health promotion. *Dairy Council Digest, 75*(3).

Diabetes Prevention Program Research Group. (2003). Reduction in the incidence of type 2 diabetes with lifestyle intervention or metformin. *New England Journal of Medicine, 346,* 393–403.

Dietary Guidelines Advisory Committee. (2000). *Report of the Dietary Guidelines Advisory Committee on the Dietary Guidelines for Americans.* Washington, DC: U.S. Department of Agriculture. Retrieved October 20, 2009, from http://www.cnpp.usda.gov/DGAs2000Guidelines.htm

Dietary Guidelines Advisory Committee. (2005). *Report of the Dietary Guidelines Advisory Committee on the Dietary Guidelines for Americans.* Washington, DC: U.S. Department of Agriculture. Retrieved October 20, 2009, from http://www.cnpp.usda.gov/DGAs2005Guidelines.htm

Dietary Guidelines Alliance. (1996). Do it yourself: Crafting consumer tips. In *Reaching Consumers with Meaningful Health Messages.* Washington, DC: Dietary Guidelines Alliance.

Doll, R., & Peto, R. (1981). The causes of cancer: Qualitative estimates of avoidable risks of cancer in the U.S. today. *Journal of the National Cancer Institute, 66,* 1191–1308.

Elo, S. L., & Caltrop, J. B. (2002). Health promotive action and preventive action model (HPA model) for the classification of healthcare services in public health nursing. *Scandinavian Journal of Public Health, 30,* 200–208.

Ernst, N. D., Sempos, S. T., Briefel, R. R., & Clark, M. B. (1997). Consistency between U.S. dietary fat intake and serum total cholesterol concentrations: The National Health and Nutrition Examination Surveys. *American Journal of Clinical Nutrition, 66,* 965S–972S.

Eyre, H., Kahn, R., & Robertson, R. M. (2004). Preventing cancer, cardiovascular disease, and diabetes. *Diabetes Care, 27,* 1812–1824.

Finkelstein, E. A., Flebelkorn, I. C., & Wang, G. (2003). National medical spending attributable to overweight and obesity: How much and who's paying. *Health Affairs,* W3-219–226.

Flegal, K. M., Carroll, M. D., Ogden, C. L., & Johnson, C. L. (2002). Prevalence and trends of obesity among U.S. adults, 1999–2000. *Journal of the American Medical Association, 288,* 1723–1727.

Food and Nutrition Science Alliance (FANSA). (2004). Diet and cancer prevention in the United States. Retrieved July 7, 2004, from www.eatright.org

Franz, M. J., Bantle, J. P., Beebe, C. A., Brunzell, J. D., Chiasson, J. L., Garg, A., et al. (2004). Nutrition principles and recommendations in diabetes. *Diabetes Care, 27,* S36.

Frazao, E. (1999). The high costs of poor eating patterns in the U.S. In E. Frazao (Ed.), *America's Eating Habits: Changes and Consequences.* AIB750. Retrieved October 20, 2009, from http://www.ers.usda.gov/publications/aib750/

Glanz, S. A., & Parmely, W. W. (1995). Passive smoking and heart disease: Mechanism and risk. *Journal of the American Medical Association, 272,* 1047–1053.

Goldberg, J. P. (1992). Nutrition and health communication: The message and the media over half a century. *Nutrition Review, 50,* 71–77.

Grundy, S. M., Cleeman, J. I., Merz, C. N., Brewer, Jr., H. B., Clark, L. T., Hunninghake, D. B., et al. (2004). For the coordinating committee of the National Cholesterol Education Program. Implications of recent clinical trials for the National Cholesterol Education Program Adult Treatment Panel III Guidelines. *Circulation, 110,* 227–239.

He, J., Whelton, P. K., Appel, L. J., Charleston, J., & Klag, M. J. (2000). Long-term effects of weight-loss and dietary sodium restriction on incidence of hypertension. *Hypertension, 35,* 544–549.

Heany, R. P. (2002). The importance of calcium intake for life-long skeletal health. *Calcified Tissue International, 70,* 70–73.

Jeffrey, R. W., Drewsiowski, A., Epstein, L. H., Stunkard, A. J., Wilson, G. T., Wing, R. R., et al. (2000). Long-term maintenance of weight-loss: Current status. *Health Psychology, 1*(Suppl.), 5–16.

Kannel, W. B., Dawber, T. R., & McGee, D. L. (1980). Perspectives on systolic hypertension: The Framingham Study. *Circulation, 61,* 1179–1182.

Kassiger, J. P., & Angell, M. (1998). Losing weight: An ill-fated New Year's resolution. *New England Journal of Medicine, 1338,* 52–54.

Kaufman, M. (Ed.). (1990). *Nutrition in Public Health: A Handbook for Developing Programs and Services.* Rockville, MD: Aspen.

Key, T. J., Allen, N. E., Spencer, E. A., & Travis, R. C. (2002). The effect of diet on risk of cancer. *Lancet, 360,* 861–868.

Koplan, J. P., & Dietz, W. H. (1999). Caloric imbalance and public health policy. *Journal of the American Medical Association, 282,* 1579–1581.

Krauss, R. M., Eckel, R. H., Howard, B., Appel, L. J., Daniels, S. R., Deckelbaum, R. J., et al. (2000). AHA dietary guidelines: Revision 2000. A statement for healthcare professionals from the Nutrition Committee of the American Heart Association. *Circulation, 102,* 2284–2299.

Kris-Etherton, P., Daniels, S. R., Eckel, R. H., Engler, M., Howard, B. V., Krauss, R. M., et al. (2001). Summary of the scientific conference on dietary fatty acids and cardiovascular health. Conference summary from the Nutrition Committee of the American Heart Association. *Circulation, 103,* 1034–1039.

Kuczmarski, R. J., & Flegal, K. M. (2000). Criteria for definition of overweight in transition: Background and recommendations for the United States. *American Journal of Clinical Nutrition, 72,* 1074–1081.

Mandelson, M. T., Oestreicher, N., Porter, P. L., White, D., Finder, C. A., Taplin, S. H., et al. (2000). Breast density as a predictor of mammographic detection: Comparison of interval- and screen-detected cancers. *Journal of the National Cancer Institute, 92,* 1081–1087.

McCullough, M. L., Feskanich, D., Stampfer, M. J., Giovannucci, E. L., Rimm, E. B., Hu, F. B., et al. (2002). Diet quality and major chronic disease in men and women: Moving toward improved dietary guidance. *American Journal of Clinical Nutrition, 76,* 1261–1271.

McGinnis, J. M., & Foege, W. H. (1993). Actual causes of death in the United States. *Journal of the American Medical Association, 270,* 2207–2212.

McRobbie, M. A., & Kolbe, L. J. (2009). The academy's pivotal role in supporting public-private partnerships to prevent chronic diseases. *Preventing Chronic Disease, 6*(2), A73.

Mokdad, A. H., Bowman, B. A., Ford, E. S., Vinicor, F., Macks, J. S., & Koplan, J. C. (2001). The continuing epidemics of obesity and diabetes in the U.S. *Journal of the American Medical Association, 286,* 1195–1200.

Mokdad, A. H., Ford, E. S., Bowman, B. A., Nelson, D. E., Engelgau, M. M., Vinicor, F., et al. (2000). Diabetes trends in the U.S.: 1990–1998. *Diabetes Care, 23,* 1278–1283.

Mokdad, A. H., Marks, J. S., Stroup, D. F., & Gerberding, J. L. (2004). Actual causes of death in the U.S., 2000. *Journal of the American Medical Association, 291,* 1238–1245.

Mokdad, A. H., Marks, J. S., Stroup, D. F., & Gerberding, J. L. (2005). Correction: Actual causes of death in the United States, 2000. *Journal of the American Medical Association, 293,* 293–294.

Narayan, K. M., Boyle, J. P., Geiss, M. A., Saaddine, J., Thompson, T. J. (2006). Impact of recent increase on incidence on future diabetes burden: U.S., 2005–2050. *Diabetes Care, 29,* 2114–2116.

National Center for Health Statistics (NCHS). (1997). Report of the final mortality statistics, 1995. *Monthly Vital Statistics Report, 5*(Suppl. 2).

National Center for Health Statistics (NCHS). (2003). *Health.* Washington, DC: Government Printing Office.

National Center for Health Statistics (NCHS). (2007). High serum total cholesterol—an indicator for monitoring cholesterol-lowering efforts: U.S. adults, 2005–06; *NCHS Data Brief,* (2), 1–8.

National Heart, Lung, and Blood Institute (NHLBI). (1995). *Consumer Awareness Surveys.* Press conference. Bethesda, MD: NHLBI. Available at http://www.faqs.org/abstracts/Health/Change-in-cholesterol-awareness-and-action-Results-from-national-physician-and-public-surveys.html

National Heart, Lung, and Blood Institute (NHLBI). (1998). *Morbidity and Mortality: 1998 Chartbook of Cardiovascular, Lung, and Blood Diseases.* Rockville, MD: U.S. Department of Health and Human Services, National Institutes of Health.

National Heart, Lung, and Blood Institute (NHLBI). (2004). National High Blood Pressure Education Program [program description]. Retrieved October 20, 2009, from http://www.nhlbi.nih.gov/about/nhbpep/index.htm

National Institute of Diabetes and Digestive and Kidney Diseases (NIDDK). (2004). Diabetes prevention program. Retrieved October 20, 2009, from http://diabetes.niddk.nih.gov/dm/pubs/preventionprogram/

National Institute of Diabetes and Digestive and Kidney Diseases (NIDDK). (2007). *National Diabetes Statistics.* NIH Publication No. 08-3892. Retrieved October 20, 2009, from http://diabetes.niddk.nih.gov/dm/pubs/statistics/index.htm

National Institutes of Health (NIH). (2001). Consensus Development Panel on osteoporosis. *Journal of the American Medical Association, 285,* 785.

National Institutes of Health (NIH). (2008). *Osteoporosis and related bone diseases, National Resource Center.* Retrieved October 15, 2009, from http://www.niams.nih.gov/Health_Info/Bone/

National Institutes of Health (NIH) Consensus Development Panel on Physical Activity and Cardiovascular Health. (1996). Physical activity and cardiovascular health. *Journal of the American Medical Association, 276,* 241–246.

National Institutes of Health (NIH) & the National Heart, Lung, and Blood Institute (NHLBI). (1998). Clinical guidelines on the identification, evaluation, and treatment of overweight and obesity in adults—the evidence report. *Obesity Research, 6,* 1105.

National Institutes of Health (NIH) Technology Assessment Conference Panel. (1993). Methods for voluntary weight loss and control. Consensus development conference. March 30–April 1, 1992. *Annals of Internal Medicine, 119,* 764–770.

National Osteoporosis Foundation. (2008). Osteoporosis, disease statistics. Retrieved July 12, 2004, from www.nof.org

National Research Council, Committee on Diet and Health. (1989). *Diet and Health: Implications for Reducing Chronic Disease Risk.* Washington, DC: National Academy Press.

Ogden, C. L., Carroll, M. D., & Flegal, K. M. (2008). High body mass index for age among U.S. children and adolescents, 2003–2006. *Journal of the American Medical Association, 299* (20), 2401–2405.

Ogden, C. L., Carroll, M. D., McDowell, M. A., & Flegal, K. M. (2007). Obesity among adults in the United States—no change since 2003–2004. NCHS data brief no. 1. Hyattsville, MD: National Center for Health Statistics. Retrieved June 14, 2009, from www.cdc/nchs/

Pate, R. R., Pratt, M., Blair, S. N., Haskell, W. L., Macera, C. A., Bouchard, C., et al. (1995). Physical activity and public health: A recommendation from the Centers for Disease Control and Prevention and the American College of Sports Medicine. *Journal of the American Medical Association, 273,* 402–407.

Pavlou, K. N., Krey, S., & Stefee, W. O. (1989). Exercise as an adjunct to weight loss and maintenance in moderately obese subjects. *American Journal of Clinical Nutrition, 49,* 1115–1123.

Pender, N. J. (1996). *Health Promotion in Nursing Practice* (3rd ed.). Stamford, CT: Appleton & Lange.

Psatsy, B. M., Smith, N. L., Siscovick, D. S., Koepsell, T. D., Weiss, N. S., Heckbert, S. R., et al. (1997). Health outcomes associated with antihypertensive therapies used as first-line agents. A systematic review and meta-analysis. *Journal of the American Medical Association, 277,* 739–745.

Resnicow, K., Orlandi, M., Vaccaro, D., & Wynder, E. (1989). Implementation of a pilot school-site cholesterol reduction intervention. *Journal of School Health, 59,* 74–78.

Ries, L., Eisner, M., Kosary, C., Hankey, B. F., Miller, B. A., Clegg, L., et al. (Eds.) (2003). *SEER: Cancer Statistics Review, 1975–2000.* Bethesda, MD: National Cancer Institute.

Sacks, F. M., Syerkey, L. P., Vollmer, W. M., Appel, L. J., Bray, G. A., Harsha, D., et al. (2001). Effects on blood pressure of reduced dietary sodium and Dietary Approaches to Stop Hypertension (DASH) diet. DASH-Sodium Collaborative Research Group. *New England Journal of Medicine, 344,* 3–10.

Serdula, M. K., Gillespie, C., Kettel-Khan, L., Farris, R., Seymour, J., & Denny, C. (2004). Trends in fruit and vegetable consumption among adults in the United States: Behavioral Risk Factor Surveillance System, 1994–2000. *American Journal of Public Health, 94,* 1014–1018.

Shamansky, S. L., & Clausen, C. (1980). Levels of prevention: Examination of the concept. *Nursing Outlook, 28,* 104–108.

Sharlin, J., Posner, B. M., Gershoff, S., Zeitlin, M., & Berger, P. (1992). Nutrition and behavioral characteristics and determinants of cholesterol levels in men and women. *Journal of the American Dietetic Association, 92,* 434–440.

Standing Committee on the Scientific Evaluation of Dietary Reference Intakes, Food and Nutrition Board, Institute of Medicine. (1997). *Dietary Reference Intakes for Calcium, Phosphorus, Magnesium, Vitamin D, and Fluoride.* Washington, DC: National Academy Press. Retrieved October 20, 2009, from http://www.nap.edu/catalog.php?record_id=5776

Stewart, S. L., King, J. B., Thompson, T. D., Friedman, C., & Wingo, P. (2004). Cancer mortality surveillance—United States, 1990–2000. National Center for Chronic Disease Prevention and Health Promotion. *Morbidity and Mortality Weekly Report, 53*(S503), 1–108.

Systolic Hypertension in the Elderly Program (SHEP) Cooperative Research Group. (1991). Prevention of stroke by antihypertensive drug treatment in older persons with isolated systolic hypertension. Final results of the SHEP. *Journal of the American Medical Association, 265,* 3255–3264.

Trials of Hypertension Prevention Collaborative Research Group. (1997). Effects of weight-loss and sodium reduction intervention on blood pressure and hypertension incidence in overweight people with high-normal blood pressure. The Trials of Hypertension Prevention, Phase 11. *Archives of Internal Medicine, 157,* 657–667.

U.S. Department of Agriculture (USDA). (1998). *USDA Continuing Survey of Food Intakes by Individuals (CSFII), 1994–1996.* Washington, DC: U.S. Department of Agriculture. Available from http://www.ars.usda.gov/Services/docs.htm?docid= 14531

U.S. Department of Agriculture (USDA). (2004). Scientific update of food guidance presented to the Dietary Guidelines Committee [news release]. Retrieved June 29, 2004, from www.usda.gov

U.S. Department of Agriculture (USDA) & U.S. Department of Health and Human Services (USDHHS). (1992). *The Food Guide Pyramid.* Washington, DC: Authors.

U.S. Department of Health and Human Services (USDHHS). (1990). *The Health Benefits of Smoking Cessation: A Report of the Surgeon General.* Public Health Service, Centers for Disease Control, Center for Chronic Disease Prevention and Health Promotion, Office on Smoking and Health. DHHS Publication No. (CDC) 90-8416.

U.S. Department of Health and Human Services (USDHHS). (1996). *Physical Activity and Health: A Report of the Surgeon General, 1996.* Centers for Disease Control and Prevention, National Center for Chronic Disease Prevention and Health Promotion. Retrieved October 20, 2009, from http://www.cdc.gov/nccdphp/sgr/ataglan.htm

U.S. Department of Health and Human Services (USDHHS). (1998). *The Surgeon General's Report on Nutrition and Health* (PHS Publication No. 88-50210). Washington, DC: U.S. Department of Health and Human Services.

U.S. Department of Health and Human Services (USDHHS). (2000a). Diabetes. In *Healthy People 2010: Understanding and Improving Health* (2nd ed., pp. 5–34). Washington, DC: U.S. Government Printing Office.

U.S. Department of Health and Human Services (USDHHS). (2000b). *Healthy People 2010: Understanding and Improving Health* (2nd ed.). 2 vols. Washington, DC: U.S. Government Printing Office.

U.S. Department of Health and Human Services (USDHHS). (2000c). Heart disease and stroke. In *Healthy People 2010: Understanding and Improving Health* (2nd ed., pp. 12–23). Washington, DC: U.S. Government Printing Office.

U.S. Department of Health and Human Services (USDHHS). (2000d). HIV. In *Healthy People 2010: Understanding and Improving Health* (2nd ed., pp. 13–27). Washington, DC: U.S. Government Printing Office.

U.S. Department of Health and Human Services (USDHHS). (2000e). Nutrition and overweight. In *Healthy People 2010: Understanding and Improving Health* (2nd ed., pp. 19–49). Washington, DC: U.S. Government Printing Office.

U.S. Department of Health and Human Services (USDHHS). (2000f). Physical activity and fitness. In *Healthy People 2010: Understanding and Improving Health* (2nd ed., pp. 22–26). Washington, DC: U.S. Government Printing Office.

U.S. Department of Health and Human Services (USDHHS). (2002). *Health, United States* (DHHS Publication No. 2002-1232). Hyattsville, MD: National Center for Health Statistics.

U.S. Department of Health and Human Services (USDHHS). (2004). *The Health Consequences of Smoking: A Report of the Surgeon General.* Atlanta: Centers for Disease Control and Prevention, National Center for Chronic Disease Prevention and Health Promotion, Office on Smoking and Health.

U.S. Department of Health and Human Services (USDHHS), Centers for Disease Control and Prevention (CDC), & National Center for Health Statistics (NCHS). (2003). *National Health Interview Survey (NHIS).* Retrieved May 26, 2004, from www.cdc.gov/nchs/

U.S. Department of Health and Human Services (USDHHS) & National Heart, Lung, and Blood Institute (NHLBI). (2001). *Third Report of the Expert Panel on the Detection, Evaluation, and Treatment of High Blood Cholesterol in Adults (Adult Treatment Panel III)* (NIH Publication No. 01-367). Retrieved October 20, 2009, from http://www.nhlbi.nih.gov/guidelines/cholesterol/index.htm

U.S. Department of Health and Human Services (USDHHS) & National Heart, Lung, and Blood Institute (NHLBI). (2007). *National High Blood Pressure Education Program.* Retrieved May 26, 2004, from http://www.nhlbi.nih.gov/about/nhbpep/

U.S. Department of Health and Human Services (USDHHS), National Institutes of Health (NIH), & National Heart, Lung, and Blood Institute (NHLBI). (2003). *Seventh Report of the Joint National Committee on Prevention, Detection, Evaluation, and Treatment of High Blood Pressure* (NIH Publication No. 04-5230).

U.S. Department of Health and Human Services (USDHHS) & the Office of the Surgeon General (OSG). (2006). *The Health Consequences of Involuntary Exposure to Tobacco Smoke: A Report of the Surgeon General.* Atlanta: U.S. Department of Health and Human Services, Centers for Disease Control and Prevention, Coordinating Center for Health Promotion, National Center for Chronic Disease Prevention and Health Promotion, Office on Smoking and Health. Retrieved June 15, 2009, from http://www.surgeongeneral.gov/library/secondhandsmoke/

U.S. Department of Health and Human Services (USDHHS), Public Health Service, Office of the Surgeon General. (2001). *Surgeon General's Call to Action to Prevent and Decrease Overweight and Obesity.* Washington, DC: U.S. Department of Health and Human Services.

U.S. Preventive Services Task Force. (2003). *Guide to Clinical Preventive Services* (3rd ed.). Washington, DC: U.S. Department of Health and Human Services.

Vollmer, W. M., Sacks, F. M., Ard, J., Appel, L. J., Bray, G. A., Simons-Morton, D. G., et al. (2001). Effects of diet and sodium intake on blood pressure. Subgroup analysis of the DASH–sodium trial. *Annals of Internal Medicine, 135,* 1019–1028.

Whelton, S. P., Chin, A., Xin, X., & He, J. (2002). Effect of aerobic exercise on blood pressure: A meta-analysis of randomized, controlled trials. *Annals of Internal Medicine, 136,* 493–503.

Willett, W. (1996). Diet and nutrition. In D. Schottenfield & J. F. Frammeni, Jr. (Eds.), *Cancer Epidemiology and Prevention* (2nd ed., pp. 438–461). New York: Oxford University Press.

Wimbush, F. B., & Peters, R. M. (2000). Identification of cardiovascular risk: Use of a cardiovascular-specific genogram. *Public Health Nursing, 17,* 148–154.

Xin, X., He, J., Frontini, M. G., Ogden, L. G., Motsamai, O. I., & Whelton, P. K. (2001). Effects of alcohol reduction on blood pressure. A meta-analysis of randomized controlled trials. *Hypertension, 38,* 1112–1117.

Xu, J., Kochanek, K. D., Tajada-Vera, B. (2007, August 19). Deaths: Preliminary data for 2004. DHHS Publication No. 2009-1120. National Center for Health Statistics. *National Vital Statistics Reports, 58,* no. 1. Retrieved October 13, 2009, from http://www.cdc.gov/nchs/products/nvsr.htm

Special Topics in Adult Nutrition: Physical Activity and Weight Management

Stella Lucia Volpe, PhD, RD, LDN, FACSM

CHAPTER OUTLINE

Definitions of Obesity and Overweight

Total Energy Expenditure
Basal Metabolic Rate • Thermic Effect of Food • Thermic Effect of Exercise • Nonexercise Activity Thermogenesis

Physical Activity and Obesity Prevention
Definitions of Physical Activity and Exercise • Weight Loss Goals • How Much Exercise or Physical Activity Is Enough?

• Physical Activity Interventions and Weight Loss • Physical Activity and Weight Loss in the Primary Care Setting • How Can People Be Successful at Maintaining Weight Loss?

Reader Objectives

After studying this chapter and reflecting on the contents, you should be able to

1. Describe the differences between overweight and obese and their implications for risk of disease.
2. Explain the components of energy balance and how they can impact weight management.
3. Describe the role of physical activity in maintaining a healthy body weight in adults based on scientific evidence.

Obesity has become a worldwide epidemic. Every country, despite its economic status, has shown some increase in body weight in its population. In the United States it has been estimated that more than 50% of adults and more than 30% of children are overweight and/or obese, and these numbers continue to rise. Many factors contribute to this rise in overweight status, and they include, but are not limited to, genetics, decrease in the thermic effect of food, environmental factors, and the effects of some medications. Nonetheless, although our genes have not changed in over hundreds of years, people are consuming more energy than before and, subsequently, becoming more sedentary. This imbalance in total energy expenditure can explain the greatest reason for this obesity epidemic.

The purpose of this chapter is to present research in the areas of physical activity, exercise, and weight management. Before the discussion of physical activity and weight management, basic definitions of overweight and obesity are described as well as a basic description of the components of total energy expenditure.

Definitions of Obesity and Overweight

Obesity: The universal definitions of overweight and obesity have been established using body mass index (BMI; kg of body weight/height [m²]). For adults, a BMI between 25 and 29.9 kg/m² is considered overweight, whereas a BMI of 30 kg/m² or greater is defined as obese. Note that this is not the best definition for individuals.

"Overweight" and "obesity" are terms used to describe ranges of body weight that are above what is regarded as healthy for a given height (Centers for Disease Control and Prevention [CDC], 2006). Obesity and overweight also define ranges of body weight that increase the risk of chronic disease (CDC, 2006). There are a number of definitions of overweight and obesity. The universal definitions of overweight and **obesity** have been established using body mass index (BMI; kg of body weight/height [m²]). For adults a BMI between 25 and 29.9 kg/m² is considered overweight, whereas a BMI of 30 kg/m² or greater is defined as obese (CDC, 2006) **(Table 11.1)**. BMI is a good tool to assess the rates of overweight status and obesity in a population, but it is not as good a tool to assess overweight status and obesity in individuals. Thus, a person should be cautious when using BMI in a clinical setting. For most of the population, which is sedentary, BMI correlates well with percent body fat, but it is not a measure of percent body fat. Therefore, individuals who may be "overweight" but not "over fat," such as athletes, are not considered to be overweight or obese because they have more muscle mass (on average) (CDC, 2006).

Because of this discrepancy between BMI and percent body fat, other definitions of obesity and overweight are based on a percentage above ideal body weight or percent body fat. In general, a person is considered overweight if his or her body weight is 20% above ideal body weight.

Underwater (hydrostatic) weighing or dual-energy x-ray absorptiometry is an ideal method of estimating a person's

TABLE 11.1	Body Mass Index Categories
Category	**Body Mass Index (kg/m²)**
Underweight	<18.5
Normal weight	18.5–24.9
Overweight	25–29.9
Obese	≥30

Adapted from U.S. Department of Health and Human Services (USDHHS); National Institutes of Health; National Heart, Lung, and Blood Institute (2006). Retrieved November 29, 2006; from http://www.nhlbisupport.com/bmi/bmicalc.htm

The ideal body weight of a person is typically assessed using the Hamwi equation. The Hamwi equation for ideal body weight in women is calculated as follows:

100 pounds for 5 feet, plus 5 pounds for every inch over 5 feet, or minus 5 pounds for every inch under 5 feet

The Hamwi equation for men is calculated as follow:

106 pounds for 5 feet, plus 6 pounds for every inch above 5 feet, and minus 6 pounds for every inch under 5 feet

For men and women, subtract or add 10%, respectively, if a person is considered small or large framed.

CRITICAL Thinking

What do you think is the major cause of obesity? Make a list of each cause (making sure that decreased energy expenditure, the topic of this chapter, is one of them), and find at least one recent (within the year) research article that pertains to each item on your list. If your list is short, find two to three research articles. From there, make a theoretical framework where you describe, based on the research, how these components are related and how they impact one another. Use thicker arrows for those components that have a greater impact on other components and thinner arrows for those that have less of an impact. If there is no relationship between one component or another, then no arrows are used.

percent body fat and, hence, determining if they are overweight due to fatness or lean body mass. However, in most situations body fat assessment, even via skinfold measures or bioelectrical impedance measures, is impractical. Thus, for the average population, BMI predicts overweight status and obesity fairly well. It does not predict overweight status and obesity well if someone is muscular and/or has dense bones. When a person who is obviously fit is said to have a high BMI, their exercise habits and body composition must be considered.

Total Energy Expenditure

Total **energy expenditure** has three main components: basal energy expenditure (or basal metabolic rate [BMR]), the thermic effect of food, and the thermic effect of activity. A fourth component, which has had a bit more attention paid to it in recent years, is nonexercise activity thermogenesis, which is also described. The measurement of total energy expenditure in humans is necessary to assess the metabolic needs of a person in relation to the aforementioned components of total energy expenditure (Levine, 2005).

Energy expenditure:
Kilocalories expended during the day. Total energy expenditure comprises basal metabolic rate, dietary-induced thermogenesis, and the thermic effect of activity. A fourth component is nonexercise activity thermogenesis (NEAT).

● **Learning Point** A rough method to assess BMR is to multiply a person's body weight by 10. Thus if someone weighs 150 pounds, their BMR is 1,500 kcal (150 × 10). Although this method is not precise, it is a good rough estimate of a person's BMR.

Basal Metabolic Rate

Basal energy expenditure and BMR are measured in kilocalories (kcal) per day, kcal/kg body weight/day, or kcal/kg fat free mass/day. Basal energy expenditure (BMR) is defined as the energy required to maintain circulation, respiration, and so forth at rest. Sometimes basal energy expenditure is referred to as resting energy expenditure or resting metabolic rate (RMR). Although resting energy expenditure and RMR are interchangeable, BMR and RMR are actually not exactly the same, because RMR is typically about 5% greater than BMR. This is because with BMR, the individual being assessed via direct or indirect calorimetry does not have to travel to a site and therefore does not have an increased heart rate before the measurement. With RMR, however, the individual typically travels to a site to have his or her RMR assessed. More recent research (Levine, 2005), however, has shown that when given 10 to 15 minutes' rest, RMR and BMR are virtually the same. Furthermore, Ventham and Reilly (1999) reported that the measurement of RMR is highly reproducible in children 6 to 11 years of age, even when children were provided only 5 to 10 minutes of rest before indirect calorimetry measurements. Regardless, both RMR and BMR are measured when an individual has fasted for 8 to 12 hours.

RMR or BMR can be assessed via indirect calorimetry, direct calorimetry, or doubly labeled water. Although direct calorimetry and doubly labeled water provide more accurate evaluations of energy expenditure, indirect calorimetry is the most often used method because of cost, but it too provides a high source of accuracy (Levine, 2005). Furthermore, doubly labeled water allows the investigator to assess only the total energy expenditure, rather than just RMR or BMR. When resources are limited and/or high accuracy is not required, noncalorimetric methods and total collection systems may be used; however, the limitations of these systems must be noted (Levine, 2005). A more holistic and accurate approach to measuring total energy expenditure is to combine any of the described methods with daily log entries of activity (Levine, 2005).

Thermic Effect of Food

The thermic effect of food is another component of the total energy expenditure equation. The thermic effect of food, also known as dietary-induced thermogenesis, is the amount of energy required for absorption and digestion of food. Using indirect calorimetry, the thermic effect of food is measured for a 4-hour period postprandially, with about 5 to 10 minutes given as a break to the individual at the end of each hour. The thermic effect of food makes up about 10% of total energy expenditure. Obese individuals may have a slightly lower thermic effect of food than 10%.

Thermic Effect of Exercise

The thermic effect of exercise is perhaps the most variable component of the total energy expenditure equation. It can be as low as 10% in very sedentary individuals and as high as 100% in Olympic athletes or professional athletes, who work out from 6 to 10 hours per day. **Table 11.2** shows activity factors that are used to estimate thermic effect of activity.

TABLE 11.2	Activity Factors Used to Estimate Thermic Effect of Activity
Activity	Multiple of Basal Energy Expenditure
Resting	= Basal energy expenditure
Very light (sitting, standing)	0.1
Light (leisure, housework)	0.25
Moderate (3.5–4.0 mph)	0.5
Heavy (fast walk +)	0.7

Nonexercise Activity Thermogenesis

Nonexercise activity thermogenesis (NEAT) is defined as "the energy expenditure of all physical activities other than volitional sporting-like exercise. NEAT includes all the activities that render us vibrant, unique, and independent beings such as working, playing, and dancing" (Levine, Vander Weg, Hill, & Klesges, 2006). This has been shown to account for up to 2,000 kcal/day, depending on the amount of NEAT a person accumulates throughout each day (Levine, Vander Weg, et al., 2006). It has been reported that lean individuals stand and move more than obese individuals, indicating that lean individuals have greater amount of NEAT than obese individuals (Levine, Lanningham-Foster, et al., 2005). Even after lean and obese individuals gained weight, NEAT was still significantly greater in lean individuals, indicating central and humoral meditators that drive sedentary behaviors in obese individuals (Levine, Lanningham-Foster, et al., 2005).

Obese individuals appear to have a natural predisposition to be seated for 2.5 hours a day more than their sedentary lean counterparts. If obese individuals could simply incorporate more NEAT into their daily routine and become more "NEAT-o-type" (Levine, Vander Web, et al., 2006), they could expend about 350 more kcal per day, which could lead to a 15-kg weight loss over a year (Levine, Lanningham-Foster, et al., 2005). Levine, Vander Weg, et al. (2006) stated that obesity reflects the surfacing of a "chair-enticing environment," where those who have a natural predisposition to sit have done so and, hence, have become obese. As a society, we need to assist individuals by promoting standing more often and becoming more active throughout the day. This can be done by reconfiguring work, school, and home environments to result in more active life-styles (Levine, Vander Weg, et al., 2006).

Lower NEAT in obese individuals could be a result of a decreased production of neuromedin U (NMU), which has been associated with the control of energy intake and expenditure (Novak, Zhang, & Levine, 2006). NMU appears to affect the hypothalamic nuclei of the brain. Novak et al. (2006) applied varying doses of NMU directly into the paraventricular and arcuate hypothalamic nuclei of Sprague-Dawley rats. They reported increased physical activity and NEAT when NMU was applied to either nu-

Nonexercise activity thermogenesis (NEAT): The energy expenditure of all physical activities other than volitional sporting-like exercise. NEAT includes such activities as working, playing, and dancing.

cleus; increased doses resulted in increased activity (Novak et al., 2006). Interestingly, they also reported that NMU decreased energy intake and body weight. Although the study of NMU is in its early stages, this peptide shows promise in combating obesity.

Despite the cause of a lower NEAT in obese individuals, a great deal of attention in the clinical setting and fitness industry has not been placed on NEAT. Nonetheless, focusing on NEAT would be a realistic and simple approach to help obese individuals incorporate more activity into their daily lives, lose weight, and then begin to incorporate physical activity and exercise into their daily routines, after some initial weight has been lost, giving them more confidence to actually exercise.

Physical Activity and Obesity Prevention

Physical activity and exercise interventions, as well as a combination of physical activity/exercise and diet interventions, have been well researched in the area of obesity prevention. In 2005 the Dietary Guidelines for Americans listed physical activity and weight management as two of its nine key recommendations (U.S. Department of Health and Human Services [USDHHS] and U.S. Department of Agriculture, 2005). The main focus of this chapter is to present recent research in physical activity and a combination of physical activity and diet interventions and discuss the main outcomes of these trials. Although the most recent research is highlighted, some key older studies are also presented to lay the groundwork of where research in this area has been and where it will be moving toward. See the 2010 Dietary Guidelines for Americans at www.dietaryguidelines.gov for updates.

Definitions of Physical Activity and Exercise

Before discussing research in the areas of physical activity and exercise and nutrition, it is important to define the differences between physical activity and exercise. **Physical activity** is defined as "bodily movement that is produced by the contraction of skeletal muscle and that substantially increases energy expenditure" (USDHHS, 1996). Common categories of physical activity include occupational, household, leisure time, and transportation (USDHHS, 1996). Occupational, household, and transportation physical activities are also known as "utilitarian" physical activities. In 2001 the Behavioral Risk Factor Surveillance System reported that in the United States from 28% to 55% of individuals performed leisure time physical activity (CDC, 2003). **Exercise** is defined as planned, structured, and repetitive bodily movement done to improve or maintain one or more components of physical fitness (USDHHS, 1996).

> **Physical activity:** Body movement produced by the contraction of skeletal muscle and that substantially increases energy expenditure. Common categories of physical activity include occupational, household, leisure time, and transportation.
>
> **Exercise:** Planned, structured, and repetitive bodily movement done to improve or maintain one or more components of physical fitness.

● **Learning Point** The five components of physical fitness are cardiorespiratory endurance, muscular endurance, muscular strength, flexibility, and body composition (Ward, 1999). It has been reported that only about 20% of individuals in the United States exercise on a regular basis (three or more times per week, for at least 20 minutes per session).

Weight Loss Goals

Despite so few people participating in physical activity or exercise on a regular basis, individuals significantly ($p < 0.05$) overestimate their energy expenditure and underestimate their energy intake by approximately 500 kcal and 1,000 kcal, respectively (Lichtman et al., 1992). In addition, it has been reported that obese individuals have unrealistic weight loss goals. Before participating in a weight loss trial, individuals stated that a 38% reduction from their initial body weight (e.g., from an average of 218 pounds to an average of 135 pounds) would be their "dream weight" and that if they lost only 17% of their initial body weight (e.g., from 218 pounds to 180 pounds) they would be "disappointed" (Foster, Wadden, Vogt, & Brewer, 1997). In reality, individuals in most weight loss studies lose an average of about 15% of their initial body weight, which would be below their "disappointed" body weight loss.

Wadden et al. (2003) evaluated whether notifying obese participants that they would lose only a modest amount of body weight would then guide them to agree to more reasonable weight loss goals. At the baseline interview, Wadden and colleagues (2003) interviewed 53 obese women who stated that, on average, they expected to lose about 28% of their initial body weight after the first year of treatment with a weight loss medication. Before initiation of the trial, it was explained to the women, both in writing and verbally, that they should expect to lose about 5% to 15% of their initial body weight (Wadden et al., 2003). Regardless of this prior information, the women did not alter their weight loss expectations throughout the trial. These unrealistic expectations may be one of the many reasons for the high rate of recidivism after weight loss trials.

How Much Exercise or Physical Activity Is Enough?

In 1995 the Surgeon General, the CDC, and the American College of Sports Medicine established that individuals should accumulate at least 30 minutes or more of exercise per day for cardiovascular fitness. However, this amount of exercise, which on average represents about 150 minutes per week, may not be enough for weight loss. In 2005 the National Academy of Sciences of the Institute of Medicine established Dietary Reference Intakes for physical activity and exercise. In brief, the Dietary Reference Intake recommendation states that individuals should exercise at least 30 minutes per day at a high intensity or at least 60 minutes per day at a low intensity (Food and Nutrition Board, Institute of Medicine, National Academy of Sciences, 2005).

In 2001 the American College of Sports Medicine published their position on effective weight loss methods (Jakicic, Clark, et al., 2001). They stated, "the American College of Sports Medicine recommends that the combination of reductions in energy intake and increases in energy expenditure, through structured exercise and other forms of physical activity, be a component of weight loss intervention programs."

Physical Activity Interventions and Weight Loss

The research in the area of physical activity and weight loss has covered many types of study designs. In an effort to assess if multiple bouts of physical activity result in weight loss similar to one longer bout of physical activity, Jakicic, Wing, and colleagues (1995) conducted a 20-week study of 56 overweight sedentary women, about 40 years of age, with a BMI of 34 kg/m^2. The long-bout group was told to walk 40 minutes per day in one session, whereas the short-bout group was told to walk for 40 minutes in two to four shorter sessions per day. Thus, total exercise time remained the same between the two groups. The women wore accelerometers to assess energy expenditure. They were also told to maintain an energy intake of between 1,200 to 1,500 kcal/day, with about 20% of total energy intake derived from fat. Jakicic, Wing, et al. (1995) reported significant ($p < 0.05$) and similar weight loss for both groups of women and significant increases in cardiorespiratory fitness in both groups. It appears from this research that exercise in multiple bouts could be an encouraging method to increase physical activity in individuals; however, the study was only 20 weeks in duration, and therefore longer-term research is required to evaluate if the participants would continue with this exercise regimen.

Jakicic, Winters, and coworkers (1999) conducted a longer-term study that somewhat paralleled the aforementioned research. They compared the effects of intermittent exercise with traditional long-bout exercise on weight loss, but they also added another component: They examined the effects of intermittent exercise with that of using home exercise equipment. The participants were 148 sedentary overweight women (BMI = 32.8 ± 4.0 kg/m^2, 36.7 ± 5.6 years of age). The study was 18 months in duration, and the subjects were randomly assigned to one of three groups: long-bout exercise, multiple short-bout exercise, or multiple short-bout exercise with home exercise equipment (SBEQ) using a treadmill. Their primary aims were to assess the differences among these three groups in body weight, body composition, cardiorespiratory fitness, and exercise adherence.

They reported that all three groups improved their cardiorespiratory fitness, with no difference among groups. Weight loss was significantly greater ($p < 0.05$) in participants in the SBEQ group compared with participants in the short-bout group, with no differences in weight loss seen between the long-bout group and either SBEQ or the short-bout group (-7.4 ± 7.8 kg [SBEQ], -3.7 ± 6.6 kg [short-bout group], -5.8 ± 7.1 kg [long-bout group]).

Two interesting findings resulted from this study. First, the SBEQ group was able to sustain a significantly greater intensity of exercise than subjects in the short-bout and long-bout groups ($p < 0.05$). In addition, Jakicic et al. (1999) found a clear and significant ($p < 0.05$) dose–response relationship of the amount of exercise to the amount of weight loss. Thus participants who exercised more than 200 minutes per week for the 18-month intervention had significantly greater weight loss than individuals who exercised from 150 to 200 minutes per week and compared with individuals who exercised less than 150 minutes per week (-13.1 ± 8.0 kg [200 min/wk], -8.5 ± 5.8 kg [150 to 200 min/wk], $<3.5 \pm 6.5$ kg [-150 min/wk]). They concluded

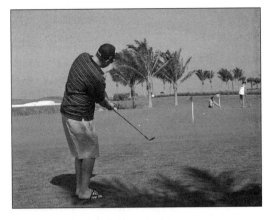

that access to home exercise equipment may assist in exercise adherence, resulting in weight loss in the long term. Furthermore, the dose–response relationship they reported, which would seem intuitive, clearly indicates that the greater the energy expenditure, the more body weight the person will lose.

Physical Activity and Weight Loss in the Primary Care Setting

The primary care setting is becoming a more popular place to conduct research on weight loss, because the patients, for the most part, have developed a relationship with their primary care practitioners. Booth et al. (2006) evaluated the effect of primary care physicians writing prescriptions that recommended life-style changes to their patients. They called this the "active nutrition script," which included five nutrition messages and personalized exercise advice for the prevention of weight gain. This was a pilot study whereby family physicians were asked to write 10 active nutrition scripts over a 4-week period to 10 adult patients who had a BMI between 23 and 30 kg/m^2. The physicians recorded the patients' body weight, height, waist circumference, gender, date of birth, type and frequency of exercise prescribed, and nutrition messages on each script. Booth et al. (2006) reported that 19 family physicians (63% of them were women) provided approximately nine active nutrition scripts over a 4-week period. A total of 145 patients (57% were women) received the active nutrition scripts (54 ± 13.2 years of age, mean BMI = 31.7 ± 6.3 kg/m^2). Seventy-eight percent of the time the physicians wrote the active nutrition scripts for weight loss. Of the physicians interviewed by the researchers (17 of 19 physicians were interviewed), they all stated that the active nutrition script messages were clear and easy to deliver. Although the physicians found this script easy to deliver, they prescribed it mainly for weight loss instead of prevention of weight gain. This research needs to be taken to the next step, where body weight and BMI are actually measured over time in the patients who receive the active nutrition scripts. Although this was a pilot study, the primary care setting may be one of the best places for prevention of weight gain and for weight loss.

McQuigg et al. (2005) conducted a study in the United Kingdom in 80 primary care settings with the primary aim to improve the management of obese adults in a primary care setting. The participants had a BMI ≥ 30 kg/m^2 or a BMI ± 28 kg/m^2 with at least one obesity-related comorbidity. This counterweight program consisted of four phases: audit and project development, practice training and support, nurse-led patient intervention, and evaluation. For the intervention portion, evidence-based pathways and incorporated approaches were used to empower the health care providers and patients in weight management. This program also had weight management advisers who were dietitians specializing in obesity.

McQuigg et al. (2005) reported that a large number of intervention practices had been trained (almost 94%), and they recruited 1,549 patients. At 1 year after implementation, 33% of the patients achieved a weight loss of 5% or more, which is clinically significant, because even just a small amount of weight loss has been shown to reduce the risk of chronic disease. It has been reported that for every kilogram of weight lost, there is a 16% reduction in the risk of type 2 diabetes mellitus (Hamman et al., 2006).

Although the aforementioned programs were successful, Morrato and colleagues asked the question, "Are health care professionals advising patients with diabetes or at risk for developing diabetes to exercise more?" Although the focus of this chapter is on physical activity and weight loss, one of the primary comorbidities developed as a result of obesity is type 2 diabetes mellitus. Morrato et al. (2006) accessed the Medical Expenditure Panel Survey, to which more than 26,000 adults in the United States responded in 2002. They found that 73% of the adults with type 2 diabetes mellitus were told by a health care professional to exercise more, compared with 31% without diabetes mellitus. In addition, the number of people receiving exercise guidance increased as the amount of diabetes risk factors increased. These researchers reported that BMI and cardiovascular disease risk factors were the strongest predictors for practitioners to give exercise recommendations. They did report, however, that as the diabetes risk factors decreased, exercise advice to patients decreased, resulting in "missed opportunities for disease prevention" (Morrato et al., 2006). Despite the exercise advice, the patients did not always change behavior, which is still the most difficult part of the equation to change (Morrato et al., 2006).

How Can People Be Successful at Maintaining Weight Loss?

The maintenance of weight loss is probably the most difficult phase of any weight loss program. After a person feels successful losing weight, he or she often returns to eating the amount of foods consumed before weight loss and decreases physical activity. Although there may be many psychological, and even perhaps physiological, reasons behind this, there are practical ways people can incorporate physical activity into their day, which can help to increase energy expenditure and maintain weight loss and/or prevent weight gain.

● Learning Point Although a small percentage of individuals in the National Weight Control Registry reported consuming a low-carbohydrate diet, the main factors that allowed these individuals to maintain weight loss over time remain the same: consumption of a low-energy diet, moderate fat intake, limited consumption of fast food, and high amounts of physical activity or exercise (Phelan et al., 2006).

Two studies (Hill, 2006, and Hill and colleagues, 2006) found that small changes can lead to big effects on the prevention of weight gain. They stated that reducing energy balance by a mere 100 kcal/day could lead to a large reduction in the obesity epidemic. People could achieve this small energy deficit simply by walking 15 minutes per day (and multiple bouts would be effective) and/or eating just a few less bites of food at each meal. These small changes are not daunting and may result in greater adherence to weight loss and maintenance.

Although the obesity epidemic is considered a gene–environment interaction (i.e., the human genotype is predisposed to ecologic influences that affect energy intake and expenditure), it is mostly a problem of energy balance (Hill, 2006). The most successful interventions are those that impact energy balance (increase expenditure and decrease intake) but that also take into consideration behavioral and environmental factors that play a big role in why individuals do not exercise or eat higher amounts of total energy (Hill, 2006). Hill (2006) stated the following:

> Our best strategy for reversing the obesity epidemic is to focus on preventing positive energy balance in the population through small changes in diet and physical activity that take advantage of our biological systems for regulating energy balance. Simultaneously we must address the environment to make it easier to make better food and physical activity choices. This is a very long-term strategy for first stopping and then reversing the escalating obesity rates, but one that can, over time, return obesity rates to pre-1980s levels.

Just as the primary care setting can be an ideal location to impact obesity, interventions that include the entire family could also lead to successful maintenance of weight loss. Rodearmel et al. (2006) focused on increasing steps walked per day and cereal consumption (for breakfast and snacks) as a weight reduction intervention for families. They included 105 families in their study who had at least one 8- to

12-year-old child who was at risk for becoming overweight or obese. This was a 13-week intervention, in which 82 families were randomly assigned to the family-based intervention (increase steps to 2,000 per day and consume two servings of ready-to-eat cereal per day) and 23 families were randomly assigned to the control group. The intervention groups showed significant reductions in BMI and BMI-for-age in the adults and children, respectively, especially in mother–daughter pairs. Focusing on the family is a logical and practical way for individuals to maintain weight loss and/or prevent weight gain, because all individuals are making healthful changes together and providing a support system for one another.

Perhaps the most well-known registry of successful weight loss maintenance is the National Weight Control Registry. This is a registry of individuals who had an initial weight loss average of 33.1 kg and who were able to maintain a 13.6-kg weight loss for 5.8 years before enrolling in the registry (Phelan, Wyatt, Hill, & Wing, 2006). Although many studies have been published on participants in the National Weight Control Registry, Phelan et al. (2006) evaluated whether dietary intake habits of registrants changed over the years, especially with the recent surge of low-carbohydrate diets. They included 2,708 partici-

pants who had been part of the National Weight Control Registry since 1995. They reported that from 1995 to 2003 energy from fat intake increased from 23.8% to 29.4%, with an increase in saturated fat from 12.3 to 15.4 g/day. Subsequently, energy from carbohydrate declined from 56% to 49% ($p < 0.0001$), and those who consumed less than 90 g/day of carbohydrate increased from 5.9% to 17.1% ($p < 0.0001$). Except for 1995, when physical activity was calculated at 3,316 kcal/wk, the remaining years were stable at about 2,620 kcal/wk. Phelan et al. (2006) stated that weight regain over 1 year was primarily associated with greater energy intake, more fast food consumption, increased fat intake, and lower amounts of physical activity ($p < 0.03$). **Table 11.3** lists practical ways people can incorporate more physical activity into their lives.

TABLE 11.3	Practical Ways to Incorporate More Physical Activity into the Day

Take the stairs instead of the elevator.
Park farther away from the destination.
Sit on a balance ball while working at a desk.
Exercise during commercials while watching television (if made into a family event it will be even more fun and successful!).
Have a Thera-Band™ available by desks, couches, and so on so that strength training exercises can be performed.
Dance.
Stretch during the day.
Stand up during meetings.
Do chair exercises (leg lifts, work on core strength, etc.).
Move as much as possible throughout the day—be "inefficient."

Summary

Obesity is a complex issue that requires a multifaceted approach. Although it is clearly a gene–environment interaction, the onus is still placed on greater energy expenditure combined with decreased energy intake. Increasing NEAT, multiple versus long bouts of exercise, and physical activity promotion in the primary care setting and family are all promising ways that the obesity epidemic can be reversed.

Issue to Debate

1. What are your views on bariatric surgery? Conduct a literature search to find at least one research article that shows a positive effect of bariatric surgery and one that does not. Find a recent (within a year) review article that describes each different type of bariatric surgery and when it needs to be performed. Debate both sides of this issue, providing background from your literature search. Include the pros and cons for prescribing physical activity to individuals who are morbidly obese and, hence, are candidates for bariatric surgery.

Case Studies

(Answers to all case studies are in the Instructor's Manual available at jbpub.com.)

Case Study

Don is a 34-year-old African-American who is an attorney at a large practice in Chicago. He is fairly new to this firm and wants to make partner. His job is very stressful. He works about 100 hours per week and gets little time to eat well or exercise, but he would really like to start to exercise even a few days per week.

Body weight: 225 pounds
Height: 5 feet, 8 inches
Exercises once or twice a week "when I get time"

He says, in general, that he consumes his breakfast "on the run," usually in the car on his way to work. His wife is also an attorney at a large firm, and they are both often very busy. When he does eat breakfast, it is usually something quick, like a doughnut, or he may stop at a fast food restaurant drive-through to get an egg and cheese croissant sandwich. He drinks about five to six cups of coffee per day.

For lunch, it is either something from the vending machine or, the opposite, a large meal at an expensive restaurant with one of his clients. Thus his lunch energy intake varies drastically. For dinner he and his wife often eat take-out Chinese food, pizza, submarine sandwiches, or hamburgers and French fries. They do try to eat more "normally" on weekends, but both are often in the office at least one day on the weekend.

1. Calculate Don's BMI (kg/m^2).
2. Calculate Don's total energy expenditure.
3. Based on this crude "dietary recall," provide a rough estimate of his energy intake.
4. What ideas would you give Don to help him improve his eating? Be conscious of the fact that he has little time to prepare meals.
5. How might Don be able to incorporate any physical activity in his life? Be creative!

Websites

American College of Sports Medicine http://www.acsm.org//AM/Template.cfm?Section=Home_PageandWebsiteKey=3bb8c0a3-b699-44f5-99ca-4c9e64600c5e
American Dietetic Association http://www.eatright.org/cps/rde/xchg/ada/hs.xsl/index.html
American Obesity Association http://www.obesity.org/
America on the Move http://aom3.americaonthemove.org/
American Society for Bariatric Surgery http://www.asbs.org/
Centers for Disease Control and Prevention http://www.cdc.gov/nccdphp/dnpa/obesity/resources.htm
NAASO, The Obesity Society http://www.naaso.org/
National Institutes of Health Obesity Research http://obesityresearch.nih.gov/

References

Booth, A. O., Nowson, C. A., Huang, N., Lombard, C., & Singleton, K. L. (2006). Evaluation of a brief pilot nutrition and exercise intervention for the prevention of weight gain in general practice patients. *Public Health Nutrition, 9,* 1005–1061.

Centers for Disease Control and Prevention (CDC). (2003). Prevalence of physical activity, including lifestyle activities among adults—United States, 2000–2001. *Morbidity and Mortality Weekly Reports, 52,* 764–769.

Centers for Disease Control and Prevention (CDC). (2006). Defining overweight and obesity. Retrieved November 29, 2006, from http://www.cdc.gov/nccdphp/dnpa/obesity/defining.htm

Food and Nutrition Board, Institute of Medicine, National Academy of Sciences. (2005). *Dietary Reference Intakes for Energy, Carbohydrate, Fiber, Fat, Fatty Acids, Cholesterol, Protein, and Amino Acids (Macronutrients).* Washington, DC: National Academy Press.

Foster, G. D., Wadden, T. A., Vogt, R. A., & Brewer, G. (1997). What is a reasonable weight loss? Patients' expectations and evaluations of obesity treatment outcomes. *Journal of Consulting and Clinical Psychology, 65,* 79–85.

Hamman, R. F., Wing, R. R., Edelstein, S. L., Lachin, J. M., Bray, G. A., Delahanty, L., et al. (2006). Effect of weight loss with lifestyle intervention on risk of diabetes. *Diabetes Care, 29,* 2102–2107.

Hill, J. O. (2006). Understanding and addressing the epidemic of obesity: An energy balance perspective. *Endocrine Reviews, 27,* 750–761.

Hill, J. O., Wyatt, H. R., Reed, G. W., & Peters, J. C. (2006). Obesity and the environment: Where do we go from here? *Science, 299,* 853–855.

Jakicic, J. M., Clark, K., Coleman, E., Donnelly, J. E., Foreyt, J., Melanson, E., et al. (2001). American College of Sports Medicine position stand. Appropriate intervention strategies for weight loss and prevention of weight regain for adults. *Medicine and Science in Sports and Exercise, 33,* 2145–2156.

Jakicic, J. M., Wing, R. R., Butler, B. A., & Robertson, R. J. (1995). Prescribing exercise in multiple short bouts versus one continuous bout: Effects on adherence, cardiorespiratory fitness, and weight loss in overweight women. *International Journal of Obesity and Related Metabolic Disorders, 19,* 893–901.

Jakicic, J. M., Winters, C., Lang, W., & Wing, R. R. (1999). Effect of intermittent exercise and use of home exercise equipment on adherence, weight loss, and fitness in overweight women: A randomized trial. *Journal of the American Medical Association, 282,* 1554–1560.

Levine, J. A. (2005). Measurement of energy expenditure. *Public Health Nutrition, 8,* 1123–1132.

Levine, J. A., Lanningham-Foster, L. M., McCrady, S. K., Krizan, A. C., Olson, L. R., Kane, P. H., et al. (2005). Interindividual variation in posture allocation: Possible role in human obesity. *Science, 307,* 584–586.

Levine, J. A., Vander Weg, M. W., Hill, J. O., & Klesges, R. C. (2006). Non-exercise activity thermogenesis: The crouching tiger hidden dragon of societal weight gain. *Arteriosclerosis, Thrombosis, and Vascular Biology, 26,* 729–736.

Lichtman, S. W., Pisarska, K., Berman, E. R., Pestone, M., Dowling, H., Offenbacher, E., et al. (1992). Discrepancy between self-reported and actual caloric intake and exercise in obese subjects. *New England Journal of Medicine, 327,* 1893–1898.

McQuigg, M., Brown, J., Broom, J., Laws, R. A., Reckless, J. P., Noble, P. A., et al. (2005). Empowering primary care to tackle the obesity epidemic: The Counterweight Programme. *European Journal of Clinical Nutrition, 59*(Suppl. 1), S93–S100.

Morrato, E. H., Hill, J. O., Wyatt, H. R., Ghushchyan, V., & Sullivan, P. W. (2006). Are health care professionals advising patients with diabetes or at risk for developing diabetes to exercise more? *Diabetes Care, 29,* 543–548.

Novak, C. M., Zhang, M., & Levine, J. A. (2006). Neuromedin U in the paraventricular and arcuate hypothalamic nuclei increases non-exercise activity thermogenesis. *Journal of Neuroendocrinology, 18,* 594–601.

Phelan, S., Wyatt, H. R., Hill, J. O., & Wing, R. R. (2006). Are the eating and exercise habits of successful weight losers changing? *Obesity, 14,* 710–716.

Rodearmel, S. J., Wyatt, H. R., Barry, M. J., Dong, F., Pan, D., Israel, R. G., et al. (2006). A family-based approach to preventing excessive weight gain. *Obesity, 14,* 1392–1401.

U.S. Department of Health and Human Services (USDHHS). (1996). Physical activity and health: A report of the Surgeon General. Atlanta, GA: USDHHS, and CDC, National Center for Chronic Disease Prevention and Health Promotion.

U.S. Department of Health and Human Services (USDHHS) and U.S. Department of Agriculture. (2005, 2010). Dietary Guidelines for Americans.

Ventham, J. C., & Reilly, J. J. (1999). Reproducibility of resting metabolic rate measurement in children. *British Journal of Nutrition, 81,* 435–437.

Wadden, T. A., Womble, L. G., Sarwer, D. B., Berkowitz, R. I., Clark, V. L., & Foster, G. D. (2003). Great expectations: "I'm losing 25% of my weight no matter what you say." *Journal of Consulting and Clinical Psychology, 71,* 1084–1089.

Ward, A. (1999). Exercise and exercise intervention in the prevention of coronary artery disease. In J. M. Rippe (Ed.), *Lifestyle Medicine* (pp. 90–97). Malden, MA: Blackwell Science.

Special Topics in Nutrition and the Older Adult: Diet, Life-Style, Disease, and Pharmacologic Considerations

Roschelle Heuberger, PhD, RD

CHAPTER OUTLINE

Reader Objectives

After studying this chapter and reflecting on the contents, you should be able to

1. Identify controversies surrounding the definition of an "older adult."
2. Categorize the emerging elderly population by demographics and specifically by socioeconomics.
3. Define cellular senescence and successful aging.
4. Itemize the direct and indirect determinants of aging and cellular senescence.
5. Delineate differences between biochemical/physiologic and life-style/environmental contributions toward inflammation, oxidative stress, apoptosis, and free-radical-induced damage with aging processes.
6. Discuss the processes and their determinants for disease states that accompany aging.
7. Identify issues in the hospitalized/institutionalized older adult. Relate those issues to morbidity and mortality through nutriture.
8. Describe the pharmacologic considerations in the treatment of diseases in older persons, inclusive of the issues of polypharmacy.
9. Define strategies for the treatment of obesity in an older adult, with attention to future directions for pharmacotherapeutic agents.

Older adults are a diverse and extremely heterogeneous population group. Differentiation between chronologic age and **senescence** must be taken into account. Some 70-year-old persons are more fit and less "aged" from a cellular and functional standpoint than some 40-year-olds, due to a variety of genetic and life-style characteristics. However, functional declines naturally occur with aging, and the oldest old (>85 years) generally exhibit changes associated with senescence (Singer & Manton, 1998). An overview of the older adult population and issues surrounding senescence, determinants of health and nutritional status, and consequences of aging and disease is given.

> **Senescence:** The process of aging taking into account cellular death and dysregulation leading to functional decline.

Older adults compose the most rapidly growing demographic in the United States as well as in other industrialized countries.

Life expectancies have increased as a result of a number of factors:

- Declines in mortality from infectious diseases
- Increases in technologic ability to detect disease at an early juncture
- Advent of new pharmacotherapies for a variety of acute and chronic disease states
- Increases in awareness of antecedents for disease among the general population
- Overall better access to health care
- Overall better nutriture and sanitation
- Overall technologic enhancements or preventative measures that may determine better health status over the life span (i.e., better automotive safety or stricter seat belt regulations)

As a result of the population living longer and the aging of the "baby boomers," there is a critical need for education regarding the requirements of older adults. Because of interrelationships of nutritional status with socioeconomics, life-style characteristics, environmental considerations, comorbid conditions, and genetics, all must be evaluated concurrently with dietary intake in this population.

Older Adults

Definitions of *elderly, older adult, geriatric, frail, senior,* and/or *aged* vary widely. This is problematic for the purposes of identifying or classifying individuals to determine policy or procedure. For the purposes of the government, such as with food assistance programs, taxation, and retirement, the person over age 65 is considered to be an older adult or senior. This is not the case when talking with persons trained in gerontology. In the social sciences, the definition of "aged" is related to functional status and not chronologic age. Functional ability is most often related to psychological status, ability to perform tasks of daily living (i.e., bathing, cooking), medical status, and socioeconomics.

For the subspecialty of geriatrics, which is more focused within the health professions, the terms "geriatric patient" or "frail elderly" are tied to medical status and cellular or mechanistic processes as opposed to holistic definitions (Woods et al., 2005). The term "frailty" is misrepresented in the literature, because it was most often in the past associated with being underweight with or without frank vitamin and mineral malnutrition (Sullivan, Lui, Roberson, Bopp, & Rees, 2004). There has been a recent shift to include normal or overweight persons in the category of frail, if they have **sarcopenia**, several diagnoses, poor nutritional status, and a decreased ability to function (Weinrebe, Guneysu, & Welz-Barth, 2002). This trend is a consequence of the obesity epidemic across all age groups, including elderly persons.

> **Sarcopenia:** Decrements in muscle mass that result in declining functional ability.

There is an increasing need to develop a uniform classification system for older adults, just as we have for the differing developmental stages of infants, children, and adolescents. Currently, the information regarding subgroups within the older adult population is lacking, and gross generalizations often result from research in this area. Each older adult must therefore be considered individually for preventative measures, nutritional recommendations, and treatment options based on the totality of the information available (Keller & Ostbye, 2003).

Epidemiology

The "graying" of America currently taking place with the aging of the baby boomers is considered to be a health care crisis, with insufficient practitioners, facilities, and accommodations for the changing demographics.

There will be fewer working adults and an enormous drain on the economy with large numbers of poor elderly persons requiring extended care. Efforts to promote a healthy aging agenda for the population are beginning to get under way, despite the fact that this national campaign should have commenced three decades ago to maximize effects in late life.

Characteristics of the U.S. population over the age of 65 include a number of regional differences, and warmer climate states usually have an over-representation of certain segments of the elderly population. Florida has the highest percentage of older adults, at nearly 20% of the population. Mississippi, Alabama, Louisiana, and Puerto Rico have 15% to 20% of their older adults living under the poverty level. Older adults are among the poorest of the poor, especially older women who were homemakers and do not receive added benefits from having worked. Women also live longer than men, and when they reach the oldest old category they have depleted any resources they may have had and require more medication, health care, and assistance, which results in the need for greater fiscal resources. Minority women make up the poorest of the poor among this demographic.

> **● Learning Point** If current trends hold, by the year 2050 one in four persons in the United States will be over the age of 65. The "oldest old" are the most rapidly increasing segment of this population. Women (minority women in particular) will soon be the dominant demographic in this oldest old category (National Institute on Aging, 2005; U.S. Bureau of the Census, 2005).

The number of elderly that live alone is estimated at 10%, and households containing an elderly person are above 23%. Asian and Hispanic descent is correlated with increased numbers of elderly as part of households, whereas African-American and white descent correlates with increased numbers of elderly living alone. Details of the national averages are shown in **Table 12.1**.

Epidemiologic data on older adults are available from a number of federal, state, local, nonprofit, and private sector sources. The federal government National Health and Nutrition Examination Survey, which has been ongoing, collected data on an over-sampling of the elderly population in the United States. A variety of statistics are available regarding socioeconomics, blood values, and dietary data. Medical and behavioral measures were also obtained for the older population in the National Health and Nutrition Examination Survey series. Behavioral Risk Factor Surveillance Studies have also included older

TABLE 12.1	Demographic Characteristics (United States)[a]			
Unadjusted Percentages for the U.S. Population		Male	Female	
Over the age of 65 in the U.S. (2005)		5.3%	7.2%	
Persons over the age of 85 in the U.S. (2005)		1.7%	1.7%	
Persons over the age of 65 in the U.S. with activity limitation due to chronic health problem (2008)				33% (total)
Projected increases in the over-85 age range among the elderly population in the U.S. by 2010		+1.5%	+3.5%	
Older adults with a disability		57.7%	70.5%	
Older adults widowed		14%	44%	
Oder adults married		71%	41%	

[a]U.S. Census. Retrieved June 26, 2009, from www.census.gov

adults. Conducted at the state level, these assessments are available for specific samples of elderly in most of the 48 contiguous states. Variables regarding demographics, health risk factors, and some dietary information are available.

The National Institute on Aging, a branch of the National Institutes of Health, promotes epidemiologic inquiry on older Americans, and organizations such as the American Association for Retired Persons and the Association on Aging also routinely collect information on the over 65 population. In addition, a number of gerontologically focused educational institutions across the nation have centers on aging and conduct aging research.

Health maintenance organizations and corporations that deal with the elderly also have available data sets. Corporate data from assisted living facilities or long-term care are extremely useful as an index of the utilization of different providers and resources for the aged population and, more important, provide critical data for the oldest old, who are routinely under-represented in governmental monitoring because of those initiatives being targeted at the noninstitutionalized (free-living) population in the United States.

Information on the oldest old has been sparse in the past, but due to the increasing numbers of this demographic, new directives have been issued to try to capture as much information as possible on this age group to enhance care and better understand issues of concern for health care providers, family, and the oldest old themselves.

Assessment Methodology

A number of methods for assessing the older adult on a large scale, such as with national nutritional monitoring systems or in community studies, have been used over the years. Quick screening tools such as the DETERMINE (Disease, Eating poorly, Tooth loss/mouth pain, Economic hardship, Reduced social contact, Multiple medications, Involuntary weight loss or gain, Needs assistance in self care, Elder years > 80) checklist and the Mini Nutritional Assessment have been shown to be useful in large-scale surveillance and in small-scale clinical settings (see http://www.aafp.org and http://www.mna-elderly.com/index.htm to access these screening tools). Both instruments have been shown to be effective for flagging older adults with issues related to nutritional status and health. The Mini Nutritional Assessment in particular has been the subject of recent research; it is being tested in a variety of populations and languages (Gazzotti, Albert, Pepinster, & Petermans, 2000; Beck, Ovensen, & Schroll, 2001).

National Health Objectives

The National Institute on Aging has reported that levels of disability among the older adult population in the United States have been falling since 1982 because of a variety of factors, such as better technology and increased access to health care. However, the National Institute on Aging proposed the following initiatives with regard to national efforts toward bettering the quality of life of the older segment of United States society:

- Sustain decreases in disability, maintaining health and function in older adults.
- Improve strategies for promoting healthy behaviors among the older population, including:
  - Diet
  - Smoking
  - Alcohol abuse
  - Safety
  - Exercise
  - Evaluation of hormone replacement therapy
  - Evaluation of dietary supplements
  - Improved interaction with the health care system
  - Reduction in caregiver and family stress
  - Improvement in individual coping with chronic disease

Each area was identified as being critical to maintaining the current decline in morbidity and mortality, despite the increasing numbers of older adults within the population (http://www.nia.nih.gov/initiatives.html). These recommendations for researchers and health care professionals were borne out of the epidemiologic evidence collected over the past few decades. In addition, public health campaigns, such as Healthy People 2010, have provided general objectives for improvement that target the lay person over the age of 65. Other groups have also targeted the lay older adult, including the American Diabetes Association and the American Cancer Society, with media campaigns specifically targeting elderly diabetics and cancer survivors.

Aging

Aging Theories

Theories regarding aging include population-based, organ-system-based, and cellular-based theories. Population-based theories involve type I, or "rate of living," and type II, or the collagen theories, of aging. Rate of living theories assume that the time it takes for development and maturity determines how long one lives. Collagen theories state that collagen cross-linking over time results in decreased longevity (Morley, Glick, & Rubenstein, 1995).

Organ system theories involve endocrine, immune, and "pacemaker" errors increasing over time and thus decreasing life span. In endocrine theories, hormonal changes or decrements result in decreased viability of organs and systems. In immune theories, failure of immunocompetence results in aging and death, and the pacemaker of aging theory involves predetermined organ system failure as a result of the body's own life clock ticking down (Morley et al., 1995).

Cellular aging theories have the most experimental evidence to back them. "Wear and tear" theories, as they are sometimes called, state that continuous use coupled with decreases in the division and maturation of new cells causes aging and ultimately death. **Apoptosis** eventually results in decreased numbers of viable cells. Somatic mutation, error catastrophe, free radical, glycation, and alteration of genetic code theories are encompassed in this category. The somatic mutation theory involves mutations that are present in cells that, over time, cause malfunction on a system-wide level, leading to death. Error catastrophe theory states that over time the number of cellular errors increases until a threshold is reached that results in catastrophe and death. The free radical theory of aging involves cumulative damage as a result of natural free radical oxidative changes, which over time result in increased antigenicity, protein changes, and oxidative DNA damage.

The sum of these processes results in cellular senescence and organ system failure, ending in death. Glycation theory assumes that posttranslational protein modification by the linking of glucose to lysine residues results in diminished protein functionality, which in turn decreases organ system viability and

Apoptosis: Preprogrammed cell death.

ends in death. The "alterations in genetic coding theory" proposes that aging is the result of changes in protein synthesis and messenger RNA processing. Chemical alterations in DNA over time, coupled with translational aberrations, are the cause of aging and death (Morley et al., 1995; Rimkus, Melinchok, McEvoy, & Yeager, 2005).

Caloric restriction, with adequate vitamin and mineral nutriture, has been associated with longevity. This is thought to be the result of decreases in oxidative stress, less metabolic free radical generation, and decrements in the abnormal compounds generated as a result of redox damage. The underlying mechanisms have yet to be fully established, but fewer glycation products, less lipid peroxidation, and fewer genetic anomalies with improved genetic expression over time seem to be causal in delayed cellular senescence (Warner, Fernandes, & Wang, 1995; Roth, Ingram, & Lane, 1999).

Determinants

Determinants of successful aging with little disease or disability involve many factors. Dietary considerations across the life span, such as increased intake of fiber, antioxidants, and minerals or caloric restriction, have been correlated with increased longevity and decreases in morbidity. Patterns of intake have also shown relationships to successful aging. Characteristics such as small, frequent meals, sitting down with family, having a glass of wine with dinner, and eating until 80% full seem to have beneficial effects over the long term.

Life-style characteristics such as maintenance of a normal body weight, decreased exposure to known carcinogens such as tobacco or heavy metals, and better coping mechanisms for stress seem to promote healthy aging. Adequate exercise and sleep are also important. Drug and alcohol use along with life-course levels of stress have been shown to have significant impact on cellular senescence.

There are other indirect determinants of successful aging with decreased cellular senescence. Some of these include mental status, mental activity, pet ownership, and social interaction. Sociodemographic characteristics also play a role, such as marital status, level of education, income, race, and ethnicity. Quality of life and perceptions of the quality of life along with spirituality, civic engagement, and coping abilities are moderating influences on the mechanisms involved in healthy longevity. Ultimately, genetic makeup and the propensity toward maintaining cellular protection against environmental influences determine the course of the individual's life span (De Groot, Verheijden, de Henauw, Schroll, & van Staveren, 2004; Bamia, 2005).

Diet

Dietary determinants of successful aging include issues with both macro- and micronutrient intake. Caloric content across the life span, adequate (but not excessive) protein intake with moderate to high bioavailability, and high complex carbohydrate consumption are all associated with decreases in morbidity and mortality (Millward, 2004; Jungjohann, Luhrmann, Bender, Blettner, & Neuhäuser-Berthold,

2005). Decreased total fat intake, with greater proportions of monounsaturates, long chain mega-3 fatty acids, and low trans/saturated fats, are associated with decrements in vascular anomalies and chronic disease with mortality (Hjerkinn et al., 2005). Micronutrient content of the diet across the life span is directly related to disease and indirectly, but ultimately, related to mortality.

Healthy aging has been associated with increased intake of antioxidants, including phytochemicals; selenium (part of glutathione peroxidase); vitamins C, E, and A; the carotenoids; and zinc (as part of metallothionein) (Gonzalez et al., 2004; Chernoff, 2005; Faure, Ducros, Couzy, Favier, & Ferry, 2005) **(Figure 12.1)**. In addition, bone health is improved with increased calcium, vitamin D, vitamin K, adequate magnesium, and lower intakes of phosphorus dur-

Figure 12.1   Fruits and vegetables.

© Denis Pepin/Dreamstime.com

ing the course of the life span (Bischoff-Ferrari et al., 2004; Ryan-Harshman & Aldoori, 2004). Increased dietary potassium and lower levels of sodium are important for blood pressure and vascular health, and the B vitamins are critical for decrements in homocysteine levels (Hamilton & Hamilton, 1997; Demingné, Sabboh, Rémésy, & Meneton, 2004; Gori et al., 2005).

Macronutrients

In older adults, adequate protein intake is essential for the prevention of muscle mass losses, pressure ulcers, and decreased immunocompetence. Sarcopenia in the elderly is associated with poor outcome, frailty, and falls. Investigations into the roles of essential amino acids in prevention of the above have shown that adequate protein intake is important to replacement of aging muscle tissue as well as in the maintenance of bone health. In conjunction with weight-bearing exercise, essential amino acids can increase the concentrations of insulin-like growth factor I, which has a permissive effect on bone and muscle cellular repair and, to some extent, replication. It should be noted that protein consumption is related to calcium intake, which mediates the relationships seen between protein intake and bone health (Devine, Dick, Islam, Dhaliwal, & Prince, 2005; Gori et al., 2005).

Other variables related to protein adequacy are socioeconomics and institutionalization. Poor and institutionalized elderly have reduced high-quality protein intakes and often have other factors that impact muscle mass, bone health, and wound healing, which cloud direct relationships in the research, such as decreased access to health care, altered mental status, and long-standing chronic disease. The provision of protein supplements to these populations has been shown to be beneficial in decreasing morbidity (Ginty, 2003; Collins, Kershaw, & Brockington, 2005; Milne, Potter, & Avenell, 2005).

Fiber intake in older persons is important for decreasing constipation, which results from enteromuscular changes consistent with aging. Both soluble and insoluble fiber sources are needed to slough abnormal cells from the gut, increase stool quality and frequency, and trap bilious cholesterol, drug metabolites, and carcinogens. In addition, fiber sources reduce calories and improve blood glucose level stability (Marlett, McBurney, & Slavin, 2002).

Fiber from whole foods is also rich in micronutrients, but this form of intake is often reduced in older persons, especially in those with poor dentition. Edentulous older persons often cannot chew high-fiber whole foods and therefore avoid them. Poorer older persons may not be able to afford fresh, high-fiber, whole foods, such as produce, which can be more expensive. Older persons who have not had dietary patterns consistent with high-fiber foods are reluctant to introduce them in late life and often exclude fruits, vegetables, legumes, and whole grains. Older adults may also have issues with fresh high-fiber foods because of their gas-forming potential. The addition of soluble and insoluble fiber sources to the diet of the older adult should be gradual. The use of bulking agents or fiber supplements may provide an acceptable option, and the untoward effects may be reduced by the addition of a supplemental form of normal gut flora, such as Bifidobacterium or other probiotics (Zunft et al., 2004).

Blood glucose control is important for decreasing glycation products, which according to theory is a contributing factor to senescence. Antioxidants from high-fiber fruits and vegetables are important for controlling free radical damage. Another theory regarding cellular senescence and the decrease in caloric content seen in high-fiber diets is associated with the maintenance of normal body weight, another factor in healthy aging and longevity. In addition, the sloughing of abnormal cells **(Figure 12.2)** with high-fiber intake reduces carcinogenesis and dis-

Figure 12.2 Abnormal cells.

Courtesy of Janice Carr/CDC

ease, and trapping cholesterol by fiber reduces atherosclerotic tendencies, which again is associated with healthier aging.

Cholesterol, trans fats, saturated fats, and total fat intake over the life span have been shown to impact morbidity and mortality in the aged (Anderson, Suchindran, Kritchevsky, & Barrett-Connor, 2004). In terms of overall macronutrient intake, these compounds have been shown to interact with genetic predisposition to increase vascular adverse events and morbidity more than any other dietary constituent. Inflammatory processes that mediate the effects involve a multitude of eicosanoids, **cytokines**, blood constituents such as platelets, hormones, and other cellular signals. In addition, body weight, energy expenditure, and environmental exposure serve to moderate the progression of disease in the face of increased intake (Okuyama, Ichikawa, Fujii, Ito, & Yamada, 2005). Cellular senescence as a result of increased fat and cholesterol intake may be related to free radical and nitric oxide generation and decrements in cellular repair with continued inflammatory response. Inflammatory markers such as C-reactive protein, sP-selectin, and sICAM-1 decrease with low fat intake over time.

> **Cytokines:** A class of cellular chemical messengers often involved in cascade reactions such as with inflammatory response.

Micronutrients

Several vitamins and minerals have been linked to healthy aging. The associations between maintenance of normal cellular function and vitamin or mineral status are also moderated by cumulative oxidative stress and inflammatory response. Antioxidants from fruits, vegetables, and whole grains prevent oxidative damage. Because oxidative stress is related to disease state from atherosclerosis as well as bone and joint health, investigations into the use of foods versus vitamin and mineral supplementation have been performed (Ganesan, Teklehaimanot, Tran, Asuncion, & Norris, 2005; Lichtenstein & Russell, 2005).

> **● Learning Point** Nutritional supplementation should be used when intake cannot provide fresh whole foods high in nutrient density (Dawson-Hughes, 2004). For certain fat-soluble vitamins like D and E or minerals such as calcium, there may be benefits of supplementation over whole foods, when dairy or fatty foods are not advisable due to the macronutrient content of the product (Deplas, Debiais, Alcalay, Bontoux, & Thomas, 2004; Nieves, 2005).

Eating whole fresh foods is preferable to increasing antioxidant capabilities because so many additional compounds are contained within the food in forms that make them potentiate the action of select micronutrients. The ancillary compounds in foods include organic acids, sulfur and nitrogenous compounds that aid in uptake, and activation and utilization of vitamins and minerals, in addition to their own direct benefits (Boudville & Bruce, 2005).

The relationships of the B vitamins to indices of cellular senescence have been the focus of recent research. Because homocysteine has been related to oxidative damage and diseases ranging from cardiovascular disease to neurodegenerative diseases of aging like Alzheimer's disease, vitamin B12, vitamin B6, and folate have been studied for their impact on disease over the life span (Bottiglieri & Diaz-Arrastia, 2005). Although **neurodegenerative disease** is thought to have a genetic component that makes the individual more susceptible with the appropriate environmental and dietary stimuli, dietary components have been shown to turn on select genes in a wide variety of models (Lewis et al., 2005).

Neurodegenerative diseases, which involve atherosclerotic changes such as vascular dementia, are also linked through the cycle involving methionine conversion, with methylmalonate, homocysteine, and S-adenosyl-methionine intermediates, each playing a role in cellular dysregulation and changes to DNA blueprinting (Quadri et al., 2004).

> **Neurodegenerative disease:** Diseases that involve malfunction of the central and peripheral nervous tissue. These are often diseases that progress slowly but insidiously and result in progressive loss of function and eventual mortality. Examples include Alzheimer's and Parkinson disease.

Homocysteine is also thought to be a modifiable risk factor for neurodegenerative diseases because of its direct neurotoxicity at high levels. Alterations in the **methylation reactions** essential for normal neurotransmitter synthesis are impaired at high levels of homocysteine and its metabolites (Tucker, Qiao, Scott, Rosenberg, & Spiro, 2005). High homocysteine levels are a result of low folate levels, and low folate levels are thought to be endemic in the elderly population in areas where mandatory folate fortification is not practiced (Wolters, Hermann, & Hahn, 2005). Decreased B_{12} absorption is also common in elderly persons who have atrophic gastritis or some other risk for the reduction of intrinsic factor production from the parietal cells lining the stomach. Older adults are also more vulnerable to B vitamin insufficiency due

> **Methylation reactions:** The process of attaching a methyl group to an existing compound through 1 C transfer by several vitamin/mineral cofactor.

to dietary choices and medication usage, which potentially interferes with bioavailability (Ravaglia et al., 2005). Cellular uptake and conversion of folates and cyanocobalamin may also be diminished as a function of aging. Receptor function and transporter capabilities naturally decline with aging. **Transcobalamin** synthesis and IF-complex reception decline, and conversion enzymes for methyl-tetrahydrofolate are diminished.

Transcobalamin: Transport protein classes for cyanocobalamin in blood and tissues.

Supplementation with B vitamins or the addition of B vitamins to foods as with fortification may be an option for elderly persons (Dhonukshe-Rutten et al., 2005). In the absence of severe decrements in transport and absorption, oral supplementation can raise levels of serum B vitamins in an older adult, thus decreasing **hyperhomocystinemia**. Additional benefits of increasing the vitamin B_{12}, folate, and pyridoxine vitamin content of foods include decreasing other ailments for which the elderly are more susceptible, such as pernicious anemia, decrements in immune function, and depressive disorders. These B vitamins are essential to cellular division and successful replication (Pfeiffer, Caudill, Gunter, Osterloh, & Sampson, 2005). Rapidly dividing cells, such as the red and white blood cells, are impacted by the insufficiency, hence the benefit from additional oral intake (Woodman, Ferrucci, & Guralnik, 2005).

Hyperhomocystinemia: Elevated blood levels of homocysteine, the sulfur-containing amino acid metabolite.

In regard to depressive symptoms, the B vitamins (folate in particular) are related to the ability to synthesize de novo methionine and S-adenosylmethionine (SAM-e). SAM-e is a universal methyl donor. Methylation reactions are essential for the synthesis of neurotransmitters such as serotonin in the brain and throughout the body. Serotonin receptors are not exclusive to the brain, and there are colonies of serotonin receptors throughout every organ system in the body. Serotonin is a chemical mediator for many homeostatic processes, including but not limited to mood. SAM-e has been shown to have potential as an antidepressant. Folate is necessary for SAM-e participation in methylation reactions, and elevated SAM-e production can be achieved through supplementation of folate in older adults (Ramos, Allen, Haan, Green, & Miller, 2004).

Dietary intake and functional B vitamin status are thus linked to cellular senescence through a number of pathways. The impact of hyperhomocystinemia on increasing oxidative stressors, with concomitant inflammatory response, is a modifiable risk factor for aging and cellular pathology. B vitamins are essential to the regulation of homocysteine. Therefore, B vitamin status is thought to be of importance to healthy aging.

Dietary Patterns

Dietary patterns are important to aging processes and cellular senescence, albeit indirectly. Differences have been investigated in the relationship between consumption patterns and inflammatory response in older persons, and the indirect relationships seem to have an effect on the progression of cellular dysregulation and ultimately disease. This can be seen in the advent of type 2 diabetes, where patterns of intake high in refined sugars and processed foods have been tied to inflammatory markers. Intake of high levels of sugared soft drinks, refined grains, diet drinks, lunch meat, and processed foods with low intake of vegetables is thought to increase CRP (C-reactive protein), interleukin-6, and **tumor necrosis factor-alpha** (Schulze et al., 2005).

Tumor necrosis factor-alpha: An indicator of inflammatory response and a mediator of several cascade mechanisms involved in immune function and homeostasis.

A Westernized dietary pattern of highly processed, high-fat foods has also been linked to morbidity through inflammatory processes and oxidative stress. Acculturation and the transition of other peoples to this consumption pattern has resulted in an increase of cellular changes and chronic diseases of aging as they move away from traditional dietary patterns of fresh whole foods (Iso, Date, Noda, Yoshimura, & Tamakoshi, 2005). Increases in patterns of consumption with fish as the dietary protein staple or of omega-3 oils from other sources have been shown to modify inflammation through the eicosanoids and their mediating influences on the inflammatory cascade (Payet et al., 2004). This decrement in inflammation over time with omega-3 fatty acid intake is directly related to cellular senescence through prolonged accumulation of oxidative stressors.

Increased low-fat dairy consumption has also been shown to be a healthful dietary pattern. Increased levels of several regulatory nutrients, not just calcium and vitamin D, may be obtained from dairy foods (McCabe et al., 2004). Encouraging older adults to consume low-fat dairy products as part of an overall dietary pattern is important. A caveat is that lactose intolerance increases with age, and arrangements must be made for use of lactose-free products, many of which are unfamiliar to older adults and may be rejected because of novelty or taste differences.

Immune function declines also occur in old age and are mediated by nutritional status. Increased infection results in increased oxidative stress. Cellular damage occurs with decrements in the immune system's ability to ward off pathologic changes such as in cancer or autoimmune disease.

Iron deficiency anemia in older adults may be due to other factors, such as the anemia of chronic disease, blood loss, or impaired absorption due to **achlorhydria**. However, regardless of the etiology, more iron is needed for red blood cell synthesis and tissue oxygenation, and poor iron status due to increased needs ultimately results in impaired immunity. Iron deficiency results in decreases in cell-mediated immune function, with decrements in T-cell proliferation and T-lymphocyte function (Ahluwalia, Sun, Krause, Mastro, & Handte, 2004).

Phagocytosis and **bacteriostatic** capabilities are diminished. Inflammatory response cytokines increase with poor iron status. It should also be noted that iron in and of itself is a potent **pro-oxidant** and must be bonded to a carrier or incorporated into a compound such as hemoglobin, because it cannot travel freely without inducing free radical damage. Therefore, carrier proteins and compounds such as myoglobin and hemoglobin must be synthesized correctly and in adequate amounts. Protein must be adequate to synthesize these components, and all cofactors for cellular differentiation and maturation must also be available in addition to the iron.

Similarly, older adults are also more susceptible to poorer zinc status. Zinc-containing foods are more expensive and may be prohibitive for older adults in lower socioeconomic strata. Zinc needs may be elevated in older adults suffering from comorbid conditions. Zinc malabsorption may take place because of gastrointestinal changes associated with aging, or deficiencies may result from dietary choices that are low in zinc. Metallothionein, the transporter for zinc, must be synthesized at optimal levels, which requires adequate protein, kilocalories, and other micronutrients. Because zinc is so tightly controlled in human serum through negative feedback homeostasis, it is often difficult to determine if older adults are deficient. Tests for zinc lack sensitivity and **specificity**. Zinc is inherently involved in the genetic upregulation of immune component synthesis. Because zinc is so closely tied to immune function, there are rapid changes in cellular components such as lymphocytes and inflammatory factors such as interleukin-2 and interleukin-6 (Andree et al., 2004). Representations of red and white cell types are shown in **Figures 12.3** through **12.7**.

Dietary intake of vitamins such as folate and vitamin C and adequacy of macronutrient intake are also essential to normal immune function. Because immunity is tied to cellular senescence through inflammatory responses, oxidative stressors, and glycation products, protein, total kilocalories, carbohydrates, and vitamins such as folate and C are essential to healthy **normative** aging. Provision of adequate micro- and macronutrients to older adults has been shown to increase immune response, regardless of form. Dietary intake of nutrient-dense whole foods is always preferable, but supplementation with enriched products also produces desirable increases in immune function (Wouters-Wesseling et al., 2005).

Nutritional status impacts morbidity and mortality in older adults. Mediating factors for cellular senescence and overall homeostasis include dietary pattern, macro- and micronutrient intake and impact on cumulative oxidative stressors, increases in glycation, and damage induced by free radical production over time. Successful aging with improved long-term outcome is inherently attributable to macro- and micronutrient availability (Donini et al., 2004).

Life-Style

Life style characteristics of an individual can have a marked impact on cellular senescence, when interacting with genetic predisposition. Many life-style attributes have been investigated in this regard:

● Learning Point Immunity and host defense are directly related to the ability to produce white blood cells, **chemokines**, and other cellular components, which ultimately depend on minerals such as iron and zinc and vitamins such as folate, in addition to other micro- and macronutrients.

Chemokines: A class of chemical messengers that constitute cellular signals that respond to very specific levels of a particular compound in a defined area of tissue.

Achlorhydria: Absence or decrement in the level of hydrochloric acid due to decreased production of the parietal cells in the fundus of the stomach.

Phagocytosis: The ability to engulf foreign bodies by white blood cells.

Bacteriostatic: The ability of immune cells to incapacitate bacterial invaders through engulfing, dissolution, or direct toxicity.

Pro-oxidant: A compound that normally has the potential to act as a free radical in its present oxidative state.

Specificity: The ability to precisely measure the component that is of interest.

Normative: Based on a normal distribution of a population, representing the "average" or normal individual within a given set of parameters.

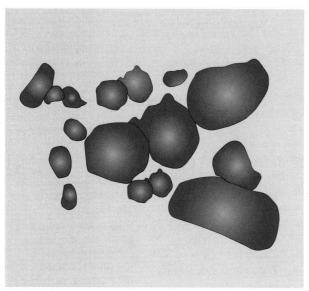

Figure 12.3   Megaloblastic cell. Immature red blood cells are often associated with nutritional deficiency and anemia. This is especially deleterious for an older person, who may be experiencing age-related declines in absorption and utilization of micronutrients.

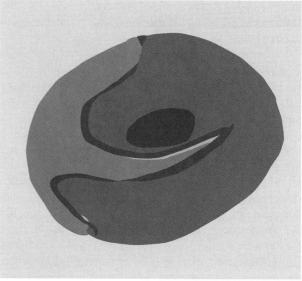

Figure 12.4   Red blood cells. Normal red blood cells are enucleated and have a life span of approximately 3 to 4 months. Their normal development requires several macronutrients, including vitamins A, K, and E; all the B vitamins; and iron, copper, and zinc. Anemia is common in older adults because of a variety of factors, including decreased micronutrient intake, absorption, distribution, and utilization.

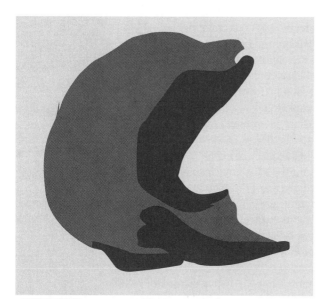

Figure 12.5   Abnormal red blood cells. Abnormal red blood cell production, activation, and destruction are important contributors as well as indices of disease. There are several diseases or circumstances in which abnormalities in erythropoiesis are present, besides nutritional deficiency. Some of these include autoimmune disease, environmental contaminant exposure with lead or mercury, or marrow failure as in cancer or prolonged sepsis.

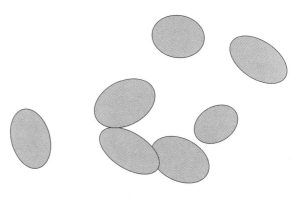

Figure 12.6   Normocytic cell. Normal cell size and shape as well as full maturation of the cell with normal functional capabilities are important tools in the evaluation of an older adult. Nutritional anemias (as well as a variety of other factors) influence cell size, shape, and activity.

- Physical activity
- **Body habitus**
- Environmental contaminant exposure
- Alcohol use
- Methylxanthine use
- Cigarette smoking
- Oral health
- Pet ownership
- Reproductive hormone levels
- Marital status
- Mental status
- Mental activity
- Socioeconomics
- Education
- Social support

Body habitus: The size and shape of the body; may also include perceptions of the size and shape of the body.

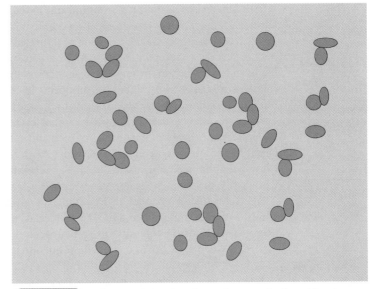

Figure 12.7   Cell size. Microcytic cells can be a result of nutritional anemias in the older adult but must be differentiated from other causes for interrupted maturation of blood cells, such as from medications, carcinogenesis, or heavy metal exposure.

This is a noncomprehensive listing of variables that all mediate and/or moderate successful aging. The interactions that occur are extremely complex, and it is extremely difficult to assess the level of impact for any one of these factors alone. Therefore, research efforts have opted to use these variables as a means of broadly classifying risk for morbidity and mortality (Brach, Simonsick, Kritchevsky, Yaffe, & Newman, 2004). The more risk factors per individual, the greater the cumulative effects in terms of cellular damage through oxidative stress, glycation, and free radical production.

Physical Activity
Physical activity over the life span is important to healthy aging, preventing functional decline. Improvements in balance, decrements in the sarcopenia of old age, and better mood and sleep are all important to overall health in the aged. It should be noted that increased physical activity is associated with increased oxidative stress, normally a result of oxygen utilization in aerobic metabolism. However, physical activity is also associated with improved ability to combat the increases in free radical production, and sustained lifelong activity improves counterregulation of oxidative cellular damage. Physical activity should be encouraged throughout the life span, thus improving appetite, enhancing weight control, decreasing visceral adiposity, and improving immune responsivity and glycemic control (Nied & Franklin, 2002; Lee et al., 2004).

Body Habitus
Visceral adiposity is an extremely strong risk factor for disease, and metabolic syndrome associations have been well studied (Wannamethee, Shaper, Morris, & Whincup, 2005). Android (apple shape) versus gynoid (pear shape) obesity has been investigated in terms of the cellular contributions this adipose tissue makes to disease over time. Body habitus, displaying an "apple" deposition, plays a role in the dysregulation of fatty acid flux from adipocytes located in and around the visceral organs that are fed by portal circulation. Increased free fatty acid flux, with resultant increases in lipoprotein transport, increased synthesis of cholesterol, and increased redistribution of triglycerides in portal circulation, is thought to increase inflammatory response (Farin, Abbasi, & Reaven, 2006). This has been shown through increased levels of mitochondrial leakage of superoxides and higher levels of serum isoprostanes, indicative of increased oxidative stress. Oxidation products and the deposition of oxidized low-density lipoprotein cholesterol into vessel endothelia dysregulate many of the ancillary feedback mechanisms for homeostatic control. One of these includes insulin responsivity (Weinbrenner et al., 2006).

Insulin resistance increases over time due to the increased levels of macronutrients in blood and alterations of the fluidity of membranes on cells that hold the receptors for insulin, among others (Jaques, Moeller, & Hankinson, 2003). Insertion of saturated fats into the membrane lipid bilayer results in stiffness and decreased receptor ability to lock onto its substrate. Insulin resistance results in higher levels of blood glucose, which in turn results in an increase in glycation products, another factor associated with cellular senescence. Gluteal femoral adiposity, in contrast, does not result in the same changes and is thought to be more "protective" in terms of disease risks (Snijder, Visser, & Dekker, 2005).

The caveat to the present knowledge is that less research has been done in this area on the frail elderly and little is known about the profiles of these older adults. In the past, the term "frailty" was believed to be antithetical to visceral obesity in an older adult, because frail elderly were thin and fragile (Kennedy, Chok-kalingham, & Srinivasan, 2004). The terminology is slowly changing to include older persons who may be obese but are still fragile (Gause-Nilsson & Dey, 2005).

A factor that determines healthy aging is body habitus. Efforts to reduce visceral obesity in older adults, both men and women, should be undertaken. The risk for increased visceral adipose accumulation increases postmenopause for women, such that it mirrors the risk for men at the same age (Z. Chen et al., 2005). Estrogen production in women serves to increase gluteal femoral deposition over android deposition, thus protecting women to some extent from swift development of metabolic syndrome (syndrome X) in the absence of other risk. It should be noted that BMI does not account for body habitus, and **skinfold thickness measures** have not been shown to be effective for assessing visceral adiposity (Snijder, Visser, & Dekker, 2002). These measures are very widely used despite these known issues because they are easy, inexpensive, and historical. There are population standards for these measures, so practitioners can evaluate their patients against known cut-off points. Pathologic processes stemming from visceral deposition result in increased cellular senescence, morbidity, and ultimately mortality. Therefore, assessment of abdominal stores should be routine for older persons. Waist circumference data are now being standardized for a variety of age, sex, and race groups (Snijder et al., 2005). Waist circumference may be a better predictor of health risk than waist-to-hip ratio in older persons (Welch & Somwers, 2000).

Skinfold thickness measures: Measurements done with the use of calipers; historically used and standardized for the measurement of subcutaneous adiposity from a variety of target points, such as the triceps area, the scapula, and the waist.

Environmental Contaminant Exposure

It has been shown that environmental contaminants contribute to morbidity through carcinogenesis, mutation, and inflammation. Known risks include asbestos, heavy metals, and ambient air pollution, among others. The mutagenesis, metabolic dysregulation, oxidative stress, and inflammation lead to alterations in cellular development, function, and homeostasis. Environmental contaminant exposure is therefore thought to be a **permissive effect** of cellular senescence. Coupled with other risk factors, long-term exposure is indirectly related to morbidity, aging, and cellular senescence (Pope et al., 2004).

Permissive effect: Factors that aid in the pathologic effect of another factor or set of antecedents.

Alcohol Use

Alcohol intake is highly controversial with respect to morbidity, mortality, and aging in general. Differences in drinking patterns and the type of alcohol consumption have varied risks associated with them. Those risks are significantly different between races, gender, and age and interact with life-style issues across the board. An example is a person who drinks one glass of red wine with dinner several nights per week for many years versus a person who engages in **binge drinking** of distilled spirits late in life as a result of depression or loss. The former is considered a healthy behavior; the latter is unhealthy and associated with morbidity. The interactions between alcohol intakes at a variety of levels with diet, exercise, and other issues are extremely complex. Because older adults are at risk for falls, take many different medications, and already suffer from many different conditions, it is best to recommend that alcohol intake be avoided in advanced age.

Binge drinking: The consumption of five or more standardized ethanol equivalents in one sitting. A standardized ethanol equivalent is 12 ounces of beer, 4 ounces of wine, or 1.5 ounces of distilled spirits.

Ethanol is broken down in a healthy liver to a variety of metabolites, all with known oxidative properties. Liver function declines in advanced age, and the metabolites, such as acetaldehyde, are thought to take more time for disposal. The use of the dehydrogenases, catalase,

$$CH_3-CH_2-OH \dashrightarrow CH_3-CH=O \dashrightarrow CH_3-COO^- \dashrightarrow CH_3-C=O-S-CoA$$

(Ethanol) Alcohol dehydrogenase (Acetaldehyde) Acetaldehyde dehydrogenase (Acetate) NAD/acylCoA synthetase (Acetyl-CoA)

Figure 12.8 Induced oxidative stress.

and the MEOSAQ2 systems for ethanol catabolism detract from these enzymes' abilities to deal with other reactions essential for drug disposition, nutrient activation, and toxin removal. Increased levels of circulating ethanol, acetaldehyde, and other intermediates are known to induce oxidative stress **(Figure 12.8)** (Lieber, 1992).

Methylxanthine Use

Methylxanthines, such as theobromine, theophylline, and caffeine, are consumed in increased amounts over the life span. These compounds are found in coffee, tea, chocolate, and cocoa as well as in over-the-counter preparations such as pain relievers and cold remedies. Methylxanthines alter neurotransmission and, ultimately, vascular response. They are inhibitors of adenosine reception and permissive for sympathetic nervous system firing. They require catabolism, and the intermediates are pro-oxidants (Shils, 2005). These compounds profoundly affect hydration and water homeostasis. They are diuretics and increase urinary calcium losses, ultimately affecting bone density in older women in particular (Shils, 2005). Methylxanthines also interact with a variety of medications used by older adults. There have been concerns regarding interactions with prescribed diuretics for blood pressure control, **sympathomimetic** drugs used to treat neurodegenerative conditions, and drugs that influence calcium uptake and disposition (Watson, 2001).

Sympathomimetic: Having the effect of upping sympathetic response, mimicking sympathetic response or acting synergistically with sympathetic response.

Cigarette Smoking

Cigarettes, chewing tobacco, and even pipe smoking are all considered deleterious to health over the long term. Known carcinogens are present in these preparations and interact with a variety of other factors to influence cellular senescence, morbidity, and mortality. Increased pro-oxidant status plus effects of contaminants contained in tobacco (such as cadmium) of smokers requires the diversion of available antioxidant mechanisms toward interruption of the pathologic changes induced by tobacco products (Y. C. Chen, Pu, & Lin, 2001). Even with adequate antioxidant capabilities, the number of oxidative events eventually surpasses response, and carcinogenic and inflammatory processes cause cellular alteration with continued tobacco use. Over time, an increase in a variety of disease states can be seen in tobacco users. Cancer, cardiovascular disease, stroke, and osteoporosis are significantly correlated with tobacco product usage; extent, duration, and type of usage should always be assessed in the older adult (Kato, Toniolo, Zeleniuch-Jacquotte, Shore, & Koenig, 2000). Other variables impact these tobacco effects in a **synergistic** manner; thus, poor diet quality, lack of exercise, body habitus, and heavy drinking elevate risk for morbidity. These variables are often seen clustered in an individual, creating a profile that is very strongly correlated with risk. Those with less education, lower economic status, and high stress often exhibit this variable profile (Burke et al., 2001).

Synergistic: The outcome of two influential factors is greater than the sum of each alone (e.g., $1 + 1 = 3 \times$ the effect).

Oral Health

Oral health is important for being able to consume foods and provide adequate nutriture. Nutritionally dense foods such as fruits and vegetables are not consumed in adequate amounts by persons with dentition problems or periodontal disease. Decreased salivation, ill-fitting dentures, and mouth sores or pain are just some of the factors involved in poor nutritional status due to decrements in oral intake. In addition to the lack of antioxidants, vitamins, minerals, and proteins are not adequately consumed. Other factors include the relationship between oral health and systemic inflammatory response (Avcu et al., 2005). The oral cavity is home to many different species of bacteria.

Increases in the chemokine response are associated with increased oxidative effects and inflammatory cascades. All-cause mortality rises with poor oral health, although much research has focused on heightened vascular infiltration and plaque formation with cardiovascular disease (Nakashini, Fukada, Takatorige, & Tatara, 2005).

Pet Ownership

Evidence of the positive effects of pet ownership on health have been documented with respect to lowering of blood pressure, decreased risk of cardiovascular disease, decreased depression and loneliness, and overall desensitization to antigens with decreases in immune and inflammatory response. Community-dwelling older adults may also see a significant impact of pets, especially dog ownership, in terms of heightened social interaction, increased physical activity, and indirectly toward better nutritional status **(Figure 12.9)** (McNicholas et al., 2005). Alternatively, studies on cohorts of persons in specific geographic areas have found anecdotal support for these findings but no statistically significant evidence (Parslow, Jorm, Christensen, Rodgers, & Jacomb, 2005). Three potential relationships exist to explain the benefits of pet ownership on health in older people:

Figure 12.9 Benefits of pet ownership.

Courtesy of Judith Sharlin

1. Pet ownership is associated with specific personality traits, age, and economic status, and it is these associated traits that mediate the positive effects of pet ownership on human health.
2. Pet ownership enhances social interactions and leads to decreased social isolation, thus providing an indirect mechanism for increased health.
3. Pet ownership itself reduces stress, increases physical activity, and changes levels of hormones involved in the inflammatory process **(Figure 12.10)**. These direct effects may also interact with the indirect effects previously outlined.

Pet ownership and its effects on overall health may require additional research to statistically obviate findings, but it should not be overlooked as a contributing factor to healthy aging.

Reproductive Hormone Levels

Declines in circulating sex steroids are known to alter inflammatory mediators such as cytokines and acute phase proteins. Several inflammatory mediators, including tumor necrosis factor-alpha, interleukin-6, and interleukin-8, are modulated by sex steroids. Aging and its declines in sex steroid production may indirectly influence cellular senescence via increased oxidative stress. In addition, the protective effects of sex steroid hormones have long been documented in terms of bone health for women, with postmenopausal women showing increased bone density losses. It has also been shown that the sex steroids in premenopausal women are protective for coronary artery disease, which can be seen in numerous surveys that

Figure 12.10 Pet ownership. Pet ownership may offer more companionship to an elderly person living alone. Pets may alleviate depression, decrease inflammatory process, and elevate nutritional intake.

Courtesy of Judith Sharlin

have corrected for other variables known to influence risk (Krabbe, Pederson, & Brüünsgaard, 2004).

Hormone replacement therapy has become increasingly widespread among postmenopausal women, and it is also thought that gluteal femoral adiposity is favored in these women and visceral adiposity is not. This may be a mediating relationship in the hypothesis that estrogen and other female sex steroids reduce oxidative risk in older women.

Age-related inflammatory cytokine increases may have multiple etiologies and may interact with a number of other compounds through a variety of mechanisms. The upshot is that inflammation increases morbidity and mortality in older adults through partial mediation by declines in the sex steroid hormones (Brüünsgaard & Pedersen, 2003).

Marital Status

Marital status is thought to have a moderating influence on healthy aging, especially in older men. Some of the reasons may involve decreased social isolation; spousal aid in procuring foods, cooking, and serving meals; or increased caregiving in general (Schone & Weinick, 1998). Widowhood is associated with increased morbidity and mortality in both older men and women and is associated with greater disability (Hokby, Reimers, & Laflamme, 2003; Iwashyna & Christakis, 2003). Nutritional status among older men is also associated with marital status, with unmarried or widowed men having poorer intakes and living alone without caregiver support being associated with poorer dietary intake in both genders (Larrieu et al., 2004).

Mental Status

Depression, declines in cognitive function, and neurodegenerative disease have profound effects on the nutritional status of the older adult (Salerno-Kennedy & Cashmanl, 2005). These conditions also impact morbidity, mortality, and cellular senescence, although the exact mechanisms are not fully understood (Robertson & Montagnini, 2004). There are probably a number of factors that are moderators of this effect, including decreased physical activity, increased stress hormone production, and alterations in neurotransmission leading to metabolic dysregulation, among others (Yaffe et al., 1999; Loucks, Berkamn, Gruenewald, & Seeman, 2005). Loneliness, social isolation, and depression can result in poor dietary intake, frank anorexia, self-neglect, and debilitation in an older person (Abrams, Lachs, McAvay, Keohane, & Bruce, 2002; Ferry, Sidobre, Lambertin, & Barberger-Gateau, 2005).

Mental Activity

Mental activity is thought to delay the progression of age-related cognitive declines and improve mood. The benefits of "psychological well-being" on morbidity and mortality have been documented in the elderly, but the exact mechanisms are not yet fully understood (Depp & Jeste, 2006). The role of mental activity in delaying cellular senescence is thought to involve the effects of nonspecific immune and inflammatory factors, which decline with improved mood, increased physical activity, more social integration, and better nutritional and life-style characteristics (Fortes et al., 2003). Having multiple roles, motivation, "personal projects," and varied activities and having one's basic needs met have been shown to impact aging, disability, disease, and mortality (Adelman, 1994; Herzog, Regula, Markus, & Holmberg, 1998; Powell, Moss, & Winter, 2002; Blazer & Sachs-Ericsson, 2005).

Socioeconomics

Socioeconomics impacts nutritional status and overall health, especially in the aged. Lack of access to health care, less money available to purchase foods, and fewer resources to procure, prepare, and consume nutritious foods are all consequences. The elderly make up some of the poorest poor, with increasing costs for medications and fixed incomes dedicated to paying for housing and other basic needs (U.S. Department of Health and Human Services, 2003). Declines in nutrient-dense food intake among the elderly result in deficiencies in calcium, iron, zinc, vitamin B_{12}, and vitamin E. Foods high in these particular micronutrients are also more expensive and are often protein sources as well (Drewnowski & Schultz, 2001). Socioeconomic hardship is associated with poorer outcome in terms of nutritional status, morbidity, and mortality.

Education

Education may be a surrogate for socioeconomic standing or may in and of itself be related to general health and nutritional status. Increased education is associated with more successful aging, perhaps through more informed dietary choices and life-style characteristics, better access to health care, or increased mental activity. Less-educated minority persons have been shown to have increased risks for nutritional deficiency as well as poorer overall health. Increased educational attainment is also associated with increased social and psychological resources, which may also mediate the relationships (Ross & Mirowsky, 1999).

Social Support

Social support and networks of friends, relatives, community resources, and religious organizations are associated with improved health and decreased disability, morbidity, and mortality among the elderly. This may be related to the provision of care by others, increased mental activity, healthier life-style, more physical activity, and less social isolation. Improved nutritional status with an extended network is also probable, with more resources for the procurement and provision of nutritious foods. In addition, place within a social hierarchy may also provide benefit, just by virtue of increased resources available (Lavis, McLeod, Mustard, & Stoddard, 2003). In older adults there are benefits to increased social networks and support on mental status, nutritional status, functional status, and overall successful aging (Koukouli, Vlachonikolis, & Philalithis, 2002; Yeh & Liu, 2003; Kirby, Coleman, & Daley, 2004).

Disease

Older adults with multiple conditions often require continuous care. Whether acute or chronic, comorbidity in the aged presents challenges in terms of health care costs and availability of facilities and staffing. The processes involved in cellular senescence along with overt disease often result in the need for hospitalization, institutionalization, or prolonged rehabilitation, because the older person does not have the recuperative capacity of a younger adult.

Malnutrition is correlated with institutionalization, hospitalization, and rehabilitative care. Poor nutritional status is a major risk factor for complications and delayed recovery. Unintentional weight loss, disease-related malnutrition, and depression-related anorexia rates are estimated to be up to 45% for older adults in the acute or subacute care setting (Brantervik, Jacobsson, Grimby, Wallén, & Bosaeus, 2005). Falls and functional decline with hospitalization often result in further complications, including sarcopenia, and constitute the sixth leading cause of death in persons over 65 years of age. This is due in part to malnutrition, reduced physical activity, reduction in sex hormone levels, and impairment in growth and insulin-like growth hormones (Borst, 2004).

Hospitalized elderly have increased rates of **nosocomial** infections with malnutrition and decrements in immune function consistent with aging. Inflammation results in hypermetabolic state, which increases needs while intakes remain marginal. Length of hospitalization worsens these effects, and the outcomes are generally poorer with longer duration of stay (Kyle, Genton, & Pichard, 2005). Generally, the type of institution also plays a role in the declines experienced by the ailing older adult. Larger institutions and/or institutions with more resources tend to offer more comprehensive care and have improved or cutting-edge practices that decrease the level of the malnutrition and improve the outcome of elderly patients.

Nosocomial: Hospital-acquired infection, usually with an antibiotic-resistant strain of organism.

Skilled nursing facilities also differ in the amount of resources and staff provided to ill elderly residents. Recent advances in low-cost formulations that are high in protein, supplemented with vitamins and minerals, and easily digested have made it easier and more feasible to deal with nutritional support in this population; however, these advances do not address the fundamental problem of poor oral feeding and the quality of life issues regarding eating of pleasurable foods (Levinson, Dwolatzky, Epstein, Adler, & Epstein, 2005). Holistic treatment of the issues regarding hospitalized or institutionalized frail older adults is essential, and clinical outcome in terms of morbidity and mortality should not be the only endpoints. Quality of life should be considered, and it comprises health and physical, social, and emotional functioning, both measured and perceived (Keller, 2004).

Hospitalization or institutionalization of the frail older person results in decrements in nutritional status just by virtue of changes to the eating environment. Institutional surroundings and lack of attention to the appearance or preparation of foods impact intake and dietary choices (Gibbons & Henry, 2005). Intake of several key macro- and micronutrients, such as vitamin D, zinc, calcium, and protein, is affected (Meydani, 2001; Pepersack et al., 2001). In the case of vitamin D, less exposure to sunlight complicates vitamin D and calcium nutriture in the geriatric patient (Lyman, 2005). Smaller macro- and micronutrient-enriched meals, properly prepared and nicely presented, may aid in improving nutritional status and preventing further debilitation among the institutionalized elderly (Kannus, Uusi-Rasi, Palvanen, & Parkkari, 2005; Lorefält, Wissing, & Unosson, 2005).

Common problems in comorbid hospitalized or institutionalized elderly include aspiration, infection due to aspiration or nosocomial acquisition, and pressure ulcers (Kikawada, Iwamoto, & Takasaki, 2005). All are inherently tied to nutriture and to increases in inflammatory response and cellular senescence. It is extremely difficult to treat these conditions, and they often result in further debilitation and ultimately in increased mortality (Mathus-Vliegen, 2004; Loeb & High, 2005). Several strategies have been used to augment treatment in the compromised older adult in these environments, including nutritional support with added select amino acids, such as glutamine or arginine; use of appetite enhancers such as megestrol; and single supplement augmentation of oral intake with zinc, chromium, copper, manganese, or antioxidant vitamins such as A and C (Rabinovitz et al., 2004; Reuben, Hirsch, Zhou, & Greendale, 2005; Stechmiller, Langkamp-Henken, & Childress, 2005).

Benefits of these artificial feeding and hydration strategies have met with mixed results, and the use of nutrition support or supplementation must be weighed against quality of life issues, such as pleasurable eating at the end of life. Implementation of best practice for nutrition in the frail older adult must be considered, taking into account personal preferences, involvement of a multidisciplinary health care team approach to oral intake, permissivity of the diet order, and incorporation of social interaction into mealtimes (Booth, Leadbetter, Francis, & Tolson, 2005). Continuous improvement of the approach to provision of nutrition to the institutionalized or hospitalized geriatric patient is essential (Pepersack, 2005). It is also important to accept that mortality is inevitable, and provision of nutrition and fluids at the end of life may not be in the best interest of the patient.

Indicators of whether or not to provide additional support to the geriatric patient may be evaluated using a number of tools, including laboratory indices, the Mini Nutritional Assessment, the minimum data set, anthropometry, and assessment of unintentional weight loss or gain (Salva, Corman, Andrieu, Salas, & Vellas, 2004; Zulkowski & Coon, 2004; Ranhoff, Gjoen, & Mowé, 2005). Regardless of physical state, the older adult should be granted autonomy in health care decisions; if the older adult is unable to make decisions due to mental status issues, a legally appointed guardian should be allowed to direct continuance of care. The wishes of the older adult should always be in the forefront when making decisions regarding medical procedures and feeding and hydration at the end of life (Stuck et al., 2005).

Artificial feeding and provision of fluids not by oral means is a burden in terms of health care costs, inefficient use of medical resources, and increased patient suffering in an elderly person at the end of life. Artificial provision of food and fluids in this stage is thought to cause continued pain and discomfort. Complications resulting from nasogastric tubes, total parenteral nutrition, or tube feeding include increases in infection, aspiration, and inflammation. Patients often have to be restrained so they do not dislodge tubes, and restraint in and of itself increases distress even in a patient with severely altered mental state (Slomka, 2003).

Dying from dehydration is a pain-free, natural, and peaceful process. Dry mouth is the only symptom associated with this course of action and is easily treated with lip balm and ice chips. Death through dehydration reduces nausea, diarrhea, and urinary output with concomitant urinary tract infection or bedsores from catheterization, wet bed sheets, and use of bedpans. Pulmonary secretions decrease, resulting in less discomfort from shortness of breath, choking, coughing, and congestion. Measures of physical pain show that in persons who are dying there is significantly less pain and in most cases mild euphoria with dehydration (Hoefler, 2000). It is unfortunate that societal norms are such that death is viewed as something that must be staved off at all costs, and the medical community has done little to inform itself and the public of the burden of keeping a dying older adult alive through artificial measures, even in situations where the individual's own wishes are overturned.

Pharmacologic Considerations

Polypharmacy is common among older persons. In addition to prescribed medications, older adults report more frequent use of over-the-counter preparations and herbal supplements **(Figure 12.11)**. Nonvitamin nonmineral supplement use complicates the interactions between over-the-counter, prescribed

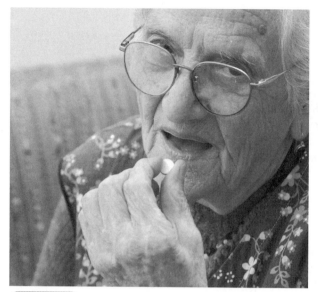

Figure 12.11 Supplements. Many supplements are marketed specifically to older adults. Several formulations exist for many herbal and other supplements with minimal standardization of dose or active ingredient. These products are largely uncontrolled by governmental agencies, and it is the burden of manufacturers to prove purity, efficacy, and legitimacy of any health claims.

© Sandor Kasco/Dreamstime.com

Figure 12.12 Drugs. Many older persons take a variety of medications every day. Average estimate of numbers of drugs taken by elderly persons, both prescribed and over-the-counter, are greater than eight per day in 70+-year-olds in the United States.

© Elena Eliseeva/Dreamstime.com

● **Learning Point** The number of prescribed medications taken by community-dwelling elderly is estimated at three or more per day, with almost half taking additional over-the-counter and supplemental products. The number of medications taken by institutionalized elderly persons is estimated at six or more per day (Bales, Ritchie, & Russell, 2004).

Dicoumarol

Warfarin

Figure 12.13 Warfarin. Coumadin, dicoumarol, and warfarin are potent inhibitors of the vitamin K-aided clotting cycles with gamma glutamic acids.

medications, and nutrients derived from oral intake or vitamin and mineral preparations **(Figure 12.12)**.

The use of herbals, botanicals, and amino acid supplements is significantly under-reported by older adults and is thought to interact with a variety of other preparations, especially the vitamin K antagonist anticoagulants, such as warfarin, Coumadin, and dicoumarol **(Figure 12.13)** (Archer, 2005). Compounds from herbals such as garlic, ginkgo biloba, Co-Q10, and others mediate the clotting cascade by the same mechanisms as the vitamin K antagonists. In addition, several botanicals have known interactions with the inflammatory cascade with potent lymphocytic activation **(Figure 12.14)**.

Aging is associated with increases in chronic and acute disease, for which multiple medications are prescribed (Soini, Routasalo, & Lagstrom, 2005). Nutritional status is often impaired as a result of the use of a variety of medications and other preparations (Eriksson, Dey, Hessler, Steen, & Steen, 2005). Polypharmacy is defined as "the use of excessive drugs or compounds with drug-like effects" or "the prescription of multiple medications given at one time" (Pugh, 2000). Current trends include the movement away from the use of nutritionally dense foods as a means of preventing or treating age-related concerns to the use of drugs, supplements, or herbal products in their stead (Solomons, 2005). Over 250 different medications alter food intake due to sensory side effects, and hundreds more have direct effects on the absorption, disposition, and utilization of nutrients.

Polypharmacy involves a complex set of problems in that foods alter drug disposition, drugs alter other drug disposition, and drugs alter nutrient disposition through a variety of mechanisms. The addition of cellular senescence, organ system deterioration, and alterations in catabolic potential for compounds, such as medications or herbal supplements, result in reductions in total homeostatic control in an older person (Bauer, 2001). Several classes of compounds are known for their interactions and nutritional effects:

- *Anticholinergic medications:* impair sensory perception, leading to declines in intake and increased gastrointestinal distress
- *Glycosides:* alter nutrient absorption, increase gastrointestinal distress and anorexia, and promote electrolyte disturbances
- *Diuretics:* affect mineral excretion, hydration, and electrolyte balance

Figure 12.14 Lymphocyte, white blood cell. Inflammation and the resultant chemokine response are intertwined with the immune system and its components. Lymphocytic activity correlates well with increases in response that increase risk for cellular senescence.
Courtesy of CDC

- *Beta-adrenergic antagonists:* alter gastrointestinal function, cause gastrointestinal distress, and impair glycogen metabolism
- *Vasodilators:* interact with B vitamins such as pyridoxine, cause gastrointestinal distress, and depress food intake
- *Antiarrhythmic agents:* cause gastrointestinal distress, anorexia, dysgeusia, dysosmia, and dry mouth
- *Anticoagulants:* cause gastrointestinal distress and interact with vitamins K and E and calcium
- *Hypolipidemics:* may alter the absorption of fat-soluble vitamins and cause gastrointestinal distress and severe constipation
- *Central nervous system or psychotherapeutic agents:* interact with a wide range of amino acids, vitamins, and minerals in addition to altering sensory perception, depressing or increasing appetite (depending on the drug), causing gastrointestinal disturbance, and altering the disposition of many metabolic intermediates (Mallarkey, 1999; Bauer, 2001).

Older adults use more than 30% of all medications prescribed, and one in three older persons has been prescribed an unnecessary, ineffective, or potentially dangerous medication. Among Medicare patients there has been documentation of more than 1,500 adverse events in a single year. Most adverse events are the result of interactions, and the estimated incidence of interaction increases from 6% in persons taking two or more drugs to 50% in persons taking five medications per day (Wootan & Galavis, 2005). Polypharmacy has also been linked to falls, worsening cognitive status, and poorer overall outcomes in both free-living and institutionalized older adults (Perr et al., 2005; Ziere et al., 2006). Because of the plethora of medications, each with its own set of drug–drug and drug–nutrient interactions, it is impossible to cover the entire spectrum of available information. There are several guides available for interactions between nutrients and drugs, herbals and drugs, and drugs and other drugs.

As a result of the increasing obesity problem in the United States, there has been an effort to assess excessive weight and obesity in the elderly population, with or without frailty. The prevalence of obesity is thought to increase to about 40% in 2010 in the oldest age groups, bringing with it an increase in cellular senescence, morbidity, and mortality along with increasing health care costs and fiscal burden in the United States (Arterburn, Crane, & Sullivan, 2004; Boyle & Holben, 2006). Drug treatment of obesity is due to come into the forefront for older adults, who will be prescribed drugs to decrease the effects of visceral adiposity, delaying metabolic syndrome complications and improving obesity-related disease (Hoekstra, Geleijnse, Schouten, Kok, & Kluft, 2005).

Pharmacotherapeutic Intervention in Obesity

In light of the changing demographics in the United States, the issues of weight and weight control in older persons will become increasingly important, and little is known about the treatment efficacy of anorexigenic drugs in this population or the likelihood of interactions between these drugs and other medications, nutrients, or herbal products. More is known about appetite stimulation in this population (Lee et al., 2005). Intuitively, this population would be better served by using diet, exercise, and nutrient density as a first response to weight change (Keller, Hadley, Hadley, Wong, & Vanderkooy, 2005). Unfortunately, societal propensity to medicate and health professionals' response to prescribe may result in an overuse of anorexigenics in older persons in the near future.

Several drugs have been used to treat obesity with limited success. The "phen/fen" regimen came under scrutiny when mitral valve abnormalities and primary pulmonary hypertension were identified as adverse events with prolonged use. Subsequently, fenfluramine was removed from the market. Phentermine (Ionamin), an amphetamine-like compound that reduces appetite through hypothalamic mediation, is still available. Phentermine is an older drug, available since the late 1970s, and is infrequently prescribed because of inconsequential long-term weight loss and ineffective weight maintenance with increased interactions with other drugs (Heuberger, 1998).

Xenical or Orlistat, a lipase inhibitor, has recently been approved for sale over the counter. It causes malabsorption of fat-soluble nutrients, without stellar weight loss. Because of the action of Orlistat on the gastrointestinal tract, there is considerable potential for steatorrhea, anal leakage, flatulence, bloating, nausea, and vomiting. Because of age-related declines in gut function, the impact of lipid malabsorption on vitamins E, D, and K are extreme. In addition, there may be loss of several minerals, through entrapment in the undigested materials in the gut, with subsequent elimination. In older persons, the prescription of a drug that causes malabsorption of key nutrients with gastrointestinal distress is not recommended (Kasper et al., 2005).

Serotonin reuptake inhibitors have also been used. Fluoxetine (Prozac) and sertraline (Zoloft) are just two examples. The weight change can go up or down, and decrements are not substantial or sustained when weight declines. Sibutramine, which affects norepinephrine, dopamine, and serotonin, has also been shown to have undesirable side effects and minimal efficacy for substantial loss and maintenance of weight loss over time. Sibutramine works through central reuptake inhibition of these neurotransmitters, which in turn affects heart rate and blood pressure and is unsuitable for use in older patients. Newer generations of endogenous hypothalamic 5-hydroxy-tryptophan medications are being developed to specifically target receptors for satiety (Fairburn & Brownell, 2002; Halford, Harrold, Lawton, & Blundell, 2005; Kasper et al., 2005).

Several targets have been identified as having an influence on weight and appetite. New drugs that either reduce food intake or increase oxygen consumption and energy expenditure are being tested. Beta-3 agonists that increase energy expenditure and uncoupling proteins to convert white to brown fat that result in elevated thermogenesis have been undergoing evaluation. Both result in increased oxidative stress and elevations in blood pressure, resting heart rate, and other side effects, making future use in elderly unlikely. Alternatively, drugs that act hypothalamically to induce satiety and reduce cravings are also of interest (Sidahaye & Cheskin, 2006).

There are a variety of these drugs under investigation, which include compounds that affect the endocannabinoid receptor systems in the brain and are thought to decrease appetite and cravings for specific macronutrients along with decreasing the desire for nicotine and smoking. The endocannabinoids are endogenous lipids that bind to specific receptors in the hypothalamic portions of the brain, including CBAQ2, CB-1AQ2, CB-2AQ2, and others. These receptors are also present in the gastrointestinal tract and peripherally in both soft tissue and adipocytes. Blocking these receptors decreases the inherent rewards of eating (Kirkham, 2005; Pagotto, Vincenati, & Pasqual, 2005).

Recent evidence also points to the influence of stimulation of these CBAQ2 receptors on fatty acid synthesis through synthetase expression. Blockage would result in decreased hepatic lipogenesis, and that in turn modulates metabolic homeostasis for weight and feeding, as well as oxidative stress (Di Marzo & Matias, 2005; Osei-Hyiaman et al., 2005). These compounds are still in clinical trial but show promise in terms of the reduction of body weight and long-term weight-loss maintenance among subjects, with few adverse effects. Rimonabant™ is one such CB-1AQ2 receptor antagonist (Boyd & Fremming, 2005).

Investigations into receptor agonists for NPYAQ2, a protein inherently tied to body weight stability and satiety, have been done with rodent models with mixed results (Boggiano et al., 2005). Lipoprotein lipase activation is also under consideration in animal models. NO-1886AQ2 increases the expression of uncoupling protein, thermogenin, with concomitant decreases in fat pads in obese animals (Kusunoki, Tsutsumi, & Iwata, 2005). Research is being conducted on drugs that will induce apoptosis in white adipose tissue, including extracts from green tea and fenugreek seeds (Handa, Yamaguchi, Sono, & Yazawa, 2005; Nelson-Dooley, Della-Fera, Hamrick, & Baile, 2005). It is unknown what the adverse potential of these novel compounds is or whether they will ever come to clinical trial in humans.

Obesity in older adults presents unique challenges, but the treatment of obesity warrants even greater concern. Most pharmacotherapeutic interventions for obesity in the older adult are contraindicated, with the elderly having multiple conditions and polydrug use. It remains to be seen if drug treatment can play a significant role in the upcoming obesity epidemic among older persons in the United States.

Summary

The concept of "successful" or "healthy" aging involves many factors. Some of these include complex interactions among nutritional status, genetics, life-style, and environmental considerations. Nutritional adequacy with caloric restriction over the life span is thought to be critical to the expression of genetic tendencies toward apoptosis or cellular senescence. Mediation of oxidative stresses and apoptotic events is thought to include exposure to environmental contaminants as well as alcohol, drug, and tobacco use. Other moderating factors that may directly or indirectly influence senescence include mental status, mental activity, pet ownership, marital status, economics, education, and parity, among others. Health conditions and acute or chronic disease requiring medication each impact the aging process. Body habitus and obesity with their concomitant influences on disease and cellular senescence are inherently tied to overall morbidity and mortality. In summary, healthy aging involves multiple factors, each with its own set of complex interactions. Older adults must be evaluated holistically, accounting for the multitude of factors that influence overall quality of life and longevity.

Issues for Debate

1. Discuss examples of health factors that have affected older people you have known.
2. How could some of these health factors have been improved?
3. What will be the impact of health factors on the aging baby boomer population?

References

Abrams, R. C., Lachs, M., McAvay, G., Keohane, D. J., & Bruce, M. L. (2002). Predictors of self-neglect in community-dwelling elders. *American Journal of Psychiatry, 159,* 1724–1730.

Adelman, P. K. (1994). Multiple roles and psychological well-being in a national sample of older adults. *Journal of Gerontology, 49,* 277S–285S.

Ahluwalia, N., Sun, J., Krause, D., Mastro, D., & Handte, G. (2004). Immune function is impaired in iron-deficient, homebound, older women. *American Journal of Clinical Nutrition, 79,* 516–521.

Anderson, J. J., Suchindran, C. M., Kritchevsky, S. B., & Barrett-Connor, E. (2004). Macronutrient intakes of elderly in the Lipid Research Clinics Program Prevalence Study. *Journal of Nutrition, Health, and Aging, 8,* 395–399.

Andree, K. B., Kim, J., Kirschke, C. P., Gregg, J. P., Paik, H., Joung, H., et al. (2004). Investigation of lymphocyte gene expression for use as biomarkers for zinc status in humans. *Journal of Nutrition, 134,* 1716–1723.

Archer, S. L. (2005). Nonvitamin and nonmineral supplement use among elderly people. *Journal of the American Dietetic Association, 105,* 63–64.

Arterburn, D. E., Crane, P. K., & Sullivan, S. D. (2004). The coming epidemic of obesity in elderly Americans. *Journal of the American Geriatric Society, 52,* 1907–1912.

Avcu, N., Ozbek, M., Kurtoglu, D., Kurtoglu, E., Kansu, O., & Kansu, H. (2005). Oral findings and health status among hospitalized patients with physical disabilities, aged 60 or above. *Archives of Gerontology and Geriatrics, 41*, 69–79.

Bales, C. W., Ritchie, C. S., & Russell, R. M. (2004). *Handbook of Clinical Nutrition and Aging* (pp. 214–271). Totowa, NJ: Humana Press.

Bamia, C. (2005). Dietary patterns among older Europeans: The EPIC-Elderly study. *British Journal of Nutrition, 94*, 100–113.

Bauer, L. A. (2001). *Applied Clinical Pharmacokinetics* (pp. 226–229). New York: McGraw-Hill.

Beck, A. M., Ovesen, L., & Schroll, M. (2001). A six-month prospective follow up of 65 and older patients from general practice classified according to nutritional risk by the MNA. *European Journal of Clinical Nutrition, 55*, 1028–1033.

Bischoff-Ferrari, H. A., Dietrich, T., Orav, E. J., Hu, F. B., Zhang, Y., Karlson, E.W., et al. (2004). Higher 25-hydroxyvitamin D concentrations are associated with better lower-extremity function in both active and inactive persons aged > 60 y. *American Journal of Clinical Nutrition, 80*, 752–758.

Blazer, D. G., & Sachs-Ericsson, N. H. (2005). Perception of unmet needs as a predictor of mortality among community-dwelling older adults. *American Journal of Public Health, 95*, 299–304.

Boggiano, M. M., Chandler, P. C., Oswald, K. D., Rodgers, R. J., Blundell, J. E., Ishii, Y., et al. (2005). PYY3-36 as an anti-obesity drug target. *Obesity Review, 6*, 307–322.

Booth, J., Leadbetter, A., Francis, M., & Tolson, D. (2005). Implementing a best practice statement in nutrition for frail older people: Part 2. *Nursing Older People, 17*, 22–24.

Borst, S. E. (2004). Interventions for sarcopenia and muscle weakness in older people. *Age and Ageing, 33*, 548–555.

Bottiglieri, T., & Diaz-Arrastia, R. (2005). Hyperhomocystinemia and cognitive function: More than just a casual link? *American Journal of Clinical Nutrition, 82*, 493–494.

Boudville, A., & Bruce, D. G. (2005). Lack of meal intake compensation following nutritional supplements in hospitalised elderly women. *British Journal of Nutrition, 93*, 879–884.

Boyd, S. T., & Fremming, B. A. (2005). Rimonobant—A selective CB-1 antagonist. *Annals of Pharmacotherapy, 30*, 684–690.

Boyle, M. A., & Holben, D. H. (2006). *Community Nutrition in Action: An Entrepreneurial Approach* (4th ed., pp. 135–140). Belmont, CA: Thomson Wadsworth.

Brach, J. S., Simonsick, E. M., Kritchevsky, S., Yaffe, K., & Newman, A. B. (2004). The association between physical function and life-style activity and exercise in the health, aging and body composition study. *Journal of the American Geriatrics Society, 52*, 502–509.

Brantervik, A. M., Jacobsson, I. E., Grimby, A., Wallén, T. C., & Bosaeus, I. G. (2005). Older hospitalized patients at risk of malnutrition: Correlation with quality of life, aid from the social welfare system and length of stay? *Age Aging, 34*, 444–449.

Brüünsgaard, H., & Pedersen, B. K. (2003). Age-related inflammatory cytokines and disease. *Immunology and Allergy Clinics of North America, 23*, 15–39.

Burke, G. L., Arnold, A. M., Bild, D. E., Cushman, M., Fried, L. P., Newman, A., et al. (2001). Factors associated with healthy aging: The cardiovascular health study. *Journal of the American Geriatrics Society, 49*, 254–262.

Chen, Z., Bassford, T., Green, S. B., Cauley, J. A., Jackson, R. D., LaCroix, A. Z., et al. (2005). Postmenopausal hormone therapy and body composition—a substudy of the estrogen plus progestin trial of the Women's Health Initiative. *American Journal of Clinical Nutrition, 82*, 651–656.

Chen, Y. C., Pu, Y. S., & Lin, R. S. (2001). Blood and urine levels of cadmium in relation to demographic and life style in middle age and elderly men. *Bulletin on Environment Contamination Toxicology, 66*, 287–294.

Chernoff, R. (1999). *Geriatric Nutrition: Health Professional's Handbook* (2nd ed., pp. 356–368). Gaithersburg, MD: Aspen Publishers.

Chernoff, R. (2005). Micronutrient requirements in older women. *American Journal of Clinical Nutrition, 81*, 1240S–1245S.

Collins, C. E., Kershaw, J., & Brockington, S. (2005). Effect of nutritional supplements on wound healing in home-nursed elderly: A randomized trial. *Nutrition, 21*, 147–155.

Dasgupta, M., Sharkey, J. R., & Wu, G. (2005). Inadequate intakes of indispensable amino acids among homebound older adults. *Journal of Nutrition for the Elderly, 24*, 85–99.

Dawson-Hughes, B. (2004). Racial/ethnic considerations in making recommendations for vitamin D for adult and elderly men and women. *American Journal of Clinical Nutrition, 80*, 1763S–1766S.

De Groot, L. C., Verheijden, M. W., de Henauw, S., Schroll, M., & van Staveren, W. A. (2004). Life-style, nutritional status, health, and mortality in elderly people across Europe: Our view of the longitudinal results of the SENECA study. *Journals of Gerontology. Series A, Biological Sciences and Medical Sciences, 59*, 1277–1284.

Demingné, C., Sabboh, H., Rémésy, C., & Meneton, P. (2004). Protective effects of high dietary potassium: Nutritional and metabolic aspects. *Journal of Nutrition, 134*, 2903–2906.

Deplas, A., Debiais, F., Alcalay, M., Bontoux, D., & Thomas, P. (2004). Bone density, parathyroid hormone, calcium and vitamin D nutritional status of institutionalized elderly subjects. *Journal of Nutrition, Health, and Aging, 8*, 400–404.

Depp, C. A., & Jeste, D. V. (2006). Definitions and predictors of successful aging: A comprehensive review of larger quantitative studies. *American Journal of Geriatric Psychiatry, 14*, 6–20.

Devine, A., Dick, I. M., Islam, A. F., Dhaliwal, S. S., & Prince, R. L. (2005). Protein consumption is an important predictor of lower limb bone mass in elderly women. *American Journal of Clinical Nutrition, 81*, 1423–1428.

Dhonukshe-Rutten, R. A., van Zutphen, M., de Groot, L. C., Eussen, S. J., Blom, H. J., & van Staveren, W. A. (2005). Effect of supplementation with cobalamin carried either by a milk product or a capsule in mildly cobalamin–deficient elderly Dutch persons. *American Journal of Clinical Nutrition, 82*, 568–574.

Di Marzo, V., & Matias, I. (2005). Endocannibinoid control of food intake and energy balance. *Nature Neuroscience, 8*, 585–589.

Donini, L. M., De Bernardini, L., De Felice, M. R., Savina, C., Coletti, C., & Cannella, C. (2004). Effect of nutritional status on clinical outcome in a population of geriatric rehabilitation patients. *Aging Clinical and Experimental Research, 16*, 132–138.

Drewnowski, A., & Schultz, J. M. (2001). Impact of aging on eating behaviors, food choices, nutrition and health status. *Journal of Nutrition, Health, and Aging, 5*, 75–79.

Eriksson, B. G., Dey, D. K., Hessler, R. M., Steen, G., & Steen, B. (2005). Relationship between MNA and SF-36 in a free-living elderly population aged 70 to 75. *Journal of Nutrition, Health, and Aging, 9,* 212–220.

Fairburn, C. G., & Brownell, K. D. (2002). *Eating Disorders and Obesity: A Comprehensive Handbook* (2nd ed., pp. 555–559). New York: Guilford Press.

Farin, H. M., Abbasi, F., & Reaven, G. M. (2006). Body mass index and waist circumference both contribute to differences in insulin-mediated glucose disposal in nondiabetic adults. *American Journal of Clinical Nutrition, 83,* 47–51.

Faure, P., Ducros, V., Couzy, F., Favier, A., & Ferry, M. (2005). Rapidly exchangeable pool study of zinc in free-living or institutionalized elderly women. *Nutrition, 21,* 831–837.

Ferry, M., Sidobre, B., Lambertin, A., & Barberger-Gateau, P. (2005). The SOLINUT study: Analysis of the interaction between nutrition and loneliness in persons aged over 70 years. *Journal of Nutrition, Health, and Aging, 9,* 261–268.

Fortes, C., Farchi, S., Forestiere, F., Agabiti, N., Pacifici, R., & Zuccaro, P. (2003). Depressive symptoms lead to impaired cellular immune response. *Psychotherapy and Psychosomatics, 72,* 253–260.

Ganesan, K., Teklehaimanot, S., Tran, T. H., Asuncion, M., & Norris, K. (2005). Relationship of C-reactive protein and bone mineral density in community-dwelling elderly females. *Journal of the National Medical Association, 97,* 329–333.

Gause-Nilsson, I., & Dey, D. K. (2005). Percent body fat estimation from skinfold thickness in the elderly. Development of a population-based prediction equation and comparison with published equations in 75-year-olds. *Journal of Nutrition, Health, and Aging, 9,* 19–24.

Gazzotti, C., Albert, A., Pepinster, A., & Petermans, J. (2000). Clinical usefulness of the mini-nutritional assessment (MNA) scale in geriatric patients. *Journal of Nutrition, Health, and Aging, 4,* 176–181.

Gibbons, M. D., & Henry, C. J. (2005). Does eating environment have an effect on food intake in the elderly? *Journal of Nutrition, Health, and Aging, 9,* 25–29.

Ginty, F. (2003). Dietary protein and bone health. *Proceedings of the Nutrition Society, 62,* 867–876.

Gonzalez, S., Huerta, J. M., Alvarez-Uria, J., Fernandez, S., Patterson, A. M., & Lasheras, C. (2004). Serum selenium is associated with plasma homocysteine concentrations in elderly humans. *Journal of Nutrition, 134,* 1736–1740.

Gori, A. M., Corsi, A. M., Fedi, S., Gazzini, A., Sofi, F., Bartali, B., et al. (2005). A proinflammatory state is associated with hyperhomocystinemia in the elderly. *American Journal of Clinical Nutrition, 82,* 335–341.

Halford, J. C., Harrold, J. A., Lawton, C. L., & Blundell, J. E. (2005). Serotonin drugs: Effects on appetite expression and the use for the treatment of obesity. *Current Drug Targets, 6,* 201–213.

Hamilton, B. P., & Hamilton, J. H. (1997). Hypertension in elderly persons. *Endocrine Practice, 3,* 29–41.

Handa, T., Yamaguchi, K., Sono, Y., & Yazawa, K. (2005). Effects of fenugreek seed extract in obese mice fed a high fat diet. *Bioscience, Biotechnology, and Biochemistry, 69,* 1186–1188.

Herzog, A., Regula, F., Markus, H., & Holmberg, D. (1998). Activities and well-being in older age: Effects of self-concept and educational attainment. *Psychological Aging, 13,* 179–185.

Heuberger, R. A. (1998). *Combination Drug Treatment of Obesity.* Ann Arbor, MI: UMI Publications.

Hjerkinn, E. M., Seljeflot, I., Ellingsen, I., Berstad, P., Hjermann, I., Sandvik, L., et al. (2005). Influence of long-term intervention with dietary counseling, long chain n-3 fatty acid supplements, or both on circulating markers of endothelial activation in men with long-standing hyperlipidemia. *American Journal of Clinical Nutrition, 81,* 583–589.

Hoefler, J. M. (2000). Making decisions about tube feeding for severely demented patients at the end of life: Clinical, legal and ethical considerations. *Death Studies, 24,* 233–254.

Hoekstra, T., Geleijnse, J. M., Schouten, E. G., Kok, F. J., & Kluft, C. (2005). Relationship of C-reactive protein with components of the metabolic syndrome in normal-weight and overweight elderly. *Nutrition, Metabolism, and Cardiovascular Disease, 15,* 270–278.

Hokby, A., Reimers, A., & Laflamme, I. (2003). Hip fractures among older people: Do marital status and type of residence matter? *Public Health, 117,* 196–201.

Iso, H., Date, C., Noda, H., Yoshimura, T., & Tamakoshi, A. (2005). Frequency of food intake and estimated nutrient intake among men and women: The JACC Study. *American Journal of Epidemiology, 15*(Suppl. 1), S24–S42.

Iwashyna, T. J., & Christakis, N. A. (2003). Marriage, widowhood and health care use. *Social Science and Medicine, 57,* 2137–2147.

Jaques, P. F., Moeller, S. M., & Hankinson, S. E. (2003). Weight status, abdominal adiposity, diabetes and early age related lens opacities. *American Journal of Clinical Nutrition, 78,* 400–405.

Jungjohann, S. M., Luhrmann, P. M., Bender, R., Blettner, M., & Neuhäuser-Berthold, M. (2005). Eight-year trends in food, energy and macronutrient intake in a sample of elderly German subjects. *British Journal of Nutrition, 93,* 361–378.

Kannus, P., Uusi-Rasi, K., Palvanen, M., & Parkkari, J. (2005). Non-pharmacological means to prevent fractures among older adults. *Annals of Medicine, 37,* 303–310.

Kasper, D. L., Fauci, A. S., Longo, D. L., Braunwald, E., Hauser, S. L., & Jameson, J. L. (2005). *Harrison's Principles of Internal Medicine* (16th ed., pp. 428–429). New York: McGraw-Hill.

Kato, I., Toniolo, P., Zeleniuch-Jacquotte, A., Shore, R. E., & Koenig, K. L. (2000). Diet, smoking and anthropometric indices and postmenopausal bone fractures: A prospective study. *International Journal of Epidemiology, 29,* 85–92.

Keller, H. H. (2004). Nutrition and health-related quality of life in frail older adults. *Journal of Nutrition, Health, and Aging, 8,* 245–252.

Keller, H. H., Hadley, M., Hadley, T., Wong, S., & Vander-kooy, P. (2005). Food workshops, nutrition education, and older adults: A process evaluation. *Journal of Nutrition for the Elderly, 24,* 5–23.

Keller, H. H., & Ostbye, T. (2003). Nutritional risk and time to death: Predictive validity of SCREEN. *Journal of Nutrition, Health, and Aging, 7,* 274–279.

Kennedy, R. L., Chokkalingham, K., & Srinivasan, R. (2004). Obesity in the elderly: Who should we be treating, and why, and how? *Current Opinion in Clinical Nutrition and Metabolic Care, 7,* 3–9.

Kikawada, M., Iwamoto, T., & Takasaki, M. (2005). Aspiration and infection in the elderly: Epidemiology, diagnosis and management. *Drugs and Aging, 22,* 115–130.

Kirby, S. E., Coleman, P. G., & Daley, D. (2004). Spirituality and well-being in frail and non-frail older adults. *Journal of Gerontology, 59,* 123–129.

Kirkham, T. C. (2005). Endocannibinoids in the regulation of appetite and body weight. *Behavioral Pharmacology, 16,* 297–313.

Koukouli, S., Vlachonikolis, I. G., & Philalithis, A. (2002). Sociodemographic factors and self-reported functional status: The significance of social support. *BMC Health Service Research, 2,* 20.

Krabbe, K. S., Pedersen, M., & Brüünsgaard, H. (2004). Inflammatory mediators in the elderly. *Experimental Gerontology, 39,* 687–699.

Kusunoki, M., Tsutsumi, K., & Iwata, K. (2005). NO-1886 (Ibrolipim), an LPL activator, increases expression of UCP-3 in skeletal muscle and suppresses fat accumulation in high-fat diet-induced obesity in rats. *Metabolism: Clinical and Experimental, 54,* 1587–1592.

Kyle, U. G., Genton, L., & Pichard, C. (2005). Hospital length of stay and nutritional status. *Current Opinion in Clinical Nutrition and Metabolic Care, 8,* 397–402.

Larrieu, S., Letenneur, L., Berr, C., Dartigues, J. F., Ritchies, K., & Alperovitch, A. (2004). Sociodemographic differences in dietary habits in a population-based sample of elderly subjects: The 3C study. *Journal of Nutrition, Health, and Aging, 8,* 497–502.

Lavis, J. N., McLeod, C. B., Mustard, C. A., & Stoddard, G. I. (2003). Is there a gradient in lifespan by position in the social hierarchy? *American Journal of Public Health, 93,* 771–773.

Lee, J. S., Kritchevsky, S. B., Harris, T. B., Tylavsky, F., Rubin, S. M., & Newman, A. B. (2005). Short-term weight changes in community-dwelling older adults: The Health, Aging, and Body Composition Weight Change Substudy. *American Journal of Clinical Nutrition, 82,* 644–650.

Lee, J. S., Kritchevsky, S. B., Tylavsky, F. A., Harris, T., Everhart, J., Simonsick, E. M., et al. (2004). Weight-loss intention in the well-functioning, community-dwelling elderly: Associations with diet quality, physical activity, and weight change. *American Journal of Clinical Nutrition, 80,* 466–474.

Levinson, Y., Dwolatzky, T., Epstein, A., Adler, B., & Epstein, L. (2005). Is it possible to increase weight and maintain the protein status of debilitated elderly residents of nursing homes? *Journals of Gerontology. Series A, Biological Sciences and Medical Sciences, 60,* 878–881.

Lewis, M. S., Miller, L. S., Johnson, M. A., Dolce, E. B., Allen, R. H., & Stabler, S. P. (2005). Elevated methylmalonic acid is related to cognitive impairment in older adults enrolled in an elderly nutrition program. *Journal of Nutrition for the Elderly, 24,* 47–65.

Lichtenstein, A. H., & Russell, R. M. (2005). Essential nutrients: Food or supplements? Where should the emphasis be? *Journal of the American Medical Association, 294,* 351–358.

Lieber, C. (1992). *Medical and Nutritional Complications of Alcoholism.* New York: Plenum.

Loeb, M., & High, K. (2005). The effect of malnutrition on risk and outcome of community-acquired pneumonia. *Respiratory Care Clinics of North America, 11,* 99–108.

Lorefält, B., Wissing, U., & Unosson, M. (2005). Smaller but energy- and protein-enriched meals improve energy and nutrient intakes in elderly patients. *Journal of Nutrition, Health, and Aging, 9,* 243–247.

Loucks, E. B., Berkamn, L. F., Gruenewald, T. L., & Seeman, T. E. (2005). Social integration is associated with fibrinogen concentration in elderly men. *Psychosomatic Medicine, 67,* 353–358.

Lyman, D. (2005). Undiagnosed vitamin D deficiency in the hospitalized patient. *American Family Physician, 71,* 299–304.

Mallarkey, G. (1999). *Drug Treatment Considerations in the Elderly* (pp. 61–64). Hong Kong: Adis International.

Marlett, J. A., McBurney, M. I., & Slavin, J. L. (2002). Position of the American Dietetics Association: Health implications of dietary fiber. *Journal of the American Dietetic Association, 102,* 993–1000.

Marshall, J. A., Lopez, T. K., Shetterly, S. M., Morganstern, N. E., Baer, K., Swenson, C., et al. (1999). Indicators of nutritional risk in a rural elderly Hispanic and non-Hispanic white population: San Luis Valley Health and Aging Study. *Journal of the American Dietetic Association, 99,* 315–322.

Mathus-Vliegen, E. M. H. (2004). Old age, malnutrition, and pressure sores: An ill-fated alliance. *Journals of Gerontology. Series A, Biological Sciences and Medical Sciences, 59,* M355–M360.

McCabe, L. D., Martin, B. R., McCabe, G. P., Johnston, C. C., Weaver, C. M., & Peacock, M. (2004). Dairy intakes affect bone density in the elderly. *American Journal of Clinical Nutrition, 80,* 1066–1074.

McNicholas, J., Gilbey, A., Rennie, A., Ahmedzai, S., Dono, J., & Ormerod, E. (2005). Pet ownership and human health: A brief review of evidence and issues. *British Medical Journal, 331,* 1252–1254.

Meydani, M. (2001). Nutrition interventions in aging and age-associated disease. *Annals of the New York Academy of Sciences, 928,* 226–235.

Millward, D. J. (2004). Macronutrient intakes as determinants of dietary protein and amino acid adequacy. *American Society for Nutritional Sciences, 134,* 1588S–1596S.

Milne, A. C., Potter, J., & Avenell, A. (2005). Protein and energy supplementation in elderly people at risk from malnutrition. *Cochrane Database System Review,* CD003288.

Mojon, P., Budtz-Jorgensen, E. R., & Henri, C. (1999). Relationship between oral health and nutrition in very old people. *Age and Aging, 28,* 463–468.

Morley, J. E., Glick, Z., & Rubenstein, L. Z. (1995). *Geriatric Nutrition: A Comprehensive Review* (2nd ed.). New York: Raven Press.

Nakashini, N., Fukada, H., Takatorige, T., & Tatara, K. (2005). Relationship between self-assessed masticatory ability and 9-year mortality in a cohort of community-residing elderly people. *Journal of the American Geriatrics Society, 53,* 54–58.

National Institute on Aging. (2005). Strategic plan research goals. Retrieved December 22, 2005, from www.nia.nih.gov

Nelson-Dooley, C., Della-Fera, M. A., Hamrick, M., & Baile, C. A. (2005). Novel treatments for obesity and osteoporosis: Targeting apoptotic pathways in adipocytes. *Current Medicinal Chemistry, 12,* 2215–2225.

Nied, R. J., & Franklin, B. (2002). Promoting and prescribing exercise for the elderly. *American Family Physician, 65,* 419–426.

Nieves, J. W. (2005). Osteoporosis: The role of micronutrients. *American Journal of Clinical Nutrition, 81,* 1232S–1239S.

Okuyama, H., Ichikawa, Y., Fujii, Y., Ito, M., & Yamada, K. (2005). Changes in dietary fatty acids and life style as major factors for rapidly increasing inflammatory diseases and elderly-onset diseases. *World Review of Nutrition and Dietetics, 95,* 52–61.

Osei-Hyiaman, D., DePetrillo, M., Pacher, P., Lui, J., Radaeva, S., & Batkai, S. (2005). Endocannabinoid activation at hepatic

CB1 receptors stimulates fatty acid synthesis and contributes to diet-induced obesity. *Journal of Clinical Investigation, 115,* 1298–1305.

Pagotto, U., Vincenati, V., & Pasquali, R. (2005). The endocannabinoid system and the treatment of obesity. *Annals of Medicine, 37,* 270–275.

Parslow, R. A., Jorm, A. F., Christensen, H., Rodgers, B., & Jacomb, P. (2005). Pet ownership and health in older adults. *Gerontology, 51,* 40–47.

Payet, M., Esmail, M. H., Polichetti, E., Le Brun, G., Adjemout, L., Donnarel, G., et al. (2004). Docosahexaenoic acid-enriched egg consumption induces accretion of arachidonic acid in erythrocytes of elderly patients. *British Journal of Nutrition, 91,* 789–796.

Pepersack, T. (2005). Outcomes of continuous process improvement of nutritional care program among geriatric units. *Journals of Gerontology. Series A, Biological Sciences and Medical Sciences, 60,* 787–792.

Pepersack, T., Rotsaert, P., Benoit, F., Willems, D., Fuss, M., Bourdoux, P., et al. (2001). Prevalence of zinc deficiency and its clinical relevance among hospitalized elderly. *Archives of Gerontology and Geriatrics, 33,* 243–253.

Perr, M., Menon, A. M., Deshpande, A. D., Shinde, S. B., Jiang, R., Cooper, J. W., et al. (2005). Adverse outcomes associated with inappropriate drug use in nursing homes. *Annals of Pharmacotherapy, 39,* 405–411.

Pfeiffer, C. M., Caudill, S. P., Gunter, E. W., Osterloh, J., & Sampson, E. J. (2005). Biochemical indicators of B vitamin status in the US population after folic acid fortification: Results from the National Health and Nutrition Examination Survey. *American Journal of Clinical Nutrition, 82,* 442–450.

Pope, A. C., Hansen, M. L., Long, R. W., Meilsen, K. R., Eatogh, N. L., & Wilson, W. E. (2004). Ambient air pollution, heart rate variability and blood markers of inflammation in a panel of elderly subjects. *Environmental Health Perspective, 112,* 339–345.

Powell, L. M., Moss, M. S., & Winter, L. H. (2002). Motivation in later life: Personal projects and well being. *Psychological Aging, 17,* 539–547.

Pugh, M. B. (2000). *Stedman's Medical Dictionary* (27th ed.). Philadelphia: Lippincott Williams & Wilkins.

Quadri, P., Fragiacomo, C., Pezzati, R., Zanda, E., Forloni, G., Tettamanti, M., et al. (2004). Homocysteine, folate, and vitamin B-12 in mild cognitive impairment, Alzheimer's disease, and vascular dementia. *American Journal of Clinical Nutrition, 80,* 114–122.

Rabinovitz, H., Friedensohn, A., Leibovitz, A., Gabay, G., Rocas, C., & Habot, B. (2004). Effect of chromium supplementation in elderly patients. *International Journal for Vitamin and Nutrition Research, 74,* 178–182.

Ramos, M. I., Allen, L. H., Haan, M. N., Green, R., & Miller, J. W. (2004). Plasma folate concentrations are associated with depressive symptoms in elderly Latina women despite folic acid fortification. *American Journal of Clinical Nutrition, 80,* 1024–1028.

Ranhoff, A. H., Gjoen, A. U., & Mowé, M. (2005). Screening for malnutrition in elderly acute medical patients: The usefulness of MNA-SF. *Journal of Nutrition, Health, and Aging, 9,* 221–225.

Ravaglia, G., Forti, P., Maioli, F., Martelli, M., Servadei, L., Brunetti, N., et al. (2005). Homocysteine and folate as risk factors

for dementia and Alzheimer disease. *American Journal of Clinical Nutrition, 82,* 636–643.

Reuben, D. B., Hirsch, S. H., Zhou, K., & Greendale, G. A. (2005). The effects of megestrol acetate suspension for elderly patients with reduced appetite after hospitalization: A phase II randomized clinical trial. *Journal of the American Geriatrics Society, 53,* 970–975.

Rimkus, A., Melinchok, M. D., McEvoy, K., & Yeager, A. K. (2005). *Thesaurus of Aging Terminology* (8th ed.). Washington, DC: AARP.

Robertson, R. G., & Montagnini, M. (2004). Geriatric failure to thrive. *American Family Physician, 70,* 343–350.

Ross, C. E., & Mirowsky, J. (1999). Refining the association between education and health: The effects of quantity, credential, and selectivity. *Demography, 36,* 445–460.

Roth, G. S., Ingram, D. K., & Lane, M. A. (1999). Calorie restriction in primates: Will it work and how will we know? *Journal of the American Geriatric Society, 47,* 896–903.

Ryan-Harshman, M., & Aldoori, W. (2004). Bone health: New role for vitamin K? *Canadian Family Physician, 50,* 993–997.

Salerno-Kennedy, R., & Cashmanl, K. D. (2005). Relationship between dementia and nutrition-related factors and disorders: An overview. *International Journal for Vitamin and Nutrition Research, 75,* 83–95.

Salva, A., Corman, B., Andrieu, S., Salas, J., & Vellas, B. (2004). Minimum data set for nutritional intervention studies in elderly people. *Journals of Gerontology. Series A, Biological Sciences and Medical Sciences, 59,* M724–M729.

Schone, B. S., & Weinick, R. M. (1998). Health-related behaviors and the benefits of marriage for elderly persons. *Gerontologist, 38,* 618–627.

Schulze, M. B., Hoffmann, K., Manson, J. E., Willett, W. C., Meigs, J. B., Weikert, C., et al. (2005). Dietary pattern, inflammation, and incidence of type 2 diabetes in women. *American Journal of Clinical Nutrition, 82,* 675–684.

Shils, M. E. (2005). *Modern Nutrition in Health and Disease* (10th ed.). Philadelphia: Lippincott Williams and Wilkins.

Sidahaye, A., & Cheskin, L. J. (2006). Pharmacologic treatment of obesity. *Advances in Psychosomatic Medicine, 27,* 42–52.

Singer, B. H., & Manton, K. G. (1998). The effects of health changes on projections of health service needs for the elderly population of the United States. *Proceedings of the National Academies of Sciences of the United States, 95,* 15618–15622.

Slomka, J. (2003). Withholding nutrition at the end of life: Clinical and ethical issues. *Cleveland Clinic Journal of Medicine, 70,* 548–552.

Snijder, M. B., Visser, M., & Dekker, J. M. (2002). The prediction of visceral fat by dual x-ray absorptiometry in the elderly: A comparison with computed tomography and anthropometry. *International Journal of Obesity and Related Metabolism Disorders, 26,* 984–993.

Snijder, M. B., Visser, M., & Dekker, J. M. (2005). Low subcutaneous thigh fat is a risk factor for unfavorable glucose and lipid levels independent of high abdominal fat. The Health ABC study. *Diabetologia, 48,* 301–308.

Soini, H., Routasalo, P., & Lagstrom, H. (2005). Nutritional status in cognitively intact older people receiving home care services—A pilot study. *Journal of Nutrition, Health, and Aging, 9,* 249–253.

Solomons, N. W. (2005). Nutritional dilemmas of long-term health: Implications of evolution and ageing for policies and food industry practices affecting chronic diseases. *Asia Pacific Journal of Clinical Nutrition, 14*(Suppl.), S1–S9.

Stechmiller, J. K., Langkamp-Henken, B., & Childress B. (2005). Arginine supplementation does not enhance serum nitric oxide levels in elderly nursing home residents with pressure ulcers. *Biology Research in Nursing, 6,* 289–299.

Stuck, A., Amstad, H., Baumann-Hölzle, R., Fankhauser, A., Kesselring, A., Leuba, A., et al. (2005). Treatment and care of elderly persons who are in need of care: Medical-ethical guidelines and recommendations. *Journal of Nutrition, Health, and Aging, 9,* 288–295.

Sullivan, D. H., Liu, L., Roberson, P. K., Bopp, M. M., & Rees, J. C. (2004). Body weight change and mortality in a cohort of elderly patients recently discharged from the hospital. *Journal of the American Geriatric Society, 52,* 1696–1701.

Tucker, K. L., Qiao, N., Scott, T., Rosenberg, I., & Spiro III, A. (2005). High homocysteine and low B vitamins predict cognitive decline in aging men: The Veterans Affairs normative aging study. *American Journal of Clinical Nutrition, 82,* 627–635.

U.S. Bureau of the Census. (2005). Retrieved December 22, 2005, from www.census.gov

U.S. Department of Health and Human Services. (2003). Health, United States, 2003: Special excerpt: Trend tables on 65 and older population. Hyattsville, MD: Centers for Disease Control and Prevention.

Wannamethee, S. G., Shaper, A. G., Morris, R. W., & Whincup, P. H. (2005). Measures of adiposity in the identification of metabolic abnormalities in elderly men. *American Journal of Clinical Nutrition, 81,* 1313–1321.

Warner, H. R., Fernandes, G., & Wang, E. (1995). A unifying hypothesis to explain the retardation of aging and tumorigenesis by caloric restriction. *Journals of Gerontology. Series A, Biological Sciences and Medical Sciences, 50,* B107–B109.

Watson, R. R. (2001). *Alcohol and Coffee Use in the Aging.* Boca Raton, FL: CRC Press.

Weinbrenner, T., Schroder, H., Escurriol, V., Fito, M., Elosua, R., Vila, J., et al. (2006). Circulating oxidized LDL is associated with increased waist circumference independent of BMI in men and women. *American Journal of Clinical Nutrition, 83,* 30–36.

Weinrebe, W., Guneysu, S., & Welz-Barth, A. (2002). Low muscle mass of the thigh is significantly correlated with delirium and worse functional outcome in older medical patients. *Journal of the American Geriatric Society, 50,* 1310–1311.

Welch, G. W., & Somwers, M. R. (2000). The interrelationship between body topology and body composition varies with age among women. *Journal of Nutrition, 130,* 2371–2377.

Wolters, M., Hermann, S., & Hahn, A. (2005). Effect of multivitamin supplementation on the homocysteine and methylmalonic acid blood concentrations in women over the age of 60 years. *European Journal of Nutrition, 44,* 183–192.

Woodman, R., Ferrucci, L., & Guralnik, J. (2005). Anemia in older adults. *Current Opinion in Hematology, 12,* 123–128.

Woods, N. F., LaCroix, A. Z., Gray, S. L., Aragaki, A., Cochrane, B. B., Brunner, R. L., et al. (2005). Frailty: Emergence and consequences in women aged 65 and older in the Women's Health Initiative Observational Study. *Journal of the American Geriatric Society, 53,* 1321–1330.

Wootan, J., & Galavis, J. (2005). Polypharmacy: Keeping the elderly safe. *RN, 68,* 44–51.

Wouters-Wesseling, W., Vos, A. P., Van Hal, M., De Groot, L. C., Van Staveren, W. A., & Bindels, J. G. (2005). The effect of supplementation with an enriched drink on indices of immune function in frail elderly. *Journal of Nutrition, Health, and Aging, 9,* 281–286.

Yaffe, K., Blackwell, T., Gore, R., Sands, L., Reus, V., & Browner, W. S. (1999). Depressive symptoms and cognitive decline in non-demented elderly women. *Archives of General Psychiatry, 56,* 425–430.

Yeh, S. C., & Liu, Y. Y. (2003). Influence of social support on cognitive function in the elderly. *BMC Health Service Research, 3,* 9.

Ziere, G., Dieleman, J. P., Hofman, A., Pols, H. A., vander Cammen, T. J., & Stricker, B. H. (2006). Polypharmacy and falls in the middle age and elderly population. *British Journal of Clinical Pharmacology, 61,* 218–223.

Zulkowski, K., & Coon, P. J. (2004). Comparison of nutritional risk between urban and rural elderly. *Ostomy/Wound Management, 50,* 46–58.

Zunft, H. J., Hanisch, C., Mueller, S., Koebnick, C., Blaut, M., & Dore, J. (2004). Symbiotic containing *Bifidobacterium animalis* and insulin increases stool frequency in elderly healthy people. *Asia Pacific Journal of Clinical Nutrition, 13*(Suppl.), S112.

Special Topics in Age-Related Risks: Unique Nutrition Issues in the Older Adult

Karen M. Funderburg, MS, RD, LD, and Migy K. Mathews, MD

CHAPTER OUTLINE

Age-Related Risks for Malnutrition

Impaired Appetite • Physiologic Changes • Cognitive Changes • Psychosocial Changes • Medication Use

Interventions for Impaired Appetite

Oral Health Problems • Swallowing Problems • Dry Mouth

Malnutrition and Nutrient Deficits

Weight Loss • Energy and Caloric Intake • Protein-Energy Malnutrition • Vitamin D • Thiamin • Vitamin B_6 • Vitamin B_{12} • Fluid

Nutrition-Related Health Problems

Cardiovascular Disease • Peripheral Vascular and Cerebrovascular Disease • Incontinence • Visual Function • Osteoporosis

Special Considerations for the Older Woman

Reader Objectives

After studying this chapter and reflecting on the contents, you should be able to

1. List the unique physiologic changes that occur with aging that affect nutrient intake and nutritional status.
2. List key psychosocial changes associated with aging that can affect the desire or ability to consume an adequate diet.
3. Discuss the impact that age-related changes have on nutritional status and quality of life.
4. Understand the consequences of age-related malnutrition and nutrient deficiencies on overall health status and quality of life.
5. Identify nutrition interventions that can improve nutritional status and enhance quality of life.

Quality of life: Personal sense of physical and mental health and the ability to react to physical and social environments.

The older adult is faced with physiologic and social changes that are unique to aging. These changes lead to a wide array of conditions that impair appetite, the ability to eat, and the utilization of nutrients, resulting in an increased risk for malnutrition, nutrition-related health problems, and decreased **quality of life,** This chapter focuses on the unique and complex nutrition issues facing the older population. Malnutrition, key nutrient deficiencies, impaired appetite, eating ability, osteoporosis, and other nutrition-related health problems are discussed. The roles of nutrition interventions that improve nutritional status and enhance quality of life are presented.

Age-Related Risks for Malnutrition

The demographic challenge of the growing population of older adults calls for solutions to reduce chronic diseases and compress morbidity. Diet presents itself as a key part of the solution. Age-related changes in physiology and metabolism affect all organ systems, with the response of the older adult often differing from that of a younger counterpart (Kinney, 2004). In addition, this age group faces socioeconomic changes that can impact availability of food and desire to eat. Nutritional status surveys of the older population have shown a relatively low prevalence of frank nutrient deficiencies but a marked increase in risk of malnutrition and evidence of subclinical deficiencies with a direct impact on function (Blumberg, 1997). In this section we discuss key changes that increase the risk of malnutrition in the older individual; in the next section we suggest nutritional interventions and strategies to reduce the chances that an inadequate diet will be consumed.

> **CRITICAL Thinking**
>
> **How Are Appetite and Hunger Similar and Different?**
>
> *Appetite* is defined as "any of the instinctive desires necessary to keep up organic life; especially the desire to eat." *Hunger* is defined as "a craving or urgent need for food or a specific nutrient; an uneasy sensation occasioned by the lack of food."
>
> Compare loneliness to social isolation. Relate these conditions to health and nutritional status in the older adult. *Loneliness* is sadness from being alone or separation from a loved one. *Social isolation* is characterized by the lack of pleasant companionship. A state of being alone is thought of as being imposed by others and seen as negative.

Impaired Appetite

At all ages in the life cycle appetite is associated with physiologic well-being. The intake of food not only provides necessary nutrients but is an important part of special occasions such as holidays, birthdays, weddings, and anniversaries. The intake of food is a daily contributor to social, cultural, and psychological quality of life. Changes in the gastrointestinal tract, decreased taste and smell acuity, medication side effects, diet modifications, depression, and altered mental status are just a few conditions that can take away the desire to eat. **Table 13.1** provides a comprehensive list of factors than may affect appetite. A diminishing appetite can lead to smaller meals, skipping meals, and poor food choices. A decline in intake of total calories and essential nutrients leads to increased risk of illness and infections. Infections may lead to a higher metabolic rate and increased nutritional needs, affecting weight and nutritional status. Ultimately, an impaired appetite may lead to significant risks to overall health and well-being (American Dietetic Association [ADA], 2005b). Early detection and creative strategies are needed to combat appetite loss and prevent serious health complications.

Appetite Assessment

Declining food intake and **anorexia** are predictors for undernutrition in older adults in community and institutional settings (ADA, 2005b). Early detection is necessary to prevent compromised nutritional status and decreased quality of life. Nutrition screening tools designed for the older population exist and screen for a variety of nutrition risk factors. The Determine Your Nutritional Health Checklist screens for number of meals eaten per day, diet modifications, prescription drug use, and social interaction at mealtime (Nutrition Screening Initiative, 1991). The Mini Nutritional Assessment looks at declining food intake, psychological stress, neuropsychological problems, medication use, and number of full meals consumed per day (Nestle Clinical Research, 1998). The main objective of both screening tools is to determine nutritional risk. Because a decline in appetite may indicate or lead to serious health problems, tools designed specifically to assess appetite are important. When a problem is identified, early detection and treatment may prevent weight loss and improve health outcomes (Wilson et al., 2005).

TABLE 13.1	Conditions That May Affect Appetite

Decreased or altered taste
Decreased smell
Decreased thirst acuity
Hypochlorhydria
Early satiety
Dyspepsia
Decreased caloric needs
Lack of hunger
Eating impairment
Diet modifications
Dining environment
Limited food choices
Lack of control over food choices
Medication side effects
Dementia
Depression
Loneliness
Social isolation

Anorexia: Diminished appetite.

An appetite self-assessment tool was used in seven countries during the Survey in Europe on Nutrition and the Elderly, a Concerted Action (SENECA) study (Mathey, de Jong, de Groot, de Graaf, & Van Staveren, 2001). The SENECA study was a three-part study with the last phase occurring in 1999, when the protocol used the Appetite, Hunger, Sensory Perception (AHSP) questionnaire (de Jong, Mulder, de Graaf, & Van Staveren, 1999). (The questionnaire consists of 29 items that estimate energy intake, appetite and hunger sensations, and taste and smell perceptions in the elderly. Before the European study, the tool had been validated as reliable in providing accurate descriptive data on elderly self-assessment of appetite.) In the SENECA study the researchers used the AHSP in three population groups. They wanted to determine if the tool could distinguish differences in sensations of appetite, hunger, and sensory perception between healthy elderly people living independently, frail elderly living independently, and nursing home residents (Mathey et al., 2001). As a subset of the SENECA study, data from the Dutch population were analyzed. Results of the Dutch study revealed that appetite is related to the health status of the elderly. In healthy subjects appetite was a good indicator of body weight. In the frail subjects disease state rather than appetite affected body weight (Mathey et al., 2001).

The Council for Nutritional Strategies in Long-Term Care developed another appetite assessment tool. The Council was formed in 1998 and is an interdisciplinary panel composed of experts from academia and the medical community, including geriatricians, dietitians, pharmacists, and nurse practitioners. The Council's charge is to examine issues related to diagnosis, prevention, and treatment of undernutrition in older adults and to identify evidence-based recommendations for the treatment of undernutrition in long-term care (Wilson et al., 2005). They developed the Council of Nutrition Appetite Questionnaire (CNAQ), which scores eight questions to determine a person's risk for anorexia. The questionnaire addresses appetite, hunger, early satiety, taste perception and changes, gastrointestinal tolerance of food intake, mood, and frequency of meals. The total points scored on the questionnaire identify a person's risk for impaired appetite.

Researchers at St. Louis University conducted a study to determine the reliability and validity of the CNAQ. Study subjects were residents in nine long-term care facilities and community-dwelling elderly. Subjects were asked to complete the simple short CNAQ and the longer questionnaire used in the European study, the AHSP tool. Because the AHSP had been validated, the researchers used it to facilitate validation of the CNAQ. During data analysis, the reliability analysis indicated that questions 3, 5, 7, and 8 were reliability reducers. Therefore questions 1, 2, 4, and 6 were separated out to form the Simplified Nutritional Appetite Questionnaire (SNAQ). In this study the CNAQ and SNAQ were validated for use in older adults to identify persons at risk for significant weight loss. Use of the CNAQ and the SNAQ as clinical tools can promptly identify problems and facilitate early intervention. Because the researchers found the SNAQ to have comparable reliability to the CNAQ, its four-question length may be preferred in a clinical setting (Wilson et al., 2005).

Diet Modification

In December 2005 the ADA released an updated position paper that stated, "Food is an essential component of quality of life; an unacceptable or unpalatable diet can lead to poor food and fluid intake, resulting in weight loss and undernutrition and a spiral of negative health effects" (ADA, 2005a, p. 1955).

A previously prescribed dietary restriction may no longer be necessary based on the person's current health, age, and dietary intake. The need for diet modifications should be carefully evaluated. In the face of declining appetite, the decision to restrict choices may do more harm than good. Diet prescriptions should be as liberal as possible for optimum intake and quality of life. According to the ADA position paper, "Overall health goals may not warrant the use of a therapeutic diet because of the possible negative effect on quality of life. Often, a more liberalized nutrition intervention allowing a resident to participate in his or her diet-related decisions can provide for nutrient needs and allow alterations contingent on medical conditions while simultaneously increasing the desire to eat and enjoyment of food" (ADA, 2005a, p. 1956). Diet modifications along with other conditions that affect appetite may result in limited food enjoyment and compromised food intake, potentially leading to unintentional weight loss and malnutrition (ADA, 2003b).

> ● **Learning Point** Special diets that alter texture or consistency because of poor dentition or disease are often unpalatable. Restriction of certain nutrients, such as sodium or fat, can also create an unacceptable diet. The insult of a restrictive diet may lead to poor intake, depression, and malnutrition.

Physiologic Changes

Food intake decreases even in healthy older adults as physical activity and metabolic rate decline. This decrease is often called anorexia of aging (ADA, 2005a). Physiologic changes can reduce hunger and lead to early satiety. Body composition changes result in decreases in muscle mass, bone density, total body water, and metabolic rate. Older adults are generally less active than in their younger years, causing a further reduction in energy requirements. These changes reduce caloric need without reducing nutritional needs, making food selection more challenging than for the younger adult.

Changes in the gastrointestinal tract are common with aging and may include problems with **dentition**, oral health, swallowing, diarrhea, constipation, and decreased hydrochloric acid in the stomach. The decrease in acid may diminish hunger and decrease vitamin B_{12} absorption. Medications that reduce stomach acid may have the same effect. Other gastrointestinal changes may cause alteration in food selections as the patient attempts to compensate for losses in gastrointestinal function or chewing and swallowing abilities.

Dentition: The natural teeth, as considered collectively.

Presbyosmia: Loss of the sense of smell.

Sensory loss is common in the aging process (ADA, 2005a). Appetite is stimulated by the sight and aroma of food. Taste and smell are intertwined and significant contributors to recognizing flavors and the enjoyment of food and beverages. Aging, chronic health problems, and medications can alter olfactory and taste perceptions (Morley, 2001). Smell sensation that declines with aging is called **presbyosmia**. According to the National Institutes of Health, Senior Health Website (www.nihseniorhealth.gov), problems with the sense of smell occur in about 30% of Americans between the ages of 70 and 80. The problem increases to two of three persons over the age of 80 (National Institute on Deafness and Other Communication Disorders, 2006). Smell plays a key role in food enjoyment. A smell disorder can decrease the appreciation of food flavors and the desire to cook and consume a variety of foods. Food taste, temperature, texture, and aroma combine to create the perceived flavor of food. Like smell, the loss of taste sensitivity can cause a loss of appetite.

The older adult is at greater risk for food-borne illness due to the physiologic changes of aging. Risk factors for food-borne illness are decreased taste and smell, diminished immune function, **hypochlorhydria**, and altered mental status (ADA, 2003a). Food safety education targeted for seniors is available from the Food Safety Inspection Service of the U.S. Department of Agriculture and other government agencies such as the U.S. Food and Drug Administration and the National Institutes of Health.

> **Hypochlorhydria:** Presence of an abnormally small amount of hydrochloric acid in the stomach.

Additional physiologic changes come in the form of disabilities and diseases. Accumulating disease and disability may rob a patient of his or her independence. The loss of the ability to shop, cook, and even eat may decrease the desire to eat. For many people disability leads to a more sedentary life-style often accompanied by social isolation (ADA, 2005b).

Cognitive Changes

Impaired mental health can have an impact on food intake and appetite. Persons may forget to eat, may have no desire to eat, or may have difficulty swallowing due to stroke, Alzheimer's disease, or other diseases such as Parkinson disease or cancer. Impaired cognition may decrease the ability to self-feed, alter appetite, impair movement, and affect memory. The loss of family members and friends can lead to loneliness, isolation, and depression. Persons who eat most of their meals alone are at increased risk for malnutrition. Depression, anxiety, and bereavement may result in a loss of interest in food and may trigger substance abuse.

One form of **dementia** is Alzheimer's disease. The Alzheimer's Association provides tips to improve intake on their website (www.alz.org). Decreasing distraction at mealtime, providing easy-to-use dishes and utensils, serving finger foods, and limiting food choices to one or two items at a time are some helpful tips (Alzheimer's Association, 2006).

> **Dementia:** The loss, usually progressive, of cognitive and intellectual function.

The Mini Mental State Examination is widely used to assess the cognitive impairment of the older adult. Eleven items measure orientation, registration, attention and calculation, recall, and language. It is an effective screening tool for older adults in all settings (Kurlowitz & Wallace, 1999).

Psychosocial Changes

Nutritional risk is associated with economic hardship and loneliness. Objectives of the Elderly Nutrition Program include combating these two barriers to nutritional health. The Administration on Aging of the U.S. Department of Health and Human Services is responsible for providing funding for congregate and home-delivered meals through state-run elderly nutrition programs. The funds are authorized under Title III and Title IV of the Older Americans Act. Programs are provided through a local Area Agency on Aging or Tribal Senior Services. Participants can build an informal support system and develop friendships and receive a well-balanced lunch meal, educational programs, and health screenings. Persons that qualify for homebound status can have a lunch meal delivered 5 days per week. The program participants are primarily at high nutritional risk. The success of the Elderly Nutrition Program is well documented (U.S. Administration on Aging, n.d.-b).

A study was done by Gollub and Weddle (2004) to determine if the addition of breakfast as a second home-delivered meal could improve the well-being of at-risk older adults. Most study participants lived alone, were low income, and had trouble shopping or preparing food. A demonstration project, the Morning Meals on Wheels Program, delivered breakfast 5 days per week to subjects who also received home-delivered lunch meals for at least 6 months. A comparison group received only the 5 home-delivered lunch meals each week. Both groups received the same lunch items, which provided one-third of the Dietary Reference Intake. The breakfast meals also provided one-third of the Dietary Reference Intake. Several surveys were used to assess participants' perceived global quality of life, health, loneliness, food security, enjoyment of food, and depression. The study found that breakfast participants had greater energy and nutrient intakes, less food insecurity, and less depressive days than the other group. The addition of the breakfast meal reduced malnutrition risk and improved appetite, perceived health, and outlook on life (Gollub & Weddle, 2004).

Medication Use

Increased disease leads to increased medication use. Many medications have side effects such as dry mouth, altered taste sensation, sedation, diarrhea, constipation, and decreased appetite. Medications that sedate patients may decrease waking active hours and affect mealtimes and intake.

Medications that stimulate appetite and produce weight gain continue to be explored. Current medications are megestrol, dronabinol, oxandrolone, testosterone, metoclopramide, and cyproheptadine. More research is needed to verify the benefits of these drug therapies.

Interventions for Impaired Appetite

Treating impaired appetite requires an individual approach. The first step is to determine the root causes or factors contributing to a decreased desire to eat. Using tools that aid in assessing appetite and mental status can assist in discovering the most significant problems. Providing choices in food selection, decreasing meals eaten alone, providing assistance with meals, maintaining independence, and using flavor enhancers are first-line strategies. Exploring medication options to decrease negative side effects should also be a part of the action plan. **Table 13.2** provides a list of strategies to increase food and nutrient intake.

Multiple factors and conditions result in decreased food intake in the older adult. Often these go hand-in-hand with impaired appetite and are just as complex. Impaired eating ability can have significant negative effects on nutritional status and quality of life. **Table 13.3** lists the common problems associated with decreased eating ability that include poor oral health and dentition, swallowing problems, and altered physical ability due to decreased motor skills, mental status, visual impairment, and range of motion.

TABLE 13.2 Strategies to Increase Food and Nutrient Intake
Allow liberalized diet
Allow freedom in food selection
Encourage eating with others
Provide for congregate meals or home-delivered meals
Provide assistance
Provide specialized utensils
Provide finger foods
Use flavor enhancers
Add nutrients to food
Add nutrient-dense snacks
Add commercial supplements
Ensure pleasant eating environment with minimal distractions
Provide praise and encouragement
Provide appetite stimulants

Oral Health Problems

Oral health problems can lead to pain, tooth loss, and alterations in the diet and have a significant impact on quality of life (Ritchie, 2002). National Health and Nutrition Examination Survey (NHANES) data from 1999 to 2002 confirm that oral health is an increasing problem with age and is compounded by poor income status and lower education level (National Center for Chronic Disease Prevention and Health Promotion, 2005). Information on tooth decay revealed that only 9% of adults aged 20 to 39 years had decay on the roots of their teeth, compared with 32% in adults 60 years or older. Forty-one percent of low-income adults (100% federal poverty level) had untreated tooth decay, as compared with 16% in the higher income group (.200% federal poverty level). Edentulousness was also affected by income. The prevalence was 15% in adults below 100% of the federal poverty level, compared with only 5% in the higher income group (.200% federal poverty level).

Education level also was shown to have a significant impact on oral health. Forty-one percent of adults who had less than a high school education had tooth decay, compared with 14% of adults who had a higher than high school education. Fourteen percent of adults who had not completed high school were **edentulous**, compared with 9% with a high school education and 4% with a post–high school education.

Other interesting oral health data from NHANES showed that smoking increases tooth decay. The data showed that 13% of current smokers were edentulous, compared with 8% of former smokers and 5% of people who had never smoked. The greatest disparities in the prevalence of root caries were seen for current smokers. Twice as many current smokers (28%) as nonsmokers (14%) had root caries (National Center for Chronic Disease Prevention and Health Promotion, 2005).

Persons who wear dentures may avoid certain foods because they are hard to chew. Dietary quality and nutrient intake can be compromised, particularly in persons who perceive that their dentures are ill-fitting (Sahyoun & Krall, 2003). An analysis of dietary quality and selection was conducted by Sahyoun and Knall (2003) using data from 4,466 NHANES III participants. Dietary intake, dietary quality, and serum nutrient values were analyzed for denture wearers and compared with participants with natural teeth. A denture wearer is someone who wears at least a full denture on the upper or lower jaw. As part of NHANES III data collection, denture wearers completed a four-item questionnaire to assess their perception of denture use and fit. The results showed that denture wearers had significantly lower serum levels of vitamins C and E, beta-carotene, lycopene, and lutein zeaxanthin than the dentate group. Participants who believed they had ill-fitting dentures consumed fewer fruits and vegetables and had less variety in their diet than the participants who perceived they had good-fitting dentures or participants who had at least 18 natural teeth.

Data from 181 rural residents of Pennsylvania enrolled in a managed-risk Medicare program were surveyed regarding mouth pain and chewing and swallowing problems. Participants were surveyed twice with a year between surveys. Twenty-two participants reported persistent oral health problems. Results of analysis revealed that these participants had significantly greater medical problems than the participants who reported no oral health problems. They were also more likely to have lower intakes of fiber and vitamins C, A, and B_6. There was no significant difference in carbohydrate, protein, and fat between the groups (Bailey, Ledikwe, Smiciklas-Wright, Mitchell, & Jensen, 2004).

Oral hygiene after each meal can reduce oral health problems. Brushing, flossing, and using antimicrobial mouthwashes can help maintain oral health and prevent tooth decay, periodontal disease, and halitosis. Residents in long-term care facilities have multiple barriers to daily oral care. They frequently have functional decline due to chronic diseases or disabilities that make routine brushing and flossing difficult or not possible (Ship, 2002). Medication side effects such as dry mouth (**xerostomia**) can also impact oral health. Residents may have ill-fitting dentures due to weight loss or bone loss. Every resident of long-term care should have access to routine dental examinations and treatment.

Decreases in tooth extraction due to dental caries or periodontal disease are addressed in Healthy People 2010 in Focus Area 21, Oral Health (Office of Disease Prevention and Health Promotion, n.d.). Two objectives specifically target the older adult. Objective 21-4 is to reduce the proportion of adults aged 65 to 74 who have had all their natural teeth extracted. The baseline data from 1997 showed that 26% of adults in this age group had full mouth extractions. The 2010 objective calls to reduce the number to 20%. Objective 21-11 aims to increase the proportion of long-term care residents who use the oral health

TABLE 13.3	Problems That Affect Eating Ability

Tooth loss
Edentulousness
Dentures
Mouth pain
Xerostomia
Dysphagia
Visual impairment
Impaired motor skills
Arthritis
Altered mental status

Edentulous: Toothless; having lost the natural teeth.

Cultural Diversity:
Non-Hispanic whites in the NHANES study had a great prevalence of tooth decay (93%) compared with African-Americans (85%) and Mexican-Americans (84%). However, the percentage of untreated decay was the lowest in non-Hispanic whites at 18%, followed by 36% in Mexican-Americans and 41% in African-Americans. Edentulousness was highest in African-Americans, at 10%, and lowest in non-Hispanic whites, at 6% (National Center for Chronic Disease Prevention and Health Promotion, 2005).

Xerostomia: A dryness of the mouth.

care systems each year. The target is 25% versus 19% from the 1997 baseline data. Federal regulations require long-term care facilities that receive Medicare and/or Medicaid funds to ensure that each resident attains and maintains the highest practicable physical, psychosocial, and mental well-being (National Center for Chronic Disease Prevention and Health Promotion, 2005).

Ironically, Medicare does not cover dental services, regardless of cause or complexity, unless the procedure itself requires inpatient hospitalization or is necessary for another medical treatment. Coverage is not based on the value or the necessity of dental care but rather on the service required. Oral care that involves treatment, removal, or replacement of teeth or structures supporting teeth, removal of diseased teeth in an infected jaw, or preparing the mouth for dentures is not covered (Centers for Medicare and Medicaid Services, n.d.). If a person has a nondental medical condition, such as a tumor, that requires teeth to be extracted, Medicare does not cover the cost of dental appliances or dentures, even though the covered medical service resulted in the need for the teeth to be repaired or replaced. The exclusion from the Social Security Act can be found on the Center for Medicare Services website (www.cms.hhs.gov). The dental exclusion was included as part of the initial Medicare Program. Congress did not limit the exclusion to routine dental services but included a blanket exclusion of dental services.

The expense of dental services and artificial teeth can be prohibitive for many people in their older years. Like other income barriers, a lack of dental care can profoundly affect a person's ability to eat and thus their nutritional status. Prevention and treatment programs for older adults are needed and should be incorporated as an interdisciplinary team approach. Further research is needed to determine the consequences of poor oral health on overall health and nutritional status.

Swallowing Problems

Swallowing problems can result from a variety of etiologies. Dementia, stroke, neurologic disease such as Parkinson disease, muscle disease such as multiple sclerosis, head and neck surgery, and weakened muscles due to aging are among the conditions that may require precautionary measures to prevent choking and **aspiration**. Impaired swallowing may lead to decreased food intake, malnutrition, dehydration, and decreased quality of life.

Aspiration: Inhalation into the airways of fluid or foreign body; when food or liquid actually enters the lungs.

Dysphagia: Difficulty in swallowing.

The assessment and diagnosis of a swallowing problem is usually triggered by signs and symptoms in the person experiencing difficulty. These include coughing before, during, or after swallowing; frequent throat clearing; hoarse breathy voice; drooling; pocketing of food; and attempting to swallow multiple times with each bite (Deering, Russell, & Womack, 2001). Silent aspiration can occur in which no warning signs are present.

If **dysphagia** is suspected, then a swallowing evaluation by a swallowing therapist, such as a speech pathologist, should be obtained. A videofluoroscopic study or barium swallow can identify specific swallowing problems (Deering et al., 2001). The results of testing are used to determine what diet modifications are the most beneficial in protecting the person from aspiration.

Modifying food and beverage consistency and positioning during swallowing are the most common interventions. Before the introduction of the National Dysphagia Diet (NDD) in 2002, there was no standardized language regarding diet consistency and thickened liquids. NDD provides a multilevel approach to diet consistency and liquid viscosity (National Institute of Dental and Craniofacial Research, 2005). Dysphagia pureed (NDD1), dysphagia mechanically altered (NDD2), and dysphagia advanced (NDD3) identify three levels of food textures that range from pudding-like to nearly normal texture solids. The four liquid viscosities are "thin," "nectar-like," "honey-like," and "spoon thick." It is vital that foods and liquids have the appropriate texture and consistency for the swallowing ability of the impaired person or aspiration can occur. Unfortunately, texture, consistency, and viscosity modifications make food less appealing and lead to decreased intake. Persons who require thickened liquids may not consume adequate liquids. Dysphagia increases the risk for dehydration and malnutrition.

Dry Mouth

Saliva plays an important role in chewing and swallowing. It also protects teeth from decay and fights mouth infections (National Institute of Dental and Craniofacial Research, 2005). Although xerostomia is not a normal part of aging, it is often the result of certain medication side effects. Common medications used for urinary incontinence, allergies, high blood pressure, and depression can alter the function of the salivary glands. Over 400 prescription and over-the-counter medications can produce this side effect. Dry mouth can also be the result of a medical condition such as diabetes, Parkinson disease, **Sjögren syndrome,** or head and neck radiation therapy or chemotherapy (National Institute of Dental and Craniofacial Research, 2005).

Sjögren syndrome: Dryness of mucous membranes.

The first step in treating dry mouth is to identify the cause. Once the cause is known, a course of treatment can be implemented. Eating moist foods and drinking water or sugarless beverages with meals are frontline solutions. Sucking on sugarless candy can stimulate the salivary glands, and keeping a water bottle close by can help moisten the mouth between meals (National Institute of Dental and Craniofacial Research, 2005).

Malnutrition and Nutrient Deficits

In the United States it is estimated that 40% of nursing home residents and 50% of hospitalized elderly patients are malnourished (Chen, Schilling, & Lyder, 2001). In the literature there are two clinical approaches to define malnutrition in the older adult. The first definition characterizes malnutrition as any insufficient dietary intake among essential nutrients. The second approach refers to malnutrition as protein–energy undernutrition. Protein–energy undernutrition is the progressive loss of both lean body muscle mass (**sarcopenia**) and adipose tissue resulting from insufficient consumption of protein and energy, although one or the other may play the dominant role in the elderly (Chen et al., 2001).

● **Learning Point** Malnutrition in the older individual affects muscle mass even more than in younger individuals with the same degree of weight loss; also, correcting malnutrition in the older person is more difficult than in the younger person with a similar degree of weight loss. The importance of prevention should therefore be stressed (Kinney, 2004).

Sarcopenia: Progressive reduction in muscle mass with aging.

Anthropometrics: Measurements of the human body.

From the literature, three measurement systems have been used in identifying malnutrition in the older population, including dietary intake, biochemical indices, and **anthropometrics**. Most nutritional assessment instruments also use all three aspects of measurement plus some clinical assessment such as anorexia or comorbid conditions. The Mini Nutritional Assessment is an example of this mixing of measurement systems. It should be noted that to date, no single measurement has emerged as optimal in defining malnutrition in the older person (Chen et al., 2001).

Weight Loss

The older adult must be evaluated periodically for unintended weight loss. Weight and height should be obtained at each visit using the same scale and without shoes. Body mass index is a ratio of body weight in kilograms divided by the height in square meters. The body mass index can guide the health care provider in determining the overall weight status of the patient. A body mass index of less than 18.5 kg/m^2 is considered underweight, 18.5 to 24.9 kg/m^2 is normal, 25 to 29.9 kg/m^2 is overweight, and higher than 30.0 kg/m^2 is considered obese (Amin, Kuhle, & Fitzpatrick, 2003).

Weight loss exceeding 5% in 1 month or 10% in 6 months deserves a complete evaluation, including a detailed physical examination, review of age-indicated preventive measures, pertinent screening tools, psychosocial assessment, review of medications, medical history, and laboratory and radiologic testing when indicated. Risk factors for poor nutritional status and subsequent weight loss are listed in **Table 13.4**.

TABLE 13.4 Risk Factors for Weight Loss
Alcohol or substance abuse
Cognitive dysfunction
Depression
Functional limitations
Inadequate financial resources
Limited education
Limited mobility
Transportation issues
Chronic medical illness
Poor dentition
Restricted diet
Poor eating habits
Social isolation

Energy and Caloric Intake

Numerous studies have shown energy intake declines with age, making a nutritionally adequate diet more difficult to achieve. A reduction in **basal metabolic rate** is partly responsible for this decline in energy and caloric intake, but a reduction in lean body mass and decreased physical activity appear to be the major causes (Wahlqvist & Savige, 2000).

Protein-Energy Malnutrition

Protein plays an important role in the maintenance of the elderly person's health. Illness or inadequate intake may result in protein–energy malnutrition, a condition more common among elderly patients, especially those in institutionalized care (Wahlqvist & Savige, 2000). Chronic deficiency of protein in the elderly person's diet may result in poor wound healing, **decubitus ulcer** development, depressed immune function, osteoporosis, and loss of muscle strength (Chrnoff, 1996). Protein foods are rich in other essential nutrients as well; their inclusion in the elderly individual's diet should be encouraged.

Vitamin D

Vitamin D deficiency has special implications for the elderly, especially those who are institutionalized or homebound. Although dietary consumption of vitamin D through fortified dairy products, sardines, and egg yolks can provide part of the daily allowance, natural sunlight is another important source. Aging skin, deteriorating renal function, and physical inactivity (with the possible consequence of less sunlight exposure) are factors that contribute to a greater likelihood of vitamin D deficiency in older adults, thus making them more susceptible to osteoporosis (Wahlqvist & Savige, 2000). The Dietary Reference Intake for vitamin D is 15 mg, three times higher than that of the younger adult (National Academy Press, n.d.).

Thiamin

Thiamin intakes vary considerably among different elderly populations. Thiamin deficiency is usually associated with poor intakes rather than an increased need, although some studies have shown that the biochemical status of older adults can indicate the presence of thiamin deficiency despite seemingly adequate intakes (Wahlqvist & Savige, 2000). Thiamin deficiency is often responsible for symptoms of peripheral neuropathy.

Vitamin B_6

A number of studies have suggested that age-related changes occur in both the absorption and metabolism of this vitamin, and as a consequence, aged adults may have a higher requirement. Vitamin B_6 is commonly found in meat and leafy greens, and deficiency of this vitamin often leads to impaired immune function and impaired cognitive function.

Vitamin B_{12}

Vitamin B_{12} deficiency is more common among older adults because of the prevalence of pernicious anemia and atrophic gastritis, which appear to increase with age. Also, the prevalence of *Helicobacter pylori* increases with age and has been shown to be associated with vitamin B_{12} malabsorption, possibly because it contributes to gastric atrophy. Deficiency of vitamin B_{12} increases the risk of irreversible neurologic damage and can likely contribute to homocysteine concentrations that are associated with vascular disease (Wahlqvist & Savige, 2000).

Fluid

Aging adults are more susceptible to the risk of dehydration due to alterations in thirst responses, decreasing renal function, and certain medical conditions. Moreover, a reduction in total body water with age also increases the susceptibility of elderly people to dehydration (Wahlqvist & Savige, 2000).

Nutrition-Related Health Problems

Although nutrition-related health problems can occur at any age, the older adult is at risk for accumulation of health problems due to years of life. In this section, vascular conditions, incontinence, visual function, and osteoporosis are discussed.

Cardiovascular Disease

Cardiovascular disease is the most common cause of death and disability in the developed world. Dietary habits may contribute to or provide protection against the risk factors associated with cardiovascular disease (Wahlqvist & Savige, 2000). Diet influences the pathogenesis of coronary artery disease in a variety of ways. The principal mechanism by which fat and cholesterol ingestion translate into increased cardiovascular risk is the induced elevation of serum lipoproteins, especially low-density lipoprotein. The initial development of fatty streaks in coronary arteries is mediated by serum lipid levels and free radical oxidation, both of which are modified by nutrients (Katz, 2000).

An inverse relationship was found between fish consumption and coronary heart disease mortality. Also, excess alcohol consumption is associated with hypertension, a risk factor for cardiovascular disease, yet moderate consumption may be protective against cardiovascular disease through its favorable effect on high-density lipoprotein cholesterol. Elevated homocysteine levels have been identified as an independent risk factor for cardiovascular disease, and it was found that elderly adults with better folate status had lower homocysteine levels. Foods that have high amounts of folate include breakfast cereal, fruit, orange juice, and leafy green vegetables.

Dietary counseling is an essential component in the primary prevention of heart disease. It is also an essential component in the clinical management of all patients with established coronary heart disease and in those with risk factors (Katz, 2000).

Peripheral Vascular and Cerebrovascular Disease

The dietary recommendations for the prevention and modification of cardiovascular risk generally are pertinent for peripheral vascular disease and cerebrovascular disease. Peripheral vascular disease is associated with elevated plasma homocysteine levels and, therefore, may be amenable to treatment with B vitamin and folate supplementation in certain patients. Also, elevated postprandial insulin levels appear to be an independent risk factor, suggesting that dietary intervention to improve glycemic control may play a role in the prevention and control of peripheral vascular disease (Katz, 2000).

The predominant risk factor for stoke is hypertension, which can be prevented and modified by dietary interventions. Dietary sodium restriction and generous intake of potassium, magnesium, and calcium may lower blood pressure (Katz, 2000).

Incontinence

Urinary and fecal **incontinence** are common and often debilitating conditions in older people. Urinary incontinence is reported to afflict approximately half the elderly living in institutions and 15% to 30% of community-based elderly (Wahlqvist & Savige, 2000). Dietary interventions that encourage an adequate intake of fluid and a variety of plant foods that are a good source of dietary fiber may assist in alleviating some of the problems that can cause incontinence (Wahlqvist & Savige, 2000).

Incontinence: Inability to control the discharge of urine or feces.

Cataract: Complete or partial opacity of the ocular lens.

Macular degeneration: An eye disease that affects the macula, a part of the retina.

Visual Function

Cataracts and age-related **macular degeneration** are common causes of visual impairment in older adults. Nutrients may play a very important role in vision; for example, the antioxidants alpha-tocopherol, beta-carotene, and ascorbic acid may help to prevent cataract formation and macular degeneration (Wahlqvist & Savige, 2000). Therefore, a diet rich in fruits and green leafy vegetables should be recommended as primary prevention of age-related eye disease. In those over the age of 50 or with less than judicious diets, supplementation with vitamin C 500 mg, vitamin E 400 to 800 IU, and zinc may be helpful in the prevention of age-related eye disease (Katz, 2000).

Osteoporosis

Osteoporosis: Reduction in the quantity of bone.

According to the 2004 Surgeon General's report on bone health and osteoporosis, the cost of caring for bone fractures from osteoporosis is $18 billion each year (U.S. Department of Health and Human Services, 2004). According to the National Institute of Arthritis and Musculoskeletal and Skin Diseases (2006), **osteoporosis** affects more than 10 million adults in the United States, and millions more are at risk for the disease. Risk factors for osteoporosis are numerous and include gender, ethnicity, and lifestyle. **Table 13.5** provides a comprehensive list.

> **● Learning Point** Sodium, caffeine, and alcohol have been associated with bone loss. Specific nutrients that may play an important role in maintaining bone health include protein, vitamin D, calcium, vitamin K, and boron (Wahlqvist & Savige, 2000).

TABLE 13.5 Risk Factors for Osteoporosis

Age
Ethnicity
  Asian-American
  White
Female gender
Early menopause
Family history
Low body weight
Medications
Smoking
Sedentary life-style
Heavy alcohol consumption
Poor calcium intake for years
Poor vitamin D intake

Dietary management is fundamental to the primary and secondary prevention of osteoporosis. The origins of osteoporosis are in childhood and adolescence, during which time adequate physical activity and dietary calcium are particularly important. Peak bone density is reached by around the end of the third decade (Katz, 2000). Many dietary factors have implications for bone health.

Dietary recommendations should focus on diversity in the diet, consumption of low-fat dairy products, calcium- and vitamin D–fortified foods, avoiding or quitting smoking, limiting alcohol intake, and engaging in consistent weight-bearing physical activity, at least some of which should be outdoors in sunlight. In older adults at risk, vitamin D supplementation with 400 to 600 IU and calcium intake of about 1,500 mg/day is advisable (Katz, 2000).

Special Considerations for the Older Woman

Women face unique challenges with aging, partially due to their long life expectancy. According to the Centers for Disease Control and Prevention, a female born in 2003 has a life expectancy of 80.1 years, compared with 74.8 years for a male born in the same year. White women have a longer life expectancy than African-American women, reported at 80.5 years compared with 76.1 years, respectively (National Center for Health Statistics, n.d.). Disease and disability increase with advanced aging. Women live longer but have more chronic

health conditions than men. These conditions include osteoporosis, depression, Sjögren syndrome, rheumatoid arthritis, and other autoimmune diseases (U.S. Department of Health and Human Services, n.d.-a). Older women are also more likely than older men to live in poverty, live in long-term care, or live alone (ADA, 2005b).

One of the conditions unique to women is menopause. Like adolescence, it is a natural process in a woman's life span. A woman is in menopause when she has not had a menstrual cycle for 12 consecutive months. Although normally this occurs in the late forties or early fifties, a younger woman who has had her ovaries surgically removed will experience the physiologic condition.

For many women menopause brings unpleasant side effects such as hot flashes, mood swings, sleep disturbances, night sweats, depression, and weight gain. Menopause can also bring serious health concerns because it increases the risk for bone loss and heart disease. Eighty percent of adults with osteoporosis are women (National Institute of Arthritis and Musculoskeletal and Skin Diseases, 2006). Historically, hormone replacement therapy has been used to prevent bone loss and to treat the symptoms of menopause. This practice has known benefits for bone health but has been linked to breast, uterine, and ovarian cancer and heart disease. Prescribing hormone replacement therapy is no longer routine, and recommendations are based on the woman's family history and degree of symptoms. Soy isoflavones, exercise, vitamin supplements, and stress reduction techniques are some alternatives for women who choose to forgo hormone replacement therapy due to the risks.

Summary

Aging brings unique challenges that encompass physical, mental, social, and financial changes. Special attention to food selection is important to meet the demands of the aging process and accompanying health issues. The ultimate goal of maintaining the highest quality of life possible through the life span is as important in the older adult as with any other age. Independence, dignity, well-being, and social interaction are desired by all human beings. Regular nutrition screening with early interventions, when problems are identified, can enhance the quality of life of the older adult.

Issue to Debate

Hormone Replacement Therapy: Benefits and Risks

Perimenopause and the transition to menopause are marked by a time in a woman's life when progesterone and estrogen levels are changing in response to an aging body. These changes are companied by symptoms ranging from mild to severe that can disrupt a woman's daily life. Unfortunately, other "silent" but significant changes are occurring. Bone mineral density can be lost during this time, placing the woman at risk for fractures, tooth loss from declining jawbone, pain, and disability.

The National Heart, Lung, and Blood Institute and the National Cancer Institute, parts of the National Institutes of Health, sponsored the Women's Health Initiative Hormone Program that examined the effects of hormone replacement therapy on women's health. Researchers conducted two studies on the use of hormone therapy. One study involved estrogen alone and the other tested estrogen plus progestin. The estrogen plus progestin study was stopped in 2002 when researchers determined that the risks of heart disease, stroke, blood clots, and breast cancer outweighed the benefits. The estrogen alone study was stopped in 2004 due to increased risk of stroke and blood clots. Researchers found no significant effect on the risk of breast or colorectal cancer in the estrogen-only group (National Institute on Aging, 2005).

Hormone replacement therapy can assist in preserving bone loss, reduce the risk of colorectal cancer, and assist in managing unpleasant symptoms of menopause.

1. Considering the known risks and benefits of hormone replacement therapy, how should a woman choose which course to take?

Case Studies

(Answers to all case studies are in the Instructor's Manual available at jbpub.com.)

Case Study

A 79-year-old woman was evaluated in an outpatient clinic. She lives with her 81-year-old husband, who is her primary caregiver. He reports that approximately 2 years ago his wife began to lose interest in the

Continues

things she enjoyed, like shopping, cooking, and sewing. Gradually, she become less interested in food and has lost 18 pounds in the past year. He has tried commercial nutritional supplements but has not been successful in getting her to consume them. He stated he is not much of a cook but has been trying his best. He is frustrated and concerned about his wife's weight loss and lack of appetite. He believes he is constantly trying to get her to eat. He does not have any family support because he and his wife never had children. Her medical evaluation revealed cognitive impairment using the Mini Mental State Examination. She does not appear to have any chewing or swallowing problems but has not seen a dentist in over 3 years. She takes one prescription medication for her arthritis.

1. What questions would you like to ask her husband?
2. What strategies might be appropriate for her treatment plan?
3. Do you have concerns about her husband and his ability to care for her?

Case Study

Mrs. Walker is a 74-year-old non-Hispanic white woman. She is 62 inches tall and weighs 112 pounds. She has lost 2 inches in height in the past 20 years. She smokes half a pack of cigarettes a day and has been a smoker for 54 years. About 18 months ago she began to experience mouth pain. A dental examination revealed several loose teeth due to severe gum disease. She has had significant dental work in the past year, which has resulted in five extracts. A partial plate with false teeth was attempted but due to continued mouth pain was not worn regularly. Mrs. Walker has altered her diet due to her poor dentition. She no longer eats fresh fruits, salad, steak, nuts, or other hard-to-chew foods. She rarely eats out anymore. It takes her twice as long to eat as a few years ago. She plans to have a full upper jaw extraction and be fitted for a full denture when she has the money. Since her dental problems began, she has lost 11 pounds. She is depressed and frustrated by the changes she has had to make in her diet. Eating has become a chore and has lost the pleasure it once had.

1. What risk factors does Mrs. Walker have for developing malnutrition?
2. What concerns you the most about this case?
3. What suggestions do you have for Mrs. Walker?

Websites

Administration on Aging www.aoa.gov
Alzheimer's Association www.alz.org
Centers for Disease Control and Prevention www.cdc.gov
Centers for Medicare and Medicaid Services www.cms.hhs.gov
Food Safety Information for Seniors www.foodsafety.gov
National Institute on Deafness and Other Communication Disorders www.nidcd.nih.gov
Nestle Nutrition; Mini Nutritional Assessment http://www.mna-elderly.com
National Osteoporosis Foundation www.nof.org
NIH Senior Health www.nihseniorhealth.gov
Women's Health Information www.womenshealth.gov

References

Alzheimer's Association. (2006). Fact sheet: Eating. Retrieved May 12, 2009, from http://www.alz.org

American Dietetic Association (ADA). (2002). *The National Dysphagia Diet Task Force. The National Dysphagia Diet: Standardization for Optimal Care.* Chicago: American Dietetic Association.

American Dietetic Association (ADA). (2003a). Position of the American Dietetic Association: Food and water safety. *Journal of the American Dietetic Association, 103,* 1203–1217.

American Dietetic Association (ADA). (2003b). Position of the American Dietetic Association: Oral health and nutrition. *Journal of the American Dietetic Association, 103,* 615–623.

American Dietetic Association (ADA). (2005a). Position of the American Dietetic Association: Liberalization of the diet prescription improves quality of life for older adults in long-term care. *Journal of the American Dietetic Association, 105,* 1955–1965.

American Dietetic Association (ADA). (2005b). Position of the American Dietetic Association: Nutrition across the spectrum of aging. *Journal of the American Dietetic Association,* *105,* 616–633.

Amin, S. H., Kuhle, C. L., & Fitzpatrick, L. A. (2003). Comprehensive evaluation of the older woman. *Mayo Clinic Proceedings, 78,* 1157–1185.

Bailey, R. L., Ledikwe, J. H., Smiciklas-Wright, H., Mitchell, D. C., & Jensen, G. L. (2004). Persistent oral health problems associated with comorbidity and impaired diet quality in older adults. *Journal of the American Dietetic Association, 104,* 1273–1276.

Blumberg, J. B. (1997). Nutritional needs of seniors. *Journal of the American College of Nutrition, 16,* 517–523.

Centers for Medicare and Medicaid Services. (n.d.). *Medicare Dental Coverage.* Retrieved March 18, 2009, from http://www.cms.hhs.gov/MedicareDentalCoverage

Chen, C. C., Schilling, L. S., & Lyder, C. H. (2001). A concept analysis of malnutrition in the elderly. *Journal of Advanced Nursing, 36,* 131–142.

Chernoff, R. (1996). Nutrition. In D. Jahnigen & R. Schrier (Eds.), *Geriatric Medicine* (2nd ed.). Cambridge, MA: Blackwell Science.

Council for Nutritional Strategies in Long-Term Care. (n.d.). *Council on Nutrition Appetite Questionnaire.* Retrieved March 18, 2009, from http://medschool.slu.edu/agingsuccessfully/pdfsurveys/appetitequestionnaire.pdf

Deering, C., Russell, C., & Womack, P. (2001). *Perspectives on Dysphagia: A Continuing Education Self-Study Guide for Dietetics Professionals.* Chicago: American Dietetic Association.

de Jong, N., Mulder, I., de Graaf, C., & Van Staveren, W. A. (1999). Impaired sensory functioning in elders: The relationship with its potential determinants and nutritional intake. *Journals of Gerontology. Series A, Biological Sciences and Medical Sciences, 54,* B324–B331.

Gollub, E. A., & Weddle, D. O. (2004). Improvement in nutritional intake and quality of life among frail homebound older adults receiving home-delivered breakfast and lunch. *Journal of the American Dietetic Association, 104,* 1227–1235.

Katz, D. L. (2000). *Nutrition in Clinical Practice.* Philadelphia: Lippincott Williams and Wilkins.

Kinney, J. M. (2004). Nutritional frailty, sarcopenia and falls in the elderly. *Current Opinion in Clinical Nutrition and Metabolic Care, 7,* 15–20.

Kurlowitz, L., & Wallace, M. (1999). *The Mini Mental State Examination (MMSE). Best Practices in Nursing Care to Older Adults.* New York: Hartford Institute for Geriatric Nursing.

Mathey, N., de Jong, C. P. G. M., de Groot, C., de Graaf, W. A., & Van Steveren (2001). Assessing appetite in Dutch elderly with the Appetite, Hunger, Sensory Perception (AHSP) questionnaire. *Journal of Nutrition, Health, and Aging, 5,* 22–28.

Morley, J. E. (2001). Decreased food intake with aging. *Journals of Gerontology. Series A, Biological Sciences and Medical Sciences, 56,* 81–88.

National Academy Press. (n.d.). National Academy of Science. Dietary Reference Intake tables. Retrieved May 12, 2009, from www.nap.edu

National Center for Chronic Disease Prevention and Health Promotion. (2005). *Fact sheet: Key findings from NHANES 1999–2002.* Retrieved March 18, 2009, from http:// www.cdc.gov/OralHealth/publications/factsheets/nhanes_findings.htm

National Center for Health Statistics. (n.d.). Life expectancy at birth, at 65 years of age, and at 75 years of age according to race and sex, United States selected years, 1900–2003. Retrieved June 30, 2009, from http://www.cdc.gov/nchs/data/hus/hus05.pdf#027

National Eye Institute. (2005). Age-related macular degeneration. Retrieved on May 14, 2009, from http://nihseniorhealth.gov/agerelatedmaculardegeneration/toc.html

National Institute of Arthritis and Musculoskeletal and Skin Diseases. (2006). Osteoporosis. Retrieved on May 12, 2009, from www.nihseniorhealth.org

National Institute of Dental and Craniofacial Research. (2005). Dry mouth. Retrieved on May 14, 2009, from http://www.nihseniorhealth.org/drymouth/toc.html

National Institute on Aging. (2005). Hormones after menopause. Retrieved on May 14, 2009, from http://www.nia.nih.gov/healthinformation/publications/hormones.htm

(National Institute on Deafness and Other Communication Disorders, 2006) .

Nestle Clinical Research. (1998). Mini Nutritional Assessment. Retrieved on May 14, 2009, from http://mna-elderly.com

Nutrition Screening Initiative. (1991). *Determine Your Nutritional Health Checklist.* Retrieved on February 25, 2009, from http://www.aafp.org/x17367.xml

Office of Disease Prevention and Health Promotion, U.S. Department of Health and Human Services. (n.d.). *Healthy People 2010.* Retrieved on March 18, 2009, from www. healthy people.gov

Ritchie, C. S. (2002). Oral health, taste, and olfaction. *Clinics in Geriatric Medicine, 18,* 709–717.

Sahyoun, N. R., & Krall, E. (2003). Low dietary quality among older adults with self-perceived ill-fitting dentures. *Journal of the American Dietetic Association, 103,* 1494–1499.

Ship, J. A. (2002). Improving oral health in older people. *Journal of the American Geriatrics Society, 50,* 1454–1455.

U.S. Administration on Aging. (n.d.-a). Addressing diversity. Retrieved May 14, 2009, from http://www.aoa.gov/prof/adddiv/adddiv.asp

U.S. Administration on Aging. (n.d.-b). *The Elderly Nutrition Program.* Retrieved June 30, 2009, from http://www.aoa.gov/AoA_Root/press_room/elderly_nutrition_program.pdf

U.S. Department of Health and Human Services. (n.d.-a). Sex differences in autoimmune disease. Retrieved on May 14, 2009, from http://www.womenshealth.gov

U.S. Department of Health and Human Services. (n.d.-b). Sex differences in musculoskeletal health. Retrieved on May 14, 2009, from http://www.womenshealth.gov

U.S. Department of Health and Human Services. (2004). The 2004 Surgeon General's report on bone health and osteoporosis: What it means to you. Retrieved on May 14, 2009, from http://www.surgeongeneral.gov

Wahlqvist, M. L., & Savige, G. S. (2000). Intervention aimed at dietary and lifestyle changes to promote healthy aging. *European Journal of Clinical Nutrition, 54,* S148–S156.

Wilson, M. M., Thomas, D. R., Rubenstein, L. Z., Chibnall, J. T., Anderson, S., Baxi, A., et al. (2005). Appetite assessment, simple appetite questionnaire predicts weight loss in community-dwelling adults and nursing home residents. *American Journal of Clinical Nutrition, 82,* 1074–1081.

Special Topics Related to the Registered Dietitian and Older Adults: Roles and Responsibilities of the Registered Dietitian in Long-Term Care

*Victoria Hammer Castellanos, PhD, RD, and
Angela Sader, RD, LD, MBA*

CHAPTER OUTLINE

Reader Objectives

After studying this chapter and reflecting on the contents, you should be able to

1. Discuss the fundamental differences between nutrition care delivery in the long-term care setting compared with other care settings, including prioritization of resident quality of life and a regulatory environment that drives patient care.

2. Describe the clinical and management responsibilities that regularly fall to the dietitian within the long-term care setting.

3. Identify the management opportunities for long-term care dietitians within the areas of clinical care, food service management, survey management, and **risk management**.

Risk management:
Identification of areas where harm may occur to an individual, such as in the case of a fall with injury. Taking precautions to limit the number of times this situation may occur is the responsibility of facility management.

Unique Characteristics of Long-Term Care

Approximately 1.5 million older adults currently reside in long-term care (LTC) facilities. A number of factors set apart the delivery of nutrition care in nursing homes, which have their own unique culture and challenges compared with other care settings (Castellanos, 2004). The nursing home environment has the following characteristics:

- The facility is considered to be the resident's home. Although some residents stay in the facility for only a few weeks or months, many residents live out the remainder of their lives in this setting.
- A large segment of the population is both very old and quite frail. However, a growing number of residents are somewhat younger adults who are suffering from an acute illness or injury and who expect to return home after a period of recovery or rehabilitation.
- Usually, both long-term and short-term stay residents suffer from a host of chronic and acute disease conditions.
- The resident's physical ability to eat enough food is often greatly reduced because of aging and/or disease processes.
- Nutrition care is both driven and hindered by the regulatory environment. The characteristics of skilled nursing facilities and the residents themselves make nutritional well-being difficult to achieve in this setting but present a rare opportunity for the nutrition professional to significantly impact both the health outcomes and quality of life of a significant number of people.

Types of LTC Centers

LTC is a designation given to any facility-based operation that has accepted the responsibility of caring for patients deemed to require some form of 24-hour-a-day supervision to meet their care-related needs. The types of LTC centers are described in **Table 14.1**. The goals of all LTC facilities are similar; each is expected to help the patients under their care reach the highest level of living and activity possible through the administration of nonskilled and/or skilled services.

Whether or not a person is qualified to reside in an LTC facility primarily depends on a certified physician recommending that individual for LTC services. There are state and **federal regulations** that provide guidance to the physicians regarding placement decisions. The acuity level of LTC residents varies from residents who have a relatively small need for services to residents who require extensive observation, care, and oversight to ensure quality care.

Significant cost is associated with LTC. There are programs designed to reduce the personal financial burden, including Medicare (federally funded), Medicaid (state indigent care

Federal regulations:
Documents published by the Centers for Medicare and Medicaid Services for use in the survey process for long-term care facilities.

TABLE 14.1	Types of LTC Centers

Facility Type	Function
Skilled nursing facilities (SNFs, pronounced "sniffs")	Facilities approved to accept Medicaid and Medicare for payment when the resident qualifies. The resident population of most SNFs represents a variety of payer sources—i.e., Medicaid, Medicare, insurance, hospice, and self-pay
Hospital-based facilities	LTC facilities under the umbrella of a hospital organization. These are usually SNFs but may be private placement or government sponsored. Because the billing mechanism is quite different in an acute care hospital from that of an LTC facility, the RD employed in this environment will be required to keep careful track of hours spent in each unit.
Private placement facilities, also called private pay facilities	Facilities in which the resident assumes all responsibility for payment of stay, either through insurance or self-pay.
Government-sponsored facilities	Facilities that are Medicaid certified but not Medicare certified.

funds), Medicare Part B (federally funded), Veterans Administration (federally funded), insurance, and hospice (federally funded). All these payer sources are designed to help individuals requiring LTC services to receive those benefits even if personal funds are not available.

LTC facilities range in size from a few to over 200 residents. Depending on their business classification, facilities may be designated as "for profit," "not for profit," "privately owned," or "publicly traded." Expectations for resident care are similar across business classifications, but internal rules and policies may vary depending on acuity of residents, number of residents involved, and reimbursement from external sources.

The exact cost of care in an LTC facility varies depending on many factors. Pricing is affected by the number of associates the individual requires to assist them with care (i.e., does it require one or two persons to move them?), room size, age of facility, services offered, the level of care, acuity of the resident, and many other factors. It is common practice for a daily rate sheet to be provided to a potential resident that lists the services covered for a flat daily fee. This varies from facility to facility. Additional services must be reimbursed by the resident's personal funds. For example, the daily rate may not cover the cost of services provided by the beautician, cable television, and so on. Although residents receive similar care regardless of payer source, out of consideration for the resident, it is important that registered dietitians (RDs) are aware of services that may cause a financial burden to the resident. For example, if a resident is not covered under Medicare or if he or she does not have private insurance, the resident is responsible for the cost of goods and services such as adaptive eating devices and laboratory blood work. Where possible, the RD should strive to achieve positive results with care approaches that are not a financial burden to the resident or family (e.g., recommend that additional blood work be completed only when the results of the laboratory analysis are clearly necessary to determine whether or not the current plan of care should be modified).

Nursing Home Regulation Drives Nutrition Care

The regulatory environment has a tremendous impact on nutrition care in the LTC setting. Nursing homes are heavily regulated at both the federal and state levels. This is in contrast to community-based care and other types of LTC that are regulated only by the states; regulations for community-based care are generally sparse. The **Centers for Medicare and Medicaid Services** enforces many specific regulations related to food and nutrition care delivery in nursing homes (American Health Care Association, 2005). The Centers for Medicare and Medicaid Services normally contracts with state health departments to complete the surveys according to federal regulations (i.e., "state survey"). Each state has additional regulations that must also be followed and are enforced by the state surveyors.

One cannot underemphasize the extent to which the state and federal regulations drive nutrition care delivery in the nursing home setting. Success as an LTC practitioner requires one to become intimately familiar with these regulations. To help drive this point home, we have referred to some of the relevant federal nursing home regulations throughout this chapter. A summary of the **Federal Nursing Home Regulation for Nutrition Services** can be found at the American Health Care Association website at www.ahcancal.org.

> **Centers for Medicare and Medicaid Services:** The federal agency responsible for nursing home regulations and their enforcement. The Centers for Medicare and Medicaid Services is part of the U.S. Department of Health and Human Services.
>
> **Federal Nursing Home Regulation for Nutrition Services:** Documents published by the Centers for Medicare and Medicaid Services for use in the survey process for long-term care facilities that focus on the nutritional oversight of and delivery to the residents in the facility.

Structure of the Nutritional Services Department

The nutritional services department is composed of the RD, the dietary service manager (DSM), the dietetic technician, and all staff involved in food production and service. It is the standard division of responsibilities in most nursing homes that the nutritional services department is responsible for getting the appropriate food and drinks to the resident's dining area, whereas it is the responsibility of the nursing staff to feed the resident. Licensed nurses are responsible for supervising the provision of food and fluid to residents by certified nursing assistants. During their training, certified nursing assistants are taught techniques to assist and/or feed residents with various kinds of health problems, including dysphagia (swallowing disorders). Federal regulation also allows for paid feeding assistants to help feed residents at low risk for choking, although not all states allow paid feeding assistants.

The basis for nutritional services staffing in the LTC facility begins with regulations F361 and 362, which state that the facility must have adequate personnel to provide dietary services and that a qualified dietitian is utilized in planning, managing, and implementing dietary service activities. The RD staff is then expanded to meet the requirements of the residing state and the needs of the facility residents.

State staffing requirements are highly variable. A particular state may go so far as to define the components of a nutritional assessment and identify the professionals appropriate to complete the task as a whole or parts of the task. A state may also specify the minimum number of hours an RD must be present in a facility to provide services or dictate the number of RD hours based on facility census or the number of nursing stations. Some states have requirements related to the dietary manager that affect both DSM and RD staffing. For example, if a state requires that the DSM complete an approved course by the Dietary Managers Association to become a "certified dietary manager," completion of the course requires oversight and training of the DSM by the RD. The assignment of responsibilities within the nutritional services department varies depending on facility characteristics and state regulations.

> **● Learning Point** The RD is responsible for reviewing the menu (for nutritional adequacy, appropriate therapeutic combinations, serving sizes, etc.), providing staff education, and providing residents with medical nutrition therapy (MNT) through assessment and appropriate intervention.

Facilities frequently use a DSM to manage department staffing, meal production, procurement, food service sanitation, and the budget. As per regulation the DSM must be under the oversight of an RD. In a smaller facility, and if state regulation allows, it is not uncommon for the DSM to be the staff member responsible for the collection of subjective and objective resident information to be used by the RD in his or her resident assessment. In this scenario, it is the responsibility of the RD to review the DSM's completion of the aforementioned activities. If a facility is larger or if a state requires that a licensed/registered health care practitioner complete documentation in the medical record, the facility may hire a dietetic technician to assist with clinical documentation. Various other staffing scenarios are also possible.

After meeting the regulatory requirements, RD staffing in a facility is largely determined by the facility census, the level of care provided, and the average number of admissions per week. Individual facilities usually have a predetermined number of beds set aside for Medicare (i.e., short-term) versus long-term residents. Residents who are admitted under Medicare after discharge from an acute care facility are usually more medically complex than long-term-stay residents. These residents are more likely to be on dialysis, have pressure ulcers, require enteral therapy, or require other types of MNT. Further, Medicare beds turn over more frequently, and with each new admission it is necessary for the RD to spend a significant amount of time on the initial nutritional assessment and development of comprehensive **care plans.**

For example, it is a common mistake to assume that nutritional services staffing should be the same for equivalently sized facilities (e.g., 120 beds) in the same state. The facility with 25 Medicare beds (resulting in an average of 7 new admissions per week) and 10 residents receiving enteral feeding requires more RD time for admission assessments, MNT documentation, and enteral therapy follow-up than a facility with only 4 Medicare beds and 2 residents receiving enteral feeding.

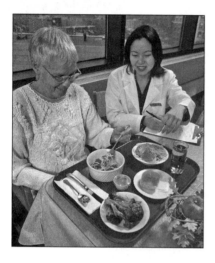

Roles of the Dietitian Within the Nutritional Services Department

Whether the services of an RD are provided by a consultant dietitian or regular employee of the company, the role of the RD in the LTC setting is central to the health and well-being of the residents and goes far beyond the responsibility of patient assessment. The RD's time in the facility is spent not only on MNT but in review of the nutritional services department and all the processes related to providing nutrition care to the residents. In the LTC setting the RD must be prepared to use skills in staff and patient education, quality management, menu planning, food production, food safety, product selection and purchasing, emergency planning, and budget management, including labor utilization.

One of the most critical functions of the dietitian in the nursing home setting is to make sure that the facility is meeting both federal and state regulations relevant to nutrition services. The nutrition professional in the nursing home setting will use a wide variety of skills and training to assist a facility in maintaining compliance with regulations and provide appropriate care to residents.

Clinical Care Delivery in the LTC Setting

Regulations require nursing facilities to meet the nutritional needs of residents (F325–327 and F360–367) while maintaining their dignity and quality of life (F240 and F241). This is also the ethical responsibility of providers. After all, the LTC facility is "home" for this population of older adults.

Residence in a nursing home is unlike a brief admission to a hospital, where limited choice and reduced quality of life are justified by short-term clinical goals. But, like a hospital, decisions regarding the menu and the exact nature of meal and snack service are made on a facility-wide basis. The implications for LTC residents are that each food, dining environment, and staffing decision made at the facility level will serve to either limit or expand the nutrition and eating pleasure available to that individual for a significant portion of his or her life.

Although such decisions bring with them significant responsibility, they also afford tremendous opportunity for the care provider. That is to say that the nursing home has both the infrastructure and consistency of client contact that make it possible to move beyond a reactive medical model and to adopt a proactive, prevention-focused, home-like approach to nutrition care. For example, weight loss and pressure ulcer prevention committees are often created in facilities. These committees meet frequently to review individual residents who have risk factors for weight loss or pressure ulcers and to initiate interventions designed to prevent weight loss or wounds from developing.

The nutritional needs of nursing home residents are likely to be affected by both illness and advanced age. Most nursing home residents are medically frail, with at least five chronic health conditions, and suffer intermittent bouts of acute illnesses, such as infection and diarrhea. These disease states tend to increase nutrient needs. Further, some aspects of institutional living may affect nutritional needs; for example, little or no exposure to sunlight makes residents highly dependent on dietary and supplemental sources of vitamin D (Institute of Medicine, 1997).

Most nutrition-related problems in nursing homes are a consequence of undernutrition. These may include unintended weight loss, protein–energy malnutrition, pressure ulcers, and dehydration (American Dietetic Association [ADA], 2005). A host of additional nutrient deficiencies are likely to occur as an accompaniment to inadequate food intake, including vitamin and mineral deficiencies. For most nursing home residents, the risk of morbidity and mortality related to undernutrition exceeds the potential for adverse outcomes of chronic disease (ADA, 2005). Having said this, there are few data on which to base standards of nutrition care for the frail oldest adults.

There are few published data regarding the food and fluid intake patterns of LTC residents. Some reports suggest that LTC residents consume a greater proportion of their breakfast meal than they do of other meals, especially dinner (Chapman, Samman, & Liburne, 1993; Endres, Welch, Ashraf, Banz, & Gower, 2000; Simmons & Reuben, 2000; Young, Binns, & Greenwood, 2001; Castellanos, Surloff, & Giordan, 2003c); however, there is typically a smaller quantity of food served at breakfast than at lunch and dinner. A study by Young et al. (2001) found that older adults with dementia tend to eat less food as the day progresses. Also, a study looking at snack interventions found that residents consumed significantly less during the evening snack period than during the morning or afternoon snack (Simmons & Schnelle, 2004).

Inadequate hydration is a significant issue in the LTC setting (Chidester & Spangler, 1997; Kayser-Jones, Schell, Porter, Barbaccia, & Shaw, 1999). Older adults in nursing facilities are likely to be unwell, have limited access to palatable fluids, and are at greater risk for suboptimal hydration than other older people (Chidester & Spangler, 1997). Inadequate water intake can contribute to acute confusion, urinary tract infections, pressure ulcers, constipation, and adverse drug responses (American Medical Directors Association, 2002). These problems can lead to increased morbidity and mortality and can escalate health care costs (Chidester & Spangler, 1997; American Medical Directors Association, 2002).

Older people do not always feel thirsty, even when they are dehydrated (Rolls & Phillips, 1990). It may be difficult or impossible for older people with neurologic or musculoskeletal disabilities to obtain or consume liquids independently. In addition, it is not uncommon for nursing home residents to have medical conditions (diarrhea, vomiting, and dysphagia) or to be prescribed treatments (diuretic medications) that put them at increased risk for dehydration. Fortunately, systems put in place to ensure adequate resident assistance with eating are likely to have the added benefit of supporting adequate intake of fluids. For example, one study found that verbal prompting increased fluid intake in 71% of residents, with the range of increase of 5 to 20 oz/day (Simmons, Alessi, & Schnelle, 2001). Also, hydration programs can be implemented to ensure that fluids offered between meals or with medications are of significant volume, frequency, and palatability to appreciably increase overall fluid intake.

LTC facilities are also filled with people suffering from acute and medically complex illnesses that were once found only in hospitals. For example, knee and hip replacement therapy is now occurring in the LTC facility instead of the hospital. At one time hospitalized people stayed in the hospital until they were well enough to be discharged home. In the current health care system these "patients" are becoming "residents" of skilled nursing facilities. Thus the LTC facility must also have the clinical staff and infrastructure to provide adequate care to severely ill people who often do not eat or drink enough to meet their nutritional needs.

Nutrition Care Process and Timeline

It is important to identify current nutrition problems and the risk of future nutrition problems in a timely fashion. This requires a logical and preplanned sequence of screening, assessments, and reviews. Many of the timeframes are dictated by federal standards, but an individual facility may choose to monitor its residents more closely than required. The policy and procedure manual in the facility should outline the timeframe for all phases of nutrition care.

Within 24 hours of admission to the facility, a member of the nutritional services department should conduct an initial interview to greet the resident, confirm the diet prescription, identify meal preferences

Nutrition assessment: A thorough evaluation of the resident's food and eating preferences, medical and nutritional status, estimation of nutritional needs, and identification of medical conditions/treatments and other factors that might make the resident at risk of developing malnutrition in the future. This information is used to develop the individualized plan of nutrition care for the resident.

Nutrition screening: A quick review to determine if the resident meets any known factors for nutrition risk that would require an immediate assessment by a registered dietitian.

Reassessment: A resident assessment that takes place after a significant change in the resident's status or after 4 months, whichever comes first. The purpose is to determine if the current nutritional regimen is adequate to meet the resident's nutritional needs.

Minimum data set (MDS): An electronic summary of the medical status of each resident mandated by the Centers for Medicare and Medicaid Services.

Resident assessment protocols: Protocols developed by the Centers for Medicare and Medicaid Services to be used for guiding resident assessment after a "trigger" on the minimum data set. These protocols have been developed for a number of nutrition-related issues.

and food dislikes, screen the resident for nutrition risk, and introduce the resident to the food service system. The DSM, dietetic technician, or RD may conduct this interview. A brief chart note should be written, and the note should state that the diet order has been confirmed and the resident has been interviewed and screened. Many times, this type of note will conclude by stating that a complete **nutrition assessment** will follow.

A **nutrition screening** is a quick review to determine if the resident meets any known factors for nutrition risk. Each facility should outline a screening process to identify which residents need immediate assessment and which residents should be given a chance to settle into the facility before the assessment takes place. Typically, a nutrition screening ascertains weight history, albumin level, diagnosis, the presence of feeding tubes, and skin condition. The nutrition screening or interview process should be sensitive enough to identify new residents with feeding tubes, intravenous lines, a diagnosis of malnutrition or dehydration, and other significant nutrition problems. An immediate assessment is warranted with certain diagnoses or the presence of a feeding tube.

Per regulations (F272 and F276), a complete nutrition assessment should be conducted within the first 14 days of admission. Many facilities improve on this standard and make it a policy to complete the assessment by the seventh day of admission. It is often advisable to wait until the resident has been in the facility for several days before completing an assessment. This short delay allows time for the resident to become accustomed to the new surroundings and for body weight and baseline laboratory data to be obtained, dining location secured, and hospital records copied for the nursing home chart. There are a number of resources available to assist the RD in making the complete assessment. The ADA described in detail the components of the nutritional assessment, which is an essential part of the nutrition care process (Lacey & Pritchett, 2003). In addition, the ADA practice group, Consultant Dietitians in Health Care Facilities, developed written resources that are specifically designed to support the assessment process in the LTC setting (http://www.cdhcf.org).

A **reassessment** of each resident must be performed a minimum of every 3 months (i.e., quarterly). A quarterly review is not as in-depth as a full initial assessment but should determine if the current nutritional regimen is adequate to meet the resident's nutritional needs. If the resident has had a change in medical condition or suffers a significant weight loss, a reassessment must be done even if it is not scheduled. A full assessment, equivalent to the initial assessment, must be completed at the end of each year of residency.

One unique component of the medical record in nursing homes is the **minimum data set (MDS)**. The MDS is an electronic summary of the medical status of each resident. The MDS Section K, Oral/Nutritional Status, is usually completed after the initial nutrition assessment is complete. It is helpful to complete the MDS as soon after the assessment as possible while the information is easily accessible and memorable. It is recommended that the same person who completes the nutrition assessment also completes the MDS. Often, facilities will use an MDS coordinator to complete the entire MDS, but it is preferable that the nutrition care professional be responsible for completing the nutrition section. In some cases the MDS Section K may be completed by the DSM because it is just the gathering of objective data from the chart. In this case the MDS coordinator, either a registered nurse or RD, reviews and signs off that Section K was completed accurately.

Dietitians within the facility use the MDS as one way to identify residents who may be experiencing a nutritional problem or who are at risk for a nutritional problem. The use of the MDS in identifying individuals at nutrition risk was validated by Blaum et al. (1997). Once a resident has been identified as being at nutritional risk, the clinician must follow up using **resident assessment protocols**. The resident assessment protocol for malnutrition is "triggered" if any of the following are indicated on the MDS: resident has a weight loss or gain of 5% or more in past 30 days or 10% or more in past 180 days; complains about the taste of many foods; leaves 25% or more food uneaten at most meals; receives a parenteral/intravenous feeding; receives a mechanically altered, syringe (oral feeding), or therapeutic diet; or has a pressure ulcer for which the highest stage is 2, 3, or 4. Once a resident assessment protocol for malnutrition is triggered, the problem must be evaluated and the response documented. This evaluation must be completed by a licensed professional, because it requires clinical judgment as to whether a problem actually exists that would need to be addressed through a care plan. After the assessment a determination is sometimes made that a care plan is not necessary. For example, a resident assessment protocol may be triggered because the MDS indicates a resident requires a texture-modified diet. However, subsequent assessment by the RD reveals that the resident has no difficulties eating the texture-modified food that is being provided, her dentures are in good repair, her intake is adequate to meet her needs, and her weight is stable. Because the resident is not experiencing a nutritional problem, there is no need for a care plan.

Care plans are required to be complete by the 21st day of admission. The care planning process is an interdisciplinary process, and the nutrition team member should initiate those who directly relate to nutrition and contribute to nursing care plans. The nutritional department usually writes care plans that involve weight loss, dehydration, tube feedings, and nutritional deficiencies, with other disciplines adding their approaches as necessary. Nutrition interventions should be found on all care plans that involve any diet-related approaches. For example, nutrition plays a role in many care plans seen as nursing issues, such as hypertension, pressure ulcers, congestive heart failure, and risk of aspiration. Care plans should be updated whenever there is a new intervention or, otherwise, at least quarterly.

Clinical RD Accountability in the LTC Setting

What is expected of the clinical dietitian, including what is written in the medical record, is significantly different in a nursing home compared with an acute care facility. The paradigm is fundamentally different due to the length of time the person spends in the facility, the regulatory environment of an LTC facility, and the central role the resident and the resident's family play in determining what care will be provided.

The average length of stay in an acute care facility is days to weeks, which compares with an average length of stay of about 2.5 years in an LTC facility (ElderWeb, n.d.). This extended stay provides significantly more opportunity for the RD to have an impact on the resident's health but brings with it a proportional increase in the RD's accountability for resident care and outcomes. In the LTC setting there is sufficient opportunity to identify the full extent of the resident's nutritional issues, as well as other factors that contribute to a resident's nutritional risk, and there is a higher expectation that each nutritional issue and risk factor will be addressed. At the same time invasive assessment and treatment methods that are used in the acute setting, such as frequent laboratory blood analysis, may be limited unless the outcome of the procedure is expected to result in a change in care that will improve the resident's quality of life.

The LTC regulations also go much further in specifying the details of clinical care. The interpretive guidelines, which have been developed to assist surveyors in evaluation and providers to comply with the intent of the federal regulations, are often quite specific regarding how care for various conditions should be provided: "Unless contraindicated, nutritional goals for a resident with nutritional compromise who has a pressure ulcer or is at risk of developing pressure ulcers should include protein intake of approximately 1.2–1.5 gm/kg body weight daily (higher end of the range for those with larger, more extensive, or multiple wounds)" (American Health Care Association, 2005). This is very different from the approach used by the Joint Commission on Accreditation of Healthcare Organizations, the accrediting body for hospitals, which does not identify such specific standards of care for various conditions. Thus it is incumbent upon the LTC RD to have a detailed knowledge of the interpretive guidelines and other regulatory language and to conduct assessments and to provide care in a manner that is consistent with them.

There is also an expectation that the dietitian will be proactive and intervene before a problem becomes significant. For example, an RD should recognize when a resident has a nutrition risk factor and bring the issue to the care team so it can be addressed before nutritional status is compromised.

Another aspect of LTC that is different from acute care is the care plan process. In LTC, the care plans for an individual resident should be as much the resident's and family's plan of care as it is the provider's (i.e., it should be individualized to meet the needs and desires of the resident and be interdisciplinary in nature). If a resident or a responsible family member refuses some aspect of care, relevant conversations with family members must be documented, including documentation that the risks and benefits have been explained. It is also the case that the members of the care plan team (nurses, therapists, dietitians, social workers, etc.) have significantly more authority in the LTC setting than they would in the acute care setting. The care planning team can, and often does, make recommendations to the physician based on their assessments.

Discharge Education

Discharge education occurs in the LTC facility less often than in an acute care setting but is needed for individuals who will discharge to a setting that provides a lower level of care, after either rehabilitation or strengthening. The dietitian needs to make sure that educational materials are available and that training is provided to both nursing staff and the DSM so that, in the dietitian's absence, discharge education may be provided to the resident, family, or other caregivers. Materials often are taken from the diet manual of the facility or are available through other resources, such as the ADA, the American Heart Association, or the National Dairy Council.

Modified Diet Menu Writing and Approval and Modified Diet Prescriptions

The nutrition care for the resident begins with a menu made up of standardized recipes in an accepted regional pattern to meet the nutritional needs of the general elderly population. Federal regulation requires that the meals meet the needs of residents in accordance with the Recommended Dietary Allowances and that planned menus are followed (F363). A complete understanding of menu and recipe mechanics and the systems related to them are key to the RD's ability to help a facility succeed in meeting its clinical and operational goals. A menu must be nutritionally sound to have a chance of meeting clinical goals, and the financial impact of a poorly planned menu is enormous. Before altering or building a menu for a facility, an RD should become familiar with the procurement process, products available through the process, nutritional content of the foods available, the budget around labor and food cost, staff skill set, equipment available, the diet manual adopted, the ADA's position on therapeutic diets, and the facility's goals regarding customer satisfaction.

If the RD is serving in the capacity of a consultant, his or her involvement in menu creation will vary based on the operational support provided by the facility—for example, whether menus are available from a corporate office, if menus are purchased from a vendor, if diets are software available, and whether purchasing programs are set up with a vendor. The assistance needed by the facility may include all or part of the following:

- Writing the entire menu, including finding recipes for texture modifications and therapeutics such as dialysis diets
- Writing the occasional combination diet for which there is no menu extension, such as a puree diet that is also a consistent carbohydrate diet
- Approving menu changes in response to facility/resident preferences or a food availability issue
- Reviewing disaster menus and plans or creating disaster menus and plans for multiple scenarios, such as no electricity, partial electricity, or evacuation to a local school or church

Many resources are available regarding disaster planning, including information in diet manuals and from consultant companies.

As discussed previously, the LTC facility is viewed as the resident's home, and the approaches should be the same as they would be at home: to maintain health and to have the highest quality of life possible. One area where this philosophy dramatically affects care is in the area of therapeutic diet prescriptions. Although there may be an occasion where a therapeutic restriction is necessary, the position of the ADA (2005) is: "the quality of life and nutritional status of older residents in the LTC facility may be enhanced by liberalization of the diet prescription." Food consumption is frequently compromised because of a combination of acute and chronic disease conditions, such that any additional restrictions that would reduce food acceptability and intake would be counterproductive to achieving the care goals.

In addition to making diet recommendations intended to maintain each resident's health and quality of life, the RD in the LTC setting also has the responsibility to evaluate the success of those recommendations over time. Because the facility provides care to most residents over a period of weeks to months, the RD must regularly reassess the resident and determine whether the current diet prescription is resulting in significant clinical progress or is otherwise meeting the resident's care goals.

Increasing and Maintaining Resident Food Intake

Dining is much more than just the consumption of food; it is the smells, sounds, conversations, and anticipation and recall of memories that inspire us to eat (Beverly Healthcare, 1999).

● **Learning Point** One of the most important contributions of the RD is to make sure the dining environment is one that optimizes resident food intake

A multifacility study conducted by the UCLA Borun Center examined the relationships between 16 nutrition care processes and prevalence of weight loss in nursing facilities (Simmons, Garcia, et al., 2003). There were no identifiable differences in the RD medical record documentation between the low-weight-loss and the high-weight-loss facilities. Instead, the major difference between the high- and low-weight-loss facilities was the dining environment. The staff at the low-weight-loss nursing homes consistently provided verbal prompting and social interaction during meals to a greater proportion of the residents, including those most at risk for weight loss. These data suggest that it is in the area of meal service and dining that the expertise of the RD may not be fully utilized in many LTC facilities.

The provision of feeding assistance at meals (social interaction throughout the mealtime period, graduated verbal prompting that enhances self-feeding capabilities, and physical assistance to the degree required) has been found to have a dramatic effect on food intake. One study found that 50% of residents previously identified as having low food intake responded to feeding assistance by increasing their food intake more than 10%. A subset of the residents (39%) in this study were identified as "highly responsive" to the intervention and increased their meal intake over 2 days from 48% to an average of 74% consumed (Simmons, Lam, Rao, & Schnelle, 2001b). Three studies, Simmons, Alessi, and Schnelle (2001), Simmons, Osterweil, and Schnelle (2001), and Simmons and Schnelle (2004) consistently found that 40% to 50% of residents who had one-on-one feeding assistance significantly increased their oral food and fluid intake during mealtime.

Similarly, some residents have responded to additional feeding assistance with snacks, and enhancing between-meal snack programs is one alternative for increasing dietary intake (Rahman & Simmons, 2005). A study by Simmons and Schnelle (2004) found that 70% of the residents who were not responsive to increased feeding assistance at meals did significantly increase their between-meal intake when targeted for additional attention and assistance during snacks. With the snacking intervention, calories consumed between meals (supplement 1 snacks) increased to 380 kcal/day from 96 kcal/day under usual care (Simmons & Schnelle, 2004). The second and third most preferred nutrition interventions among family members of residents were improved feeding assistance and the provision of multiple small meals and snacks, respectively (Simmons, Lam, et al., 2003).

Most family members of nursing home residents prefer an intervention that includes the provision of more nutritious food (Simmons, Lam, et al., 2003). This is often referred to by dietitians as a "food first" approach, and many facilities have a policy for such an offering. There is some evidence that the energy and nutrient intakes of nursing home residents can be significantly increased by increasing the energy/nutrient density of several foods across two or more meals each day (Olin, Osterberg, et al., 1996; Barton, Beigg, Macdonald, & Allison, 2000; Castellanos et al., 2003c; Olin, Armyr, et al., 2003),

● **Learning Point** Providing residents with a choice of preferred foods and drinks has been found to significantly increase food and fluid intake, particularly in residents who are cognitively intact (Simmons et al., 2001a).

where the energy density of a food is defined as the energy content per weight or volume of food served (Kral & Rolls, 2004). Increasing the nutrient density of the foods residents are already choosing to eat, instead of providing substitute foods or supplements, also allows residents both choice and control over their environment (Castellanos, Surloff, & Giordan, 2003; Simmons, Lam, et al., 2003). Further, research has shown that food preferences and acceptability are important determinants of amounts consumed (de Jong, Chin-A-Paw, de Graff, de Groot, & van Staveren, 2001), particularly for residents who are cognitively intact (Simmons, Alessi, et al., 2001). Often, the enhanced items are varied or rotated to limit the chance of taste fatigue for the resident.

Provision of liquid nutrition supplements is one of the nutrition interventions least preferred by residents' family members (Simmons et al., 2003b). Although the data are limited, studies suggest that some residents are willing to consume supplements and do benefit from them (Johnson, Dooley, & Gleick, 1993). However, as many as 40% of residents do not consume the liquid supplements they are provided (Johnson et al., 1993; Ross, 1999). Dietitians, however, perceived supplemental products to be second only to tube feedings in terms of effectiveness for increasing intake (Cluskey & Kim, 1997). It should be noted that there is some evidence that supplements consumed with meals cause early satiation (reduce intake of other foods provided in the meal) (Wilson, Purushothaman, & Morley, 2002); thus the greatest benefit to residents is likely to occur when liquid supplements are provided between meals. For residents with poor appetite, replacing restrictive diets with a wider range of food choices may also improve intake and quality of life (ADA, 2005).

Medications thought to stimulate appetite are sometimes used to improve food intake and weight status, but their use is controversial. It is a common belief that some older people eat better when they are provided with "small portions." Here a note of caution is warranted. Although the impact of portion size on food intake in older people has not been thoroughly studied, the few studies that do speak to this issue have found that some LTC residents eat less, whereas others are unaffected when portion sizes are reduced (Cluskey & Dunton, 1999; Young et al., 2001; Castellanos, Georgian, & Wellman, 2003). That is to say, there is no evidence that smaller portions enhance food intake in this population. This is consistent with a large number of studies in younger people showing that food intake decreases when smaller portions are served (Kral & Rolls, 2004).

Cultural Diversity in LTC Facilities

LTC facilities are distinctly different from both acute care and community settings in that they are both residential and institutional. That is to say that the facility is "home" to the client for at least a few weeks, and many residents live out the remaining months or years of their lives in this care setting. At the same time the provider, not the individual resident, is in the position to make decisions regarding the nature of the food that is available, the manner of food service, and the timing of resident access to food. It is not difficult to imagine that these factors can have a tremendous impact, either negatively or positively, on the quality of life of the residents.

For example, the availability of culturally acceptable foods can impact a resident's food and nutrient consumption, affecting both health and quality of life. Staple foods are very culture specific, and people from a given culture prefer to eat their particular staple food (e.g., tortillas, bread, rice, beans, or pasta) many times a week, if not several times a day. If a resident is not able to regularly obtain the foods that are staples of his or her culture and instead receives the staples of another culture (e.g., an Asian immigrant who receives bread at most meals instead of rice), the menu is unlikely to be acceptable to that individual. Further, the standard of a well-planned menu is determined by the cultural perspective of the evaluator. For example, a menu writer of northern European descent may not think twice that bread is served at every evening meal but would never develop a menu where rice and beans are served at every evening meal. However, this same menu writer may be responsible for a facility with a large number of Hispanic residents. Some Hispanics, depending on their country of origin, would expect to eat rice and beans at almost every noon and evening meal. They may also perceive different beans and legumes (e.g., black, white, red, garbanzo, etc.) as entirely different foods and consider beans served on rice as entirely different from beans cooked with rice. In short, planning a single menu for a group of residents from varying cultures can be a challenging task.

Also making food provision in the LTC setting more complicated is the fact that people reside in facilities because they suffer from a number of acute and chronic diseases such that they cannot be cared for at home. Federal regulations require that food be served in a form and nutrient content to meet individual needs and to support treatment and plan of care. Further, this population is known to be at high risk for deficiencies in energy, protein, fiber, and water, as evidenced by the high prevalence of unintended weight loss, compromised protein status, constipation, and dehydration. Unfortunately, any resident provided a culturally unacceptable menu is unlikely to eat well, which is likely to result in weight loss and undernutrition and a spiral of negative health effects.

Federal regulation specifies the facility's responsibilities toward creating and maintaining an environment that humanizes and individualizes each resident, including how each resident is treated at mealtime. This is consistent with the position of the ADA that nutrition care in LTC facilities must promote quality of life. Because of this, it is standard practice for LTC facilities to provide menus that are consistent with regional and cultural norms (e.g., rice and beans may be on the menu frequently in Miami but will be rarely if ever served in Kansas City). Facilities are also adopting new attitudes toward providing care, as described by the ADA (2005). A "resident-centered" or "person-centered" care approach involves residents in decisions about schedules, menus, and dining locations. This approach is one way to honor the relationship between food and culture in the LTC setting while at the same time meeting the intent of the federal statutes.

Qualified dietitians should be responsible for managing facility-wide dining and snack programs and should optimize menus to meet the unique needs of this population. It is both a necessity and an opportunity for the nutrition professional to take responsibility for all the processes and systems in the facility that support adequate food and fluid intake of residents.

Food Preparation

Food preparation and service are critical functions in the LTC facility, yet they often receive insufficient attention from the RD. Tags F362 to F365, F368, and F369 address various aspects of the proper-preparation and service of food, and the dietitian is responsible for ensuring that the facility is in compliance. However, the health and well-being of the residents and the financial viability of the company are both equally important reasons for dietitians to give adequate time and attention to the food service operation.

From both the financial and the resident outcomes points of view, the most expensive meal to a facility is the one that is not consumed. Food and dining are important quality of life issues for residents, and food of poor nutritional quality or food that is not consumed in adequate amounts results in a decline in the health and nutritional status of residents. Further, food service operations are resource intensive, and if the food service in an LTC facility is poorly managed, scarce resources available for resident care will be wasted. However timely and thorough a dietitian may be in completing clinical assessments and care plans, if the food leaving the kitchen is not nutritionally adequate or if it is not consumed by residents (because is unpalatable, not served at an acceptable temperature, not in the proper form, or served at an acceptable time), then the documentation in the medical record is of little use.

RDs have tremendous opportunities to assist the facility in improving resident care through their expertise in staff management, food preparation, food service systems, training skills, and financial management. For example, to verify the use of standardized recipes and instructions and compliance with the menu, the dietitian can periodically observe food preparation. Staff can be reminded or educated in regard to cooking methods that preserve nutritional quality and texture, such as limiting water when heating vegetables and batch cooking. The tray line can also be observed periodically to verify that the menu is being followed for therapeutic diets and that alternates are available. Further, the RD can minimize food waste by making sure that items on the tray line are portioned correctly according to the recipes (e.g., correct pan size and the number of cuts per pan) and the menu (e.g., use of a no. 8 scoop for 1/2-cup servings). Food safety and palatability are always of paramount importance, and the RD can spot check to verify that tray line temperatures meet both **Hazard Analysis Critical Control Point (HACCP)** process and palatability requirements. Although the DSM and/or the cook should observe a dining room at every meal to determine resident acceptance, the RD should also routinely observe dining to identify any issues with the service of the meal, the dining environment, the provision of feeding assistance, and meal acceptance.

> **Hazard Analysis Critical Control Point (HACCP):** A process used in cooking to identify steps and points in food preparation that are deemed as critical in preventing food-borne illness.

Food Safety and Sanitation

The most common deficiency in LTC surveys is F371: Store, prepare, distribute, and serve food under sanitary conditions. Over 40% of LTC facilities are cited for deficient practice under this tag. Per the federal guidelines, the intent of this regulation is "to prevent the spread of food-borne illness and reduce those practices, which may result in food contamination and compromise food safety in nursing homes. Food-borne illness is often fatal to nursing home residents and can and must be avoided" (American Health Care Association, 2005).

Food Code: Published by the U.S. Food and Drug Administration, this is a model that assists food control jurisdictions at all levels of government by providing them with a scientifically sound technical and legal basis for regulating the retail and food service segments of the industry.

The federal guidelines suggest the use of the U.S. Food and Drug Administration **Food Code** as a resource, but the regulation does not mandate its use. Since the advent of this guideline, several states have adopted the Food Code, and several counties are mandating its use, especially in reference to HACCP. HACCP is a process used in cooking to identify steps and points in food preparation deemed critical in preventing food-borne illness. Although all chapters of the Food Code are relevant, chapters 1 through 4 tend to be the most applicable to LTC settings. The Food Code is one of the most heavily used reference books in the LTC industry, and a copy should be placed in every nutritional services department and should be the foundation for all sanitation training. It should be noted that the Food Code is updated approximately every 2 years, and it is common for a state to adopt a specific version of the Food Code and not recognize newer versions (e.g., a state may use the 2002 Food Code instead of the 2005 version). Thus it is important for a facility RD to be aware of and follow the version of the Food Code that his or her state uses.

Because F371 is such a problem in LTC settings, most facility administrators and nursing home companies focus efforts on avoiding this citation. These stakeholders look to the RD to assist them in making sure the facility practices help them achieve that goal.

A study by the RD Council for Quality Nursing Home Care identified the three most common surveyor observations associated with F371 in 95 surveys across nine different LTC companies (Nevins, Gluch, Castellanos, & RD Council for Quality Nursing Home Care, 2003):

- In 45.3% of F371 citations, surveyors observed problems with soiled equipment.
- In 41.1% of F371 citations, surveyors observed problems with food storage. This included a range of problems from food not labeled and dated to improper thawing and cooling of food.
- In 35.8% of F371 citations, surveyors observed problems with the cleanliness and condition of the physical structure of the kitchen. This covers dirty walls and surfaces, broken floor tiles, and holes in screens or gaps in windows.

A dietitian can significantly improve a facility's ability to achieve compliance with F371. On a routine basis the RD should review cooling and thawing practices, educate staff on proper procedures, and conduct spot checks in the kitchen. The RD should regularly inspect equipment sanitation, assist the facility in the use of cleaning schedules, and provide training on the proper use and cleaning of equipment. The RD should also make sure there is an effective system for the fulfillment of maintenance requests and completion of the routine types of cleaning normally performed by facility maintenance (e.g., refrigerator fans). Finally, the RD can review facility policies to make sure they are consistent with the Food Code currently being used by that state.

Survey Management

Numerous times in this chapter we have referenced the regulations the LTC facility must follow when caring for its residents. An annual survey to determine the facility's compliance with the regulations occurs a minimum of once every 18 months. Other surveys do occasionally take place, such as a "complaint survey" for review of a complaint made to the state about the facility. A **state survey** team can enter the facility at any time, including the middle of the night or on weekends. Occasionally, a federal survey team, whose job it is to review the state team's results for accuracy, follows them a few days later. At times the federal survey team will actually accompany the state survey team. Thus there may be anywhere from three to nine surveyors in a facility at one time. The survey teams usually include nurses, sanitarians, and social workers and may occasionally include an RD.

State survey: The process of the state department of health entering a facility to determine if the Centers for Medicare and Medicaid Services and state requirements are being met.

The survey experience can be unsettling to both residents and staff. The best way to make this experience a positive one is to plan for the survey in conjunction with the DSM and be prepared to man-

TABLE 14.2 Planning for and Managing the LTC Survey

Planning	Managing
Educating staff about the federal and state regulations, interpretive guidelines, and investigative protocols.	Identifying the contact person in the nutritional services department to communicate with the surveyor.
Educating staff regarding the procedures used by surveyors. This clarifies the expectations of the survey process and how staff should respond in anticipation of the next step in the process.	Determining who will stay with the surveyor assigned to nutritional services throughout the survey process so that resources, documentation, justifications/explanations, and so on can be provided as needed.
Ensuring systems are in place so that proper meal production and service can be practiced every day.	Responding to potential deficiency areas discovered during the survey using a predetermined approach, e.g., fix any problematic issues immediately.
Attending resident council meetings periodically and probing for issues or complaints that residents may bring to surveyors so that they can be addressed beforehand.	Holding staff meetings at the beginning and the end of the day to review issues such as surveyor comments, ingredient availability, and staffing.
Participating in the facility plan for the surveyor visit, such as determining where the surveyors will be given space to work so as to minimize interference with resident activities and planning what food and beverages will be provided to them so that those items can be on hand.	Determine a plan for management to follow up on potential issues mentioned by surveyors.

age the survey. Some steps in planning for and managing a survey are listed in **Table 14.2**. Knowledge is power and confidence. These planning steps, and many others, can be taken to give staff the tools and confidence they need to succeed under pressure. Taking steps to manage the survey helps to keep everyone calm and focused during the actual survey.

Quality Management

In most businesses, quality assessment and assurance is optional and is used for business improvement. In LTC settings quality management is required by the federal government (F520 and 521). Dietitians in the LTC setting play a critical role in ensuring that the facility meets quality care standards in both clinical care and meal production. Well-designed systems must be in place to ensure appropriate and timely nutrition assessment of residents, execution of the nutrition care plan, minimal weight loss and pressure ulcers, and proper sanitation, food preparation, and delivery of the meals. Quality assurance activities are necessary to ensure the delivery of high-quality nutritional services.

The essential elements of traditional **quality assurance** are to (1) identify potential problems that may exist that can be measured through review of data and outcomes, (2) set a

Quality assurance: A system for ensuring that quality care is being delivered and that the activities required to maintain quality are being performed at an acceptable level.

performance standard, (3) screen to ensure compliance to the performance standard, (4) gather individual feedback and identify deficiencies, (5) review systems and processes to determine where breakdown is occurring, (6) institute corrective action to achieve performance standard, and (7) emphasize health care structure, process, and outcome.

Step 5 of the quality assurance process is critical for ensuring that quality care is being delivered and that the activities required to maintain quality are being performed at an acceptable level. The efficacy of the quality assurance committee depends on their ability to evaluate the systems and processes in a facility. Although quality assurance may not be a responsibility of the dietitian in other care settings, the nature of the LTC setting demands that dietitians use a wide range of management skills to ensure that residents receive quality care during the entire length of their stay. Although the dietitian may not be in attendance for all quality assurance meetings (e.g., if the facility RD is a consultant), the RD should review the minutes of quality assurance meetings and assist the DSM in the system analysis.

The Centers for Medicare and Medicaid Services also has a focus on quality management. State and federal regulators use facility data from the MDS to monitor various **quality indicators**; the MDS Quality Indicator Report for Nutrition/Eating includes "prevalence of weight loss," "prevalence of tube feeding," and "prevalence of dehydration."

The Centers for Medicare and Medicaid Services has also made certain data available to the public so that they, the consumers, can use it to compare nursing homes. Selected MDS data from each facility are available nationally at the Nursing Home Compare website (www.medicare.gov/NHCompare/). These data, called **quality measures**, are intended to represent the quality of care provided at nursing facilities so that consumers can make an informed decision. Of particular relevance to nutrition services is the "weight loss quality measure." The quality measure reports the percentage of residents with a significant weight loss, excluding residents receiving hospice care; that is, residents who have experienced a weight loss of more than 5% of their body weight in 1 month or 10% of their body weight in 6 months.

It is appropriate that the facility RD take the lead in efforts to improve the facility's weight loss quality measure. The etiology of unintentional weight loss and undernutrition is multifactorial and is likely related to both psychological factors and physiologic changes (Morley, 2003). Studies have suggested that behavioral and environmental factors may be the most important determinants of food intake in the nursing home setting (Simmons, Alessi, et al., 2001; Simmons, Babinou, et al., 2002). It is critical that nutrition care processes focus on underlying causes and emphasize prevention of weight loss (Beck & Ovesen, 1998).

Unique Role of the Consultant Dietitian in LTC

A *consultant,* as defined by Merriam-Webster Online (http://www.merriam-webster.com/), is a person who is called on for professional or technical advice or opinions. RD consultants are in a unique position because not only do they have the clinical training necessary to provide MNT, they are also highly valued for their knowledge in the areas of food preparation, sanitation, and food service systems. If the facility RD is a consultant and not a full-time employee of the facility or company, it is important to remember that the resident is not the only customer. The clients of the consultant RD also include the facility administrator, the director of nursing services, and the DSM.

Consultants are in an LTC facility a limited number of hours per week. If the activities of a consultant are limited only to charting and pointing out sanitation or production errors, then the facility is not able to take full advantage of the expertise of the consultant in helping them to develop in-house staff and improve their performance over time. However, if the consultant takes the time to identify and understand the current issues or concerns of the facility, he or she may be able to provide relevant staff education and/or offer several possible solutions to ongoing problems. This approach allows the facility team the opportunity to develop their own competency in the area of concern and affords staff the opportunity to choose and take ownership of the solution. Staff development and buy-in are essential for long-term correction of any problem.

An example consultant report is as follows: Cross-contamination between clean and dirty dishes in the dish room is observed. An alternative consultant report that provides more information and solutions follows: At entrance conference facility expressed concern regarding sanitation. Sanitation tour completed, see attached. Provided in-service to staff on dish machine procedures. Recommend two options for change: (1) Move the hand sink closer to the dish area as discussed and/or (2) Restructure staffing to allow for one associate on each end of the dish machine, thus eliminating need to crossover from clean to dirty side.

Summary

In summary, the role of the RD in LTC settings is much more complex than it is in many other care settings. In LTC it is the expectation that the dietitian not only will be proficient in MNT but will have expertise in the regulatory environment, food preparation, sanitation, dining, and survey and quality management. The provision of nutrition care in this setting also requires a proactive and system-oriented approach, where residents' quality of life is a primary consideration in every decision, and care should be provided in the most home-like manner possible. The potential for the RD to make a significant difference in the quality of life of residents and to be valued by the facility are limited only by the aspirations of the individual practitioner.

Issues to Debate

1. Discuss the effects of being unregulated on the residents of an LTC facility.
2. Discuss the effects of making a dietitian's consultation optional to the residents of an LTC facility.
3. Discuss the potential differences between a private and public LTC facility.

Websites

American Dietetic Association www.eatright.org
American Dietetic Association Evidence Analysis Library www.adaevidencelibrary.org
American Health Care Association http://www. ahca.org/
American Society for Parenteral and Enteral Nutrition http://www.nutritioncare.org/
Centers for Medicare and Medicaid Services http://www.cms.hhs.gov/default.asp?
    fromhcfadotgov=true and http://www.cms.hhs.gov/
The Clinician's Ultimate Guide to Drug Therapy http://www.globalrph.com/
Dietary Managers Association http://www.dmaonline.org/index
Dietetics in Health Care Facilities www.cdhcf.org
Drug Bank http://redpoll.pharmacy.ualberta.ca/drugbank/
2005 Food Code http://www.fda.gov/Food/FoodSafety/RetailFoodProtection/FoodCode/FoodCode2005/default.htm
Food Insight www.ific.org
National Academies www.nas.edu/health/
National Quality Measures Clearinghouse http://www.qualitymeasures.ahrq.gov/
National Resource Center on Nutrition, Physical Activity and Aging, Long Term Care Institute
    http://nutritionandaging.fiu.edu/about_long_term.asp
Nursing Home Compare http://www.medicare.gov/NHCompare/
Nursing Home Quality Initiatives http://www.cms.hhs.gov/NursingHomeQualityInits/
UCLA Borun Center for Gerontological Research http://borun.medsch.ucla.edu/
USDA Nutrient Data Laboratory http://www.nal.usda.gov/fnic/foodcomp
U.S. Department of Agriculture, MyPyramid www.mypyramid.gov

References

American Dietetic Association (ADA). (2005). Position of the American Dietetic Association: Liberalization of the diet prescription improves quality of life for older adults in long term care. *Journal of the American Dietetic Association, 105,* 1955–1965.

American Health Care Association. (2005). *The Long Term Care Survey.* Washington, DC: Author.

American Medical Directors Association. (2002). *Clinical Practice Guidelines: Dehydration and Fluid Maintenance.* Columbia, MD: Author.

Barton, A. D., Beigg, C. L., Macdonald, I. A., & Allison, S. P. (2000). A recipe for improving food intakes in elderly hospitalized patients. *Clinical Nutrition, 19,* 451–454.

Beck, A. M., & Ovesen, L. (1998). At which body mass index and degree of weight loss should hospitalized elderly patients be considered at nutritional risk? *Clinical Nutrition, 17*, 195–198.

Beverly Healthcare. (1999). *Enhanced Dining Resources*. Little Rock, AR: Author.

Blaum, C. S., O'Neill, E. F., Clements, K. M., Fries, B. E., & Fiatarone, M. A. (1997). Validity of the minimum data set for assessing nutritional status in nursing home residents. *American Journal of Clinical Nutrition, 66*, 787–794.

Castellanos, V. H. (2004). Food and nutrition in nursing homes. *Generations, 28*, 65–71.

Castellanos, V. H., & Andrews, Y. N. (2002). Inherent flaws in a method commonly used to report food intake in long term care facilities. *Journal of the American Dietetic Association, 102*, 826–830.

Castellanos, V. H., Georgian, M. E., & Wellman, N. S. (2003). Fluid intake increased when larger portions were offered to nursing home residents with medications. *FASEB Journal, 17*, A285.

Castellanos, V. H., Silver, H. J., Gallagher-Allred, C., & Smith, T. (2003). Nutrition issues in home, community, and long-term care setting. *Nutrition Clinical Practice, 18*, 21–36.

Castellanos, V. H., Surloff, S. C., & Giordan, W. L. (2003). Systematic enhancement of food over short term increased calorie intake by residents with dementia. *Journal of the American Dietetic Association, 103*, A40.

Chapman, K., Samman, S., & Liburne, A. M. (1993). Are the guidelines for nutritional care and food service in nursing homes being implemented? *Australian Journal of Nutrition and Diet, 50*, 39–45.

Chidester, C., & Spangler, A. A. (1997). Fluid intake in the institutionalized elderly. *Journal of the American Dietetic Association, 97*, 23–28.

Cluskey, M., & Dunton, N. (1999). Serving meals of reduced portion size did not improve appetite among elderly in a personal-care section of a long-term care community. *Journal of the American Dietetic Association, 99*, 33–35.

Cluskey, M., & Kim, Y. (1997). Use and perceived effectiveness of strategies for enhancing food and nutrient intakes among elderly persons in long-term care. *Journal of the American Dietetic Association, 101*, 111–114.

de Jong, N., Chin-A-Paw, M. J., de Graff, C., de Groot, L., & van Staveren, W. A. (2001). Appraisal of 4 months' consumption of nutrient-dense foods within the daily feeding pattern of frail elderly. *Journal of Aging and Health, 13*, 200–216.

ElderWeb. (n.d.). Average length of nursing home stay. Retrieved May 1, 2006, from http://www.elderweb.com/home/node/ 2770

Endres, J., Welch, P., Ashraf, H., Banz, W., & Gower, E. (2000). Acceptance of soy foods by the elderly in a long-term care facility. *Journal of Nutrition in the Elderly, 19*, 1–17.

Gibson, R. S. (2005). *Principles of Nutritional Assessment* (2nd ed.). New York: Oxford University Press.

Institute of Medicine. (1997). *Dietary Reference Intakes for Calcium, Phosphorus, Magnesium, Vitamin D, and Fluoride*. Washington, DC: National Academy Press.

Johnson, L. E., Dooley, P. A., & Gleick, J. G. (1993). Oral nutritional supplement use in elderly nursing home patients. *Journal of the American Geriatrics Society, 41*, 947–952.

Kayser-Jones, J., Schell, E. S., Porter, C., Barbaccia, J. C., & Shaw, H. (1999). Factors contributing to dehydration in nursing homes: Inadequate staffing and lack of professional super-

vision. *Journal of the American Geriatrics Society, 47*, 1187–1193.

Kral, T. V., & Rolls, B. J. (2004). Energy density and portion size: Their independent and combined effects on energy intake. *Physiology & Behavior, 82*, 131–138.

Lacey, K., & Pritchett, E. (2003). Nutrition care process and model: ADA adopts road map to quality care and outcomes management. *Journal of the American Dietetic Association, 103*, 1061–1072.

Morley, J. E. (2003). Anorexia and weight loss in older persons. *Journal of Gerontology, 58A*, 131–137.

Nevins, D. A., Gluch, L. A., Castellanos, V. H., & RD Council for Quality Nursing Home Care. (2003). Most common causative factors for F371 deficiencies in long-term care state surveys. *Journal of the American Dietetic Association, 103*, A42.

Olin, A. O., Armyr, I., Soop, M., Jerstrom, S., Classon, I., Cederholm, T., et al. (2003). Energy-dense meals improve energy intake in elderly residents in a nursing home. *Clinical Nutrition, 22*, 125–131.

Olin, A. O., Osterberg, P., Hadell, K., Armyr, I., Jerstrom, S., & Ljungqvist, O. (1996). Energy-enriched hospital food to improve energy intake in elderly patients. *Journal of Parenteral and Enteral Nutrition, 20*, 93–97.

Rahman, A. N., & Simmons, S. F. (2005). Individualizing nutritional care with between-meal snacks for nursing home residents. *Journal of the American Medical Directors Association, 6*, 215–218.

Rolls, B. J., & Phillips, P. A. (1990). Aging and disturbances of thirst and fluid balance. *Nutrition Reviews, 48*, 137–143.

Ross, F. (1999). An audit of nutritional supplement distribution and consumption on a care of the elderly ward. *Journal of the Human Nutritional Diet, 12*, 445–452.

Shatenstein, B., & Ferland, G. (2000). Absence of nutritional or clinical consequences of decentralized bulk food portioning in elderly nursing home residents with dementia in Montreal. *Journal of the American Dietetic Association, 100*, 1354–1360.

Simmons, S. F., Alessi, C., & Schnelle, J. F. (2001). An intervention to increase fluid intake in nursing home residents: Prompting and preference compliance. *Journal of the American Geriatrics Society, 49*, 926–934.

Simmons, S. F., Babinou, S., Garcia, E., & Schnelle, J. F. (2002). Quality assessment in nursing homes by systematic direct observations: Feeding assistance. *Journal of Gerontology. Series A, Biological Sciences and Medical Sciences, 57*, M665–M671.

Simmons, S. F., Garcia, E. T., Cadogan, M. P., Al-Samarrai, N. R., Levy-Storms, L. F., Osterweil, D., et al. (2003). The minimum data set weight-loss quality indicator: Does it reflect differences in care processes related to weight loss? *Journal of the American Geriatrics Society, 51*, 1410–1418.

Simmons, S. F., Lam, H. Y., Rao, G., & Schnelle, J. F. (2003). Family members' preferences for nutrition interventions to improve nursing home residents' oral food and fluid intake. *Journal of the American Geriatrics Society, 51*, 69–74.

Simmons, S. F., Osterweil, D., & Schnelle, J. F. (2001). Improving food intake in nursing home residents with feeding assistance: A staffing analysis. *Journal of Gerontology. Series A, Biological Sciences and Medical Sciences, 56*, M790–M794.

Simmons, S. F., & Reuben, D. (2000). Nutritional intake monitoring for nursing home residents: A comparison of staff documentation, direct observation, and photography methods. *Journal of the American Geriatrics Society, 48,* 209–213.

Simmons, S. F., & Schnelle, J. F. (2004). Individualized feeding assistance care for nursing home residents: Staffing requirements to implement two interventions. *Journal of Gerontology. Series A, Biological Sciences and Medical Sciences, 59A,* 966–973.

Splett, P. L., Roth-Yousey, L. L., & Vogelzang, J. L. (2003). Medical nutrition therapy for the prevention and treatment of unintentional weight loss in residential healthcare facilities. *Journal of the American Dietetic Association, 103,* 352–362.

Wilson, M. M. G., Purushothaman, R., & Morley, J. E. (2002). Effect of liquid dietary supplements on energy intake in the elderly. *American Journal of Clinical Nutrition, 75,* 944–947.

Young, K. W., Binns, M. A., & Greenwood, C. E. (2001). Meal delivery practices do not meet needs of Alzheimer patients with increased cognitive and behavioral difficulties in a long-term care facility. *Journal of Gerontology. Series A, Biological Sciences and Medical Sciences, 56,* M656–M661.

Special Topics in Nutrition and Ethics: Nutritional and Ethical Issues at the End of Life

Judith Sharlin, PhD, RD, and I. David Todres, MD

CHAPTER OUTLINE

Reader Objectives

After studying this chapter and reflecting on the contents, you should be able to

1. Address the appropriate uses and methods for artificial nutrition and hydration and the role of the registered dietitian at the end of life.
2. Describe the benefits, risks, and burdens associated with artificial nutrition and hydration.
3. Apply an ethical framework for decision-making regarding the appropriateness of artificial nutrition and hydration.
4. Learn the legal application of ethical principles and understand two seminal cases regarding tube-feeding termination.
5. Understand the use of advanced directives and how they affect decision-making in long-term tube-feeding care.

Artificial Nutrition and Hydration: Definition, Indications, and Prevalence

Nutrition and hydration and the end of life are considered by health care professionals to be medical interventions (American Dietetic Association, 2002). It is the patient's articulated desire for extent of medical care that should be the driving force for determining the level of nutrition intervention (American Dietetic Association, 2002). Before any medical, nutritional, or ethical decisions can be made about a patient's care, however, it is important to understand the definitions of artificial nutrition and hydration. Artificial nutrition and hydration (ANH) is defined as "any nutrition and/or hydration support of an invasive nature requiring placement of a tube into the alimentary tract or parenterally via intravenous or subcutaneous means" (Burge et al., 1995). Tube feeding is used for patients with a functioning gastrointestinal tract who cannot eat or who are unable to swallow (McMahon, Hurley, Kamath, & Mueller, 2005). Tube feeding can include nasoenteric, gastrostomy, and jejunostomy tubes. Since medical advancements in the 1980s, percutaneous endoscopic gastrostomy (PEG) tubes have become the method of choice for long-term tube feeding (Ponsky & Gauderer, 1981).

The benefits of the use of the PEG tube in patients with certain diseases include that these tubes may prolong life and may help alleviate the discomfort of symptoms and enhance quality of life (Ganzini, 2006). PEG feeding tubes extend life by improving nutrition, lessening dehydration, reducing aspiration, and helping to heal pressure sores. Health care professionals, patients, and families also perceive tube feeding to be less invasive than parenteral nutrition. In addition, tube feeding has fewer complications and is less costly than parenteral nutrition (McMahon, 2004; Hurley & McMahon, 2005).

There has been a dramatic increase in the placement of PEG tubes in patients—from 61,000 in 1988 to 121,000 in 1995. About 30% of those patients receiving PEG tubes had dementia (Rabeneck, Wray, & Petersen, 1996). Studies of PEG tubes and patients with dementia have shown 30-day post-PEG mortality to be as high as 25% to 30% (Cox, 2006). The use of PEG tubes and its negative outcomes in older adults with advanced dementia has been documented. In reviewing studies from 1966 through 1999 on tube-feeding patients with advanced dementia, none of them showed any of the (previously mentioned) benefits to the patient: prolonged life, reduced risk of pressure sores or infections, preventing aspiration pneumonia, or palliative care (Finucane, Christmas, & Travis, 1999). There is also no evidence showing survival benefits with the PEG tube in patients suffering terminal diseases, including Alzheimer's disease, amyotrophic lateral sclerosis, and terminal stages of cancer (Rabeneck et al., 1996). More education is needed among health care professionals and families to alleviate conflicts around feeding problems in patients with dementia.

In many states there are financial incentives in nursing facilities for tube feeding, even though many experts believe it is more ethical and effective to spoon feed these patients (Ganzini, 2006). Many nursing home settings are, unfortunately, driven by profit and state regulations. Although it is more labor intensive to feed patients by hand (Mitchell, Buchanan, Littlehale, & Hamel, 2003), it is more nurturing for patients. Hand feeding may provide patients with appropriate social and sensory stimulation that enhances quality of life.

The major complication associated with tube feeding is aspiration. Aspiration occurs between 25% and 40% of patients who are receiving tube feeding (McClave & Chang, 2003). Major risk factors include a history of previous aspiration, depressed level of consciousness, neuromuscular disease, vomiting, and prolonged supine position (McClave, DeMeo, et al., 2002).

Dehydration

There is a current debate whether or not terminally ill patients facing imminent death benefit from dehydration. Deprivation of water causes a decrease in secretions, urinary output, edema, and ascites and increases an endogenous dynorphin that acts as a very potent opiate, which calms the patient (Printz, 1992). Dehydration also causes confusion and lethargy in dying patients secondary to hyponatremia (Sullivan, 1993). However, other researchers have shown dehydration to be isotonic in the dying patient and have discounted the hyper- and hyponatremic effects (Cox, 2006). Studies of cancer patients have shown that more than two-thirds complain of thirst or dry mouth at the end of life (Huang & Ahronheim, 2000). Contrary to healthy individuals, however, thirst in advanced cancer patients appears to be unrelated to dehydration and serum sodium and is not relieved by fluids. In fact, some terminally ill patients have experienced uncomfortable and painful effects from the administration of fluids, including increased urinary output, diarrhea, nausea, and respiratory problems (Viola, Wells, & Peterson, 1997).

Fluid overload from artificial hydration increases pulmonary and gastrointestinal secretions, urinary output, and pharyngeal secretions that could lead to the choking and gurgling sounds known as the "death rattle" (Gallagher, 1989). A study showed increased peripheral edema, ascites, and pleural effusions with modest hydration and no difference in bronchial secretion or delirium (Morita et al., 2005). Research has strongly suggested that oral disease is the main cause of thirst in terminally ill patients (Byock, 1995). Most health care professionals in palliative care promote the use of good mouth care and sips of water and ice chips, when desired (Ersek, 2003). At the end of life, a decrease in food and fluid intake seems to be part of the natural physiology of dying (Burge et al., 1995). Data from hospice health workers suggest that not eating and drinking at the end of life causes little suffering.

Meaning of Food and Drink

In patient care both food and drink have psychological and physical functions as well as many social meanings. Giving food and drink encompasses strong cultural and emotional values that are often equated with nurturing and caring. Providing nutrition and hydration is, however, not synonymous with eating or with feeding someone. Normally, people eat through the mouth with utensils. A medical intervention such as ANH is not considered socially normative (Slomka, 2003). In fact, until recently the term "tube feeding" was called "forced feeding."

In the position paper of the American Dietetic Association (2002) concerning ethical and legal issues in nutrition, hydration, and feeding, the following guidelines were proposed for oral intake (nutrition and hydration):

1. Oral feeding should be advocated whenever possible.
2. The patient's physical and emotional enjoyment of food should be the primary consideration. Staff and family members should be encouraged to assist in feeding the patient.

3. Nutrition supplements should be used to encourage oral intake and alleviate painful symptoms associated with hunger, thirst, or malnutrition.
4. Diet restrictions should be reevaluated.
5. The patient has the right to determine whether he or she wants to consume foods outside of the "diet prescription."
6. Suboptimal oral feedings may be more appropriate than tube or parenteral feeding.

Finally, it seems appropriate for the health care professional to ask the following questions: Is withholding or withdrawing ANH the same as denying food and drink? Is there a "moral imperative" required by human decency to provide nutrition and hydration (Slomka, 2003)?

Roles of the Registered Dietitian

Registered dietitians are in a unique position, because of their education and background, to work collaboratively with the health care team to make nutrition, hydration, and feeding recommendations. Registered dietitians are trained to assess patients' nutritional needs, offer nutritional counseling, and provide meals that reduce side effects of medicine and treatment. Dietitians can also encourage patients and families to suggest or supply their own favorite meals, if appropriate, and to assist in hand feeding patients. Often, a registered dietitian's familiarity with practical aspects of food and fluid at the end of life are helpful to answer families' concerns and questions about chewing, swallowing, and the cessation of thirst and hunger.

A registered dietitian may be able to best express "knowing what is wanted" by the patient because they are the main conversation partners about feeding issues with the patient and family (American Dietetic Association, 2002). They are in a position to contribute the most accurate information on nutritional value judgments. The registered dietitian is trained in medical nutrition therapy and teaching so that he or she can assume the responsibility of keeping the patient's understanding of the options and outcomes about feeding in the center of the deliberation. The registered dietitian has the responsibility to make sure all options about feeding are deliberated, rather than assuming that one strategy is obligatory. For example, a situation might occur with a patient in which tube feeding seems to be the only option when, in fact, careful hand feeding may be a better alternative for adequate nutrition. Finally, the dietitian's role, along with the rest of the health care team, is to promote a compassionate and positive experience for the patient, family, and loved ones at the end of life.

Ethical Principles as a Framework for Decision-Making

The practice of long-term tube feeding has escalated over the past two decades as a result of an aging population and new technology. Ensuring that the patient is given food and water is an important symbolic nurturing act that is deeply rooted in cultural and religious traditions. However, in special circumstances it may be morally correct to consider it inappropriate to provide ANH to the patient. This consideration raises strong emotional reactions and leads to anguished decision-making for patients, families, and health care workers. Appreciating the ethical principles underlying these decisions is helpful in ensuring that the patient's care rests on a strong moral foundation (Mueller, Hook, & Fleming, 2004; Casarett, Kapo, & Caplan, 2005; McMahon et al., 2005).

The Terri Schiavo Case

To understand the ethical issues raised in the appropriateness of long-term tube feeding, it is helpful to review the recent case of Terri Schiavo (Gostin, 1997). This case highlighted the complexities of medicine, ethics, law, and family dynamics in deciding on the appropriateness of ANH for Terri Schiavo. The patient had suffered a cardiac arrest in 1990 as a result of an electrolyte imbalance precipitated by an eating disorder. The patient had been sustained by ANH through a feeding tube for 15 years. A struggle that was fought out in the courts and the public resulted from a wish by the patient's husband to discontinue ANH and the patient's parents and siblings insisting on ANH being continued.

The facts of the case clearly demonstrated that Ms. Schiavo was in a permanent vegetative state (PVS), a state in which there is no higher cortical functioning and therefore no cognition. Initially, PVS is considered a persistent state, and after a period of 1 year this state becomes permanent. This was attested to by multiple neurologic examinations and is an important point because the facts have to be clear and consistent for a successful ethical discussion. Because there was no conscious awareness, there would be no suffering on her part. Ms. Schiavo was not in a position to state her own wishes—the principle of autonomy rooted in the precept of respect for the person—but her wishes would have been known had she left an advance directive regarding her future care. Because no advance directive was left, the principle of **substituted judgment** was applied through statements by her closest family. Legally, the designated decision-maker was Terri Schiavo's husband, who requested withdrawal of the tube feeding.

When the patient's wishes cannot be ascertained (e.g., in the case of an infant or one who has always been incompetent to rationally choose), then treatment decisions are based on the patient's best interests—that is, what a reasonable person would most likely want in the same circumstances (Annas, 2004). Ms. Schiavo's parents and siblings did not accept the diagnosis of PVS and believed the condition would improve with further rehabilitative care. The parents strongly believed that withdrawal of the feeding tube would violate their daughter's Catholic belief and be tantamount to euthanasia. This belief, that the withdrawal of feeding would be morally wrong, had the support of a recent allocution by the late Pope John Paul II, who stated that for patients in PVS, "the administration of water and food even when provided by artificial means of preserving life, [is] not a medical act . . . and as such is morally obligatory" (Pope John Paul II, 2004). According to Paris (2005), this interpretation of the Catholic position on the sanctity of life is not consistent with traditional church teaching, and Paris cites the 2001 directive of the U.S. Catholic bishops that states, "A person may forgo means that in the patient's judgment do not offer a reasonable hope or benefit and entail an excessive burden" (Paris, 2005).

There were multiple court hearings and repeated episodes of tube withdrawal and replacement. The case was also politicized, until finally it involved the president of the United States. However, in the end the judicial court ruling of withdrawal of the tube was carried out (Quill, 2005). Ms. Schiavo died a few days after the withdrawal of tube feeding.

Surveys of the attitudes of the American public regarding the Terri Schiavo case were carried out (Blendon, Benson, & Herrmann, 2005). Twelve national opinion surveys showed that most Americans opposed efforts by elected politicians to intervene in the Schiavo case. However, the public was more divided on the question of whether Schiavo's feeding tube should be removed. A substantial minority, 24% to 42%, opposed it. Of interest too is that one-third of respondents believed she could experience pain and discomfort when the feeding tube was withdrawn.

The Nancy Cruzan Case

The 1990 Nancy Cruzan case also illustrates the legal and ethical approach to withdrawal of tube feeding (*Cruzan v. Director,* 1990). Ms. Cruzan was a patient who had been diagnosed as in a PVS. Her parents brought the issue of withdrawal of tube feeding to the courts. The family was united in this. The Missouri Supreme Court noted that tube feeding could be discontinued on the basis of Nancy's right of self-determination. However, because she was in a PVS she was unable to make that decision, and the court stated that tube feeding could be stopped only if those speaking for her could produce "clear and convincing" evidence that she would refuse the tube feeding if she could speak for herself. Eventually, evidence was brought forward to this effect and the tube feeding was discontinued.

Advance Directives

The Nancy Cruzan case stimulated the public to ensure that individuals could convey personal wishes regarding their care through advance directives or assignments of durable power of attorney. The advance directive would take the form of a "living will" or designation of a health care proxy (Hanson & Rodgman, 1996; Hofmann et al., 1997; Tulsky, Fischer, Rose, & Arnold, 1998; Gillick, 2004). By 2000 every state had passed some form of living will or health care proxy law.

The optimal way in which an advance directive should be implemented is to designate one or more persons to act on our behalf to make the treatment decisions when we are unable to make them ourselves (Annas, 2004). This is done in writing using a health care proxy form. It is also important to inform the person or persons designated (often family) how one wants to be treated in specific situations, for example, "do not wish to be tube fed." Doing this verbally is acceptable, but it is preferred to have the instructions in a written letter or living will.

A living will also has its shortcomings. Interventions will be employed by the medical team that the patient may not want to have. This is often difficult to predict. However, with a trusted health care agent who is made aware of your goals of care and your values, the right decision will be made that is in your best interests. The health care proxy assumes responsibility when the patient becomes incompetent. Despite the ethical advantages of an **advance directive**, however, only one-fifth of the public have one in place (Morrison, Zayas, Mulvihill, Baskin, & Meier, 1998).

> **Advance directive:** Information in written or oral form provided by the patient that outlines the competent adult's wishes regarding medical treatment should he or she become incompetent in the future.

The Anthony Bland Case

This seminal case in Britain involved a young man, Anthony Bland, who was in a PVS for three years. The courts were asked to adjudicate the withdrawal of food and water administered by a tube. The case eventually reached the highest court in Britain, the law lords in the High Court. The overall decision was to support the withdrawal of ANH. However, of ethical interest are the different approaches by which the justices came to this decision. Some stated it would be an assault to continue to treat without his consent. Others stated that continued treatment would be futile; still others stated it could not be in his best interests to continue to provide treatment that had no prospect of improving his condition. They made the distinction that because he required assisted feeding via a tube, he was unable to feed himself. Therefore it was held that ANH was a medical treatment, which could be withdrawn on the grounds of futility (McClean & Mason, 2003).

Special Condition of Dementia

The wisdom of providing tube feeding in patients with severe dementia has come under question (Finucane et al., 1999; Mitchell, Tetroe, & O'Connor, 2001; Post, 2001; Meier, Ahronheim, Morris, Baskin-Lyons, & Morrison, 2002). Tube feeding seldom achieves its intended medical aims in this condition and rather than prevent suffering can cause it; thus it should not be recommended to patients with advanced dementia (Gillick, 2000). These patients often pull out their tubes and therefore have to be restrained, leading to further agitation and distress, with the need for pharmacologic sedation. Also, the feeding tube fails to prevent pulmonary aspiration, because this usually occurs as a result of gastric reflux and aspiration of saliva. Survival rates in patients with tube feeding are not extended (Sanders et al., 2000). Overall, there is little benefit for gastrostomy tubes and much potential for harm.

Withdrawing or Withholding Treatment

Many believe it is more acceptable to withhold a treatment than to withdraw it. This distinction is not supported by currently accepted ethical and legal reasoning (Beauchamp & Childress, 2001; Meisel & Cerminara, 2004).

Some have argued that there is an analogy between tube feeding and mechanical ventilation: Both are seen as medical treatments, and withdrawal of one has the same ethical and legal foundation as the other. Others have argued, however, that mechanical ventilation replaces the capacity to breathe, whereas a tube does not replace the capacity to digest but merely delivers food to the stomach (Keown, 2002).

With regard to withholding or withdrawing ANH from terminally ill or permanently unconscious patients, the courts have decreed that administration of ANH is like any other medical treatment and may be withdrawn if the patient refuses the treatment or, in the case of the incapacitated patient, the appropriate standard is met (Meisel, Snyder, Quill, & the American College of Physicians–American Society of Internal Medicine End-of-Life Care Consensus Panel, 2000). This followed the U.S. Supreme Court's 1990 *Cruzan* decision giving qualified approval to this practice. In this situation the death of the patient results from the patient's underlying condition, so there is no legal liability for the patient's death.

Quality of Life

Quality of life at the end of life is receiving increasing attention. In considering the patient at the end of life, the whole person's physical, psychological, social, and spiritual parts need to be considered because they significantly affect the person's experience of illness (Singer, Martin, & Kelner, 1999). It is estimated that almost 85% of Americans who continue to die in hospitals and nursing homes are denied the benefits of palliative care at this time (Rummans, Bostwick, & Clark, 2000). Modern sophisticated technologies are often accompanied by increased suffering, pain, and emotional distress. It is important for health care workers to recognize that their own biases and misconceptions can greatly influence patients' emotional, social, and spiritual distress.

Moral Distinction Between Killing and Letting Die

Of concern in the act of withdrawing tube feeding is the moral distinction between killing and letting die. It is legally and ethically acceptable to allow a patient to die when the burdens and risks of life-prolonging treatment clearly outweigh their benefits. Legally, an act of killing is murder if it was intended and is prohibited in our culture. When ANH is withdrawn the foreseen death occurs from natural

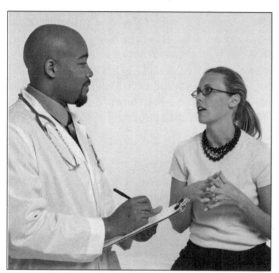

causes. There can be ambiguity around the cause of death when the feeding tube is withdrawn. Some argue that withdrawal of the tube is the cause of death. However, death is caused by the underlying failure of an organ system; the fundamental cause of death is the patient's condition, not the withdrawal of treatment. The life support has on a temporary basis postponed the death. If there is no reasonable hope of recovery, further life-sustaining treatment cannot benefit the patient, and therefore it is not in the patient's interests to continue it. When it is removed, the body's own causality results in the death (Randall & Downie, 1999).

Communication

Effective communication often helps to prevent ethical dilemmas. In communicating with the patient we need to learn the patient's values, goals, and beliefs. It is also very important that the prognosis and facts associated with the patient's condition are clearly spelled out and mutually understood. The process of informed consent should be carefully carried out, not rushed, and with a mutual understanding of the patient's goals of care (Brett & Rosenberg, 2001). Deep-rooted cultural and religious beliefs affect the patient's approach to the consideration of the appropriateness of long-term tube feeding (Orr, Marshall, & Osborn, 1995; Helman, 2000). Some patients and especially families consider removal of tube feeding as unethical because it is a state of "starvation" (Helman, 2000; Pope John Paul II, 2004).

Patients' families at times believe that lack of ANH causes suffering and will demand that "everything be done" to avoid this, including placement of PEG and long-term tube feeding. However, clinicians are not obligated to provide futile treatment (Snyder, Leffler, & the Ethics and Human Rights Committee, American College of Physicians, 2005). It is necessary to clearly define what is meant by futile. This judgment must take into account the goals of care, the proposed treatment, and the outcome so that we are virtually certain the goal cannot be achieved.

How the issue of ANH is presented to the patient and family requires compassion and appropriate choice of words that are clearly communicated. An example of this was provided by clinicians caring for amyotrophic lateral sclerosis patients based on their clinical experience. They explained that PEG had risks, such as infection at the site of the tube, disfigurement of body shape, and diarrhea or constipation that may not always be transient. They also explained that tube feeding was cumbersome and with loss of hand movement required an assistant at every meal. The clinicians told patients that to decide against tube feeding was okay and they wouldn't starve because their bodies would adjust and not feel hunger. However, many patients have stated that they wished they'd chosen it sooner (Mitsumoto & Rabkin, 2007).

Many health care workers, unfamiliar with the ethical arguments, the law in the state in which they practice, and the fact that the Supreme Court justices decreed ANH to be a form of medical treatment and could be terminated, align themselves with family concerns that their loved one would "starve to death." In a study of physicians regarding ANH appropriateness, 34% of medical attending physicians and 45% of surgical attending physicians that responded believed that even if life support in the form of mechanical ventilation of dialysis was stopped, nutrition and hydration should always be continued (Solomon et al., 1993).

Summary

The increasing use of tube feeding has led to a consideration of the appropriateness based on the benefits and burdens associated with the procedure. Studies have been carried out to assess the patients' and families' preferences and the experience of tube feeding being withheld.

When a decision is considered that enteral tube feeding is indicated, the patient is informed of the risks and benefits of the intervention and alternatives, including doing nothing. This is the basis of informed consent, and the patient demonstrates a clear understanding of the issues and appropriate decision-making capacity. Respecting the patient's choice is the principle of **autonomy** and in our culture has come to override the other principle of **beneficence**—that is, doing good (or nonmalfeasance—that is, not doing harm). The need for advanced directives is stressed as a means to ensure the patient's wishes are respected at all times. Optimal care of the patient involves a multidisciplinary approach in which the registered dietitian should play an active role in all decisions made by the health care team.

> **Autonomy:** The paramount ethical principle that states the competent adult has the right to make choices about treatment options.
>
> **Beneficence:** The ethical principle of doing good; for example, proposing a therapy that is worthwhile for the patient (patient centered). This agrees with the ethical principle of nonmalfeasance, which is "not doing any harm."

Case Studies

(Answers to all case studies are in the Instructor's Manual available at jbpub.com.)

Case Study and Issues to Debate

The patient is an 82-year-old with severe Alzheimer's dementia. He has had repeated episodes of aspiration pneumonia. He lacks decision-making capacity and had not left an advance directive as to his care wishes. Identifying the ethically relevant facts is considered under the following in this case (Jonsen et al., 2002):

1. Medical indication for long-term tube feeding: The principles of beneficence and nonmalfeasance (do no harm) are applied. Will the patient benefit from the procedures, and will the procedure hurt more than help?
2. Patient preferences: Respect for autonomy is the primary principle. Does the patient have decision-making capacity? Lacking this capacity, is there an appropriate surrogate?
3. Quality of life: The principles of beneficence, nonmalfeasance, and autonomy are considered. In this case the evidence appears to indicate no worthwhile benefits to tube feeding, whereas the procedure has significant risks.
4. Contextual features: Cultural and religious traditions need to be taken into account. If there is a conflict of interest with regard to the clinician's or institution's standards, consideration should be given to transfer to another clinician or institution.

References

American Academy of Hospice and Palliative Medicine. (2006, December 8). Statement on the use of nutrition and hydration. Retrieved July 24, 2009, from http://www.aahpm.org/positions/nutrition.html

American Dietetic Association. (2002). Ethical and legal issues in nutrition, hydration and feeding. *Journal of the American Dietetic Association, 102,* 716–726.

American Nurses Association. (1992, April 2). Position statement on foregoing nutrition and fluid. ANA Nursing World. Retrieved July 24, 2009, from http://www.nursingworld.org/EthicsHumanRights

Annas, G. J. (2004). *The Rights of Patients* (3rd ed.). New York: New York University Press.

Annas, G. J. (2005). "Culture of life" politics at the bedside: The case of Terri Schiavo. *New England Journal of Medicine, 352,* 1710–1715.

Beauchamp, T. L., & Childress, J. F. (2001). *Principles of Biomedical Ethics* (6th ed.). New York: Oxford University Press.

Blendon, R. J., Benson, J. M., & Herrmann, M. J. (2005). The American public and the Terri Schiavo case. *Archives of Internal Medicine, 65,* 2580–2584.

Brett, A. S., & Rosenberg, J. C. (2001). The adequacy of informed consent for placement of gastrostomy tubes. *Archives of Internal Medicine, 161,* 745–748.

Burge, F., Byock, I., Daniels, D., Mueller, F., Schmale, J., & William, C. (1995). Artificial hydration and nutrition in the terminally ill: A review. *Academy of Hospice Physicians.*

Byock, I. (1995). Patient refusal of nutrition and hydration: Walking an ever-finer line. *American Journal of Hospice Palliative Care, 12,* 8–13.

Casarett, D., Kapo, J., & Caplan, A. (2005). Appropriate use of artificial nutrition and hydration: Fundamental principles and recommendations. *New England Journal of Medicine, 353,* 2607–2612.

Cox, A. (2006). End-of-life nutrition and hydration: Issues and ethics. *Today's Dietitian, 7,* 35–40.

Cruzan v. Director, Missouri Department of Health, 110 S.Ct. 2841 (1990).

Ersek, M. (2003). Artificial nutrition and hydration: Clinical issues. *Journal of Hospice Palliative Care Nursing, 5,* 221–230.

Finucane, T. E., Christmas, C., & Travis, K. (1999). Tube feeding in patients with advanced dementia: A review of the evidence. *Journal of the American Medical Association, 282,* 1365–1370.

Gallagher, A. C. R. (1989). *Nutritional Care of the Terminally Ill.* Rockville, MD: Aspen Publishers.

Ganzini, L. (2006). Artificial nutrition and hydration at the end of life: Ethics and evidence. *Palliative and Supportive Care, 4,* 135–143.

Ganzini, L., Goy, E. R., Miller, L. L., Harvath, T. A., Jackson, A., & Delorit, M. A. (2003). Nurses' experiences with hospice patients who refuse food and fluids to hasten death. *New England Journal of Medicine, 349,* 359–365.

Gillick, M. R. (2000). Rethinking the role of tube feeding in patients with advanced dementia. *New England Journal of Medicine, 342,* 206–210.

Gillick, M. R. (2004). Advance care planning. *New England Journal of Medicine, 350,* 7–8.

Gostin, L. O. (1997). Deciding life and death in the courtroom: From Quinlan to Cruzan, Glucksberg, and Vacco: A brief history and analysis of constitutional protection of the "right to die." *Journal of the American Medical Association, 278,* 1523–1528.

Hanson, L. C., & Rodgman, E. (1996). The use of living wills at the end of life: A national study. *Archives of Internal Medicine, 156,* 1018–1022.

Helman, C. (2000). *Culture, Health, and Illness* (4th ed.). Oxford: Butterworth–Heinemann.

Hofmann, J. C., Wenger, N. S., Davis, R. B., Teno, J., Connors, A. F. Jr., Desbiens, N., et al. (1997). Patient preferences for communication with physicians about end of life decisions. *Annals of Internal Medicine, 127,* 1–12.

Huang, Z. B., & Ahronheim, J. C. (2000). Nutrition and hydration in terminally ill patients: An update. *Clinics in Geriatric Medicine, 16,* 313–325.

Hurley, D. L., & McMahon, M. M. (2005). Diabetes mellitus. In R. H. Rolandelli, R. Bankhead, J. I. Boulatta, & C. W. Com-

pher (Eds.), *Clinical Nutrition: Enteral and Tube Feeding* (4th ed., pp. 498–505). Philadelphia: Elsevier Saunders.

Jonsen, A. R., Siegler, M., & Winslade, W. J. (2002). *Clinical Ethics: A Practical Approach to Ethical Decisions in Clinical Medicine* (5th ed.). New York: McGraw-Hill.

Keown, J. (2002). *Euthanasia, Ethics and Public Policy.* Cambridge: Cambridge University Press.

McClave, S. A., & Chang, W. K. (2003). Complications of enteral access. *Gastrointestinal Endoscopy, 58,* 739–751.

McClave, S. A., DeMeo, M. T., DeLegge, M. H., DiSario, J. A., Heyland, D. K., Maloney, J. P., et al. (2002). North American Summit on Aspiration in the Critically Ill Patient: Consensus statement. *JPEN. Journal of Parenteral and Enteral Nutrition, 26*(6 Suppl.), 580–585.

McClean, S., & Mason, G. K. (2003). *Legal and Ethical Aspects of Health Care* (p. 165). London: Greenwich Medical Media.

McMahon, M. M. (2004). Parenteral nutrition. In L. Goldman & D. Aussiello (Eds.), *Cecil's Textbook of Medicine* (vol. 2, 22nd ed., pp. 1322–1326). Philadelphia: W. B. Saunders and Co.

McMahon, M. M., Hurley, D. L., Kamath, P. S., & Mueller, P. S. (2005). Medical and ethical aspects of long-term enteral tube feeding. *Mayo Clinic Proceedings, 80,* 1461–1476.

Meier, D. E., Ahronheim, J. C., Morris, J., Baskin-Lyons, S., & Morrison, R. S. (2002). High short-term mortality in hospitalized patients with advanced dementia: Lack of benefit of tube feeding. *Archives of Internal Medicine, 161,* 594–599.

Meisel, A., & Cerminara, K. L. (2004). *The Right to Die: The Law of End-of-Life Decision Making* (3rd ed.). New York: Aspen.

Meisel, A., Snyder, L., Quill, T., & the American College of Physicians–American Society of Internal Medicine End-of-Life Care Consensus Panel. (2000). Seven legal barriers to end-of-life care: Myths, realities, and grains of truth. *Journal of the American Medical Association, 284,* 2495–2501.

Mitchell, S. L., Buchanan, J. L., Littlehale, S., & Hamel, M. B. (2003). Tube feeding versus hand feeding nursing home residents in advanced dementia. *Journal of the American Geriatrics Society, 51,* 129–131.

Mitchell, S. L., Tetroe, J., & O'Connor, A. M. (2001). A decision aid for long-term tube feeding in cognitively impaired older persons. *Journal of the American Geriatrics Society, 49,* 313–316.

Mitsumoto, H., & Rabkin, J. G. (2007). Palliative care for patients with amyotrophic lateral sclerosis. *Journal of the American Medical Association, 298,* 207–216.

Morita, T., Hyodo, I., Yoshimi, T., Ikenaga, M., Tamura, Y., Yoshizawa, A., et al. (2005). Association between hydration volume and symptoms in terminally ill cancer patients with abdominal malignancies. *Annals of Oncology, 16,* 640–647.

Morrison, R. S., Zayas, L. H., Mulvihill, M., Baskin, S. A., & Meier, D. E. (1998). Barriers to completion of health care proxies: An examination of ethnic differences. *Archives of Internal Medicine, 158,* 2493–2497.

Mueller, P. S., Hook, C. C., & Fleming, K. C. (2004). Ethical issues in geriatrics: A guide for clinicians. *Mayo Clinic Proceedings, 79,* 554–562.

Orr, R. D., Marshall, P. A., & Osborn, J. (1995). Cross-cultural considerations in clinical ethics consultations. *Archives of Family Medicine, 4,* 159–164.

Paris, J. J. (2005). To feed or not to feed: Terri Schiavo and the use of artificial nutrition and fluids. *Southern Medical Journal, 98,* 757–758.

Ponsky, J. L., & Gauderer, M. W. L. (1981). Percutaneous endoscopic gastrostomy, a non-operative technique for feeding gastrostomy. *Gastrointestinal Endoscopy, 27,* 9–11.

Pope John Paul II. (2004). Address to the participants in the International Congress on Life Sustaining Treatments and Vegetative States: Scientific advances and ethical dilemmas. *Origins, 33,* 738–740.

Post, S. G. (2001). Tube feeding and advanced progressive dementia. *Hastings Center Report, 31,* 36–42.

Printz, L. A. (1992). Terminal dehydration, a compassionate treatment. *Archives of Internal Medicine, 152,* 697–700.

Quill, T. E. (2005). Terri Schiavo: A tragedy compounded. *New England Journal of Medicine, 352,* 1630–1633.

Rabeneck, L., Wray, N. P., & Petersen, N. J. (1996). Long-term outcomes of patients receiving percutaneous endoscopic gastrostomy tubes. *Journal of General and Internal Medicine, 11,* 287–293.

Randall, F., & Downie, R. S. (1999). *Palliative Care Ethics* (2nd ed., p. 271). Oxford: Oxford University Press.

Rummans, T. A., Bostwick, T. M., & Clark, M. M. (2000). For the Mayo Clinic cancer center quality of life working group. *Mayo Clinic Proceedings, 75,* 1305–1310.

Sanders, D. S., Carter, M. J., D'Silva, J., James, G., Bolton, R. P., & Bardhan, K. D. (2000). Survival analysis in percutaneous endoscopic gastrostomy feeding: A worse outcome in patients with dementia. *American Journal of Gastroenterology, 95,* 1472–1475.

Singer, P. A., Martin, D. K., & Kelner, M. (1999). Quality end-of-life care: Patients' perspectives. *Journal of the American Medical Association, 281,* 163–168.

Slomka, J. (2003). Withholding nutrition at the end of life: Clinical and ethical issues. *Cleveland Clinic Journal of Medicine, 70,* 548–552.

Snyder, L., Leffler, C., & the Ethics and Human Rights Committee, American College of Physicians. (2005). Ethics manual. *Annals of Internal Medicine, 142,* 560–582.

Solomon, M. Z., O'Donnell, L., Jennings, B., Guilfoy, V., Wolf, S. M., Nolan, K., et al. (1993). Decisions near the end of life: Professional views on sustaining treatments. *American Journal of Public Health, 83,* 14–23.

Sullivan, R. J. (1993). Accepting death without artificial nutrition or hydration. *Journal of General Medicine, 8,* 220–224.

Tulsky, J. A., Fischer, G. S., Rose, M. R., & Arnold, R. M. (1998). Opening the black box: How do physicians communicate about advance directives? *Annals of Internal Medicine, 129,* 441–449.

Viola, R. A., Wells, G. A., & Peterson, J. (1997). The effects of fluid status and fluid therapy on the dying: A systematic review. *Journal of Palliative Care, 13,* 41–52.

Centers for Disease Control and Prevention Growth Charts

Birth to 36 months: Boys
Length-for-age and Weight-for-age percentiles

NAME _____

RECORD # _____

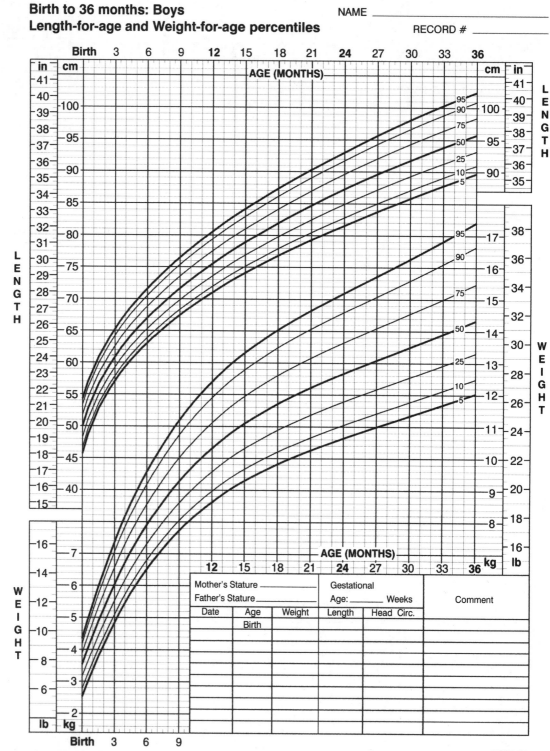

Published May 30, 2000 (modified 4/20/01).
SOURCE: Developed by the National Center for Health Statistics in collaboration with
the National Center for Chronic Disease Prevention and Health Promotion (2000).
http://www.cdc.gov/growthcharts

SAFER · HEALTHIER · PEOPLE™

Birth to 36 months: Girls
Length-for-age and Weight-for-age percentiles

NAME _____

RECORD # _____

Published May 30, 2000 (modified 4/20/01).
SOURCE: Developed by the National Center for Health Statistics in collaboration with
the National Center for Chronic Disease Prevention and Health Promotion (2000).
http://www.cdc.gov/growthcharts

CDC
SAFER · HEALTHIER · PEOPLE™

Dietary Reference Intakes (DRIs)

Dietary Reference Intakes (DRIs): Recommended Intakes for Individuals, Vitamins

Food and Nutrition Board, Institute of Medicine, National Academies

Life Stage Group	Vit A (μg/d)[a]	Vit C (mg/d)	Vit D (μg/d)[b,c]	Vit E (mg/d)[d]	Vit K (μg/d)	Thiamin (mg/d)	Riboflavin (mg/d)	Niacin (mg/d)[e]	Vit B$_6$ (mg/d)	Folate (μg/d)[f]	Vit B$_{12}$ (μg/d)	Pantothenic acid (mg/d)	Biotin (μg/d)	Choline (mg/d)[g]
Infants														
0–6 mo	400*	40*	5*	4*	2.0*	0.2*	0.3*	2*	0.1*	65*	0.4*	1.7*	5*	125*
7–12 mo	500*	50*	5*	5*	2.5*	0.3*	0.4*	4*	0.3*	80*	0.5*	1.8*	6*	150*
Children														
1–3 y	**300**	**15**	5*	**6**	30*	**0.5**	**0.5**	**6**	**0.5**	**150**	**0.9**	2*	8*	200*
4–8 y	**400**	**25**	5*	**7**	55*	**0.6**	**0.6**	**8**	**0.6**	**200**	**1.2**	3*	12*	250*
Males														
9–13 y	**600**	**45**	5*	**11**	60*	**0.9**	**0.9**	**12**	**1.0**	**300**	**1.8**	4*	20*	375*
14–18 y	**900**	**75**	5*	**15**	75*	**1.2**	**1.3**	**16**	**1.3**	**400**	**2.4**	5*	25*	550*
19–30 y	**900**	**90**	5*	**15**	120*	**1.2**	**1.3**	**16**	**1.3**	**400**	**2.4**	5*	30*	550*
31–50 y	**900**	**90**	5*	**15**	120*	**1.2**	**1.3**	**16**	**1.3**	**400**	**2.4**	5*	30*	550*
51–70 y	**900**	**90**	10*	**15**	120*	**1.2**	**1.3**	**16**	**1.7**	**400**	**2.4**[i]	5*	30*	550*
>70 y	**900**	**90**	15*	**15**	120*	**1.2**	**1.3**	**16**	**1.7**	**400**	**2.4**[i]	5*	30*	550*
Females														
9–13 y	**600**	**45**	5*	**11**	60*	**0.9**	**0.9**	**12**	**1.0**	**300**	**1.8**	4*	20*	375*
14–18 y	**700**	**65**	5*	**15**	75*	**1.0**	**1.0**	**14**	**1.2**	**400**[i]	**2.4**	5*	25*	400*
19–30 y	**700**	**75**	5*	**15**	90*	**1.1**	**1.1**	**14**	**1.3**	**400**[i]	**2.4**	5*	30*	425*
31–50 y	**700**	**75**	5*	**15**	90*	**1.1**	**1.1**	**14**	**1.3**	**400**[i]	**2.4**	5*	30*	425*
51–70 y	**700**	**75**	10*	**15**	90*	**1.1**	**1.1**	**14**	**1.5**	**400**	**2.4**[h]	5*	30*	425*
>70 y	**700**	**75**	15*	**15**	90*	**1.1**	**1.1**	**14**	**1.5**	**400**	**2.4**[h]	5*	30*	425*
Pregnancy														
14–18 y	**750**	**80**	5*	**15**	75*	**1.4**	**1.4**	**18**	**1.9**	**600**[j]	**2.6**	6*	30*	450*
19–30 y	**770**	**85**	5*	**15**	90*	**1.4**	**1.4**	**18**	**1.9**	**600**[j]	**2.6**	6*	30*	450*
31–50 y	**770**	**85**	5*	**15**	90*	**1.4**	**1.4**	**18**	**1.9**	**600**[j]	**2.6**	6*	30*	450*
Lactation														
14–18 y	**1,200**	**115**	5*	**19**	75*	**1.4**	**1.6**	**17**	**2.0**	**500**	**2.8**	7*	35*	550*
19–30 y	**1,300**	**120**	5*	**19**	90*	**1.4**	**1.6**	**17**	**2.0**	**500**	**2.8**	7*	35*	550*
31–50 y	**1,300**	**120**	5*	**19**	90*	**1.4**	**1.6**	**17**	**2.0**	**500**	**2.8**	7*	35*	550*

NOTE: This table (taken from the DRI reports, see www.nap.edu) presents Recommended Dietary Allowances (RDAs) in **bold type** and Adequate Intakes (AIs) in ordinary type followed by an asterisk (*). RDAs and AIs may both be used as goals for individual intake. RDAs are set to meet the needs of almost all (97 to 98 percent) individuals in a group. For healthy breast-fed infants, the AI is the mean intake. The AI for other life stage and gender groups is believed to cover needs of all individuals in the group, but lack of data or uncertainty in the data prevent being able to specify with confidence the percentage of individuals covered by this intake.

[a] As retinol activity equivalents (RAEs). 1 RAE = 1 μg retinol, 12 μg β-carotene, 24 μg α-carotene, or 24 μg β-cryptoxanthin. The RAE for dietary provitamin A carotenoids is twofold greater than retinol equivalents (RE), whereas the RAE for preformed vitamin A is the same as RE.

[b] As cholecalciferol. 1 μg cholecalciferol = 40 IU vitamin D.

[c] In the absence of adequate exposure to sunlight.

^{d}As α-tocopherol. α-tocopherol includes *RRR*-α-tocopherol, the only form of α-tocopherol that occurs naturally in foods, and the *2R*-stereoisomeric forms of α-tocopherol (*RRR-*, *RSR-*, *RRS-*, and *RSS*-α-tocopherol) that occur in fortified foods and supplements. It does not include the *2S*-stereoisomeric forms of α-tocopherol (*SRR-*, *SSR-*, *SRS-*, and *SSS*-α-tocopherol), also found in fortified foods and supplements.

^{e}As niacin equivalents (NE). 1 mg of niacin = 60 mg of tryptophan; 0–6 months = preformed niacin (not NE).

^{f}As dietary folate equivalents (DFE). 1 DFE = 1 μg food folate = 0.6 μg of folic acid from fortified food or as a supplement consumed with food = 0.5 μg of a supplement taken on an empty stomach.

^{g}Although AIs have been set for choline, there are few data to assess whether a dietary supply of choline is needed at all stages of the life cycle, and it may be that the choline requirement can be met by endogenous synthesis at some of these stages.

^{h}Because 10 to 30 percent of older people may malabsorb food-bound B_{12}, it is advisable for those older than 50 years to meet their RDA mainly by consuming foods fortified with B_{12} or a supplement containing B_{12}.

^{i}In view of evidence linking folate intake with neural tube defects in the fetus, it is recommended that all women capable of becoming pregnant consume 400 μg from supplements or fortified foods in addition to intake of food folate from a varied diet.

^{j}It is assumed that women will continue consuming 400 μg from supplements or fortified food until their pregnancy is confirmed and they enter prenatal care, which ordinarily occurs after the end of the periconceptional period—the critical time for formation of the neural tube.

Copyright 2004 by the National Academy of Sciences. All rights reserved.

Dietary Reference Intakes (DRIs): Recommended Intakes for Individuals, Elements

Food and Nutrition Board, Institute of Medicine, National Academies

Life Stage Group	Calcium (mg/d)	Chromium (mg/d)	Copper (mg/d)	Fluoride (mg/d)	Iodine (mg/d)	Iron (mg/d)	Magnesium (mg/d)	Manganese (mg/d)	Molybdenum (mg/d)	Phosphorus (mg/d)	Selenium (mg/d)	Zinc (mg/d)	Potassium (g/d)	Sodium (g/d)	Chloride (g/d)
Infants															
0–6 mo	210*	0.2*	200*	0.01*	110*	0.27*	30*	0.003*	2*	100*	15*	2*	0.4*	0.12*	0.18*
7–12 mo	270*	5.5*	220*	0.5*	130*	11	75*	0.6*	3*	275*	20*	3	0.7*	0.37*	0.57*
Children															
1–3 y	500*	11*	340	0.7*	90	7	80	1.2*	17	460	20	3	3.0*	1.0*	1.5*
4–8 y	800*	15*	440	1*	90	10	130	1.5*	22	500	30	5	3.8*	1.2*	1.9*
Males															
9–13 y	1,300*	25*	700	2*	120	8	240	1.9*	34	1,250	40	8	4.5*	1.5*	2.3*
14–18 y	1,300*	35*	890	3*	150	11	410	2.2*	43	1,250	55	11	4.7*	1.5*	2.3*
19–30 y	1,000*	35*	900	4*	150	8	400	2.3*	45	700	55	11	4.7*	1.5*	2.3*
31–50 y	1,000*	35*	900	4*	150	8	420	2.3*	45	700	55	11	4.7*	1.5*	2.3*
51–70 y	1,200*	30*	900	4*	150	8	420	2.3*	45	700	55	11	4.7*	1.3*	2.0*
>70 y	1,200*	30*	900	4*	150	8	420	2.3*	45	700	55	11	4.7*	1.2*	1.8*
Females															
9–13 y	1,300*	21*	700	2*	120	8	240	1.6*	34	1,250	40	8	4.5*	1.5*	2.3*
14–18 y	1,300*	24*	890	3*	150	15	360	1.6*	43	1,250	55	9	4.7*	1.5*	2.3*
19–30 y	1,000*	25*	900	3*	150	18	310	1.8*	45	700	55	8	4.7*	1.5*	2.3*
31–50 y	1,000*	25*	900	3*	150	18	320	1.8*	45	700	55	8	4.7*	1.5*	2.3*
51–70 y	1,200*	20*	900	3*	150	8	320	1.8*	45	700	55	8	4.7*	1.3*	2.0*
>70 y	1,200*	20*	900	3*	150	8	320	1.8*	45	700	55	8	4.7*	1.2*	1.8*
Pregnancy															
14–18 y	1,300*	29*	1,000	3*	220	27	400	2.0*	50	1,250	60	12	4.7*	1.5*	2.3*
19–30 y	1,000*	30*	1,000	3*	220	27	350	2.0*	50	700	60	11	4.7*	1.5*	2.3*
31–50 y	1,000*	30*	1,000	3*	220	27	360	2.0*	50	700	60	11	4.7*	1.5*	2.3*
Lactation															
14–18 y	1,300*	44*	1,300	3*	290	10	360	2.6*	50	1,250	70	13	5.1*	1.5*	2.3*
19–30 y	1,000*	45*	1,300	3*	290	9	310	2.6*	50	700	70	12	5.1*	1.5*	2.3*
31–50 y	1,000*	45*	1,300	3*	290	9	320	2.6*	50	700	70	12	5.1*	1.5*	2.3*

NOTE: This table presents Recommended Dietary Allowances (RDAs) in **bold type** and Adequate Intakes (AIs) in ordinary type followed by an asterisk (*). RDAs and AIs may both be used as goals for individual intake. RDAs are set to meet the needs of almost all (97 to 98 percent) individuals in a group. For healthy breast-fed infants, the AI is the mean intake. The AI for other life stage and gender groups is believed to cover needs of all individuals in the group, but lack of data or uncertainty in the data prevent being able to specify with confidence the percentage of individuals covered by this intake.

Sources: *Dietary Reference Intakes for Calcium, Phosphorus, Magnesium, Vitamin D, and Fluoride* (1997); *Dietary Reference Intakes for Thiamin, Riboflavin, Niacin, Vitamin B₆, Folate, Vitamin B₁₂, Pantothenic Acid, Biotin, and Choline* (1998); *Dietary Reference Intakes for Vitamin C, Vitamin E, Selenium, and Carotenoids* (2000); *Dietary Reference Intakes for Vitamin A, Vitamin K, Arsenic, Boron, Chromium, Copper, Iodine, Iron, Manganese, Molybdenum, Nickel, Silicon, Vanadium, and Zinc* (2001); and *Dietary Reference Intakes for Water, Potassium, Sodium, Chloride, and Sulfate* (2004). These reports may be accessed via http://www.nap.edu.

Dietary Reference Intakes (DRIs): Tolerable Upper Intake Levels (UL[a]), Vitamins

Food and Nutrition Board, Institute of Medicine, National Academies

Life Stage Group	Vitamin A (μg/d)[b]	Vitamin C (mg/d)	Vitamin D (μg/d)	Vitamin E (mg/d)[c,d]	Vitamin K	Thiamin	Ribo-flavin	Niacin (mg/d)[d]	Vitamin B$_6$ (mg/d)	Folate (μg/d)[d]	Vitamin B$_{12}$	Pantothenic acid	Biotin	Choline (g/d)	Caro-tenoids[e]
Infants															
0–6 mo	600	ND[f]	25	ND	ND	ND	ND	ND	ND	ND	ND	ND	ND	ND	ND
7–12 mo	600	ND	25	ND	ND	ND	ND	ND	ND	ND	ND	ND	ND	ND	ND
Children															
1–3 y	600	400	50	200	ND	ND	ND	10	30	300	ND	ND	ND	1.0	ND
4–8 y	900	650	50	300	ND	ND	ND	15	40	400	ND	ND	ND	1.0	ND
Males,															
Females															
9–13 y	1,700	1,200	50	600	ND	ND	ND	20	60	600	ND	ND	ND	2.0	ND
14–18 y	2,800	1,800	50	800	ND	ND	ND	30	80	800	ND	ND	ND	3.0	ND
19–70 y	3,000	2,000	50	1,000	ND	ND	ND	35	100	1,000	ND	ND	ND	3.5	ND
>70 y	3,000	2,000	50	1,000	ND	ND	ND	35	100	1,000	ND	ND	ND	3.5	ND
Pregnancy															
14–18 y	2,800	1,800	50	800	ND	ND	ND	30	80	800	ND	ND	ND	3.0	ND
19–50 y	3,000	2,000	50	1,000	ND	ND	ND	35	100	1,000	ND	ND	ND	3.5	ND
Lactation															
14–18 y	2,800	1,800	50	800	ND	ND	ND	30	80	800	ND	ND	ND	3.0	ND
19–50 y	3,000	2,000	50	1,000	ND	ND	ND	35	100	1,000	ND	ND	ND	3.5	ND

[a]UL = The maximum level of daily nutrient intake that is likely to pose no risk of adverse effects. Unless otherwise specified, the UL represents total intake from food, water, and supplements. Due to lack of suitable data, ULs could not be established for vitamin K, thiamin, riboflavin, vitamin B$_{12}$, pantothenic acid, biotin, carotenoids. In the absence of ULs, extra caution may be warranted in consuming levels above recommended intakes.

[b]As preformed vitamin A only.

[c]As α-tocopherol; applies to any form of supplemental a-tocopherol.

[d]The ULs for vitamin E, niacin, and folate apply to synthetic forms obtained from supplements, fortified foods, or a combination of the two.

[e]β-carotene supplements are advised only to serve as a provitamin A source for individuals at risk of vitamin A deficiency.

[f]ND = Not determinable due to lack of data of adverse effects in this age group and concern with regard to lack of ability to handle excess amounts. Source of intake should be from food only to prevent high levels of intake.

Sources: *Dietary Reference Intakes for Calcium, Phosphorous, Magnesium, Vitamin D, and Fluoride* (1997); *Dietary Reference Intakes for Thiamin, Riboflavin, Niacin, Vitamin B$_6$, Folate, Vitamin B$_{12}$, Pantothenic Acid, Biotin, and Choline* (1998); *Dietary Reference Intakes for Vitamin C, Vitamin E, Selenium, and Carotenoids* (2000); *and Dietary Reference Intakes for Vitamin A, Vitamin K, Arsenic, Boron, Chromium, Copper, Iodine, Iron, Manganese, Molybdenum, Nickel, Silicon, Vanadium, and Zinc* (2001). These reports may be accessed via http://www.nap.edu.

Dietary Reference Intakes (DRIs): Tolerable Upper Intake Levels (UL^a), Elements
Food and Nutrition Board, Institute of Medicine, National Academies

Life Stage Group	Arsenic^b	Boron (mg/d)	Calcium (g/d)	Chromium	Copper (µg/d)	Fluoride (mg/d)	Iodine (µg/d)	Iron (mg/d)	Magnesium (mg/d)^c	Manganese (mg/d)	Molybdenum (µg/d)	Nickel (mg/d)	Phosphorus (g/d)	Potassium	Selenium (µg/d)	Silicon^d	Sulfate	Vanadium (mg/d)^e	Zinc (mg/d)	Sodium (g/d)	Chloride (g/d)
Infants																					
0–6 mo	ND^f	ND	ND	ND	ND	0.7	ND	40	ND	ND	ND	ND	ND	ND	45	ND	ND	ND	4	ND	ND
7–12 mo	ND	ND	ND	ND	ND	0.9	ND	40	ND	ND	ND	ND	ND	ND	60	ND	ND	ND	5	ND	ND
Children																					
1–3 y	ND	3	2.5	ND	1,000	1.3	200	40	65	2	300	0.2	3	ND	90	ND	ND	ND	7	1.5	2.3
4–8 y	ND	6	2.5	ND	3,000	2.2	300	40	110	3	600	0.3	3	ND	150	ND	ND	ND	12	1.9	2.9
Males, Females																					
9–13 y	ND	11	2.5	ND	5,000	10	600	40	350	6	1,100	0.6	4	ND	280	ND	ND	ND	23	2.2	3.4
14–18 y	ND	17	2.5	ND	8,000	10	900	45	350	9	1,700	1.0	4	ND	400	ND	ND	ND	34	2.3	3.6
19–70 y	ND	20	2.5	ND	10,000	10	1,100	45	350	11	2,000	1.0	4	ND	400	ND	ND	1.8	40	2.3	3.6
>70 y	ND	20	2.5	ND	10,000	10	1,100	45	350	11	2,000	1.0	3	ND	400	ND	ND	1.8	40	2.3	3.6
Pregnancy																					
14–18 y	ND	17	2.5	ND	8,000	10	900	45	350	9	1,700	1.0	3.5	ND	400	ND	ND	ND	34	2.3	3.6
19–50 y	ND	20	2.5	ND	10,000	10	1,100	45	350	11	2,000	1.0	3.5	ND	400	ND	ND	ND	40	2.3	3.6
Lactation																					
14–18 y	ND	17	2.5	ND	8,000	10	900	45	350	9	1,700	1.0	4	ND	400	ND	ND	ND	34	2.3	3.6
19–50 y	ND	20	2.5	ND	10,000	10	1,100	45	350	11	2,000	1.0	4	ND	400	ND	ND	ND	40	2.3	3.6

^{a}UL = The maximum level of daily nutrient intake that is likely to pose no risk of adverse effects. Unless otherwise specified, the UL represents total intake from food, water, and supplements. Due to lack of suitable data, ULs could not be established for arsenic, chromium, silicon, potassium, and sulfate. In the absence of ULs, extra caution may be warranted in consuming levels above recommended intakes.

^{b}Although the UL was not determined for arsenic, there is no justification for adding arsenic to food or supplements.

^{c}The ULs for magnesium represent intake from a pharmacological agent only and do not include intake from food and water.

^{d}Although silicon has not been shown to cause adverse effects in humans, there is no justification for adding silicon to supplements.

^{e}Although vanadium in food has not been shown to cause adverse effects in humans, this data could be used to set a UL for adults but not children and adolescents. The UL is based on adverse effects in laboratory animals and this data could be used to set a UL for adults but not children and adolescents.

^{f}ND = Not determinable due to lack of data of adverse effects in this age group and concern with regard to lack of ability to handle excess amounts. Source of intake should be from food only to prevent high levels of intake.

Sources: *Dietary Reference Intakes for Calcium, Phosphorous, Magnesium, Vitamin D, and Fluoride* (1997); *Dietary Reference Intakes for Thiamin, Riboflavin, Niacin, Vitamin B$_6$ Folate, Vitamin B$_{12}$, Pantothenic Acid, Biotin, and Choline* (1998); *Dietary Reference Intakes for Vitamin C, Vitamin E, Selenium, and Carotenoids* (2000); *Dietary Reference Intakes for Vitamin A, Vitamin K, Arsenic, Boron, Chromium, Copper, Iodine, Iron, Manganese, Molybdenum, Nickel, Silicon, Vanadium, and Zinc* (2001); and *Dietary Reference Intakes for Water, Potassium, Sodium, Chloride, and Sulfate* (2004). These reports may be accessed via http://www.nap.edu.

Copyright 2004 by the National Academy of Sciences. All rights reserved.

Dietary Reference Intakes (DRIs): Estimated Energy Requirements (EER) for Men and Women 30 Years of Age[a]

Food and Nutrition Board, Institute of Medicine, National Academies

Height (m [in])	PAL[b]	Weight for BMI[c] for 18.5 kg/m² (kg [lb])	Weight for BMI for 24.99 kg/m² (kg [lb])	EER, Men[d] (kcal/day)		EER, Women[d] (kcal/day)	
				BMI of 18.5 kg/m²	BMI of 24.99 kg/m²	BMI of 18.5 kg/m²	BMI of 24.99 kg/m²
1.50 (59)	Sedentary	41.6 (92)	56.2 (124)	1,848	2,080	1,625	1,762
	Low active			2,009	2,267	1,803	1,956
	Active			2,215	2,506	2,025	2,198
	Very active			2,554	2,898	2,291	2,489
1.65 (65)	Sedentary	50.4 (111)	68.0 (150)	2,068	2,349	1,816	1,982
	Low active			2,254	2,566	2,016	2,202
	Active			2,490	2,842	2,267	2,477
	Very active			2,880	3,296	2,567	2,807
1.80 (71)	Sedentary	59.9 (132)	81.0 (178)	2,301	2,635	2,015	2,211
	Low active			2,513	2,884	2,239	2,459
	Active			2,782	3,200	2,519	2,769
	Very active			3,225	3,720	2,855	3,141

[a]For each year below 30, add 7 kcal/day for women and 10 kcal/day for men. For each year above 30, subtract 7 kcal/day for women and 10 kcal/day for men.

[b]PAL = physical activity level.

[c]BMI = body mass index.

[d]Derived from the following regression equations based on doubly labeled water data:

Adult man: EER = 662 − 9.53 × age (y) + PA × (15.91 × wt [kg] + 539.6 × ht [m])

Adult woman: EER = 354 − 6.91 × age (y) + PA × (9.36 × wt [kg] + 726 × ht [m])

Where PA refers to coefficient for PAL

PAL = total energy expenditure ÷ basal energy expenditure

PA = 1.0 if PAL ≥ 1.0 < 1.4 (sedentary)

PA = 1.12 if PAL ≥ 1.4 < 1.6 (low active)

PA = 1.27 if PAL ≥ 1.6 < 1.9 (active)

PA = 1.45 if PAL ≥ 1.9 < 2.5 (very active)

Dietary Reference Intakes (DRIs): Acceptable Macronutrient Distribution Ranges

Food and Nutrition Board, Institute of Medicine, National Academies

Macronutrient	Range (percent of energy)		
	Children, 1–3 y	Children, 4–18 y	Adults
Fat	30–40	25–35	20–35
n-6 polyunsaturated fatty acids[a] (linoleic acid)	5–10	5–10	5–10
n-3 polyunsaturated fatty acids[a] (α-linolenic acid)	0.6–1.2	0.6–1.2	0.6–1.2
Carbohydrate	45–65	45–65	45–65
Protein	5–20	10–30	10–35

[a]Approximately 10% of the total can come from longer-chain *n*-3 or *n*-6 fatty acids.

Source: *Dietary Reference Intakes for Energy, Carbohydrate, Fiber, Fat, Fatty Acids, Cholesterol, Protein, and Amino Acids* (2002).

Dietary Reference Intakes (DRIs): Recommended Intakes for Individuals, Macronutrients

Food and Nutrition Board, Institute of Medicine, National Academies

Life Stage Group	Total Water[a] (L/d)	Carbohydrate (g/d)	Total fiber (g/d)	Fat (g/d)	Linoleic acid (g/d)	α-Linolenic acid (g/d)	Protein[b] (g/d)
Infants							
0–6 mo	0.7*	60*	ND	31*	4.4*	0.5*	9.1*
7–12 mo	0.8*	95*	ND	30*	4.6*	0.5*	11.0[c]
Children							
1–3 y	1.3*	130	19*	ND	7*	0.7*	13
4–8 y	1.7*	130	25*	ND	10*	0.9*	19
Males							
9–13 y	2.4*	130	31*	ND	12*	1.2*	34
14–18 y	3.3*	130	38*	ND	16*	1.6*	52
19–30 y	3.7*	130	38*	ND	17*	1.6*	56
31–50 y	3.7*	130	38*	ND	17*	1.6*	56
51–70 y	3.7*	130	30*	ND	14*	1.6*	56
>70 y	3.7*	130	30*	ND	14*	1.6*	56
Females							
9–13 y	2.1*	130	26*	ND	10*	1.0*	34
14–18 y	2.3*	130	26*	ND	11*	1.1*	46
19–30 y	2.7*	130	25*	ND	12*	1.1*	46
31–50 y	2.7*	130	25*	ND	12*	1.1*	46
51–70 y	2.7*	130	21*	ND	11*	1.1*	46
>70 y	2.7*	130	21*	ND	11*	1.1*	46
Pregnancy							
14–18 y	3.0*	175	28*	ND	13*	1.4*	71
19–30 y	3.0*	175	28*	ND	13*	1.4*	71
31–50 y	3.0*	175	28*	ND	13*	1.4*	71
Lactation							
14–18 y	3.8*	210	29*	ND	13*	1.3*	71
19–30 y	3.8*	210	29*	ND	13*	1.3*	71
31–50 y	3.8*	210	29*	ND	13*	1.3*	71

NOTE: This table presents Recommended Dietary Allowances (RDAs) in **bold type** and Adequate Intakes (AIs) in ordinary type followed by an asterisk (*). RDAs and AIs may both be used as goals for individual intake. RDAs are set to meet the needs of almost all (97 to 98 percent) individuals in a group. For healthy infants fed human milk, the AI is the mean intake. The AI for other life stage and gender groups is believed to cover the needs of all individuals in the group, but lack of data or uncertainty in the data prevent being able to specify with confidence the percentage of individuals covered by this intake.

[a]Total water includes all water contained in food, beverages, and drinking water.

[b]Based on 0.8 g/kg body weight for the reference body weight.

[c]Change from 13.5 in prepublication copy due to calculation error.

Dietary Reference Intakes (DRIs): Additional Macronutrient Recommendations

Food and Nutrition Board, Institute of Medicine, National Academies

Macronutrient	Recommendation
Dietary cholesterol	As low as possible while consuming a nutritionally adequate diet
Transfatty acids	As low as possible while consuming a nutritionally adequate diet
Saturated fatty acids	As low as possible while consuming a nutritionally adequate diet
Added sugars	Limit to no more than 25% of total energy

Source: *Dietary Reference Intakes for Energy, Carbohydrate, Fiber, Fat, Fatty Acids, Cholesterol, Protein, and Amino Acids* (2002).

Dietary Reference Intakes (DRIs): Estimated Average Requirements for Groups
Food and Nutrition Board, Institute of Medicine, National Academies

Life Stage Group	CHO (g/d)	Protein (g/d)[a]	Vit A (µg/d)[b]	Vit C (mg/d)	Vit E (mg/d)[c]	Thiamin (mg/d)	Riboflavin (mg/d)	Niacin (mg/d)[d]	Vit B6 (mg/d)	Folate (µg/d)[b]	Vit B12 (µg/d)[b]	Copper (µg/d)	Iodine (µg/d)	Iron (mg/d)	Magnesium (mg/d)	Molybdenum (µg/d)	Phosphorus (mg/d)	Selenium (µg/d)	Zinc (mg/d)
Infants																			
7–12 mo		9*												6.9					2.5
Children																			
1–3 y	100	11	210	13	5	0.4	0.4	5	0.4	120	0.7	260	65	3.0	65	13	380	17	2.5
4–8 y	100	15	275	22	6	0.5	0.5	6	0.5	160	1.0	340	65	4.1	110	17	405	23	4.0
Males																			
9–13 y	100	27	445	39	9	0.7	0.8	9	0.8	250	1.5	540	73	5.9	200	26	1,055	35	7.0
14–18 y	100	44	630	63	12	1.0	1.1	12	1.1	330	2.0	685	95	7.7	340	33	1,055	45	8.5
19–30 y	100	46	625	75	12	1.0	1.1	12	1.1	320	2.0	700	95	6	330	34	580	45	9.4
31–50 y	100	46	625	75	12	1.0	1.1	12	1.1	320	2.0	700	95	6	350	34	580	45	9.4
51–70 y	100	46	625	75	12	1.0	1.1	12	1.4	320	2.0	700	95	6	350	34	580	45	9.4
>70 y	100	46	625	75	12	1.0	1.1	12	1.4	320	2.0	700	95	6	350	34	580	45	9.4
Females																			
9–13 y	100	28	420	39	9	0.7	0.8	9	0.8	250	1.5	540	73	5.7	200	26	1,055	35	7.0
14–18 y	100	38	485	56	12	0.9	0.9	11	1.0	330	2.0	685	95	7.9	300	33	1,055	45	7.3
19–30 y	100	38	500	60	12	0.9	0.9	11	1.1	320	2.0	700	95	8.1	255	34	580	45	6.8
31–50 y	100	38	500	60	12	0.9	0.9	11	1.1	320	2.0	700	95	8.1	265	34	580	45	6.8
51–70 y	100	38	500	60	12	0.9	0.9	11	1.3	320	2.0	700	95	5	265	34	580	45	6.8
>70 y	100	38	500	60	12	0.9	0.9	11	1.3	320	2.0	700	95	5	265	34	580	45	6.8
Pregnancy																			
14–18 y	135	50	530	66	12	1.2	1.2	14	1.6	520	2.2	785	160	23	335	40	1,055	49	10.5
19–30 y	135	50	550	70	12	1.2	1.2	14	1.6	520	2.2	800	160	22	290	40	580	49	9.5
31–50 y	135	50	550	70	12	1.2	1.2	14	1.6	520	2.2	800	160	22	300	40	580	49	9.5
Lactation																			
14–18 y	160	60	885	96	16	1.2	1.3	13	1.7	450	2.4	985	209	7	300	35	1,055	59	10.9
19–30 y	160	60	900	100	16	1.2	1.3	13	1.7	450	2.4	1,000	209	6.5	255	36	580	59	10.4
31–50 y	160	60	900	100	16	1.2	1.3	13	1.7	450	2.4	1,000	209	6.5	265	36	580	59	10.4

NOTE: This table presents Estimated Average Requirements (EARs), which serve two purposes: for assessing adequacy of population intakes, and as the basis for calculating Recommended Dietary Allowances (RDAs) for individuals for those nutrients. EARs have not been established for vitamin D, vitamin K, pantothenic acid, biotin, choline, calcium, chromium, fluoride, manganese, or other nutrients not yet evaluated via the DRI process.

[a] For individual at reference weight (Table 1-1). *indicates change from prepublication copy due to calculation error.

[b] As retinol activity equivalents (RAEs). 1 RAE = 1 µg retinol, 12 µg β-carotene, 24 µg α-carotene, or 24 µg β-cryptoxanthin. The RAE for dietary provitamin A carotenoids is twofold greater than retinol equivalents (RE), whereas the RAE for preformed vitamin A is the same as RE.

[c] As α-tocopherol. α-tocopherol includes *RRR*-α-tocopherol, the only form of α-tocopherol that occurs naturally in foods, and the 2*R*-stereoisomeric forms of α-tocopherol (*RRR*-, *RSR*-, *RRS*-, and *RSS*-α-tocopherol) that occur in fortified foods and supplements. It does not include the 2*S*-stereoisomeric forms of α-tocopherol (*SRR*-, *SSR*-, *SRS*-, and *SSS*-α-tocopherol), also found in fortified foods and supplements.

[d] As niacin equivalents (NE). 1 mg of niacin = 60 mg of tryptophan.

*a*As dietary folate equivalents (DFE). 1 DFE = 1μg food folate = 0.6 μg of folic acid from fortified food or as a supplement consumed with food = 0.5 μg of a supplement taken on an empty stomach.

Sources: *Dietary Reference Intakes for Calcium, Phosphorous, Magnesium, Vitamin D, and Fluoride* (1997); *Dietary Reference Intakes for Thiamin, Riboflavin, Niacin, Vitamin B*$_6$*, Folate, Vitamin B*$_{12}$*, Pantothenic Acid, Biotin, and Choline* (1998); *Dietary Reference Intakes for Vitamin C, Vitamin E, Selenium, and Carotenoids* (2000); *Dietary Reference Intakes for Vitamin A, Vitamin K, Arsenic, Boron, Chromium, Copper, Iodine, Iron, Manganese, Molybdenum, Nickel, Silicon, Vanadium, and Zinc* (2001), and *Dietary Reference Intakes for Energy, Carbohydrate, Fiber, Fat, Fatty Acids, Cholesterol, Protein, and Amino Acids* (2002). These reports may be accessed via www.nap.edu.

Body Mass Index for Adults

Body Mass Index Table

Body Weight (pounds)

Height (inches)	Normal						Overweight					Obese										Extreme Obesity														
BMI	19	20	21	22	23	24	25	26	27	28	29	30	31	32	33	34	35	36	37	38	39	40	41	42	43	44	45	46	47	48	49	50	51	52	53	54
58	91	96	100	105	110	115	119	124	129	134	138	143	148	153	158	162	167	172	177	181	186	191	196	201	205	210	215	220	224	229	234	239	244	248	253	258
59	94	99	104	109	114	119	124	128	133	138	143	148	153	158	163	168	173	178	183	188	193	198	203	208	212	217	222	227	232	237	242	247	252	257	262	267
60	97	102	107	112	118	123	128	133	138	143	148	153	158	163	168	174	179	184	189	194	199	204	209	215	220	225	230	235	240	245	250	255	261	266	271	276
61	100	106	111	116	122	127	132	137	143	148	153	158	164	169	174	180	185	190	195	201	206	211	217	222	227	232	238	243	248	254	259	264	269	275	280	285
62	104	109	115	120	126	131	136	142	147	153	158	164	169	175	180	186	191	196	202	207	213	218	224	229	235	240	246	251	256	262	267	273	278	284	289	295
63	107	113	118	124	130	135	141	146	152	158	163	169	175	180	186	191	197	203	208	214	220	225	231	237	242	248	254	259	265	270	278	282	287	293	299	304
64	110	116	122	128	134	140	145	151	157	163	169	174	180	186	192	197	204	209	215	221	227	232	238	244	250	256	262	267	273	279	285	291	296	302	308	314
65	114	120	126	132	138	144	150	156	162	168	174	180	186	192	198	204	210	216	222	228	234	240	246	252	258	264	270	276	282	288	294	300	306	312	318	324
66	118	124	130	136	142	148	155	161	167	173	179	186	192	198	204	210	216	223	229	235	241	247	253	260	266	272	278	284	291	297	303	309	315	322	328	334
67	121	127	134	140	146	153	159	166	172	178	185	191	198	204	211	217	223	230	236	242	249	255	261	268	274	280	287	293	299	306	312	319	325	331	338	344
68	125	131	138	144	151	158	164	171	177	184	190	197	203	210	216	223	230	236	243	249	256	262	269	276	282	289	295	302	308	315	322	328	335	341	348	354
69	128	135	142	149	155	162	169	176	182	189	196	203	209	216	223	230	236	243	250	257	263	270	277	284	291	297	304	311	318	324	331	338	345	351	358	365
70	132	139	146	153	160	167	174	181	188	195	202	209	216	222	229	236	243	250	257	264	271	278	285	292	299	306	313	320	327	334	341	348	355	362	369	376
71	136	143	150	157	165	172	179	186	193	200	208	215	222	229	236	243	250	257	265	272	279	286	293	301	308	315	322	329	338	343	351	358	365	372	379	386
72	140	147	154	162	169	177	184	191	199	206	213	221	228	235	242	250	258	265	272	279	287	294	302	309	316	324	331	338	346	353	361	368	375	383	390	397
73	144	151	159	166	174	182	189	197	204	212	219	227	235	242	250	257	265	272	280	288	295	302	310	318	325	333	340	348	355	363	371	378	386	393	401	408
74	148	155	163	171	179	186	194	202	210	218	225	233	241	249	256	264	272	280	287	295	303	311	319	326	334	342	350	358	365	373	381	389	396	404	412	420
75	152	160	168	176	184	192	200	208	216	224	232	240	248	256	264	272	279	287	295	303	311	319	327	335	343	351	359	367	375	383	391	399	407	415	423	431
76	156	164	172	180	189	197	205	213	221	230	238	246	254	263	271	279	287	295	304	312	320	328	336	344	353	361	369	377	385	394	402	410	418	426	435	443

Source: Adapted from Clinical Guidelines on the Identification, Evaluation, and Treatment of Overweight and Obesity in Adults: The Evidence Report.

INDEX

PHOTO CREDITS

Chapter 1
Page 16 © Photodisc; **page 17** © Denis Vrublevski/ShutterStock, Inc.; **page 18** © David Young-Wolff/PhotoEdit Inc.

Chapter 2
Page 27 © Gelpi/ShutterStock, Inc.; **page 35** Courtesy of Mead Johnson & Company; **page 40** © Fashion Studio/ShutterStock, Inc.; **page 41** © Lena S/ShutterStock, Inc.

Chapter 3
Page 50 © Nick Vedros/age fotostock; **page 56** © Monkey Business Images/Dreamstime.com; **page 60** © Monkey Business Images/Dreamstime.com; **page 61** © Losevsky Pavel/ShutterStock, Inc

Chapter 4
Page 70 © Monkey Business Images/Dreamstime.com; **page 75** © Erwin Purnomo Sidi/Dreamstime.com; **page 77** © Shawn Pecor/ShutterStock, Inc.; **page 78** © BananaStock/age fotostock

Chapter 5
Page 86 © Gert Vrey/Dreamstime.com; **page 93** © Scientifica/Visuals Unlimited

Chapter 6
Page 102 © Sonbeam/Dreamstime.com; **page 105** © Tatyana Gladskikh/Dreamstime.com; **page 110** © Hannamariah/ShutterStock, Inc.

Chapter 7
Page 133 © Bochkarev Photography/ShutterStock, Inc.; **page 134** © Djk/Dreamstime.com; **page 143** © Ivonne Wierink/ShutterStock, Inc.; **page 144** © matka wariatka/ShutterStock, Inc.

Chapter 8
Page 172 © Anetta/ShutterStock, Inc.; **page 177** © Ron Chapple Studios/Dreamstime.com; **page 187** © sima/ShutterStock, Inc.

Chapter 9
Page 200 © Lisa F. Young/Dreamstime.com; **page 212** © Kiselev Andrey Valerevich/ShutterStock, Inc.

Chapter 10
Page 224 © Regien Paassen/ShutterStock, Inc.; **page 230** © Photos.com

Chapter 11
Page 245 © David Gaylor/ShutterStock, Inc.

Chapter 12
12.1 © Denis Pepin/Dreamstime.com; **12.2** Courtesy of Janice Carr/CDC; **12.11** © Sandor Kacso/Dreamstime.com; **12.12** © Elena Elisseeva/Dreamstime.com; **12.14** Courtesy of CDC

Chapter 13
Page 284 © Ken Hammond/USDA; **page 290** © mozzyb/ShutterStock, Inc.

Chapter 14
Page 298 Photo by Scott Bauer/USDA; **page 303** © Thinkstock/age fotostock

Chapter 15
Page 314 © Monkey Business Images/ShutterStock, Inc.; **page 318** © Ron Chapple Studios/Dreamstime.com